DIABETES MELLITUS: MANAGEMENT AND COMPLICATIONS

CONTEMPORARY ISSUES IN ENDOCRINOLOGY AND METABOLISM
Volume 1

SERIES EDITOR

Jerrold M. Olefsky, M.D.

Professor of Medicine
Division of Endocrinology/Metabolism
School of Medicine
University of California, San Diego
LaJolla, California

Forthcoming Volumes in the Series

Vol. 2 Prolactinomas, Jerrold M. Olefsky, M.D., and Richard Robbins, M.D., Editors

Vol. 3 Atherosclerosis, Daniel Steinberg, M.D., Ph.D., and Jerrold M. Olefsky, M.D., Editors

DIABETES MELLITUS: MANAGEMENT AND COMPLICATIONS

Edited by

Jerrold M. Olefsky, M.D.

Professor of Medicine
Division of Endocrinology/Metabolism
School of Medicine
University of California, San Diego
LaJolla, California

Robert S. Sherwin, M.D.

Associate Professor of Medicine
Director, Diabetes Research Unit
Yale University School of Medicine
New Haven, Connecticut

CHURCHILL LIVINGSTONE
NEW YORK, EDINBURGH, LONDON, AND MELBOURNE
1985

Acquisitions editor: Gene Kearn
Copy editor: Michael Kelley
Production editor: Fred Kantrowitz
Production supervisor: Sharon Tuder
Compositor: The Maple-Vail Book Manufacturing Group
Printer/Binder: The Murray Printing Co.

Distributed in the United Kingdom by Churchill Livingstone, Robert Stevenson House, 1–3 Baxter's Place, Leith Walk, Edinburgh EH1 3AF and by associated companies, branches and representatives throughout the world.

First published 1985
Printed in USA

ISBN 0-443-08379-7

7 6 5 4 3 2 1

Library of Congress Cataloging in Publication Data
Main entry under title:

Diabetes mellitus.

(Contemporary issues in endocrinology and metabolism ; v. 1)
Includes bibliographies and index.
1. Diabetes—Complications and sequelae—Treatment.
I. Olefsky, Jerrold M. II. Sherwin, Robert S.
III. Series. [DNLM: 1. Diabetes Mellitus—complications.
2. Diabetes Mellitus—therapy. W1 CO769MQN v.1 /
WK 810 D5375293]
RC660.D455 1985 616.4'62 84-29258
ISBN 0-443-08379-7

Manufactured in the United States of America

Contributors

Andrew J.M. Boulton, M.D.
Visiting Assistant Professor of Medicine
University of Miami School of Medicine
Miami, Florida
Senior Medical Registrar
Royal Hallamshire Hospital
Sheffield, United Kingdom

John H. Bowker, M.D.
Professor
Department of Orthopaedics and Rehabilitation
Medical Director
Jackson Memorial Hospital Rehabilitation Center
Miami, Florida

Irwin M. Braverman, M.D.
Professor of Dermatology
Department of Dermatology
Yale University School of Medicine
New Haven, Connecticut

Donald R. Coustan, M.D.
Associate Professor of Obstetrics and Gynecology
Brown University
Director of Maternal-Fetal Medicine
Women and Infants Hospital of Rhode Island
Providence, Rhode Island

Jaime A. Davidson, M.D.
Medical Director of Diabetes Self-Care Program
National Medical Care Center
Clinical Assistant Professor
Department of Internal Medicine
University of Texas Health Science Center at Dallas
Southwestern Medical School
Dallas, Texas

Ralph A. DeFronzo, M.D.
Associate Professor of Medicine
Divisions of Endocrinology/Diabetes and Nephrology
Yale University School of Medicine
New Haven, Connecticut

Robert V. Farese, M.D.
Professor of Medicine
Director, Division of Endocrinology and Metabolism
College of Medicine
University of South Florida
Tampa, Florida

John A. Galloway, M.D.
Lilly Clinical Research Consultant
Lilly Laboratory for Clinical Research
Professor of Medicine
Indiana University School of Medicine
Indianapolis, Indiana

Douglas A. Greene, M.D.
Director, Clinical Research Center and Diabetes Research Laboratories
Department of Medicine
University of Pittsburgh School of Medicine
Pittsburgh, Pennsylvania

Alan M. Jacobson, M.D.
Chief, Mental Health Unit
Joslin Diabetes Center
Assistant Professor in Psychiatry
Harvard Medical School
Boston, Massachusetts

Ronald Klein, M.D., M.P.H.
Associate Professor
Department of Ophthalmology
University of Wisconsin
Madison, Wisconsin

Joan Leibovich, L.I.C.S.W.
Chief Social Worker
Joslin Diabetes Center
Boston, Massachusetts

Michael A. Pfeifer, M.D.
Director, Kentucky Comprehensive Care Diabetes Center
Department of Medicine
University of Louisville School of Medicine
Veterans Administration Medical Center
Louisville, Kentucky

Michael L. Reeves, M.D.
Assistant Professor of Medicine
University of Miami School of Medicine
Miami, Florida

Robert A. Rizza, M.D.
Associate Professor of Medicine
Mayo Medical School, Mayo Foundation
Rochester, Minnesota

David S. Schade, M.D.
Associate Professor of Medicine
Division of Endocrinology
Department of Medicine
University of New Mexico School of Medicine
Albuquerque, New Mexico

Robert S. Sherwin, M.D.
Associate Professor of Medicine
Director, Diabetes Research Unit
Yale University School of Medicine
New Haven, Connecticut

Pomeroy Sinnock, Ph.D.
Chief, Information and Training Section
Division of Diabetes Control
Center for Prevention Services
CDS
Atlanta, Georgia

Jay S. Skyler, M.D.
Associate Professor of Medicine
University of Miami School of Medicine
Miami, Florida

William V. Tamborlane, M.D.
Associate Professor of Pediatrics
Yale University School of Medicine
New Haven, Connecticut

Foreword

Contemporary Issues in Endocrinology and Metabolism is a new series which will address selected topics in the field as they relate to clinical practice. The scientific underpinning of endocrinology and metabolism has expanded enormously in recent years, and even greater advances are likely in the near future. The purpose of this new series, then, is to update the clinician on the latest advances in pathophysiology, diagnosis, and management of selected disease states and to translate the latest scientific information for use in the clinical arena.

Since this will be a regular series, publication will be far more rapid than regular textbooks, assuring that the information presented will be as up-to-date as possible. Each volume will consist of ten to twelve chapters focused around a particular disease entity or organ system, and we will have each chapter written by an acknowledged expert in the field. The subject of each volume will be selected so that a comprehensive review can be provided in a relatively concise and readable format. Each volume will synthesize new facts and new ideas which will interest a broad range of clinicians whose experiences relate to the general fields of endocrinology and metabolism. The editors hope that this format will lead to a series of timely, theme-related reviews which will provide guides to management, teaching aids, and up-to-date references.

Jerrold M. Olefsky, M.D.

Preface

Diabetes Mellitus: Management and Complications is the first volume in a new series entitled CONTEMPORARY ISSUES IN ENDOCRINOLOGY AND METABOLISM. This inaugural volume addresses a topic of broad and general interest to a wide spectrum of clinicians.

Chapter 1 reviews the central clinical question in the field of diabetes mellitus—namely, What is the relationship between hyperglycemia and chronic complications? Areas of agreement and disagreement are thoroughly discussed by the authors, and though no final answers are yet available, conclusions which have major implications for treatment strategies are drawn.

Chapter 2 provides a detailed practical guide to methods of intensive insulin management of diabetic patients. This includes multiple insulin injection regimens, insulin pump therapy, as well as suggestions for glucose monitoring. Attempts at rigorous glycemic control through intensive insulin management are not without complications and these are discussed in Chapter 3.

The next five chapters separately address, by organ system, the major complications of this disease. This includes chapters on diabetic eye problems, nephropathy, neuropathy, the diabetic foot, and dermatologic complications.

Special problems in diabetes management such as diabetes and pregnancy, diabetes in surgery, and treatment of hypertension in the diabetic are discussed in Chapters 9, 10, and 11. Finally, the psychosocial and economic impact of diabetes is discussed from several unique perspectives.

Jerrold M. Olefsky, M.D.
Robert S. Sherwin, M.D.

Contents

1 Metabolic Control and Diabetic Complications

Robert S. Sherwin
William V. Tamborlane

More than 60 years have passed since the discovery of insulin, and yet it is still not known if this therapeutic breakthrough offers the potential for minimizing or preventing the long-term vascular and neuropathic complications of diabetes. There is little doubt that insulin treatment, as currently applied, has nearly eliminated death from extreme metabolic decompensation. Nonetheless, late degenerative complications have continued to be a major source of morbidity and mortality. Clinically detectable microangiopathy involving the retina and/or kidneys can be expected in at least 80–85% of patients 20–25 years after onset. The diabetic is at increased risk for atherosclerotic vascular disease as well as peripheral and autonomic neuropathy. Children with diabetes may fail to reach their full growth potential. Unfortunately, neither the rate of appearance of complications nor the diabetic's reduced life expectancy as compared to the general population has substantially changed in recent years.

The view that diabetic complications are attributable to inadequate therapeutic correction of the metabolic abnormality formed early and has been the subject of heated debate ever since. The metabolic hypothesis is supported by conventional wisdom as well as by most experts in the field. However, some have challenged this assumption, pointing to evidence that vascular lesions may antedate the appearance of diabetes and thus be genetically determined. Furthermore, they cite those clinical studies and specific patient examples which show no clear-cut relationship between the severity of hyperglycemia and diabetic complications. Clinicians have, for the most part, taken a middle ground, implying a lack of conviction that the potential long-term benefits of attaining normal blood glucose levels justified the immediate risks (e.g., hypoglycemia) and the heavy demands made in provision of care. Earlier clinical studies that attempted to resolve this issue suffered from deficiencies in experimental design, inadequate methods for assessing diabetic control, and the lack of effective treatment regimens. As a result, direct scientific evidence linking the metabolic disturbance with complications mainly derives from experiments using animal models of diabetes. This work has focused on microangiopathic and neuropathic complications and, in general, provides strong support for the metabolic hypothesis. There is little evidence, however, that the accelerated atherosclerosis can be prevented by more effective treatment of hyperglycemia.

The introduction of improved methods for quantifying blood glucose control and delivering insulin in a more physiological manner have raised hopes that the requisite tools may now be available to test the metabolic hypothesis more directly in humans. Preliminary reports, however, have failed to provide clear-cut answers; data have been generated that support both sides of the controversy. In this review we discuss the current status of the debate. The issue involved is not simply of academic interest but has far-reaching clinical implications for the future management of diabetes.

PATHOGENESIS OF DIABETIC COMPLICATIONS: CURRENT THEORIES

Our general lack of knowledge concerning the pathogenesis of diabetic complications has contributed to the uncertainty about the potential value of improved metabolic control. It must be kept in mind that a single pathogenetic mechanism may not be operative and that the influence of the metabolic disturbance may vary among the multiple affected organ systems. Nevertheless, several general theories have emerged, each resting on the premise that hyperglycemia or some related metabolic abnormality is the primary event triggering tissue damage (Table 1–1). This has provided an attractive rationale for the metabolic hypothesis and has strengthened the argument for tighter diabetic control. Yet these theories remain untested in humans and therefore must be viewed in this context.

The observation that diabetics have increased amounts of glycosylated hemoglobin was rapidly seized upon as a means of quantifying diabetic control.[1] Glucose was shown to react nonenzymatically with the N-terminal amino group of the β-chain of the hemoglobin A molecule, eventually forming a stable ketoamine linkage that persists for the life span of the red blood cell. This negatively charged minor hemoglobin component, designated hemoglobin A_{IC}, is readily separated from hemoglobin A by a variety of methods.[2] Although it was initially thought that glycosylation might be restricted to the N-terminus of the β-chain, it was later shown that glucose forms ketoamine linkages with a variety of sites on both the α- and β-chains.[3] The relative nonspecificity of the process became apparent when it was found that nonenzymatic

Table 1-1. Postulated Mechanisms for Diabetic Complications

Protein glycosylation
Polyol pathway
Platelet/coagulation
Hemodynamic abnormalities

glycosylation also occurs with serum proteins, cell membrane proteins, low density lipoproteins (LDLs), peripheral nerve protein, and structural proteins, e.g., collagen and lens crystallins.[4] Of particular importance is the fact that increased quantities of a variety of glycosylated proteins have been demonstrated in human and experimental diabetes. This has led to the idea that hyperglycemia might induce widespread post-translational modifications of cellular and basement membrane proteins that contribute to the long-term complications of diabetes. Several recent observations are consistent with this view. It has been shown that the degradation of glycosylated LDL by cultured human fibroblasts is retarded[5] and that glycosylated albumin is preferentially taken up by isolated endothelial cells when compared to native albumin.[6] Furthermore, glycosylated collagen, which is increased in aorta and glomerular basement membrane in diabetic subjects, has been found to trigger the production of antibodies in rats that are specifically directed against the altered collagen molecule.[7] These findings imply that extensive protein glycosylation could potentially interfer with cellular function. Nevertheless, it is unclear whether the more limited degree of glycosylation that occurs in diabetic patients has any functional consequences.

Another potential biochemical mechanism through which hyperglycemia could impair cell function involves the polyol pathway. This pathway of glucose metabolism consists of two enzymatic steps: Nonphosphorylated glucose is first reduced to sorbitol by the enzyme aldose reductase, and subsequently sorbitol is converted to fructose through the action of sorbitol dehydrogenase. Polyol pathway activity is regulated by the intracellular concentration of free glucose and therefore would be expected to vary according to blood glucose levels in insulin-independent tissues containing polyol pathway enzymes, e.g., peripheral nerve Schwann cells, retinal pericytes, and lens.[8,9] Indeed, increased concentrations of sorbitol and fructose have been reported in peripheral nerve of diabetic rats.[10] It has been postulated that accumulated sorbitol (fructose is capable of leaving the cell) might exert osmotic effects which over time may lead to cell injury. The recent demonstration that aldose reductase inhibitors modestly improve nerve conduction in diabetic patients provides clinical support for this hypothesis.[11] On the other hand, evidence is lacking for excessive water accumulation in nerve cytoplasm in diabetic animals.[12] Thus if polyols actually do interfere with nerve function, they may operate through a nonosmotic mechanism. Moreover, recent evidence suggests that axonal (rather than Schwann cell) injury may be the primary event leading to diabetic neuropathy,[13] and that glucose and/or sorbitol may induce nerve dysfunction by reducing the content of myoinositol in nerve tissue.[14,15]

Alterations in platelet and/or endothelial function have been thought to contribute to the vascular complications of diabetes. The recent demonstration of microthrombi in retinal vessels of diabetic rats support this view.[16] Evidence has accumulated which suggests that platelet and endothelial alterations in diabetes may antedate clinically detectable vascular disease. These include: increased platelet aggregation, increased platelet metabolism of arachidonic acid, decreased platelet survival, decreased prostacyclin production by endothelial cells, increased von Willebrand factor, and diminished fibrinolytic activity. Although it is not entirely clear if all of these changes are directly mediated by poor metabolic control, at least some seem to be responsive to intensive insulin treatment.[17]

Recently it was proposed that hemodynamic alterations in the microcirculation of diabetic subjects may play an important role in initiating microangiopathy.[18,19] Early in the course of diabetes, particularly during poor metabolic control, blood flow is increased through the capillary beds of a wide variety of tissues, including kidney, retina, muscle, fat, and skin.[19] In the kidney the glomerular filtration rate is increased out of proportion to the changes in plasma flow, in part due to an elevation in the transglomerular pressure gradient.[20] Similar changes in capillary hydrostatic pressure may occur in other organs as well. Hostetter et al.[18] suggested that the raised glomerular pressures and flows observed early in diabetes might contribute to the development of renal disease. This hypothesis is based on the observation that single nephron hyperfiltration after partial renal ablation in the nondiabetic rat causes proteinuria and progressive glomerular damage in the remnant kidney.[21] They postulated that the hemodynamic alterations of diabetes caused transglomerular passage of proteins, and with time protein accumulation in the mesangium triggered proliferation of mesangial cells and matrix, eventually leading to glomerulosclerosis (Fig. 1-1). Those glomeruli that were less affected would develop compensatory hyperfiltration but ultimately succumb as does the remnant kidney. Studies in diabetes support this view. Glomerular changes in streptozocin diabetic rats are accentuated by unilateral nephrectomy[22] and reduced in the clipped kidney (which is protected from hypertension) of the so-

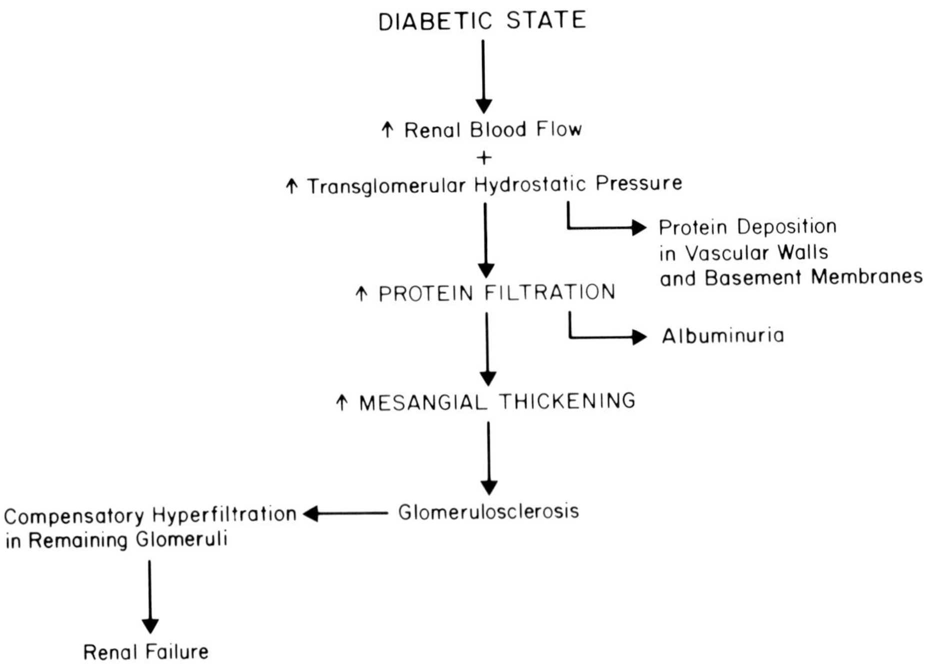

Fig. 1-1. Hemodynamic hypothesis for the pathogenesis of diabetic nephropathy. (Based on the proposal by Hostetter TH, Rennke HG, Brenner BM: The case of intrarenal hypertension in the initiation and progression of diabetic and other glomerulopathies. Am J Med 72:375, 1982.)

called two-kidney Goldblatt hypertensive model.[23] A diabetic patient with renal artery stenosis showed nodular glomerulosclerosis restricted to the kidney with the fully patent artery.[24] Parving et al.[19] suggested that the diabetes-associated increase in microcirculatory hydrostatic pressure is not limited to the kidney. If this is correct, it may account for the widespread deposition of plasma proteins in vessel walls and basement membranes as well as the generalized capillary leakage of macromolecules reported in diabetic patients.

Although the precise mechanism(s) responsible for the hemodynamic changes accompanying diabetes remain unestablished, there is little doubt that the metabolic disturbance is intimately involved. Intensive insulin treatment reduces the glomerular filtration rate toward normal[25] and diminishes albumin excretion,[26] fluorescein leakage from retinal vessels,[27] and peripheral extravasation of serum proteins in diabetic patients.[28] The importance of hyperglycemia per se is suggested by data showing that glucose infusion increases the glomerular filtration rate in normal subjects[29] and retinal blood flow in cats.[30] Other metabolic and/or hormone factors have been implicated, including glucagon, growth hormone, prostaglandins, and lactate.[18,19]

It is evident that the currently popular theories for the pathogenesis of diabetic microangiopathy would predict considerable benefits from efforts aimed at correction of the metabolic disturbance early in the disease. Whether similar effects can be expected once vascular damage has occurred is less clear. For example, extensive glycosylation of proteins with slow turnover rates, e.g., collagen, elastin, and crystallin, would not be readily affected by correction of hyperglycemia. Furthermore, the hemodynamic explanation for nephropathy would predict that once glomerulosclerosis has caused compensatory hyperfiltration progressive injury would continue in the remaining glomeruli, regardless of the prevailing metabolic state.

Animal Studies

Microangiopathy lesions resembling those seen in humans have been observed in animals with diabetes regardless of whether the disease occurs spontaneously or is induced by chemical, dietary, or viral means. Early retinal vascular changes have been reported in rats made diabetic with streptozotocin or a high-sucrose diet[31] and in dogs with chemically induced or spontaneous diabetes.[32,33] Renal glomerular lesions also appear in diabetic animals and display a number of histological features (e.g., basement membrane and/or mesangial thickening) in common with those reported in humans. Such abnormalities are documented in a wide variety of animal models including: the streptozotocin-treated[34] and pancreatectomized[35] diabetic rat; the viral-induced diabetic mouse[36]; dogs with spontaneous diabetes or who are rendered diabetic by alloxan[32,33] ; and the alloxan-induced diabetic monkey.[33] These observations imply that microangiopathy in diabetic animals is independent of the cause of diabetes and is thus linked to the metabolic disturbance. It is noteworthy, however, that the spontaneously diabetic BB Wistar rat seems to be considerably more resistant to microangiopathic changes than other rat strains thus far tested.[37]

Evidence pointing to the critical influence of metabolic control on the development of retinopathy in animals principally derives from the classic studies of Engerman et al.[32] These workers randomly assigned alloxan-diabetic dogs to either of two treatment regimens. In one group (n = 10) insulin was purposely administered in inadequate doses to allow for chronic hyperglycemia, and in other (n = 10) twice-daily insulin injections were given to minimize hyperglycemia. Both groups were then prospectively followed until sacrifice approximately 5 years later (Fig. 1-2). During the study there was clear glycemic separation between the groups: Mean plasma glucose levels varied between 350 and 400 mg/dl in the poorly controlled dogs and 90 and 180 mg/dl in the well-controlled group. After 2–3 years the inadequately treated dogs showed signs of early retinal vascular changes. By the end of the study at 5 years, each of the inadequately treated dogs developed saccular microaneurysms, hypocellular capillaries, pericyte ghosts, and retinal hemorrhage. The picture was quite different, however, in the well-controlled animals; their retinas were similar to those of nondiabetic controls, except for one animal that had died prematurely and had been less successfully treated (Fig. 1-2).

Several points deserve consideration when assessing the clinical implications of these data. First, the retinal disease was mild and did not show proliferative changes. Although neovascular lesions may have appeared if the experiments were continued longer, some questions could be raised about the relevance of the model to diabetes-

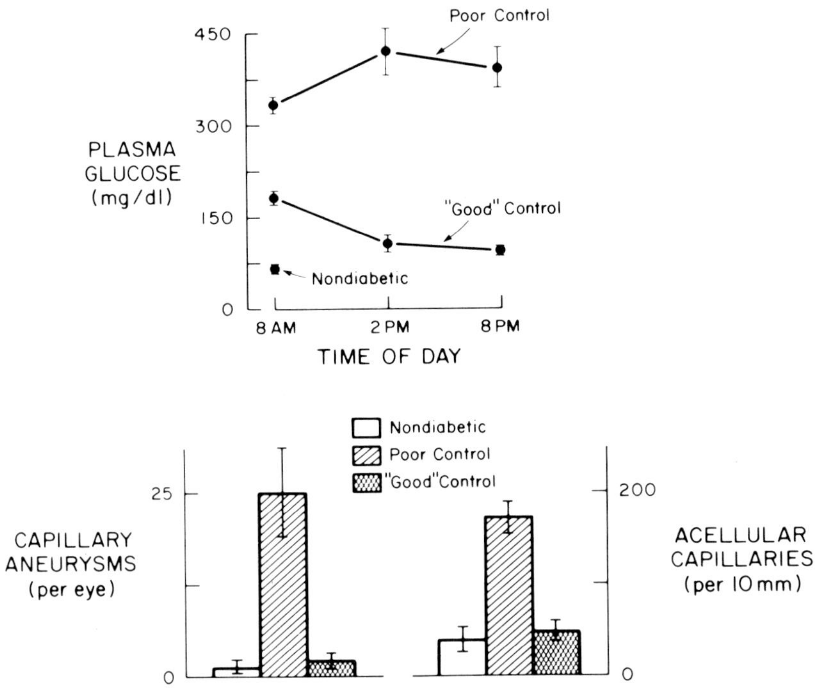

Fig. 1-2. Mean diurnal plasma glucose levels and retinal findings at autopsy after 60 months of diabetes in dogs. Results are compared in animals given insulin treatment designed to achieve either poor or good control of hyperglycemia. Data from nondiabetic control dogs are shown for comparison. (Data from Engerman R, Bloodworth JM Jr, Nelson S: Relationship of microvascular disease in diabetes to metabolic control. Diabetes 26:760, 1977.)

associated blindness. Second, the level of diabetes control achieved in the "well-controlled" group fell short of normalization and was no better than that currently attained with intensive insulin regimens. The implication is that diabetes care may now have improved sufficiently to test the metabolic hypothesis in humans. Finally, intensive treatment was initiated at the onset of disease, before the development of vascular changes. The study must therefore be viewed as a prevention trial and may have little bearing on the effect of tight metabolic control once vascular lesions have already appeared.

There are considerably more data showing the benefit of improved metabolic control on the appearance and progression of glomerular lesions in diabetic animals, particularly the rat. Rasch,[38] using a prospective randomized design, demonstrated that mesangial and basement membrane thickening does not appear in streptozotocin diabetic rats treated intensively with insulin (plasma glucose 90–180 mg/dl). Such lesions were consistently observed in poorly controlled rats over that period. It has also been reported that a less substantial blood glucose reduction reduces the appearance of glomerular lesions in diabetic rats.[39] These findings complement the retinopathy experiments in dogs (see above) and serve to strengthen the argument that greatly improved control delays or prevents microangiopathy in animals.

The elegant experiments of Mauer and co-workers also provide evidence that established glomerular lesions may be reversed. They found that transplantation of pancreatic islets into diabetic rats 6–8 months after streptozotocin administration totally reversed immunoglogulin and complement deposition in the mesangium, and either reversed or arrested the increase in mesangial matrix.[34,40] Comparable results were obtained when affected diabetic kidneys were transplanted into genetically identical nondiabetic recipients.[34] In addition, characteristic diabetic lesions appeared in normal kidneys after they were transplanted into a diabetic host.[41] Taken together, these findings suggest that reversal of microangiopathy may be possible. However, it remains unclear if this type of response requires near-complete normalization of glucose metabolism (as is achieved by islet transplantation). Furthermore, in these short-term studies, streptozotocin diabetic rats did not develop renal insufficiency. As a result, these experiments do not necessarily imply that stabilization or reversal would be attainable once diabetic glomerulopathy has become clinically apparent.

Neuropathic abnormalities have also been reported in a variety of animal models of diabetes.[14,42,43] These changes (which have been most extensively studied in the rat) resemble those seen in human diabetes and include decreased sensory and motor nerve conduction velocity, abnormal nerve content of myoinositol and sorbitol, axonal degeneration, and segmental demyelination.[10,13,14,42,43] The functional and biochemical disturbance appears early (before structural changes occur) and is rapidly ameliorated by insulin treatment.[10,14] The latter seems to be dependent on the extent that hyperglycemia is corrected.[14] It is less certain, however, that diabetic nerve lesions in the rat can also be reversed. Nevertheless, a report has appeared suggesting that the early axonal changes in diabetic rats may be prevented or delayed by intensive insulin treatment.[44] It should be noted that neuropathic signs were not monitored in any of these animal experiments. Inasmuch as clinical neuropathy may not be correlated with the severity of functional or histological changes, the clinical implications of such observations remain uncertain.

Human Studies

Although results of animal experiments relating diabetic hyperglycemia to the development of the degenerative complications are of interest, their extrapolation to human disease must be made with caution. Some changes may be, in part, due to the toxic effects of drugs used to induce diabetes. As noted earlier, neither the glomerular nor the retinal lesions seen in diabetic animals are characteristic of advanced disease in humans. Most importantly, the effects of hyperglycemia in man may be modified by hereditary or environmental factors not present in animal models of diabetes.

Unfortunately, extensive clinical experience and numerous investigations in man have so far failed to demonstrate conclusively that metabolic control affects the course of vascular and neuropathic complications of diabetes. This critically important issue remains unresolved, not because of lack of interest but because major obstacles have been encountered. Until the development of glycosylated hemoglobin assays, which provide an index of integrated plasma glucose values over many weeks,[1] human studies were hampered by the imprecision of urine glucose testing and occasional blood glucose measurements to accurately reflect glycemic control between clinic visits. This may help explain the discrepant findings in many of the early retrospective case studies.[45–47] Furthermore, even under ideal circumstances, conventional treatment with one or two insulin injections is accompanied by wide swings in plasma glucose well outside the range of normal. It is therefore not surprising that Knowles et al.[48] found that the prevalence of vascular complications in their loosely controlled insulin-dependent diabetics was similar to that of other centers where more rigid control was attempted but not necessarily achieved. Essentially, they were comparing relatively poor with worse metabolic control.

The retrospective study of Johnson[49] in 1960 is of interest because he did have contrasting treatment groups. All patients in Malmö, Sweden in whom diabetes was diagnosed before 40 years of age were reviewed for the occurrence of nephropathy and retinopathy. The patients were then subdivided into two groups. Group I (71 patients) included those diagnosed between 1922 and 1935, a period when treatment consisted of strict dietary regulation and multiple injections of rapid-acting insulin; group II (115 patients) consisted of diabetics diagnosed between 1936 and 1945 when patients were given free diets and single daily injections of long-acting insulin. Nephropathy and more severe retinopathy were more common in group II patients even though the duration of diabetes was on average 8–10 years shorter than in group I. It should be noted, however, that 24% of group I patients died early in the course of their disease and were not included in the analysis, whereas only 8% of group II patients were not analyzed.

Prospective natural history studies, e.g., those reported by Pirat[50] and others,[51,52] suffer from problems in experimental design. In the Pirat study, 4,400 patients were followed over a 25-year period. He reported a markedly reduced frequency and delayed onset of microangiopathic and neuropathic complications in those patients with lower fasting and postprandial plasma glucose values.[50] Miki and coworkers[51] examined factors influencing progression of retinopathy in 364 diabetics (less than 19 to more than 70 years of age) followed for 2–6 years. Progression of retinopathy was significantly greater in the fair- and poor-control groups judged by fasting blood sugar measurements. Takazakura et al.[52] performed serial renal biopsies (interval 24–96 months) in 23 of their diabetic patients. Poorly controlled juvenile and "intermediate" type diabetics showed rapid progression of glomerular lesions. In many of the adult-type diabetes who were well controlled, renal lesions neither developed or progressed. Conclusions concerning cause-and-effect relationships are severely limited in such studies. Patients with increased frequency of complications may have also differed with respect to the degree of insulin deficiency, prevalence of hypertension, genetic factors, or other confounding variables not taken into account. Problems in interpretation are compounded by inclusion of patients of widely varying age, age at onset, and duration of diabetes.

Job and colleagues[53] attempted to avoid some of these difficulties when they designed a study to prospectively examine whether multiple (three) daily injections of insulin might alter the progression of background diabetic retinopathy. Patients were randomly assigned to either single- or multiple-injection groups, and the change in retinopathy was assessed by serial fluorescein angiograms. After approximately 3 years of follow-up, a greater increase in microaneurysm counts was reported in the single-injection group. Although these data have been cited as proof of a beneficial effect of tight metabolic control, criticism of the study illustrates some of the difficulties that can be encountered in clinical trials. Firstly, the investigators failed to show substantial differences in metabolic control between the treatment groups using fasting blood glucose and urinary glucose measurements. Even more importantly, the number of patients was small, and fewer than half (20 of 52) remained in their assigned treatment group for the duration of the study. Patients in the single-injection group seem to have had more severe disease at the start of the study. The ophthalmologists who counted the microaneurysms were not masked with respect to treatment group. Finally, there was no attempt to localize microaneurysms in order to assess individual lesion responses to treatment or to determine if microaneurysm counts are an appropriate measure of disease progression. For example, the number of microaneurysms may decrease because of diminished perfusion and thus not be indicative of an improvement in retinal status.

In 1978 Raskin critically reviewed the available data concerning diabetic regulation and its relationship to microangiopathy.[54] He pointed out that the issue would remain moot until modes of therapy became available that restored the diabetic's blood glucose to normal levels throughout the day. During the past 5–6 years, this hope has been at least partially fulfilled. Improvements in monitoring blood glucose levels and in insulin delivery [using either multiple daily injections or continuous subcutaneous insulin (CSII)] have provided the means to achieve normal or near-normal glucose control for extended periods of time. These advances have provided new opportunities to reexamine the issue.

METABOLIC AND HORMONAL EFFECTS OF IMPROVED GLYCEMIC CONTROL

Poorly controlled type I diabetes is characterized by a variety of metabolic and hormonal abnormalities in addition to hyperglycemia. Because these abnormalities may also contribute to the vascular or neuropathic complications of diabetes, a number of studies have examined whether such alterations are corrected in conjunction with improved glucose regulation. Conversely, attention has focused on whether intensive insulin treatment has adverse metabolic effects.

Abnormalities in lipid metabolism are commonly observed in patients with type I diabetes and may be an important pathogenic factor in the accelerated atherosclerosis of diabetes. Total cholesterol and particularly triglycerides are increased. Several investigators have demonstrated a reduction in total cholesterol and triglyceride concentrations in diabetic patients after several weeks of CSII treatment.[55,56] As shown in Figure 1–3, the rapid fall in total cholesterol is primarily accounted for by a sharp reduction in LDL cholesterol, which is sustained so long as treatment is continued.[56] Conversely, high density lipoprotein (HDL) cholesterol (which may facilitate the removal of cholesterol from large vessels) increases slowly over several months.[56] It has also been reported that more rigorous glycemic control improves cellular metabolism of lipoproteins.[57] Internalization and degradation of LDL from poorly controlled diabetics by normal human fibroblasts is impaired but is restored to normal

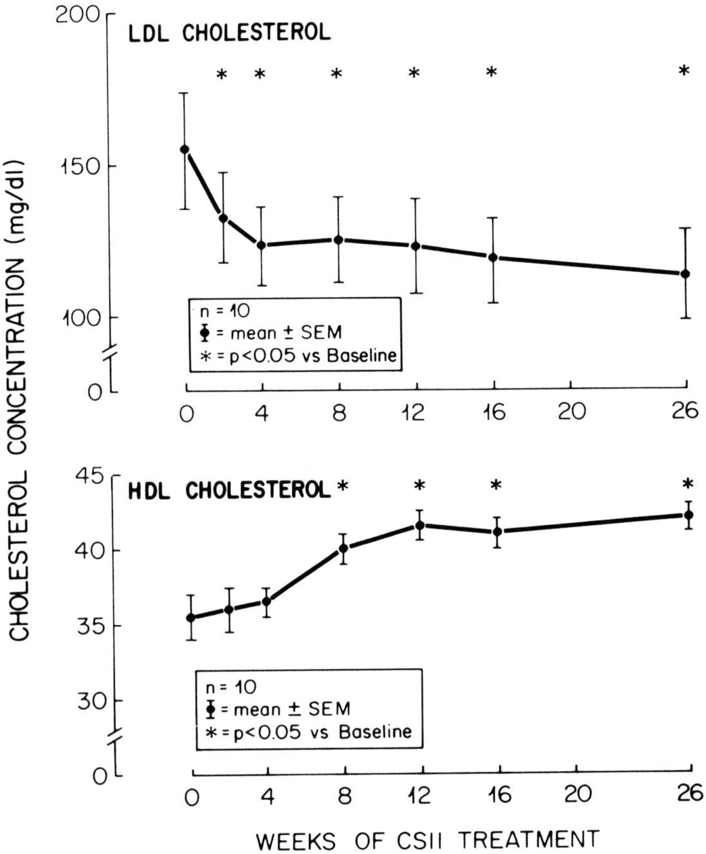

Fig. 1-3. Changes in LDL and HDL cholesterol during treatment of diabetes with continuous subcutaneous insulin infusion (CSII). (Data from Dunn R, Pietri A, Raskin P: Plasma lipid and lipoprotein levels with continuous subcutaneous insulin infusion in type I diabetes mellitus. Ann Intern Med 95:426, 1981.)

after 2 weeks of intensive insulin treatment. To the extent that lipid abnormalities contribute to the early development of atherosclerosis, these findings suggest that intensive insulin treatment may reduce the prevalence of this complication.

Elevations in growth hormone concentrations are commonly observed in patients with poorly controlled diabetes after exercise and during 24-hr monitoring.[58,59] Increased growth hormone levels have been implicated in the pathogenesis of microangiopathy, particularly retinopathy. Indeed, a reduction in growth hormone secretion was the rationale for pituitary ablation, a treatment for proliferative diabetic retinopathy in the era before laser therapy. Hansen was the first to demonstrate the reversibility of growth hormone hypersecretion by intensive treatment with multiple injections of insulin.[58] Similarly, basal and postexercise growth hormone concentrations have been restored to normal following short- and long-term CSII treatment.[60,61]

Hypersecretion of growth hormone may also help perpetuate the metabolic derangements of diabetes to a much greater extent than generally appreciated. In a recent study Press et al.[62] administered exogenous growth hormone as hourly intravenous pulses for 21–45 hr to a group of diabetics who were optimally controlled with CSII. Before growth hormone administration, mean 24-hr plasma glucose and growth hormone levels were within the range of normal. However, when serum growth hormone was raised to levels similar to those observed in poorly controlled diabetics, a marked deterioration in glycemic control was observed. Circulating fatty acids, ketones, and branched-chain amino acids were also increased. Thus growth hormone elevations can themselves reproduce the entire spectrum of poor diabetic control in spite of previously optimized insulin treatment. It follows therefore that some of the metabolic benefits of more intensive insulin regimens may be derived from their growth-hormone-lowering effects.

The use of intensive treatment has provided new insights into the hormonal basis of the impaired growth seen in uncontrolled diabetes during childhood (Mauriac syndrome). Because growth hormone levels tend to be increased rather than reduced in poorly controlled diabetes, attention turned to a possible diabetes-induced defect in other circulating growth factors, in particular insulin-like growth factor I (IGF-I). Early studies in diabetics receiving conventional treatment yielded contradictory results; normal, elevated, and reduced levels of IGF-I were reported.[63,64] These discrepancies may have resulted from differences in methodologies (i.e., bioassay versus radioimmunoassay), variability in the level of diabetic control, and failure to account for the changes in IGF-I which accompany normal growth and pubertal development. (IGF-I levels are low during infancy and peak to values in the acromegalic range during normal adolescence).[65] Recent studies using CSII, however, clearly demonstrated that insulin deficiency results in a defect in IGF-I synthesis. Not only were IGF-I levels reduced in poorly controlled diabetic patients as compared to age- and sex-matched normal controls,[66] but IGF-I levels increased by 25 percent after only 1 week of insulin pump treatment in the face of a fall in growth hormone values. A further rise in IGF-I concentrations is observed with more prolonged improvement in metabolic control.[61] These data suggest that hypersecretion of growth hormone in poorly controlled diabetes may be a compensatory response to a reduction in IGF-I levels. The rise in IGF-I values induced by intensive treatment may, in turn, cause suppression of growth hormone hypersecretion via a negative feedback mechanism.

Despite the diverse metabolic and hormonal derangements seen in conventionally treated diabetic children, a number of studies have failed to domonstrate a relationship between growth and diabetes control.[67,68] Interpretation is limited by difficulties in the assessment of growth potential as well as the failure to obtain optimal metabolic control in the population under study. Recent studies with intensive treatment regimens, however, suggest that children receiving conventional injection therapy may not reach their full growth potential. There is a sharp increase in growth velocity in diabetic youngsters with apparent normal stature and growth rates after institution of CSII or multiple-injection treatment.[69] It is reasonable to speculate that this effect on growth is mediated, at least in part, by stimulation of IGF-I production (Fig. 1-4). However, the increase in IGF-I seen with improved control may have negative clinical implications as well. Merimee and colleagues[70] reported significant elevations of IGF-I levels in type I diabetics with fulminant proliferative diabetic retinopathy.

It has been suggested that systems which utilize a peripheral rather than a portal route of insulin delivery might lower plasma glucose at the expense of hyperinsulinemia. Hyperinsulinemia might have adverse metabolic effects or contribute to insulin resistance due to down-regulation of the insulin receptor. Yet only mild elevations in basal free insulin levels have been observed with CSII, and the peak postprandial values seem to be lower than postprandial insulin concentrations in normal subjects.[71,72] Furthermore, intensive treatment does not reduce below normal the concentrations of insulin-sensitive fuels that are largely metabolized by peripheral tissues, e.g., branched-chain amino acids, free fatty acids, and ketones.[55,73] It is also

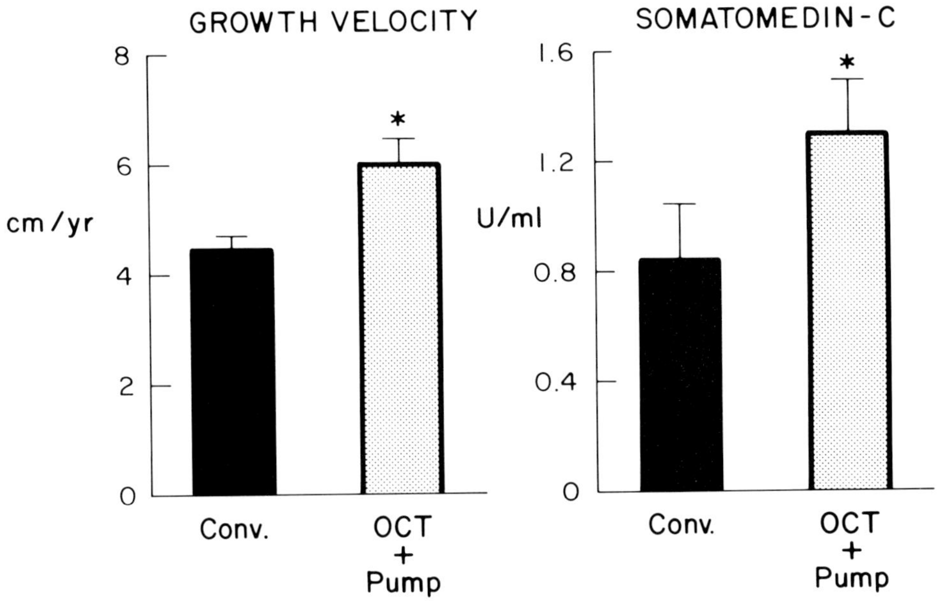

Fig. 1-4. Effect of intensive insulin treatment (either with a pump or optimized conventional therapy (OCT) for 1 year on the rate of growth and the levels of somatomedin-C (or 1GF-1) in adolescent diabetic patients.

noteworthy that CSII has not caused a reduction in either insulin binding or insulin sensitivity (as assessed by the euglycemic, insulin clamp technique).[74,75] Insulin sensitivity tends to increase but may not be totally normalized with CSII.

It is conceivable, of course, that the mild elevations of circulating insulin concentrations seen between meals with the use of subcutaneous insulin may have harmful effects that are not readily detected in short-term studies. For example, it has been theorized that peripheral hyperinsulinemia may play a role in the accelerated atherosclerosis that accompanies diabetes.[76] Concerns about the development of secondary amyloidosis with the use of insulin infusion devices has been raised by a recent study in beagle dogs.[77] Amyloid deposits were demonstrated in the liver, kidney, spleen, and pancreas in both nondiabetic and diabetic dogs receiving intravenous insulin via a portable pump for 2–8 months. The mechanism of this complication and its relevance to man are not understood. The amyloid may have resulted from the long-term use of the intravenous route or from insulin aggregates found in the insulin reservoir. It is reassuring that Koivisto et al.[78] failed to demonstrate any signs of local or systemic amyloidosis in patients treated with CSII for 3–40 months.

CAPILLARY BASEMENT MEMBRANE THICKENING

The concept that diabetic microangiopathy is largely determined by genetic (rather than metabolic) factors derives support from studies of skeletal muscle capillary basement membranes. In 1968 Siperstein et al.[79] reported that muscle biopsy specimens from a vast majority of diabetic patients have markedly thickened capillary basement membranes, a finding analogous to that found in most other tissues. The degree of basement membrane thickening in this study did not seem to be related to age or to the severity or duration of the diabetes. Even more surprisingly, similar (albeit less severe) basement membrane changes were noted in over 50 percent of subjects with a strong family history of diabetes (''prediabetes'') but with normal glucose tolerance. Furthermore, the appearance of basement membrane thickening in patients with secondary diabetes (e.g., pancreatitis) was found to be much less frequent despite marked hyperglycemia.[79] In a more recent study, Marks et al.[80] found that a significant number of parents of type I diabetic children who themselves did not have diabetes had thickened muscle capillary basement membranes. Interesting, this finding was closely associated with the presence of the HLA-DR4 haplotype. Taken together, these data imply that genetic factors may play an important role in the pathogenesis of diabetic complications.

These studies have been challenged on both technical and experimental grounds.[81] It has been suggested that the modest increase in basement membrane thickening observed in ''prediabetes'' by Siperstein et al. could be accounted for by the fact that this group was older than the nondiabetic controls to which they were compared. In normal subjects capillary basement membrane width increases with age.[81] Other studies have provided evidence that muscle capillary basement membrane thickening follows rather than precedes the development of overt diabetes and that muscle capillary basement membrane width depends on the duration of the diabetes.[81,82] In a more clinically relevant tissue, Osterby demonstrated that glomerular basement membrane width is normal at the onset of insulin-dependent diabetes and that subsequent increases in basement membrane thickness are the earliest ultrastructural lesions to become detectable in the kidney.[83] In a complementary study, Mauer and associates determined glomerular basement membrane thickness in renal allograph biopsies before and 2 years after transplantation in diabetic and nondiabetic patients.[84] Increases in glomerular basement membrane width occurred only in kidneys transplanted into diabetics.

The importance of metabolic factors in the development of muscle capillary basement membrane thickening is also supported by recent studies with intensive insulin treatment. Peterson et al.[85] showed a decrease in the width of the capillary basement membrane in six of seven diabetic patients after 8–10 months of an intensive program employing multiple daily insulin injections and blood glucose self-monitoring. An increase in basement membrane thickness was observed in the only patient who failed to lower glycosylated hemoglobin values during the study. Raskin and colleagues[86] used CSII to examine this issue (Fig. 1-5). They studied 23 type I diabetics: 13 patients received CSII, and 10 patients remained on unchanged conven-

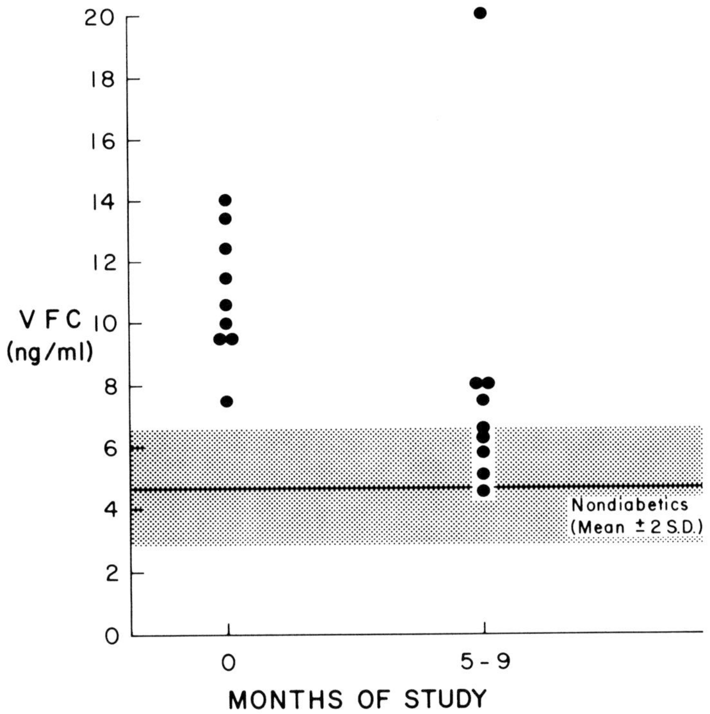

Fig. 1-5. Effect of intensive insulin treatment for 2 years on muscle capillary basement membrane thickness in type I diabetic patients. The control group was treated with conventional injection therapy. (Adapted with permission from Raskin P, Pietri AO, Unger R, Shannon WA Jr: The effect of diabetic control on the width of skeletal-muscle capillary basement membrane in patients with type I diabetes mellitus. N Engl J Med 309:1546, 1983.)

tional insulin treatment. After 2 years most patients given CSII showed a sharp reduction in both glycosylated hemoglobin levels and skeletal muscle capillary basement membrane width. No change in either of these parameters was consistently observed in the conventional treatment group. At the same time, Camerini-Davalos et al.[87] reported a reduction in basement membrane thickness in patients with impaired carbohydrate tolerance after 3 years of treatment with glipizide compared to controls given a placebo. In an accompanying editorial, Siperstein cautioned against over-interpreting these findings.[88] One cannot safely extrapolate the degree of microangiopathy in muscle to that in more clinically important sites; capillary turnover is much more rapid in skeletal muscle than in the eye and kidney. Perhaps more important, the relationship between basement membrane thickening and other more destructive lesions of the retina and glomerulous remains speculative.

EFFECT OF INTENSIVE TREATMENT ON DIABETIC MICROANGIOPATHY

Retinopathy

Functional Abnormalities. Functional changes of the retina, e.g., increased fluorescein leakage from retinal vessels[89] and decreased oscillatory potential and macular recovery time,[90] may be observed in diabetic patients either before or coincident with the appearance of mild retinopathy. These changes are thought to reflect alterations in the retina-blood barrier and in retinal performance, and may be premonitory of more advanced disease. Bleicher et al.[91] estimated retinal fluorescein leakage using the vitreous fluorophotometry technique in a group of type I diabetic patients without proliferative retinopathy who were being treated with multiple daily injections. Fluorescein leakage seemed to be related to the degree of metabolic control; vitreous fluorescein concentrations were increased only in those patients who failed to normalize HbA_{1c} levels. White and associates[27] used the same technique to measure fluorescein leakage in 11 type I diabetics before and after 5–9 months of intensive treatment. They reported a reduction in leakage in eight of nine patients without proliferative retinopathy treated with either CSII or multiple injections (Fig. 1-6). However, vitreous fluorescein concentrations were not altered in the two patients with proliferative retinopathy, and leakage increased in one patient with a concurrent deterioration of background changes.

Improvements in retinal function after 6 months of rigorous metabolic control were also noted in a preliminary report from the Steno Study Group.[90] These investigators randomized 32 type I diabetics with nonproliferative retinopathy to either unchanged conventional treatment or to CSII. In the CSII group, blood glucose and HbA_{1c} fell to near-normal values, and this was accompanied by decreased fluorescein leakage as well as increased oscillatory potential and macular recovery time. In contrast, hyperglycemic patients in the conventional treatment group showed a deterioration in all indices of retinal function. It should be emphasized, however, that these functional changes have not been definitively linked to the retinal complications of diabetes. As is commented on below, a subsequent report from the Steno Study Group

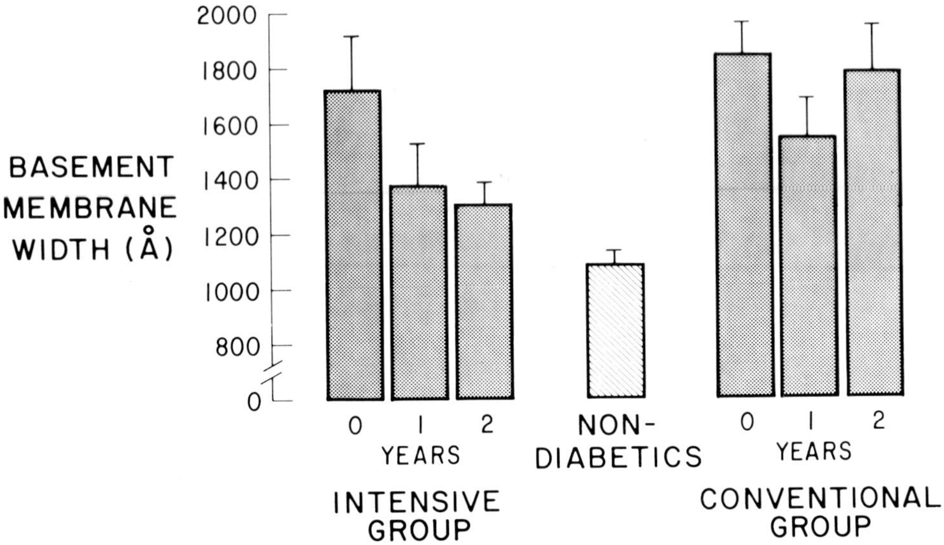

Fig. 1-6. Vitreous fluorescein concentration in the posterior chamber of diabetic patients with nonproliferative retinopathy after intravenous fluorescein injection. Results are compared 1 month before and 5–9 months after intensive insulin treatment. (Adapted from White NH, Waltman SR, Krupin T, Santiago J: Reversal abnormalities in ocular fluorophotometry in insulin-dependent diabetes after five to nine months of improved metabolic control. Diabetes 31:80, 1982.)

indicates that functional improvements may occur even in the face of worsening in clinical retinopathy as assessed by retinal photographs.[92] Given this apparent paradox, it seems prudent to rely on well-established clinical endpoints.

Established Retinopathy. It was hoped that the controversy surrounding the metabolic hypothesis would be quickly resolved when CSII therapy was used to treat patients with established microangiopathy. Interest was heightened by early individual case reports recounting the benefit of CSII on diabetic retinopathy. Unfortunately, these preliminary reports have not been confirmed. This was apparent when we analyzed the retinal photographs from the original group of diabetic patients recruited at our center for long-term outpatient CSII therapy.[93] The group consisted of 27 patients with type I diabetes who had received CSII for more than 2–3 years. They ranged in age from 13 to 46 years and had a history of diabetes for 2–29 years. Seven patients had no evidence of microvascular disease at the start of the study, whereas 20 had diabetic retinopathy of varying severity. As shown in Figure 1-7, one of the 14 eyes without retinopathy developed minimal background retinopathy; 11 of 25 eyes with background retinopathy worsened, including two eyes that developed proliferative changes; 4 of 15 eyes (27%) with proliferative changes progressed. Thus in spite of a dramatic improvement in metabolic control, diabetic retinopathy continued to progress, and in no case did it reverse.

Such results indicate the need for long-term, controlled, randomized trials. Several small-scale, single and multicenter studies (the Steno Study Group and Kroc Col-

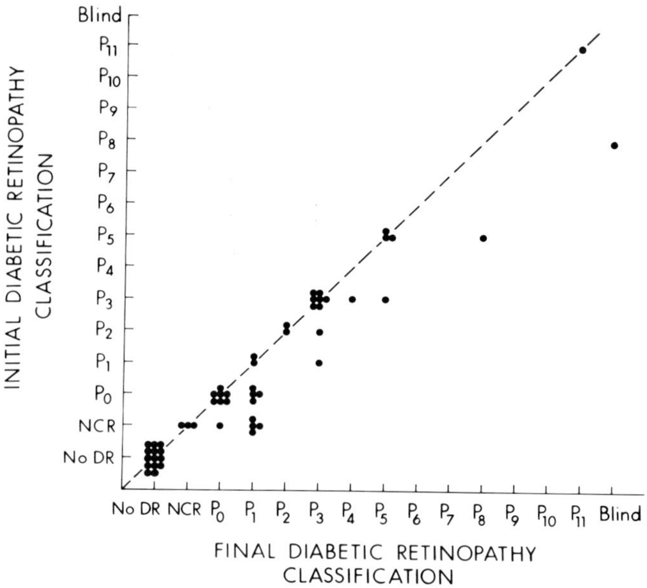

Fig. 1-7. Effect of long-term (2–3 years) CSII treatment on diabetic retinopathy. The scatter diagram plots the initial modified ETDRS classification (from retinal photographs) of each age on the ordinate with the final modified ETDRS classification on the abscissa. Dots falling on the 45° line represent no change; those below the line represent a progression of retinopathy. Eyes denoted as "no DR" showed no evidence of retinopathy, and those denoted as "NCR" showed very mild nonproliferative retinopathy that was insufficient to be classified as group Po. (Adapted with permisison from Puklin JE, Tamborlane WV, Sherwin RS: Diabetic retinopathy is not reversed by longterm insulin pump treatment. In Henkind P (ed): ACTA XXIV International Congress of Ophthalmology. Vol. 2. p. 803. Lippincott, Philadelphia, 1983.)

laborative Group studies) have already been undertaken, and the feasibility of the large Diabetes Control and Complications Trial sponsored by the National Health Institutes of Health is presently being tested. As alluded to earlier, the Steno Study Group reported improvements in retinal function after 6 months of CSII.[90] The original optimism, however, has been tempered by their less encouraging report describing the morphological changes in the retina after 1 year of follow-up.[92] The changes in the severity of diabetic retinopathy by treatment group as assessed by stereo fundus photographs and fluorescein angiograms are shown in Figure 1-8. When both treatment groups are taken together, more patients showed deterioration than showed improvement. Although the frequency of deterioration was highest in the CSII treatment group, this difference did not achieve statistical significance.

The Steno Study might be criticized because of the small number of patients studied and on the basis of the local methods used to quantitate retinopathy. The Kroc Collaborative Study was similar to the Steno Study in design, except that it was carried out at six clinical centers and involved more patients.[94] In addition, stereo fundus photographs were graded by an independent reading center not directly involved with the development of the trial. In the Kroc Study, 70 patients with early nonpro-

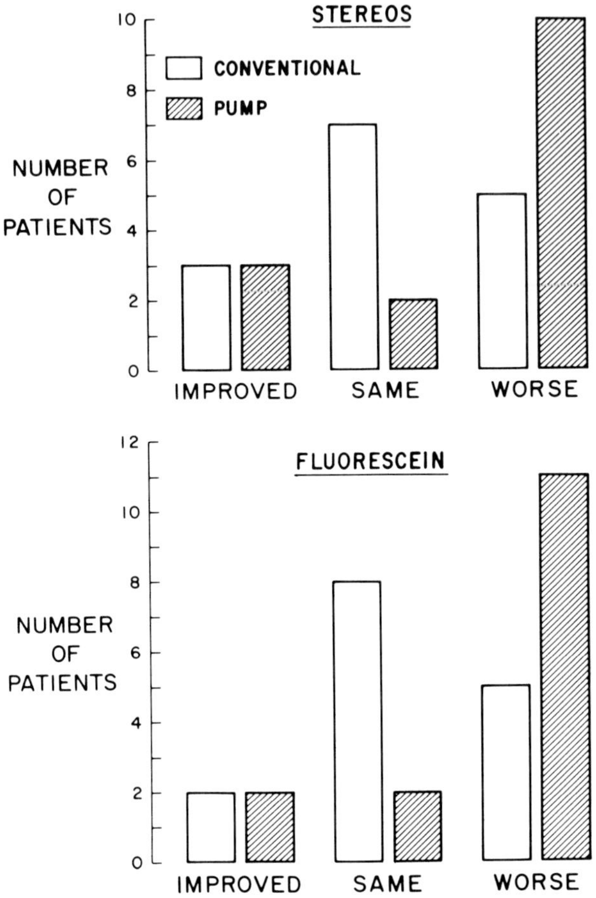

Fig. 1-8. Number of diabetic patients whose retinal stereo photographs and fluorescein angiograms improved, stayed the same, or worsened 1 year after randomization to either CSII (pump) or conventional injection therapy. (Data from Steno Study Group: Effect of 1 year of near-normal blood glucose levels on retinopathy in insulin-dependent diabetics. Lancet 1:200, 1983.)

liferative diabetic retinopathy were randomly assigned to CSII or unchanged conventional injection treatment. At the start of the study, both groups displayed similar clinical and glycemic characteristics. Over the succeeding 8 months, blood glucose and HbA_1 levels fell to near-normal values with CSII but remained elevated in the conventional treatment group. There was evidence that the retinopathy worsened in both groups over a relatively short period of time. As with the Steno Study, this occurred slightly more rapidly with CSII.

The results of the Steno and Kroc studies indicate that improvement in glycemic control for 8–12 months is ineffective in slowing the progression of established retinopathy and may cause the appearance of new lesions. In both studies the new lesions consisted mostly of soft exudates, which are thought to represent microinfarcts of the nerve fiber layer. Perhaps the metabolic improvement induced by CSII reduces retinal perfusion, which in turn causes infarction of previously compromised areas. Whatever the mechanism, the loss of localized areas of the retina may simply be the price paid for preservation of normal retinal tissue. It should be kept in mind that the long-term outcome may be quite different. Indeed, a preliminary 2-year follow-up report by the Steno Group suggests that CSII treatment may lead to lessening of the retinopathy after a more-prolonged period of observation.[95] Furthermore, it remains to be established whether intensive treatment regimens might prevent the development of retinopathy if initiated early in the course of the disease.

Nephropathy

Functional Abnormalities. Renal hypertrophy, hyperperfusion, and hyperfiltration occurs in conventionally treated type I diabetics at the onset of the disease, long before the appearance of clinical diabetic nephropathy. Furthermore, before the development of gross proteinuria, excessive urinary excretion of albumin can be detected in diabetics using sensitive radioimmunoassay techniques. Many patients with normal basal excretion rates of albumin show excessive albuminuria with exercise.[96] The potential importance of these observations is underscored by the report of Viberti et al.,[97] which suggests that elevated basal microalbuminuria is predictive of subsequent clinical nephropathy.

The group at Guy's Hospital were the first to examine the effects of CSII on microalbuminuria.[26] Seven patients with elevated albumin excretion rates on conventional treatment showed a reduction after only 1–3 days of improved metabolic control. β_2-Microglobulin excretion (an index of renal tubular reabsorptive capacity) did not change. Even more importantly, a persistent reduction in microalbuminuria to normal control values has been noted with more prolonged CSII therapy.[90] Koivisto and co-workers[98] demonstrated that the exaggerated, exercise-induced increments in albumin excretion seen in early diabetes are also blunted with improved metabolic control.

Glomerular filtration rate is increased in newly diagnosed type I diabetes and can be promptly reduced with the initiation of insulin treatment.[25] Several groups have postulated that these early hemodynamic changes may play an important role in the subsequent development of microalbuminuria and nephrosclerosis (see above). It is therefore not surprising that glomerular filtration rates were significantly reduced after 4 months of CSII in the Steno Study but increased slightly in the conventional treatment group.[90]

Clinical Nephropathy. Studies of the effect of intensive treatment in patients with established diabetic nephropathy have yielded a picture that is quite similar to that of retinopathy. In contrast to the improvement in early functional changes, studies thus far have failed to demonstrate a beneficial effect of "tight" glucose regulation on more-advanced renal disease (Fig. 1-9). Six of our original group of CSII-treated patients had proteinuria in excess of 1 g/day. Although they demonstrated an initial decline in proteinuria during the first few months of CSII treatment, this effect was not sustained and all remained proteinuric after 13–18 months.[99] Two patients have subsequently developed end-stage renal disease. Vilberti et al.[100] also examined the influence of improved metabolic control in diabetic patients whose glomerular filtration rate had already begun its usual inexorable downward slope. In spite of CSII therapy for up to 2 years, they were not able to arrest the decline in glomerular filtration rate.

The lack of response of clinical nephropathy to CSII may be related to the fail-

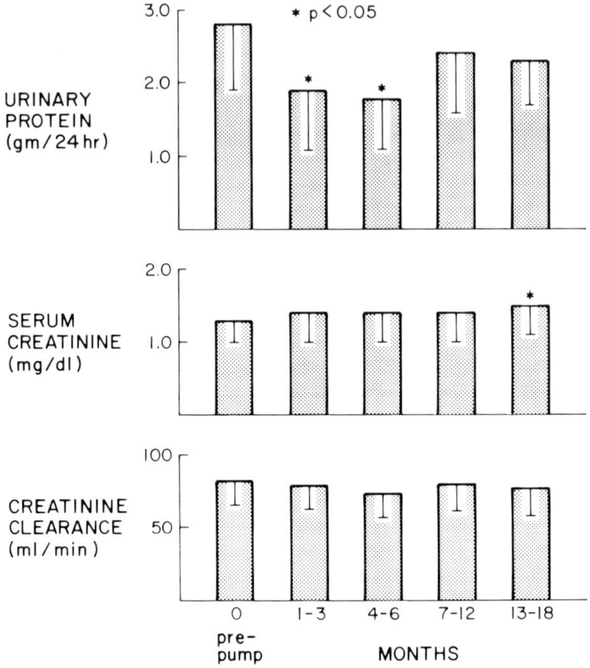

Fig. 1-9. Changes in urinary protein excretion, serum creatinine, and creatinine clearance after CSII (insulin pump) treatment in six type I diabetics with clinical evidence of nephropathy. Values are presented as the mean ±SEM. (Data from Tamborlane WV, Puklin JE, Bergman M, et al: Long-term improvement of metabolic control with the insulin pump does not reverse diabetic microangiopathy. Diabetes Care, suppl. 1, 5:58, 1982.)

ure of this therapy to totally correct the metabolic disturbance. Even in the best hands, average HbA_{1c} levels during CSII tend to settle at or just above the upper limit of the normal range. It is also possible that once overt nephropathy appears the histological lesions are so advanced that they are no longer amenable to therapy. As noted earlier, the hemodynamic theory of the pathogenesis of diabetic nephropathy would predict such an outcome. A provocative experiment in nature has shed some light on this issue by providing evidence that glomerular lesions may be reversed by restoration of normal glucose metabolism. Abouna et al.[101] transplanted the kidneys from a patient with a 17-year history of insulin-dependent diabetes into two nondiabetic recipients. At the time of death, the diabetic donor had proteinuria but normal serum creatinine. Histological examination of the kidneys showed features of established diabetic nephropathy, including diffuse glomerulosclerosis and thickening of the mesangial matrix and capillary basement membranes. Renal biopsy specimens taken 7 months after transplantation showed dramatic change, with near-complete resolution of the diabetic lesions. Furthermore, the nondiabetic recipients continued to be free of proteinuria for a further 7 months.

This observation is complemented by the report of Mauer et al.,[84] which demonstrated the appearance of diabetic glomerulopathy in normal living related donor and cadaver kidneys after transplantion into diabetic recipients. Within 2 years, each of six diabetic patients showed an increase in glomerular basement membrane thickness and mesangial widening in their new kidney: Such changes were not observed in nondiabetic transplant recipients. Taken together, these findings provide graphic support for the metabolic hypothesis and are remarkably similar to analogous studies in diabetic animals.[34,40] Enthusiasm must still be tempered because of the limited amount of data available and the fact that the histological changes occurred in a setting of normoglycemia. The latter is rarely if ever attainable, despite current improvements in diabetic care.

Neuropathy

Functional Studies. Abnormalities in nerve conduction can be detected in many diabetic patients before the onset of neuropathic signs and symptoms. Graf and associates[102] studied sensory and motor conduction velocities in type II diabetics before and after treatment with either diet, sulfonylureas, or insulin. The metabolic improvements which accompanied such therapies were associated with an increase in motor, but not sensory, conduction velocities. In addition, substantial increases in motor conduction velocities have been observed in asymptomatic type I diabetes after diabetic control was improved with CSII.[103] In a controlled trial, Holman et al.[104] observed an improvement in vibration sensory threshold in type I diabetes randomized to an intensive program, whereas this parameter deteriorated in patients in the conventional treatment group. An improvement in sensory conduction velocity with CSII has been observed by some[105] but not all investigators.[103]

The hypothesis that the polyol pathway plays a role in mediating the effects of hyperglycemia on nerve conduction is supported by a recent study using the drug sorbinil. Sorbinil, a potent aldose reductase inhibitor, was administered for 9 weeks to 39 stable diabetics without symptoms of neuropathy in a randomized, double-blind, cross-over study.[11] Medial motor and sensory and peroneal motor conduction velocities all increased even though HbA_1 levels remained unchanged. This effect was rapidly dissipated when the drug was discontinued. It should be noted, however, that the changes in conduction velocity were very small, and thus their clinical relevance can be questioned. Furthermore, it remains unclear whether the improvement in nerve conduction seen with intensive treatment can be invoked as evidence for its utility in preventing the appearance of clinically overt neuropathic symptoms.

Symptomatic Neuropathy. Boulton and colleagues recently examined whether CSII might alter the course of symptomatic polyneuropathy.[106] Nine type I diabetics were studied before and after 4 months of improved metabolic control. Symptomatic relief was noted by all patients, and this was accompanied by a significant improvement in pain scores. There was also an increase in the vibration perception threshold and the motor conduction velocity. Other case reports have suggested an improvement in symptoms of autonomic as well as peripheral neuropathy with intensive treatment.[107] However, controlled studies in large numbers of patients are needed to determine if the symptomatic changes actually result from the improvement in metabolic control. This is particularly important because neuropathic symptoms are known to wax and wane, even in the absence of changes in glucose regulation and because the treatment regimen itself could easily have had a placebo effect. Clinical experience suggests that the response of neuropathic symptoms to intensified insulin treatment is highly variable.

Atherosclerosis

In spite of the focus on microvascular complications, atherosclerosis involving the arteries of the heart, lower extremities, and brain continues to be the major cause of death from diabetes. This is especially true in the most common form of the disease, noninsulin-dependent diabetes. The atherosclerosis process is indistinguishable from that seen in the nondiabetic population but begins earlier and is more severe. The predilection to atherosclerosis is uniformly observed over the entire spectrum of diabetes: from difficult-to-control insulin-dependent patients to those patients with mild hyperglycemia not requiring insulin. For unclear reasons, the disparity between diabetic and normal subjects with respect to atherosclerosis is more pronounced in women.[108]

The explanation for the accelerated atherosclerosis in diabetes is not known. It seems to be an independent risk factor and not solely attributable to an increased frequency of the other recognized factors, e.g., hypertension, smoking, or hyperlipidemia. It is appealing to ascribe the phenomenon in some way to the metabolic disturbance. Surely there are a number of theoretical considerations that would support this view. Nonetheless, there is little, if any, clinical evidence linking the severity of the metabolic disorder to the incidence of atherosclerosis. This issue is complicated by the multifactorial nature of the disorder and its lack of specificity for diabetes. Unfortunately, animal models of diabetes have not proved useful in studying the problem; the appearance of microangiopathy in such animals is not generally accompanied by significant large-vessel disease.

There is a substantial amount of data from large population surveys indicating that the level of hyperglycemia bears little relationship to the appearance of clinically detectable large-vessel disease.[109–111] Similar conclusions were made by Pirat[50] from his long-term prospective analysis of a large group of diabetic patients. Whereas microvascular and neuropathic complications developed more commonly in individuals showing the highest glucose levels, this was not true for atherosclerotic complications.[50] One could argue that some other metabolic abnormality induced by diabetes, but which is not closely correlated with the degree of hyperglycemia, could be responsible. Although there remains no proof that this is the case, a large array of potential contributors to the atherosclerotic process have been found to be abnormal in diabetic patients (Table 1-2).

It has also been difficult to show that efforts aimed at improving metabolic con-

Table 1-2. Possible Factors Contributing to Increased Risk of Atherosclerosis in Diabetes

Lipoprotein abnormalities
Increased platelet prostaglandin synthesis
Decreased prostacyclin release
Increased platelet aggregation
Increased von Willebrand factor and fibrinogen
Decreased fibrinolysis
Increased growth hormone and epinephrine
Presence of antigen-antibody complexes
Increased blood viscosity
Hyperglycemia (sorbitol)

trol have any influcence on the course of large-vessel complications in diabetic patients. The UGDP study reported no reduction in cardiovascular mortality or morbidity in noninsulin-dependent diabetics treated with oral hypoglycemic agents.[112] More importantly, patients randomly assigned to the variable insulin therapy group failed to show a significant change in the death rate from cardiovascular causes compared to a placebo group, despite a diminution in average blood glucose levels.[113,114] There was, among the insulin-treated patients, a tendency toward less cardiovascular mortality in those patients who achieved normal fasting glucose levels the majority of the time. However, such artificial subdivisions of the data defeat the purpose of the randomization procedure and thus must be viewed with extreme caution. Yet there are theoretical reasons for anticipating some benefit from tighter metabolic control. Intensive insulin treatment has been shown to lower LDL cholesterol and very low density lipoprotein (VLDL) triglycerides, increase HDL cholesterol, improve platelet and endothelial cell function, reduce fibrinogen turnover, and reduce exercise-induced catecholamine release in humans.[17,56,60,85] Such data must be viewed as circumstantial however; the issue will only be resolved on the basis of definable clinical endpoints.

SUMMARY

It is still uncertain if the degenerative complications of human diabetes are caused by inadequate correction of the metabolic derangement and if they can be prevented or delayed by more intensive treatment regimens. Logic dictates an affirmative answer. However, the issue has never been put to formal test in man and thus continues to be a subject of heated debate. The bulk of experimental data reviewed in this chapter supports the metabolic hypothesis, at least with respect to microvascular and neuropathic complications. Surely if current theories regarding the pathogenesis of complications are correct and diabetic animals are appropriate models of human diabetes, there is little doubt that benefits would be accrued from early institution of tight metabolic control. This may not necessarily follow for established complications, however. With the exception of Mauer's data, there is little evidence from animals indicating that structural lesions can be reversed. Furthermore, it can be argued that glomerular lesions in those studies were not sufficient to have caused clinical disease and that the mode of treatment (islet transplantation) produced metabolic correction not clinically possible.

The metabolic hypothesis is supported by data in the human as well. Perhaps the most compelling evidence derives from a few experiments in nature. It is difficult to ignore the appearance of early diabetic renal lesions in normal kidneys transplanted into diabetic patients or the clearing of nephropathic changes after transplantation of a diabetic kidney into a nondiabetic host. The potential value of new improved treatment methods is suggested by evidence that functional abnormalities and muscle capillary basement membrane thickening can be reversed. Yet if the metabolic abnormalities are casually responsible, why has it not been possible to reverse or even halt progression of microangiopathic complications with intensive insulin treatment? Indeed the progression of mild nonproliferative retinopathy seems to accelerate in the short term after such treatment. Furthermore, clinical experience with more aggressive attempts at correction of hyperglycemia have not clearly demonstrated an improvement in neuropathy or a diminution in cardiovascular mortality. We have all seen patients who in spite of good control of hyperglycemia have been ravaged by diabetic complications and, conversely, poorly controlled patients with negligible problems.

How can these apparent discrepancies be resolved? Existing clinical data in no way refute the idea that the metabolic disturbance plays a critical role in *initiating* most, if not all, of the degenerative complications of diabetes. However, they do suggest that in man the story is more complicated, perhaps because individual patients display wide variation in their susceptibility to metabolic injury. The clinical data also suggest that a point may be reached when the propagation of diabetic lesions occurs independent of the metabolic disturbance. This view is not inconsistent with either current metabolic theories or animal experiments. It is noteworthy in this regard that histological damage may long antedate clinically detectable disease.

If this interpretation is correct, it implies that the degree of metabolic correction required to prevent or arrest early lesions varies among diabetic patients; the imperfect therapy available today may not be sufficient in all patients. More importantly, it would predict that intensive therapy would be most effective early, long before complications have appeared. This, of course, is easier said than done. In spite of recent advances, youngsters with diabetes continue to be the most difficult group in whom to achieve and maintain tight metabolic control.

REFERENCES

1. Keonig RJ, Peterson CM, Jones RL, et al: Correlation of glucose regulation and hemoglobin A_{1c} in diabetes mellitus. N Engl J Med 295:417, 1976
2. Bunn HF: Evaluation of glycosylated hemoglobin in diabetic patients. Diabetes 30:613, 1981
3. Shapiro R, McManus MJ, Zalut C, Bunn HF: Sites of nonenzymatic glycosylation of human hemoblogin A. J Biol Chem 255:3120, 1980
4. Bunn HF: Nonenzymatic glycosylation of protein: relevance to diabetes. Am J Med 70:325, 1981
5. Witztum JL, Mahoney EM, Branks MJ, et al: Nonenzymatic glucosylation of low-density lipoprotein alters it biological activity. Diabetes 31:283, 1982
6. Williams SK, Devenney JJ, Bitensky WM: Micropinocytic ingestions of glycosylated albumin by isolated microvesicles: possible role in pathogenesis of diabetic microangiopathy. Proc Natl Acad Sci USA 78:2392, 1981
7. Bassiouny AR, Rosenberg H, McDonald TL: Glycosylated collagen is antigenic. Diabetes 32:1182, 1983
8. Clements RS Jr, Weaver JP, Wingrad AI: The distribution of polyol: NADP oxidoreductase in mammalian tissues. Biochem Biophys Res Commun 36:1006, 1969
9. Gabbay KH, O'Sullivan JB: The sorbitol pathway in diabetes and galactosemia: enzyme and substrate localization. Diabetes 17:300, 1968
10. Ward JD, Baker RWR, Davis BH: Effect of blood sugar control on the accumulation of sorbitol and fructose in nervous tissue. Diabetes 21:1173, 1972

11. Judzewitxch RG, Jaspan JB, Polonsky KS, et al: Aldose reductase inhibition improves nerve conduction velocity in diabetic patients. N Engl J Med 308:119, 1983
12. Jakobsen J: Peripheral nerves in early experimental diabetes: expansion of the endoneurical space as a cause of increased water content. Diabetologia 14:113, 1978
13. Sidenius P: The axonopathy of diabetic neuropathy. Diabetes 31:356, 1982
14. Greene DA, Lattimer SA: Sodium- and energy-dependent uptake of myoinositol by rabbit peripheral nerve: competitive inhibition by glucose and lack of an insulin effect. J Clin Invest 70:1009, 1982
15. Greene DA, DeJesus PV Jr, Winegrad AI: Effects of insulin and dietary myoinositol on impaired peripheral motor nerve conduction velocity in acute streptozotocin diabetes. J Clin Invest 55:1326, 1975
16. Ishibashi T, Tanaka K, Taniguchi Y: Platelet aggregation and coagulation in the pathogenesis of diabetic retinopathy in rats. Diabetes 30:601, 1980
17. Colwell JA, Winocour PD, Halushka PV: Do platelets have anything to do with diabetic microvascular disease? Diabetes, suppl. 2, 32:14, 1983
18. Hostetter TH, Rennke HG, Brenner BM: The case of intrarenal hypertension in the initiation and progression of diabetic and other glomerulopathies. Am J Med 72:375, 1982
19. Parving H-H, Viberti GC, Keen H, et al: Hemodynamic factors in the genesis of diabetic microangiopathy. Metabolism 32:943, 1983
20. Hostetter TH, Tory JL, Brenner BM: Glomerular hemodynamics in experimental diabetes. Kidney Int 19:410, 1981
21. Hostetter TH, Olson JL, Rennke HG, et al: Hyperfiltration in remnant nephrons: a potentially adverse response to renal ablation. Am J Physiol 241:F85, 1981
22. Steffes MW, Brown DM, Mauer SM: Diabetic glomerulopathy following unilateral nephrectomy in the rat. Diabetes 27:35, 1978
23. Mauer SM, Steffes MW, Azar S, et al: The effects of Goldblatt hypertension on development of the glomerular lesions of diabetes mellitus in the rat. Diabetes 27:738, 1978
24. Berkman J, Rifkin H: Unilateral nodular diabetic glomerulosclerosis (Kimmelstiel-Wilson). Metabolism 22:715, 1973
25. Christiansen JS, Gammelgaard J, Tronier B, et al: Kidney function and size in diabetics before and during initial insulin treatment. Kidney Int 21:683, 1982
26. Viberti GC, Pickup JC, Jarrett RJ, Keen H: Effect of control of blood glucose on urinary excretion of albumin and β-microglobulin in insulin-dependent diabetics. N Engl J Med 300:638, 1979
27. White NH, Waltman SR, Krupin T, Santiago J: Reversal abnormalities in ocular fluorophotometry in insulin-dependent diabetes after five to nine months of improved metabolic control. Diabetes 31:80, 1982
28. O'Hara JA, Twoney BM, Ferris JB, O'Sullivan DJ: Metabolic control, hypertension, and microvascular complications independently affect transcapillary escape of albumin in diabetes. Diabetologia 22:391, 1982
29. Morgensen CE: Glomerular filtration rate and renal plasma flow in normal and diabetic man during elevation of blood sugar levels. Scand J Clin Lab Invest 28:177, 1981
30. Atherton A, Hill DW, Keen H, et al: The effect of acute hyperglycaemia on the retinal circulation of the normal cat. Diabetologia 18:233, 1980
31. Papachristodoulou D, Heath H, Kang SS: The development of retinopathy in sucrose-fed and streptozotocin-diabetic rats. Diabetologia 12:367, 1976
32. Engerman R, Bloodworth JM Jr, Nelson S: Relationship of microvascular disease in diabetes to metabolic control. Diabetes 26:760, 1977
33. Bloodworth JMB Jr, Engerman RL, Anderson PJ: Microangiopathy in the experimentally

diabetic animal. In Camerini-Davalos RA, Cole HS (eds): Vascular and Neurological Changes in Early Diabetes. p. 245. Academic Press, New York, 1973
34. Mauer SM, Sutherland DER, Steffes MW, et al: Pancreatic islet transplantation: effects on the glomerular lesions of experimental diabetes in the rat. Diabetes 23:748, 1974
35. Folgia VG, Mancini RE, Cardeza AF: Glomerular lesions in the diabetic rat. Arch Pathol 50:75, 1950
36. Kanich RE, Craighead JE, Kessler JB: Lesions of renal glomeruli in mice with virus-induced diabetes mellitus-like disease. Diabetologia 9:203, 1973
37. Brown, DM, Steffes MW, Thibert P, et al: Glomerular manifestations of diabetes in the BB rat. Metabolism, suppl. 1, 32:131, 1983
38. Rasch R: Prevention of diabetic glomerulopathy in streptozotocin diabetic rats by insulin treatment: the mesangial regions. Diabetologia 17:243, 1979
39. Hägg E: Influence of insulin treatment on glomerular changes in rats with longterm alloxan diabetes. Acta Pathol Microbiol Scand 82:228, 1974
40. Mauer SM, Steffes MW, Sutherland DER, et al: Studies of the rate of regression of the glomerular lesions in diabetic rats treated with pancreatic islet transplantation. Diabetes 24:280, 1975
41. Lee CS, Mauer SM, Brown DM, et al: Renal transplantation in diabetes mellitus in rats. J Exp Med 139:973, 1974
42. Sima AF: The development and structural characterization of the neuropathies in the spontaneously diabetic BB Wistar rat. Metabolism 32:106, 1983
43. Clements RS: Diabetic neuropathy—new concepts of its etiology. Diabetes 28:604, 1979
44. Jakobsen J: Early and preventable changes of peripheral nerve structure and function in insulin-dependent diabetic rats. J Neurol Neurosurg Psychiatry 42:509, 1979
45. Keiding NR, Root HF, Marble A: Importance of control of diabetes in prevention of vascular complications. JAMA 150:964, 1952
46. Hardin RC, Jackson RL, Johnson TL: The development of diabetic retinopathy: effects of duration and control of diabetes. Diabetes 5:397, 1956
47. Dolger H: Clinical evaluation of vascular damage in diabetes mellitus. JAMA 134:1289, 1947
48. Knowles HC, Guest GM, Lampert J: The course of juvenile diabetes treated with unmeasured diet. Diabetes 14:239, 1965
49. Johnsson S: Retinopathy and nephropathy in diabetes mellitus: comparison of the effects of two forms of treatment. Diabetes 9:1, 1960
50. Pirat J: Diabetic mellitus and its degenerative complications; a prospective study of 4,400 patients observed between 1947 and 1973. Diabetes Care 1:168, 1978
51. Miki E, Fukuda M, Kuzuya T, et al: Relation of the course of retinopathy to control of diabetes, age and therapeutic agents in diabetic Japanese patients. Diabetes 18:773, 1969
52. Takazakura E, Nakamoto Y, Hayakawa H, et al: Onset and progression of diabetic glomerulosclerosis: a prospective study based on serial renal biopsies. Diabetes 24:1, 1976
53. Job D, Eschwege E, Guyot-Argenton C, et al: Effect of multiple daily insulin injections on the course of diabetic retinopathy. Diabetes 25:463, 1976
54. Raskin P: Diabetic regulation and its relationship to microangiopathy. Metabolism 27:235, 1978
55. Tamborlane W, Genel M, Sherwin R, Felig P: Restoration of normal lipid and amino acid metabolism in diabetic patients treated with a portable insulin-infusion pump. Lancet 1:1258, 1979
56. Dunn F, Pietri A, Raskin P: Plasma lipid and lipoprotein levels with continuous subcutaneous insulin infusion in type I diabetes mellitus. Ann Intern Med 95:426, 1981
57. Lopes-Virella M, Sherer G, Lees A, et al: Surface binding, internalization and degrada-

tion by cultured human fibroblasts of low density lipoproteins isolated from type I (insulin-dependent) diabetic patients: changes with metabolic control. Diabetologia 22:430, 1982

58. Hansen AP: Normalization of growth hormone hyperresponse to exercise in juvenile diabetes after "normalization" of blood sugar. J Clin Invest 50:1806, 1971
59. Molnar CG, Taylor WF, Langworthy A, Fatourechi V: Diurnal growth hormone and glucose abnormalities in unstable diabetics: studies of ambulatory-fed subjects during continuous blood glucose analysis. J Clin Endocrinol Metab 34:837, 1972
60. Tamborlane WV, Sherwin RS, Koivisto V, et al: Normalization of the growth hormone and catecholamine response to exercise in juvenile onset diabetics treated with a portable insulin infusion pump. Diabetes 28:785, 1979
61. Tamborlane WV, Hintz RL, Bergman M, et al: Insulin infusion pump treatment of diabetes: influence of improved metabolic control on plasma somatomedin levels. N Engl J Med 305:303, 1981
62. Press M, Tamborlane WV, Sherwin RS: Importance of raised growth hormone levels in mediating the metabolic derangements of diabetes. N Engl J Med 310:810, 1984
63. Nash H: Growth failure, somatomedin and growth hormone levels in juvenile diabetes mellitus: a pilot study. Aust NZ J Med 9:245, 1979
64. Yde H: The growth hormone dependent sulfation factor in serum from patients with various types of diabetes. Acta Med Scand 186:293, 1969
65. Luna AM, Wilson DM, Wibbelsman CJ, et al: Somatomedins in adolescents: a cross-sectional study of the effect of puberty on plasma insulin-like growth factor I and II levels. J Clin Edocrinol Metab 57:268, 1983
66. Tamborlane W, Ritchey AK, Davis P, et al: Diabetic control and growth: hormonal and cellular aspects. Pediatr Res 16:265A, 1982
67. Levinsky RL, Trompeter RS, Grant DB: 24-Hour urinary glucose excretion in assessment of control in juvenile diabetes mellitus. Arch Dis Child 51:463
68. Jivani SKM, Rayner PHW: Does control influence the growth of diabetic children? Arch Dis Child 48:109, 1973
69. Rudolf MCJ, Sherwin RS, Markowitz R, et al: Effect of intensive insulin treatment on linear growth in the young diabetic patient. J Pediatr 101:333, 1982
70. Merimee TJ, Zapf J, Froesch ER: Insulin-like growth factors: studies in diabetics with and without retinopathy. N Engl J Med 309:527, 1983
71. Champion MC, Shephard GAA, Rodger NW, Dupre J: Continuous subcutaneous infusion of insulin in the management of diabetes mellitus. Diabetes 29:206, 1980
72. Verdonk C, Tamborlane W, Hendler R, et al: Does insulin pump treatment of diabetes cause hyperinsulinemia and hypoaminoacidemia? Clin Res 29:425A, 1981
73. Pickup JC, Keen H, Parsons JA, et al: Continuous subcutaneous insulin infusion: improved blood glucose and intermediary metabolite control in diabetics. Lancet 1:1255, 1979
74. Simonson D, Sherwin R, Tamborlane W, DeFronzo R: Insulin resistance in insulin-dependent diabetes mellitus is not reversible with chronic insulin pump treatment. Diabetes 31:15A, 1982
75. Del Prato S, Nosachini R, Tiengo P, et al: Insulin-mediated glucose disposal in type I diabetes: evidence for insulin resistance. J Clin Endocrinol Metab 57:904, 1983
76. Stout RW: The relationship of abnormal circulating insulin levels to atherosclerosis. Atherosclerosis 27:1, 1977
77. Williamson J, Bahoric A, Perlman K, Albisser AM: Secondary amyloidosis in (beagle) dogs receiving insulin via mechanical pumps. Diabetes, suppl. 2, 31:50A, 1982
78. Koivisto V, Teppo A, Maury P, Taskinen M-R: No evidence of amyloidosis in type I

diabetics treated with continuous subcutaneous insulin infusion. Diabetes 32:88, 1983
79. Siperstein M, Unger R, Madison L: Studies of muscle capillary basement membranes in normal subjects, diabetic and prediabetic patients. J Clin Invest 47:1973, 1968
80. Marks JF, Raskin P, Stastny P: Increase in capillary basement membrane width in parents of children with type I diabetes mellitus: association with HLA-DR4. Diabetes 30:475, 1981
81. Kilo C, Vogler N, Williamson J: Muscle capillary basement membrane changes related to aging and to diabetes mellitus. Diabetes 21:881, 1972
82. Bennett PH: The basement membrane controversy. Diabetologia 16:280, 1979
83. Osterby R: Early phases in the development of diabetic glomerulopathy: a quantitative electron microscopic study. Acta Med Scand [Suppl] 574:1, 1975
84. Mauer SM, Steffer MW, Connett J, et al: The development of lesions in the glomerular basement membrane and mesangium after transplantion of normal kidneys in diabetic patients. Diabetes 32:948, 1983
85. Peterson CM, Jones RL, Esterly JA, et al: Changes in basement membrane thickening and pulse volume concomitant with improved glucose control and exercise in insulin-dependent diabetes mellitus. Diabetes Care 3:586, 1980
86. Raskin P, Pietri AO, Unger R, Shannon WA Jr: The effect of diabetic control on the width of skeletal-muscle capillary basement membrane in patients with type I diabetes mellitus. N Engl J Med 309:1546, 1983
87. Camerini-Davalos RA, Velasco C, Glasser M, Bloodworth JMB Jr: Drug-induced reversal of early diabetic microangiopathy. N Engl J Med 309:1551, 1983
88. Siperstein MD: Diabetic microangiopathy and the control of blood glucose. N Engl J Med 309:1577, 1983
89. Cunha-Vaz J, Faria de Abreu J, Figo G: Early breakdown of the blood-retinal barrier in diabetes. Br J Ophthalmol 59:649, 1975
90. Steno Study Group: Effect of 6 months of strict metabolic control on eye and kidney function in insulin-dependent diabetics with background retinopathy. Lancet 1:121, 1982
91. Bleicher S, Lee T, Bernstein R, et al: Effect of blook glucose control on retinal vascular permeability in insulin-dependent diabetes mellitus. Diabetes Care 3:184, 1980
92. Steno Study Group: Effect on 1 year of near-normal blood glucose levels on retinopathy in insulin-dependent diabetics. Lancet 1:200, 1983
93. Puklin JE, Tamborlane WV, Sherwin RS: Diabetic retinopathy is not reversed by long-term insulin pump treatment. In Henkind P (ed): ACTA XXIV International Congress of Ophthalmology. Vol. 2. p. 803. Lippincott, Philadelphia, 1983
94. Kroc Collaborative Study Group: Near normal glycemic control does not slow progression of mild diabetic retinopathy. Diabetes, suppl. 1, 32:10A, 1983
95. Steno Study Group: Continuous subcutaneous insulin. Lancet 1:1455, 1983
96. Viberti GC, Jarrett RJ, McCartney M, Keen H: Increased glomerular permeability to albumin induced by exercise in diabetic subjects. Diabetologia 14:293, 1978
97. Viberti GC, Hill RD, Jarrett RJ, et al: Microalbuminuria as a predictor of clinical nephropathy in insulin-dependent diabetes mellitus. Lancet 1:1430, 1982
98. Koivisto VA, Huttunen NP, Vierikko P: Continuous subcutaneous insulin infusion corrects exercise-induced albuminuria in juvenile diabetes. Br Med J 282:779, 1981
99. Tamborlane WV, Puklin JE, Bergman M, et al: Long-term improvement of metablic control with the insulin pump does not reverse diabetic microangiopathy. Diabetes Care, suppl. 1, 5:58, 1982
100. Viberti GC, Bilous RS, Mackintosh D, et al: Long-term correction of hyperglycemia and progression of renal failure in insulin-dependent diabetes. Br Med J 286:598, 1983
101. Abouna GM, Al-Adnani MS, Kremer GB, et al: Reversal of diabetic nephropathy in hu-

man cadaveric kidneys after transplantation into non-diabetic recipients. Lancet 2:1274, 1983

102. Graf RJ, Halter JB, Pfeifer MA, et al: Glycemic control and nerve conduction abnormalities in non-insulin-dependent diabetic subjects. Ann Intern Med 94:307, 1981
103. Pietri A, Ehle AL, Raskin P: Changes in nerve conduction velocity after six weeks of glucoregulation with portable insulin infusion pumps. Diabetes 29:668, 1980
104. Holman RR, Dorman TL, Mayon-White V, et al: Prevention of deterioration of renal and sensory-nerve function by more intensive management of insulin-dependent patients: a two-year randomized prospective study. Lancet 1:204, 1983
105. Tamborlane WV, Sherwin RS, Bergman M, et al: Long-term outpatient management of diabetes with a portable insulin infusion pump improves sensory nerve conduction. Clin Res 28:577A, 1980
106. Boulton AJM, Drury J, Clarke B, Ward J: Continuous subcutaneous insulin infusion in the management of painful diabetic neuropathy. Diabetes Care 5:386, 1982
107. White NH, Saltman SR, Krupin T, Santiago J: Reversal of neuropathic and gastrointestinal complications related to diabetes mellitus in adolescents with improved metabolic control. J Pediatr 99:41, 1981
108. Kannel W, McGree D: Diabetes and cardiovascular disease: the Framingham study. JAMA 241:2035, 1979
109. Ostrander LD, Lamphier DE, Block WD: Biochemical precursors of atheroslerosis: studies in apparently healthy men in a general population. Ann Intern Med 134:224, 1974
110. Keen H: Glucose intolerance, diabetes mellitus, and atherosclerosis: prospects for prevention. Postgrad Med J 52:445, 1976
111. Fuller HJ, McCartney P, Jarrett R, et al: Hyperglycemia and coronary heart disease: the Whitehall study. J Chronic Dis 32:721, 1979
112. University Group Diabetes Program: A study of the effects of hypoglycemic agents on vascular complications in patients with adult onset diabetes II: mortality results. Diabetes, suppl. 2, 19:785, 1970
113. University Group Diabetes Program: A study of the effects of hypoglycemic agents on vascular complications in patients with adult-onset diabetes. VI. Supplementary report on nonfatal events in patients treated with tolbutamide. Diabetes 25:1129, 1976
114. University Group Diabetes Program: Effects of hypoglycemic agents on vascular complications in patients with adult-onset diabetes. VIII. Evaluation of insulin therapy: final report. Diabetes, suppl. 5, 31:1, 1982

2 Intensive Treatment of Type I Diabetes Mellitus

Jay S. Skyler
Michael L. Reeves

The isolation of insulin in 1922 revolutionized the treatment of insulin-dependent diabetes mellitus (IDDM). Prolongation of life permitted by insulin therapy allowed the emergence of the chronic degenerative complications of diabetes, including microangiopathy (involving the eyes and kidneys in particular), neuropathy, and accelerated atherosclerosis. The weight of currently available scientific evidence strongly suggests that the microangiopathic and neurological complications of diabetes arise as a consequence of, or are in large part influenced by, the metabolic derangements that characterize the diabetic state. This has stimulated physicians to attempt to develop therapeutic approaches that would lessen the risk of development of these complications.

A number of advances during the last few years have facilitated these efforts. Perhaps the most important of these advances has been the development of patient self-monitoring of blood glucose (SMBG) as a practical clinical tool, thus permitting the definition of treatment targets near the physiological range and providing the ability to document the level of glycemia that is attained during ordinary life. Moreover, the routine use of SMBG allows the development and implementation of a plan designed to achieve those treatment targets. Targets for an individual patient vary (as discussed in detail later in this chapter) and may be influenced by such factors as ability to recognize and respond to hypoglycemia, ability to spontaneously recover from hypoglycemia, age, the presence of other illnesses, and the use of other medications. For relatively healthy young patients who are able to recognize and respond

Table 2-1. Target Glucose Levels

Time of Sample	Ideal (mg/dl)	Acceptable (mg/dl)
Prebreakfast	70–90	70–110
Preprandial	70–105	70–130
One-hour postprandial	100–160	100–180
Two-hour postprandial	80–120	80–150
2 AM to 4 PM	≥70	≥70

to hypoglycemia, the targets outlined in Table 2-1 may be used. These include both "ideal" targets, which are defined by the glucose levels seen in nondiabetic individuals, and "acceptable" targets, which although slightly higher than glucose levels seen in nondiabetic individuals can be attained by many patients without an unacceptable frequency of hypoglycemia.

The development of assays for glycosylated hemoglobin has permitted the documentation of average glycemic control attained over several weeks. Glycosylated hemoglobin measurements serve as an independent measure of control and stand as the best single assessment tool currently available.

Studies of appropriate waveforms for automated intravenous insulin delivery and the development of portable infusion pumps for subcutaneous insulin delivery have not only provided a new approach to insulin therapy but have contributed to a renewed interest in insulin availability and the design of treatment regimens. These and other studies have served to emphasize the distinction between basal and meal-related insulin availability. In addition, the portable infusion pumps themselves have emerged as an important clinical tool.

The introduction of SMBG and the design of insulin regimens which provide both basal insulin availability and meal-related incremental insulin have permitted the development of therapeutic programs for IDDM designed to attain near-normalization of glycemia, as evidenced by both near-normal levels of glycemia and near-normal levels of glycosylated hemoglobin. Such programs have come to be known as "intensive insulin therapy." In our view, there are eight elements that constitute a program of intensive insulin therapy of IDDM. These are listed in Table 2-2.

In this chapter, we discuss the design and implementation of a program of "intensive insulin therapy," including what we deem the appropriate roles of such advances in therapy as SMBG, glycosylated hemoglobin, portable insulin infusion pumps, and emerging forms of therapy, e.g., the use of human insulin preparations.

Table 2-2. Elements of Intensive Therapy of IDDM

1. Multiple component insulin program
2. Careful balance of food intake, activity, and insulin dosage
3. Daily self-monitoring of blood glucose
4. Patient adjustments of insulin dosage and supplements according to predetermined plan
5. Defined targer glucose levels
6. Frequent contact between patient and staff
7. Patient education and motivation
8. Psychological support

INSULIN SECRETION AND THE DESIGN OF INSULIN REGIMENS

There are two major components to physiological insulin secretion in nondiabetic individuals: (1) meal-related incremental insulin secretion, responsible for utilization and storage of nutrients; and (2) basal insulin secretion between meals, responsible for modulating hepatic glucose production and metabolic homeostasis during the postabsorptive period. These two components of physiological insulin secretion are depicted in Figure 2-1. Both meal-related and basal insulin secretion are crucial for maintenance of normal intermediary metabolism. Both components are impaired in IDDM. Both need replacement.

Careful examination of Figure 2-1 reveals that in nondiabetic individuals in the basal state there is a tendency for a glucose nadir to occur at around 3:00–4:00 AM, and a tendency for a rise in basal insulin secretion between 5:00 and 8:00 AM, preceding consumption of breakfast. For illustrative purposes, both of these diurnal trends have been exaggerated in the figure. In many studies these trends fail to achieve statistical significance, yet their recurrent appearance suggests that they are real. In IDDM the tendency to diurnal variation in glycemia persists and is evidenced by: (1) a tendency to hypoglycemia at 3:00–4:00 AM at the time of the physiological glucose nadir; and (2) a tendency toward increased insulin need in the morning hours before the consumption of breakfast (and often continuing after breakfast), perhaps best demonstrated by increased insulin requirements to maintain euglycemia with a glucose-sensor-controlled insulin infusion system (''artificial endocrine pancreas''). In the absence of the provision of increased insulin during this time, progressive hyperglycemia supervenes. This has been labeled the ''dawn phenomenon.'' The mechanism responsible for the dawn phenomenon has not yet been defined. In our experience, this phenomenon attains clinical significance in approximately 20–30 percent of patients with IDDM.

There are a number of factors involved in physiological endogenous insulin secretion which impact on the design of insulin regimens for the management of IDDM. These are that physiological insulin secretion involves: (1) substrate-mediated insulin secretion, which actually is initiated by neural and gut factors prior to the hyperglycemic stimulus; (2) substrate-related cessation of insulin secretion as plasma glucose falls; (3) continuing basal insulin secretion in the postabsorptive state between meals and overnight; (4) diurnal variation in the basal insulin secretory rate, particularly

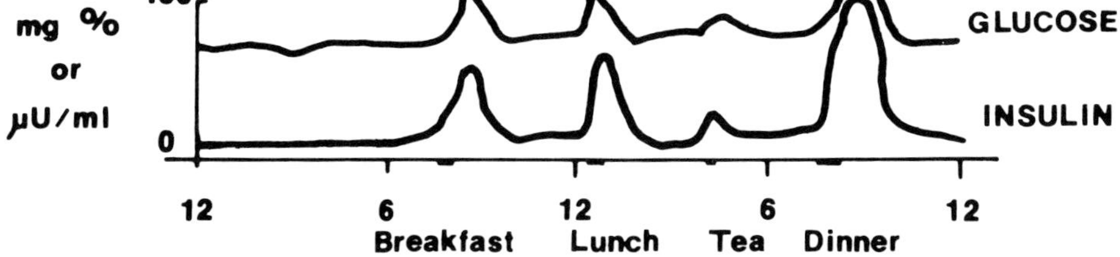

Fig. 2-1 The 24-hr plasma glucose and insulin levels in a hypothetical normal man.

during the predawn hours; (5) insulin secretion into the hepatic portal circulation such that hepatic portal insulin levels are significantly higher than systemic insulin levels; and (6) variation in insulin secretion in response to physiological or psychological stress, thus limiting consequent hyperglycemia. The ideal treatment regimen of IDDM would consider all of these elements involved in physiological insulin secretion. However, exogenous insulin therapy is generally delivered into the systemic circulation, rather than the hepatic portal circulation. Also, the availability of exogenous insulin, except in the case of a glucose-sensor-controlled insulin infusion system (artificial endocrine pancreas), is not related to substrate availability or prevailing level of glycemia. Rather, exogenous insulin availability depends on the pharmacokinetics of the insulin preparation and the route of insulin delivery. For chronic management, which generally involves subcutaneous insulin administration, a critical determinant of insulin availability is its absorption characteristics from subcutaneous tissue. Conventional subcutaneous insulin regimens are based on the assumption that insulin absorption and availability are predictable and reproducible. Yet many factors may influence insulin absorption and alter insulin availability. Nevertheless, based on the usual time courses of action of given insulin preparations, it is possible to devise a number of insulin regimens that mimic physiological insulin availability and thus facilitate the attainment of glycemic control in patients with IDDM.

If our goal is to attain glycemic control as close to physiological status as possible, insulin availability must also attempt to mimic normal physiology. It should be readily apparent that such is not possible with a single daily dose of intermediate- or long-acting insulin, with a single dose mixture of short- and intermediate-acting insulin, or with a split dose of twice-daily intermediate-acting insulin. Such regimens are unphysiological and are doomed to failure if near-normalization of glycemia is the therapeutic goal. Attempts to achieve near-normalization are complicated by hypoglycemia at the time of peak insulin action, and inadequate control may still be present during other periods of the day.

A commonality of all physiological insulin regimens is that they have multiple components of insulin availability, including components designed to coincide with each major meal and a component designed to provide sustained insulin availability during the basal state overnight. Perhaps the most popular multiple-component regimen used over the years has been the split-and-mixed regimen in which there are twice-daily injections of combinations of regular and intermediate-acting insulin, as depicted in Figure 2-2. This regimen provides insulin availability with each major meal and has a component of insulin action (the evening intermediate-acting insulin) which provides sustained insulin availability overnight. A pitfall of this regimen in some patients has become evident with attempts to produce morning euglycemia before breakfast. The evening intermediate-acting insulin has its peak action during the night, 8–10 hr after its administration. Because of this, attempts to normalize prebreakfast glucose values may result in nocturnal hypoglycemia. The diurnal variation that results in a nadir of blood glucose around 3:00–4:00 AM and in the dawn phenomenon may aggravate this risk of nocturnal hypoglycemia. There is also increased risk during pregnancy, where continuous glucose consumption by the products of conception results in a nocturnal hypoglycemic tendency even in nondiabetic women. These problems have led several authors to suggest an alternative regimen in which

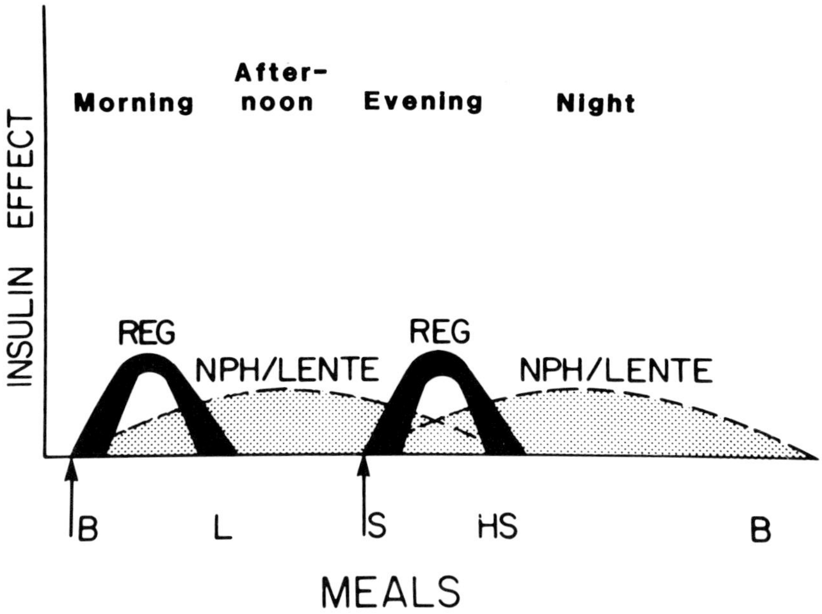

Fig. 2-2 Idealized periods of insulin effect for a "split and mixed" insulin regimen, consisting of two daily doses of regular and intermediate-acting insulin. Symbols used in Figures 2-2 through 2-6 are: B = breakfast, L = lunch, S = supper, HS = bedtime, Arrow = time of insulin injection at 30 min before meal, REG = regular or rapid-onset, short-acting insulin effect, NPH/LENTE = intermediate-acting insulin effect.

the evening intermediate-acting insulin is delayed until bedtime, as depicted in Figure 2-3. The peak effect of insulin action then coincides with the waking period, helping to obliterate the dawn phenomenon and permitting the peak insulin effect to occur at a time when the patient is awake and blood glucose can routinely be measured. With either of the regimens depicted in Figures 2-2 and 2-3, patients must eat on time, particularly lunch and supper. Delay of meal consumption may result in hypoglycemia from the intermediate-acting insulin.

An alternative multiple-component regimen is depicted in Figure 2-4. This regimen provides rapid-onset regular insulin before each meal and a bedtime dose of intermediate-acting insulin, useful for the reasons discussed above. Attempts to use a multiple-injection scheme based on four injections of regular insulin impose the risk of nocturnal hypoglycemia from the peak effect of bedtime regular insulin and fail to adequately control prebreakfast blood glucose. The multiple-injection scheme depicted in Figure 2-4 solves both problems. Moreover, patients may be more flexible in meal size without sabotaging glycemic control. Thus for a large meal they take a larger amount of preprandial regular insulin, and for a small meal they take a smaller amount of preprandial regular insulin. However, these patients must still eat on time and take their preprandial insulin on time. Delayed administration of preprandial regular insulin permits hyperglycemia to supervene.

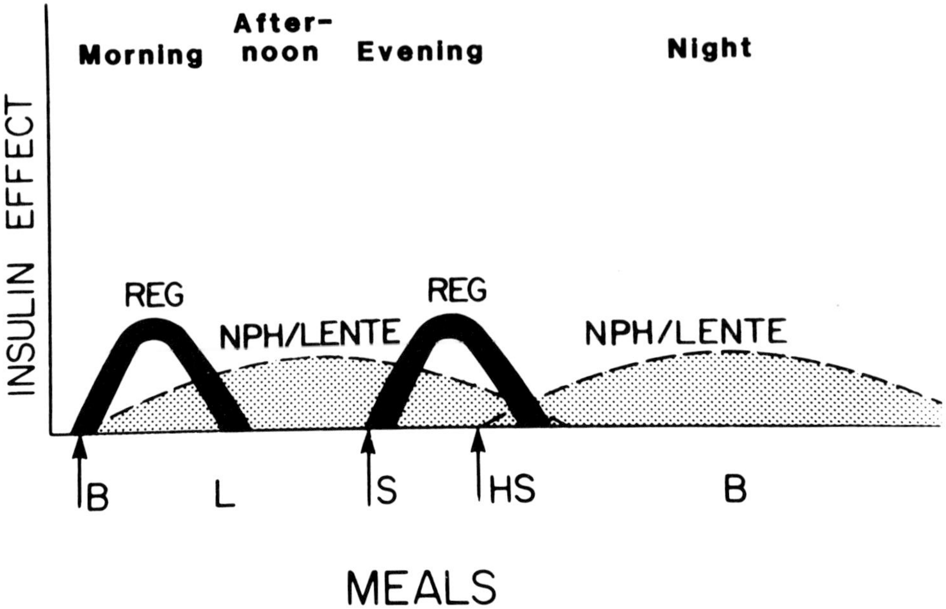

Fig. 2-3 Idealized periods of insulin effect for a "split and mixed" insulin regimen in which the evening intermediate-acting insulin is delayed until bedtime. This results in peak insulin action coinciding with prebreakfast blood glucose, which is measured. Symbols are as noted in Figure 2-2.

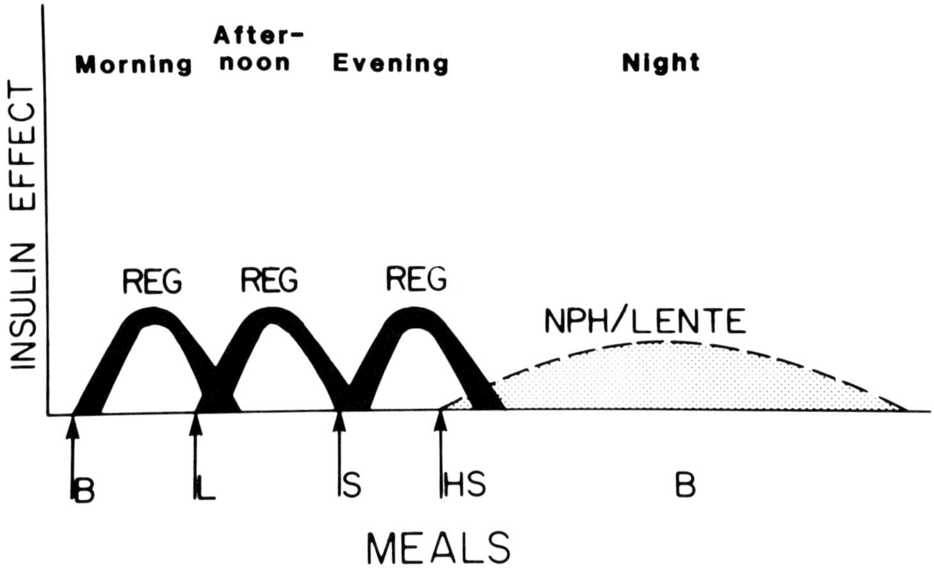

Fig. 2-4 Idealized periods of insulin effect for a multiple-dosage regimen providing four insulin injections daily. Regular insulin is given before meals. Intermediate-acting insulin is given at bedtime to ensure duration of action through the night. This results in peak insulin action coinciding with prebreakfast blood glucose, which is measured. Symbols are as noted in Figure 2-2.

An alternative multiple-injection regimen has been devised to permit flexibility in both meal size and meal timing. This regimen entails preprandial rapid-onset regular insulin to provide meal-related incremental insulinemia, coupled with the prolonged, relatively peakless action of ultralente insulin to provide basal insulinemia in order to maintain hepatic glucose production equivalent to peripheral glucose utilization. This regimen is depicted in Figure 2-5. In this regimen, again there is flexibility in meal size, with a larger amount of preprandial regular insulin being taken for a large meal and a smaller amount for a small meal. Moreover, meal timing may be varied widely, continuing to take preprandial regular insulin before consumption of each meal. This is particularly helpful for shift workers or individuals flying across time zones. In addition, meals may even be omitted, also omitting the corresponding dose of preprandial regular insulin.

As indicated in Figure 2-5, several authors have found it helpful to divide the ultralente insulin into two injections, administering half with the prebreakfast regular insulin and half with the presupper regular insulin. This takes advantage of the small peak in action seen in some patients 12–15 hr after administration, limits the total volume of injection, and has no influence on the general profile of insulin action,

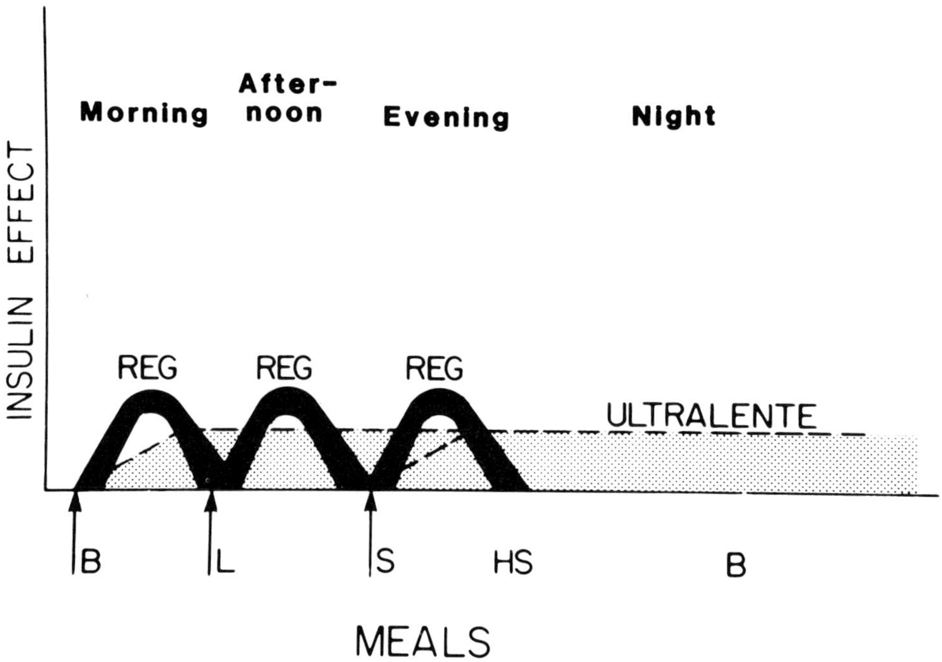

Fig. 2-5 Idealized periods of insulin effect for a multiple-dosage regimen providing preprandial regular insulin and basal insulin as long-acting, relatively peakless ultralente insulin. The ultralente insulin may be mixed with the prebreakfast regular insulin or the presupper regular insulin; or a portion of the total ultralente insulin dosage may be mixed with each. Symbols are as noted in Figure 2-2.

i.e., prolonged and relatively peakless. A disadvantage of this regimen is that there is a large subcutaneous depot present at all times. Given the vagaries of insulin absorption, this occasionally leads to protracted hypoglycemia in some patients.

One way to mimic physiological insulin availability, permit flexibility in both meal size and meal timing, yet obviate a large subcutaneous insulin depot and its variable absorption, is the use of portable infusion pumps to deliver insulin, i.e., continuous subcutaneous insulin infusion (CSII). In CSII, the pump continually delivers a basal rate of microliter amounts of regular insulin, which provides a background of insulin throughout the day and night, maintaining hepatic glucose production equivalent to peripheral glucose utilization. In addition, the pump may be activated to deliver incremental meal-related insulin boluses tailored to limit postprandial glucose excursions. The pattern of insulin availability provided by CSII is depicted in Figure 2-6.

Newer pumps are programmable, permitting variation in the basal insulin delivery rate, which may permit one to decrease this rate during the time of physiological glucose nadir (e.g., lower rate from midnight to 4:00 AM) and/or to increase the rate to counteract the dawn phenomenon (e.g., higher rate from 5:00 to 9:00 AM). The use of such programmable variable-rate pumps is the subject of ongoing investigation. Also, currently under development are implantable pumps for intraperitoneal insulin delivery, thus permitting some insulin to be absorbed directly into the portal circulation, the physiological route.

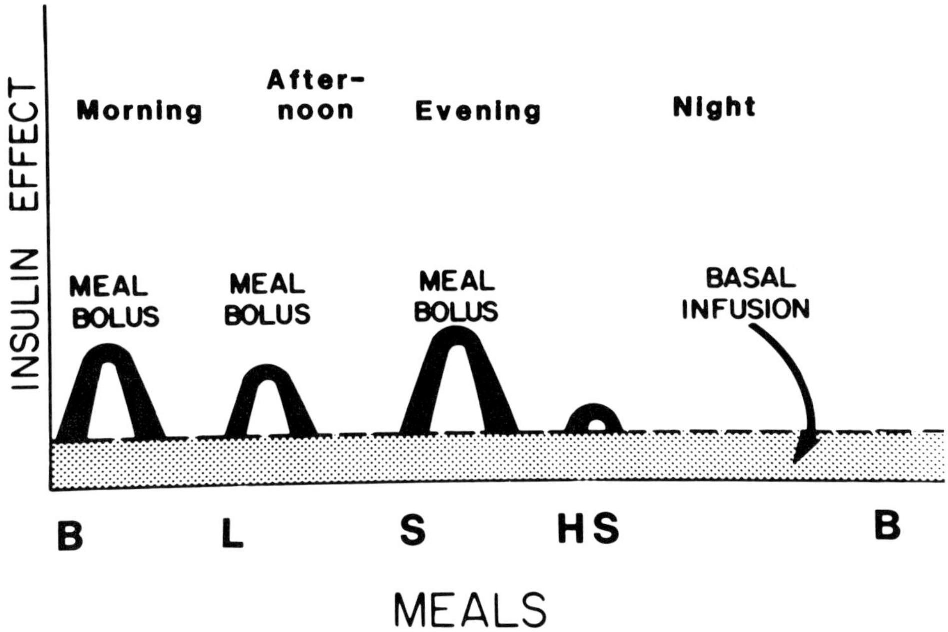

Fig. 2-6 Idealized periods of insulin effect provided by continuous subcutaneous insulin infusion. Symbols are as noted in Figure 2-2.

There is a distinct difference in life style possible with various regimens. Any regimen that uses preprandial regular insulin permits flexibility in meal size, with the insulin dose varying with the anticipated carbohydrate or calorie content of the meal. Further flexibility is possible with CSII and the ultralente-based regimens, as these provide a background of basal insulinemia during the course of the day and night. In this circumstance there can be considerable flexibility in meal timing (which is helpful for shift workers or those with varying schedules) and even omission of a meal with omission of the preprandial regular insulin. Our patients seem to recognize this, and when offered the opportunity to select whichever regimen they wish they often prefer a regimen which permits them this flexibility.

Several studies have demonstrated better glycemic control with CSII than with intensive injection programs. There may be a pharmacokinetic explanation for this. The shorter the time period of insulin absorption, the less variation there will be in time course of action and in depot size. With CSII, only rapidly absorbed regular insulin is used. Moreover, continuing absorption of infused basal insulin means that only the preprandial boluses contribute to the subcutaneous depot in patients with CSII, thus minimizing an important variable in insulin action and perhaps limiting the risk of exercise-induced hypoglycemia. In contrast, there is greater variation in insulin absorption and larger depot size when intermediate- and long-acting insulins are used. Thus for ultralente insulin, with a coefficient of variation of absorption of 25–35 percent, it can be calculated that the ultralente depot at any one time varies between 90 and 240 percent of the daily dose, a vertiable time bomb which if released could cause sustained hypoglycemia, a problem encountered in patients treated with ultralente insulin. For this reason we suspect that in the long run CSII will become the preferred form of insulin delivery for patients in whom optimal glycemic control is being sought.

INITIAL INSULIN DOSES AND DISTRIBUTION

The insulin dosage required to attain near-normalization of glycemia (e.g., the blood glucose targets listed in Table 2-1) in typical IDDM patients within 20 percent of their ideal body weight, in the absence of intercurrent infections or other periods of instability, approximates 0.5–1.0 u/kg body weight per day. (For the ultralente-preprandial regular regimen depicted in Figure 2-5, total daily doses are 20–30 percent higher, or 0.6–1.3 U/kg/day. The prolonged period of absorption of ultralente insulin, perhaps coupled with tissue degradation of insulin, decreases its relative bioavailability.) During the period of relative remission ("honeymoon" period) early in the course of the disease, insulin requirements generally are less. During periods of intercurrent illness, the dosage requirement may increase markedly. Dosage also increases during the adolescent growth spurt, and some adolescents may have a sustained increased dose requirement. Table 2-3 summarizes the insulin doses we use when initiating a program of intensive insulin therapy.

Initial insulin distribution is empirically derived from the average distribution requirements of other patients. Each patient then alters the various components individually to attain the desired control. For the twice-daily regular plus intermediate-

Table 2-3. Insulin Doses Used for Initiation of Intensive Insulin Therapy in IDDM

IDDM Status	
Newly diagnosed	0.5 U/kg/day
During "honeymoon" period	0.4 U/kg/day
Pregnant women—first 20 weeks' gestation	0.6 U/kg/day
Established IDDM—previously treated with 0.7–0.9 U/kg/day	0.7 U/kg/day
Established IDDM—previously treated with less than 0.7 U/kg/day	Previous dose unless obviously inadequate
Established IDDM—previously treated with greater than 0.9 U/kg/day	Reduce previous dose by 20–25%

For ultralente, preprandial regular regimen doses are 20–30% higher.

acting insulin regimen (Fig. 2-2) and the regimen entailing regular plus intermediate-acting insulin before breakfast, regular insulin before supper, and intermediate-acting insulin at bedtime (Fig. 2-3), initial distribution provides two-thirds of the total daily dose in the morning and one-third of the daily dose in the evening. The morning prebreakfast dose is divided as one-third regular insulin and two-thirds intermediate-acting insulin. One-half of the evening dose is given as regular insulin before supper, and one-half is given as intermediate-acting insulin either mixed with regular insulin before supper (as in Figure 2-2) or as a separate dose at bedtime (as in Figure 2-3). For the four injection scheme depicted in Figure 2-4, 20–25 percent of the total daily dose is as intermediate-acting insulin at bedtime; the remainder (regular insulin) is divided as 30–45 percent before breakfast, 25–30 percent before lunch, and 25–30 percent before supper. For the ultralente/preprandial regular regimen depicted in Figure 2-5, we initially use about 50 percent (40–60 percent) of the total daily dose as long-acting ultralente insulin (generally administering half with the prebreakfast regular and half with the presupper regular); and the remainder (regular insulin) is divided as 30–45 percent before breakfast, 25–30 percent before lunch, and 25–30 percent before supper. Some patients desire or require a small additional dose of regular insulin to cover a bedtime snack.

For CSII, depicted in Figure 2-6, we initially use the insulin doses listed in Table 2-3, with initial distribution of insulin as follows: basal infusion 40–50 percent of the total daily dose, prebreakfast bolus 15–25 percent of the total daily dose, prelunch bolus about 15–20 percent of the total daily dose, presupper bolus 15–20 percent of the total daily dose, and prebedtime snack bolus 0–10 percent of the total daily dose. Some devices have the feature of being able to program multiple basal rates (e.g., decreased basal rate from midnight to 4:00 AM, increased basal rate from 5:00 to 9:00 AM, etc.). We incorporate these features into our treatment scheme in any given patient only after initial experiences with a constant basal rate regimen. Patients must learn to use the individual infusion pump selected for them, which in some instances may involve learning to dilute insulin to appropriate concentrations.

In addition to the usual approaches to hyperglycemia (outlined later in this chapter), patients on devices must be made aware of the need to check the intactness of insulin delivery if hyperglycemia supervenes.

Obviously, unusual meal distributions may dictate a deviation from the above scheme. Preprandial injections or activation of preprandial boluses generally should occur at least 20–30 min before meal consumption.

FOOD INTAKE AND ACTIVITY PLANNING

The attainment of near-normalization of glycemia in IDDM entails careful balancing between energy expenditure (activity), energy (calorie) intake, and insulin availability. As noted earlier, modern multiple component insulin regimens may permit greater flexibility in meal size and meal timing without sabotaging glycemic control. This may lead to increased patient compliance and improved therapeutic outcome. Exercise is potentially beneficial to all patients and may be incorporated into the therapeutic program. Through understanding of basic principles and their diligent application, patients with IDDM can live a relatively normal life style in terms of their eating habits and physical activity.

Physiological insulin secretion in response to meals in nondiabetic individuals involves both substrate-mediated insulin secretion and cessation of insulin secretion as plasma glucose falls. Although amino acids and protein also influence insulin secretion, glucose seems to be the primary modulator. After meal ingestion, insulin secretion is initiated by neutral and gut factors before a change in circulating glucose concentration.

In contrast to the nondiabetic subject, the patient with IDDM has little or no beta-cell secretory capacity and is therefore dependent on exogenous insulin administration to restrain postprandial hyperglycemia and to promote efficient energy utilization. This involves predicting the exogenous insulin dose before eating in order to ensure appropriate assimilation of the meal calories. Thus for IDDM patients, nutritional planning traditionally has been based on four basic principles. These traditional principles for nutritional management of IDDM are summarized in Table 2-4 and are developed below.

Table 2-4. Nutritional Principles in IDDM

1. Develop a basic daily meal plan that is relatively consistent in terms of
   a. Total energy (calorie) intake
   b. Balance of energy-yielding nutrients (carbohydrates, fats, and proteins)
2. Provide for compensatory changes for nonbasal circumstances
   a. Extra food for extra activity
   b. Extra insulin or activity for extra food
3. Avoid hyperglycemia by
   a. Omitting rapidly absorbed simple sugars from regular meal planning
4. Avoid hypoglycemia by
   a. Reasonably consistent meal timing
   b. Provision of snacks

A Basic Meal Plan

Assuming that a given patient's activities (and energy expenditure) are relatively constant from day to day, it is possible to develop a basic meal plan to provide energy for these activities. The basic daily meal plan should also be relatively consistent in terms of total energy intake (calories) and distribution of energy-yielding nutrients (carbohydrates, fats, and proteins). In this way a basic insulin dosage can be prescribed which, together with the basic meal plan, provides a balance with the patient's energy expenditure. Different meal plans (and/or insulin dosages) may be required for different degrees of energy expenditure, which may change weekly (weekend versus weekday), monthly (with menses), seasonally (winter versus summer), or sporadically (during vacation).

Compensatory Changes

There are occasions when patients may wish to depart from their basic plan in terms of either food intake or activity routine (e.g., to play tennis, go bowling, or do spring cleaning). In order to maintain glycemic control in the face of alteration of any of the three components of therapy—food, activity, insulin—at least one other component must also be altered in a compensatory fashion. Thus in addition to developing a basic meal plan, IDDM patients must learn how to provide extra food for extra activity and how to compensate for those occasions when food intake is increased with increases in insulin or activity.

During activity that is not part of the patient's daily routine, extra food intake may be used to compensate for the increased energy expended.

Consumption of an unusually large (or small) meal should be accompanied by a corresponding increase (or decrease) in insulin dose. Obviously, patients on regimens that entail preprandial regular insulin (either as an injection or a bolus) may be permitted great flexibility in meal size, with the insulin dose varying with the anticipated carbohydrate or caloric content of the meal. Patients on regimens that do not include preprandial regular insulin for all meals may take an additional injection for a large meal but require advanced planning for a small meal.

Avoidance of Hyperglycemia

The lack of physiological glucose-mediated insulin secretion necessitates the omission of rapidly absorbed simple sugars from regular meal planning. This principally involves restriction of glucose, sucrose, and maltose consumption, except in the treatment or prevention of hypoglycemia.

Avoidance of Hypoglycemia

In patients treated with conventional injections, particularly when the regimen includes intermediate or long-acting insulins that result in prolonged absorption of exogenous insulin from its depot sites, several nutritional actions are necessary to avert hypoglycemia. First, there should be reasonable constancy in timing of meals, with particular emphasis on avoiding long delays between meals. In addition, extra feedings (snacks) are often necessary to shorten periods between calorie intake and to provide substrate at times of peak exogenous insulin action or excessive exercise. A bedtime snack is an example of the former and a midafternoon snack on a busy day is an example of the latter. In contrast, patients on regimens that include relatively constant "basal" insulin concentrations during the day as well as the night (either as a basal infusion by a portable insulin infusion pump or as long-acting ultralente insulin) have greater flexibility in meal timing than do patients on conventional programs. This is accomplished by altering both meal timing and the timing of the accompanying preprandial regular insulin. Such flexibility is particularly helpful for shift workers or those with varying schedules. These patients may even omit a meal with omission of the accompanying preprandial regular insulin bolus or dose. The background basal insulinemia is relatively constant at a level sufficient to maintain hepatic glucose production and peripheral glucose utilization at equal levels, in contrast to a regimen based on intermediate-acting insulin that results in a peak of insulin action at a particular time of day. Such peak effects may cause hypoglycemia to supervene if a patient delayed or omitted a meal.

[It is important to note that this flexibility in meal timing is not possible with the multiple-dose regimen that includes preprandial regular insulin and intermediate-acting insulin at bedtime. In that regimen it has been noted that delay of a meal and hence delay of an insulin dose results in hyperglycemia outside the target range, as sustained basal insulin availability is not provided.]

If hypoglycemic symptoms occur, patients should verify the presence of hypoglycemia by monitoring their blood glucose. Self-monitoring determines if these symptoms are attributable to some other cause (e.g., anxiety). It also helps patients previously uncontrolled to adapt to lower ambient levels of glucose without ingesting additional calories for symptoms that may be triggered by counterregulatory hormone release occurring without true hypoglycemia. If hypoglycemia is documented or a blood glucose determination cannot be obtained but hypoglycemic symptoms appear, the patient should consume rapidly absorbed simple sugar, containing about 10 g of carbohydrate. Patients should always carry or have available an acceptable source of sugar for this purpose. If meal time is more than an hour away, additional slowly absorbed food (complex carbohydrate and/or protein) should be consumed. If the hypoglycemic episode cannot be explained by an alteration in food intake or activity, the patient must also consider a reduction in insulin dosage the next day.

Implementation of the Meal Plan

In order to facilitate selection of a wide variety of food choices while remaining within a basic meal plan, the patient needs to learn a substitution system that permits equivalent amounts of food to be interchanged. A number of systems have been developed for this purpose based on calorie and/or carbohydrate and other energy-yielding nutrient content of foods. More recently it has been suggested that such systems be based on the relative degree of glycemia that occurs in response to consumption of specific foods (glycemic index). In the future, this will likely supplant the other substitution systems.

Because the nutritional plan must be used by the patient on a continuous basis, successful therapy requires that it is acceptable and understandable to, as well as compatible with the life style of the patient. The plan should be individualized for each patient based on a careful and detailed dietary history obtained by a trained dietitian or nutritional counselor. The meal plan must be reasonable and realistic, keeping in mind that it is better for it to be attractive, understood, and adhered to than to be theoretically ideal but ignored. The patient should understand the degree of precision desired in portion estimation, bearing in mind that daily energy expenditure is not always constant and thus energy requirements are not always the same. As a result of this possible variability, food intake may be modified within reason. Emphasis is placed on consumption of a wide variety of foods. Unpopular and unfamiliar foods are not recommended, as they add nothing to the nutritional plan and are not likely to be eaten anyway.

In order to improve patient compliance it is often helpful to discuss with the patient and his/her family the conceptual view that the nutritional program is one of meal planning that balances energy intake, energy expenditure, and insulin dosage. It should be noted that the meal plan is consistent with recommended dietary goals for all Americans and that the entire family may benefit from such eating habits. It is also important to emphasize that the basic meal plan should be altered to compensate for increased activity and that it is possible on special occasions to deviate from the basic meal plan, provided there are also compensatory changes in activity or insulin dosage. Furthermore, it should be pointed out to the patient that the basic meal plan itself can be adjusted or adapted as he/she grows, if his/her routine activity changes, or if he/she for any reason is not satisfied with it. The guiding principle is that the basic meal plan is a dynamic tool that facilitates diabetes management and not a static restraint interfering with the patient's life style.

Physical Activity

The physiological response to physical activity is a complex process involving circulatory, metabolic, and hormonal regulatory phenomena. The responses to acute exercise vary with both the duration and the intensity of exercise and are relatively short-lived. Long-term adaptations occur in response to physical training involving regularly performed strenuous exercise.

There is a direct relationship between physical activity and energy (calorie) requirement. As indicated earlier, if it is assumed that energy expenditure is relatively consistent from day to day, calorie intake also should be relatively consistent from day to day and in proportion to energy expenditure. Moreover, if activity varies from weekday to weekend, summer to winter, etc., then those periods may require different meal plans and different insulin doses. Thus the patient who has a predictable pattern of variable activity can be readily managed by developing an appropriate array of basic meal plans and insulin doses. In this section sporadic alterations in physical activity are discussed. Before developing management principles for this circumstance, it is necessary to briefly review some aspects of the physiology of exercise.

Sporadic Exercise. Exercise increases muscle fuel consumption 7- to 40-fold. To meet those energy needs, fuel is derived from muscle glycogenolysis, fatty acids, and glucose released by the liver. To meet the increased glucose demands of exercise, hepatic glucose output increases. Normally, the rate of glucose utilization is precisely matched by increments in glucose production so that plasma glucose concentration remains relatively constant during brief or mild exercise. When mild exercise is prolonged for several hours, there is a progressive fall in plasma glucose concentrations, although marked hypoglycemia rarely occurs in normal subjects. In addition to its effects on altering glucose metabolism, exercise increases lipolysis and thus provides an additional energy source, which is sustained during prolonged exercise. With prolonged endurance exercise, hepatic glucose production eventually declines while muscle glucose consumption continues, resulting in a tendency to hypoglycemia.

The metabolic response to exercise requires precise regulation between overall fuel utilization, muscle energy requirements, muscle glucose utilization, and hepatic glucose output. The regulatory scheme mediating this metabolic response to exercise no doubt involves a combination of hormonal, substrate, enzymatic, and neural (autonomic) mechanisms. The major hormonal alterations that occur with the onset of exercise are a suppression of insulin secretion and increased circulating levels of catecholamines (epinephrine and norepinephrine), growth hormone, cortisol, and glucagon. Glucagon and epinephrine have important effects in stimulating hepatic glucose production. Despite decreased insulin secretion and decreased plasma insulin concentration with exercise, there may be relative increased availability of insulin to exercising muscle due to increased blood flow, the opening of capillaries, and other local effects. The role of insulin in mediating the metabolic response to exercise is crucial, as the fall in insulin must be sufficient to permit both the increased hepatic glucose output in response to exercise and the peripheral mobilization of alternative energy substrate (free fatty acids) from enhanced lipolysis. Yet there must be sufficient insulin availability to modulate these processes and to facilitate the enhanced glucose uptake by exercising muscle. This is dramatically demonstrated by the acceleration of hyperglycemia, lipolysis, and ketogenesis which ensues during exercise in the presence of insulin deficiency.

Exercise also seems to enhance sensitivity to insulin, such that insulin is more biologically potent, particularly in the exercised part. Moreover, exercise also increases glucose utilization independent of insulin and substrate concentrations.

Two problems may emerge in diabetic patients. One is that, in contrast to normal physiology, circulating insulin levels fail to decline during activity, thus restraining hepatic glucose output and preventing it from providing sufficient glucose to meet the needs of increased energy expenditure. Persistent insulin absorption from its subcutaneoud depot precludes a decline in circulating insulin level. Indeed, circulating insulin levels may even increase during exercise as a consequence of exercise-induced mobilization of insulin, thus increasing the propensity to hypoglycemia. A significant advantage of continuous insulin infusion is that it obviates a subcutaneous depot except during the first few hours after a preprandial insulin bolus. Thus in theory, pump-treated patients may exercise during the postabsorptive period with little risk of hypoglycemia, particularly if the infusion is disconnected during the activity. Nevertheless, because of a delay in insulin absorption from subcutaneous tissue, the insulin binding to circulating antibodies, and other factors, free insulin concentrations may remain elevated in some diabetic patients for much of the work period, placing these individuals at risk of exercise-induced hypoglycemia.

It is necessary for patients to anticipate postprandial exercise and decrease the magnitude of the preprandial insulin dosage if hypoglycemia is to be avoided. Alternatively, extra food may be provided before or during the activity. Although the amount of food required to meet the energy demand varies with the magnitude of the activity, a rule of thumb is to provide 10–15 g carbohydrate every 30–45 min during increased activity. Blood glucose should be monitored before and after the activity to quantify the effects of such extra food, at least during the initial experience with a given exercise and until a predictable response is seen.

The second problem which may be encountered during acute exercise in diabetic patients is the progressive deterioration of the diabetic state which occurs in insulin-deficient patients. Progressive hyperglycemia seems to be a consequence of increased hepatic glucose output outstripping muscle glucose utilization. There is concomitant acceleration of lipolysis and ketogenesis disproportionate to their utilization, with resultant increased ketosis. These metabolic responses (glucagon, cortisol, and growth hormone) may be mediated in part by the increased plasma catecholamine responses to exercise that occur in insulin-deficient diabetic subjects. The absence of opposing effects of insulin (which ordinarily modulates these responses) permits the deterioration in glycemia and ketosis. Patients at risk of such deterioration are those with ambient blood glucose levels above 250–300 mg/dl, usually with at least some ketosis. Such patients should be cautioned to correct their hyperglycemia before undertaking strenuous exercise. Moreover, they should understand that one cannot use exercise as a replacement for insulin either to control hyperglycemia or to attempt to avert impending ketoacidosis.

Thus in educated patients the risk of exercised-induced hypoglycemia can be minimized, as can the potential of exacerbating hyperglycemia in the face of insulin deficiency. When deciding how to handle sporadic exercise, the patient should consider: (1) how much insulin has already been administered and at what time (if any) it is anticipated to peak; (2) when was the last meal or snack and when is the next anticipated meal or snack; (3) what is the prevailing blood glucose level before commencing the exercise; and (4) how much exercise is anticipated and what response to this type and degree of exercise has been seen in the past. Considering these factors, intelligent patients can make sensible decisions about the need for alterations in food or insulin so as to exercise without inducing hypoglycemia or exacerbating hyperglycemia.

SELF-MONITORING OF BLOOD GLUCOSE

The first reports of patient self-monitoring of blood glucose (SMBG) appeared in early 1978. They were met with skepticism on the part of many diabetes experts, who asserted that patients would not, could not, and should not measure their own blood glucose. These skeptics have been proved wrong, as the majority of patients exposed to SMBG have enthusiastically endorsed the concept. The growing use of SMBG has resulted in at least three international symposia on the subject and an explosion of technological advances. One of the most important of these has been the availability of automated, spring-operated devices that make the finger-pricking process simple and virtually painless. A variety of strips and meters are available for blood glucose testing, including several portable, battery-operated meters that patients may easily use in any setting. Some strips may be interpreted visually (without a meter), although this requires keen visual acuity and permits quantification of blood glucose only into broad ranges, unless the patient learns to interpolate color changes.

The available information about SMBG permits the following conclusions to be drawn:

1. SMBG is feasible, practical, and acceptable to patients.
2. Few technical difficulties are encountered. Patients have no difficulty in obtaining capillary blood. Blood glucose determinations are sufficiently accurate for clinical use.
3. SMBG facilitates patient understanding of diabetes. It improves and reinforces motivation.
4. Glycemic control may be improved if SMBG is used as part of an intensive therapeutic program of diabetes management involving careful balance of food, activity, and insulin.
5. Patients who can afford the cost of SMBG almost never want to return to urine glucose monitoring.

An American Diabetes Association Policy Statement, issued in 1982, states that SMBG "is preferable to urine testing in *any* insulin-requiring diabetic patient for the following reasons: (1) It facilitates the prevention of hyperglycemia that cannot be detected by urine testing. (2) It facilitates the prevention of hypoglycemia, particularly severe episodes that may occur when the patient has accumulated an overload of insulin." Although SMBG may be desirable in all insulin-treated patients for routine monitoring, not all patients are willing to use this approach. However, all insulin-treated patients should learn how to do SMBG (at least with patient-interpreted strips) and should keep finger-sticking aids and strips at home. SMBG is crucial for verifying hypoglycemia and for minitoring diabetes during intercurrent illness.

There are some categories of patients in whom SMBG is particularly useful. It is obligatory in pregnant women with diabetes, as meticulous control of maternal glycemia is the most important factor influencing fetal outcome. It also is mandatory in all patients who are using a portable insulin infusion pump or any intensive insulin program aimed at achieving excellent glucose control.

SMBG is also helpful in patients in whom hypoglycemia has been frequent or is especially to be averted (e.g., those who fail to recognize hypoglycemic symptoms, those with autonomic neuropathy, those with a coexisting seizure disorder) and in patients in whom urine glucose monitoring is unreliable or misleading (e.g., those with an altered or shifting renal threshold), impossible (e.g., anephric patients on dialysis, or color-blind patients), or difficult to perform (e.g., babies and young children still in diapers, incontinent patients). SMBG may also be helpful for problem-solving, in labile patients, and as a component in a comprehensive diabetes education program.

The frequency of monitoring depends on the reason for which SMBG is undertaken and the type of treatment program of any individual patient. As a general principle, unstable labile diabetes requires more frequent monitoring than stable diabetes. As a second principle, fasting and preprandial glucose measurements alone underestimate the extent of postprandial glucose excursions and are inadequate as the sole monitoring times if excellent control is desired.

A recent study in patients with IDDM who had attained excellent control (near-normal glycosylated hemoglobin values) demonstrated that such control deteriorated if SMBG was reduced to less than four determinations per day. Moreover, this prompted the investigators to institute a crossover study in which they demonstrated that better control was attained with four or more daily blood glucose determinations than with fewer measurements (Fig. 2-7).

For patients with IDDM embarking on a program of intensive therapy aimed at excellent control, our practice is to commence with nine or more determinations daily: prebreakfast, postprandial breakfast, prelunch, postprandaial lunch, presupper, postprandial supper, bedtime, midnight, and 2:00–4:00 AM. We reduce the frequency of monitoring when a relatively stable pattern is obtained. Then we recommend mea-

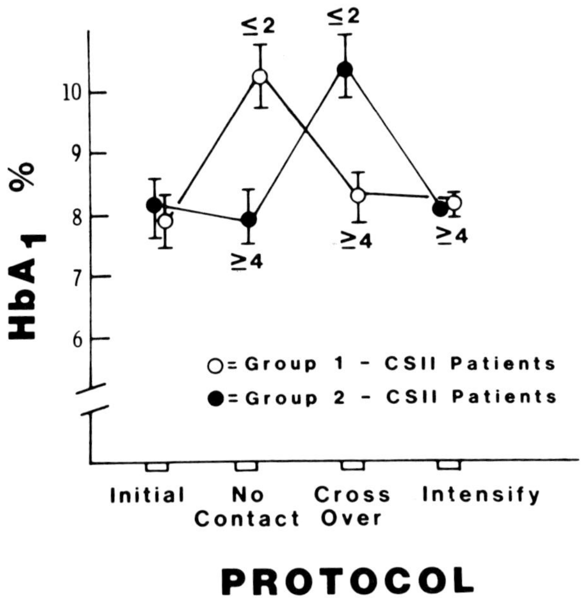

Fig. 2-7 Glycemic control, assessed by glycosylated hemoglobin (HbA_1) values, in relation to number of daily self-monitored blood glucose determinations. After 1 year of intensive therapy, HbA_1 values were near normal ("Initial"). Patients had been performing SMBG four or more times daily. During the next 6 months ("No Contact"), patients monitored their blood glucose levels at whatever frequency they wished. HbA_1 values remained unchanged in patients who continued SMBG ≥ four times daily, whereas they deteriorated in patients who reduced SMBG to ≤ two times daily. Noting this, the investigators asked patients who had been performing SMBG ≥ four times daily to reduce their frequency to ≤ two times daily during the next 3 months ("Crossover") and those who had performed SMBG ≤ two times daily to increase their frequency to ≥ four times daily during the same 3-month period. These changes resulted in a reversal of HbA_1 values. During a subsequent 3-month period ("Intensify"), all patients performed SMBG ≥ four times daily and achieved near-normal HbA_1 values. Thus in all instances near-normal HbA_1 values were associated with ≥ four monitorings of blood glucose daily and were not achieved with ≤ two monitorings daily.

surement of four samples (preprandial and bedtime) most days with a complete profile (nine determinations) monthly and 2:00–4:00 AM samples at least once weekly. Additional samples should be taken any time hypoglycemia is suspected and to measure the impact of alterations in food, activity, or insulin program.

For stable patients with non-insulin-dependent diabetes mellitus (NIDDM) after control is attained, we recommend that prebreakfast samples be measured three to seven times weekly, with a four-point (preprandial and bedtime) profile one to three times monthly, and a seven-point profile (four-point plus postprandial) monthly. Because there are prolonged postprandial glucose excursions in NIDDM, SMBG can be used to determine the interval necessary for glucose levels to be restored to their fasting level, before consumption of the next meal (generally 4–5 hr).

If glycemic control deteriorates, it is necessary to increase the frequency of monitoring. Frequent sampling is also necessary during intercurrent illness and for problem assessment.

Merely measuring blood glucose rather then urine glucose may result in a modest improvement in glucose control by provoking greater dietary adherence and/or stimulating patient motivation. The attainment of excellent glycemic control requires that the patient embark on a total program of intensive insulin therapy as defined in this chapter. SMBG alone does not dramatically alter glycemic control. On the other hand, SMBG is essential for the attainment of excellent glucose control.

The major advantage of SMBG is that it enables therapeutic goals to be clearly defined and permits assessment of glycemic control during ordinary life. In this regard, it complements glycosylated hemoglobin measurements. SMBG defines the extent of glycemic excursions whereas glycosylated hemoglobin documents average glycemic control. More importantly, SMBG determinations may be used on an ongoing basis by patients to aid in the adjustment of the therapeutic regimen. Thus in the context of an intensive program of diabetes management, SMBG becomes an integral component of treatment, facilitating the attainment of improved glycemic control.

SMBG may result in decreased hospitalizations and thus an overall saving in cost. However, careful cost-benefit studies have not been reported, with the exception of a preliminary report dealing with pregnant diabetic women. The long-term potential benefits of SMBG in facilitating glycemic control and reducing diabetic complications remain to be established. In theory, this should result. Obviously, if this is the case the benefits not only in cost-effectiveness but in human terms would be enormous.

Furthermore, SMBG obviates the disadvantages of urine glucose monitoring, which may be misleading and inadequate and which correlates poorly with glycemia (Fig. 2-8). In this context, it is interesting to note that up to two-thirds of patients incorrectly use procedures for urine glucose monitoring.

On the other hand, there are potential disadvantages of SMBG as well. There is considerable initial investment in time required on the part of both the patient and the health care team. Continuing contact between these two entities is also required if excellent glycemic control is to be achieved. Moreover, SMBG is relatively expensive. After purchase of a meter, SMBG (with determinations done four times daily) costs $750 to $1000 per year compared with less than $100 for urine glucose moni-

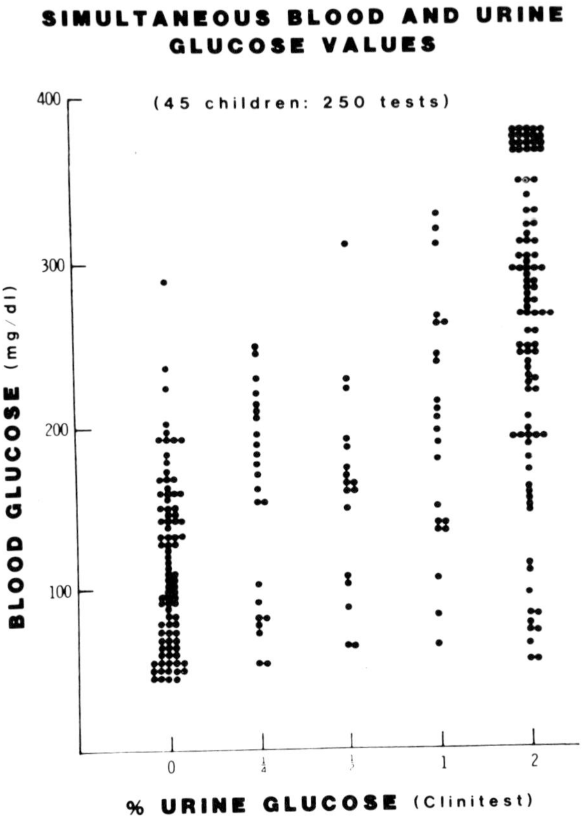

Fig. 2-8 Correlation between urine glucose concentration (conventional five-drop Clinitest) and simultaneous blood glucose concentration in 45 diabetic children. The absence of glycosuria may be associated with blood glucose concentration from 45 to over 270 mg/dl.

toring. Increased frequency of hypoglycemia is a potential complication of intense management of IDDM, although this has not been a particular problem in practice because glycemic excursions are lessened and introduction of SMBG is generally accompanied by modification of food, insulin, and activity regimens. Nevertheless, because of the potential risk of hypoglycemia, it is necessary to exercise prudence when selecting goals of therapy, appropriately monitoring blood glucose, and regulating therapy.

Infection at sites of blood-letting is not usually a problem, provided the patient washes his/her hands. An exception may be in patients who have impaired blood supply to the hands and are on immunosuppressive therapy. A recent report describes two patients who after kidney transplantation developed finger sepsis in the hand that had an arteriovenous fistula (for previous dialysis). Coarsening of the fingertips is seen, and possible loss of fine discrimination has been posed as a possible problem. This can be obviated by using the sides of the fingers for blood-letting. Other side effects, e.g., preoccupation of the patient with diabetes, may be seen. Noncompliance and/or reporting of fraudulent or inaccurate results may occur, but these problems are not unique to SMBG.

On balance, SMBG is an effective, safe clinical tool that permits patients and their physicians to define, measure, and achieve treatment targets that result in improved diabetes management.

ATTAINMENT OF EXCELLENT GLUCOSE CONTROL

The most important component of a program of intensive insulin therapy is the patient's ability to utilize the information obtained from SMBG in order to make sensible decisions concerning the balance between food intake, activity, and insulin dosage in an attempt to achieve the target blood glucose levels that he/she is striving for (e.g., those listed in Table 2-1). Acceptable blood glucose levels may vary according to a patient's progress in implementing an intensive program of treatment. Thus the initial goal may be to attain preprandial glucose levels of 100–200 mg/dl. The next goal might be preprandial levels of 100–175 mg/dl, followed by 90–150 mg/dl. Once this has been consistently achieved, the patient can aim for "acceptable" preprandial levels of 70–130 mg/dl. Some patients might then attempt to achieve the "ideal" preprandial values of 70–105 mg/dl. Blood glucose targets are set higher for patients who are prone to hypoglycemia or who fail to recognize or recover from hypoglycemia, in order to lessen their risk of hypoglycemia. For example, preprandial targets for such patients might be 120–180 mg/dl or occasionally even higher.

One reason for sequential targets is that these facilitate patient adaptation to a lower prevailing level of glycemia. An abrupt change in glycemia often results in patients feeling quite uncomfortable, manifesting headaches, and developing symptoms of hypoglycemia with normal concentrations of plasma glucose. This is accompanied by a measurable counterregulatory response and may be accounted for by an influence of chronically elevated plasma glucose in repressing glucose transport capacity across the blood-brain barrier. Health professionals and patients should be aware of the symptomatic discomfort that predictably occurs with the establishment of markedly improved glycemic control, and patients should be assured that it is a transient phenomenon generally lasting several days to a fortnight. After adaptation to normoglycemia these symptoms abate, and indeed patients usually feel better than they did in the face of chronic hyperglycemia. On the other hand, their symptoms of hypoglycemia may be different than they were with higher levels of average glycemia. Thus they should be alert for new and subtler symptoms of hypoglycemia (e.g., paresthesia around the lips).

In response to blood glucose fluctuations, the patient must learn how to take appropriate action. To this end, the patient may learn a sequence of responses predetermined by the physician. The system we use for this purpose is that of "algorithms" for insulin dose alteration.

Two general types of alteration in insulin may be defined: adjustments and supplements. Adjustments, which are modifications in the basic insulin dose, presuppose that the patient has a stable pattern of meals and activities, has no intercurrent illness, and is free from unusual stress.

Insulin supplements may be used when the pattern of meals or activities is not stable, when there is intercurrent illness or other stress, or to correct unexplained hyperglycemia. Supplements, then, are temporary insulin doses. Two types may be used:

(1) anticipatory supplements, given to limit expected hyperglycemia, e.g., before a large meal; and (2) compensatory supplements, given to overcome unusual hyperglycemia—particularly important during intercurrent illness.

Adjustments of Insulin Dose

When blood glucose levels are outside the target range, the basic insulin dosage is adjusted (Tables 2-5 through 2-8). Such adjustments should not be made if the patient has an incurrent illness or is experiencing stress. Before altering the basic insulin dose, the patient should make sure that changes in the blood glucose level are not due to alterations in food intake or activity. Before lowering the prebreakfast (postnadir) blood glucose level, the patient should verify that the blood glucose nadir

Table 2-5. Algorithms for Adjusting Insulin Doses Using a "Split-and-Mixed" Regular and NPH or Lente Insulin Regimen

A. **Target blood glucose levels**

Before breakfast	70–110 mg/dl
Before lunch, supper, and bedtime snack	70–130 mg/dl
One hour after meals	≤180 mg/dl
Two hours after meals	≤150 mg/dl
2:00 AM to 4:00 AM	> 70 mg/dl

B. **Assumptions**
1. The prebreakfast short-acting regular insulin has major action between breakfast and lunch, and its effect is reflected in the results of blood glucose tests after breakfast and before lunch.
2. The prebreakfast intermediate-acting NPH or lente insulin has major action between lunch and supper, and its effect is reflected in the results of blood glucose tests after lunch and before supper.
3. The presupper regular insulin has major action between supper and bedtime, and its effect is reflected in the results of blood glucose tests after supper and at bedtime.
4. The presupper or bedtime NPH or lente insulin has major action overnight, and its effect is reflected in the results of blood glucose tests during the middle of the night and on arising the next morning.

C. **Hyperglycemia (high blood sugar) not explained by unusual diet/exercise/insulin**
1. If prebreakfast blood glucose is greater than 110 mg/dl for 2–4 days in a row, increase your presupper or bedtime NPH or lente insulin by 1 or 2 units. (Before making such changes, verify that the blood glucose nadir, usually around 3:00–4:00 AM, is not below 70 mg/dl.)
2. If prelunch blood glucose is greater than 130 mg/dl for 2–4 days in a row, increase your prebreakfast regular insulin by 1 or 2 units.
3. If presupper blood glucose is greater than 130 mg/dl for 2–4 days in a row, increase your prebreakfast NPH or lente insulin by 1 or 2 units.
4. If bedtime blood glucose is greater than 130 mg/dl for 2–4 days in a row, increase your presupper regular insulin by 1 or 2 units.

D. **Hypoglycemia (low blood sugar) not explained by unusual diet/exercise/insulin**
1. *Prevent insulin reactions by eating meals and snacks on time.*
2. If prebreakfast blood glucose is less than 70 mg/dl or if there is evidence that hypoglycemic reactions are occurring during the night, reduce your presupper or bedtime NPH or lente insulin by 1 or 2 units.
3. If prelunch blood glucose is less than 70 mg/dl or if you have a hypoglycemic reaction between breakfast and lunch, reduce your prebreakfast regular insulin by 1 or 2 units.
4. If presupper blood glucose is less than 70 mg/dl or if you have a hypoglycemic reaction between lunch and supper, reduce your prebreakfast NPH or lente insulin by 1 or 2 units.
5. If bedtime blood glucose is less than 70 mg/dl or if you have a hypoglycemic reaction between supper and bedtime, reduce your presupper regular insulin by 1 or 2 units.

The regimens herein are depicted in Figures 2-2 and 2-3.

Table 2-6. Algorithms for Adjusting Insulin Doses Using Bedtime NPH or Lente and Three Doses of Regular Insulin Regimen

A. **Target blood glucose levels**

Before breakfast	70–110 mg/dl
Before lunch, supper, and bedtime snack	70–130 mg/dl
One hour after meals	≤180 mg/dl
Two hours after meals	≤150 mg/dl
2:00 AM to 4:00 AM	> 70 mg/dl

B. **Assumptions**
1. The bedtime intermediate-acting NPH or lente insulin has major action overnight, and its effect is primarily reflected in the results of blood glucose tests during the middle of the night and on arising the next morning.
2. The prebreakfast short-acting regular insulin has major action between breakfast and lunch, and its effect is reflected in the results of blood glucose tests before lunch.
3. The prelunch regular insulin has major action between lunch and supper, and its effect is reflected in the results of blood glucose tests before supper.
4. The presupper regular insulin has major action between supper and bedtime, and its effect is reflected in the results of blood glucose tests at bedtime.

C. **Hyperglycemia (high blood sugar) not explained by unusual diet/exercise/insulin**
1. If prebreakfast blood glucose is greater than 110 mg/dl for 2–4 days in a row, increase your bedtime NPH or lente insulin by 1 or 2 units. (Before making such changes, verify that the blood glucose nadir, usually around 3:00–4:00 AM, is not below 70 mg/dl.)
2. If prelunch blood glucose is greater than 130 mg/dl for 2–4 days in a row, increase your prebreakfast regular insulin by 1 or 2 units.
3. If presupper blood glucose is greater than 130 mg/dl for 2–4 days in a row, increase your prelunch regular insulin by 1 or 2 units.
4. If bedtime blood glucose is greater than 130 mg/dl for 2–4 days in a row, increase your presupper regular insulin by 1 or 2 units.

D. **Hypoglycemia (low blood suger) not explained by unusual diet/exercise/insulin**
1. *Prevent insulin reactions by eating meals and snacks on time.*
2. If prebreakfast blood glucose is less than 70 mg/dl or if there is evidence that hypoglycemic reactions are occurring during the night, reduce your bedtime NPH or lente insulin by 1 or 2 units.
3. If prelunch blood glucose is less than 70 mg/dl or if you have a hypoglycemic reaction between breakfast and lunch, reduce your prebreakfast regular insulin by 1 or 2 units.
4. If presupper blood glucose is less than 70 mg/dl or if you have a hypoglycemic reaction between lunch and supper, reduce your prelunch regular insulin by 1 or 2 units.
5. If bedtime blood glucose is less than 70 mg/dl or if you have a hypoglycemic reaction between supper and bedtime, reduce your presupper regular insulin by 1 or 2 units.

The regimen herein is depicted in Figure 2-4.

(usually occurring between 3:00 AM and 4:00 AM) is not in the hypoglycemic range (i.e., not below 70 mg/dl). Moreover, an attempt should be made to determine if there is an early morning rise in glucose level (see below).

Hyperglycemia. Adjustments in the relevant insulin component may be made when blood glucose levels exceed the target range. The overnight component is adjusted on the basis of the blood glucose levels at midnight, 3:00–4:00 AM, and before breakfast, as discussed below. The premeal insulin doses are adjusted to eliminate postprandial hyperglycemia and to achieve target blood glucose levels before the next meal. However, the patient should not make an adjustment on the basis of postprandial excess if the blood glucose level before the next meal is already within the ideal range. In that circumstance, several options are possible: Decrease or omit carbohydrate from the preceding meal, add fiber to that meal, alter the timing of preprandial

Table 2-7. Algorithms for Adjusting Insulin Doses Using Ultralente Insulin and Three Doses of Regular Insulin Regimen

A. **Target blood glucose levels**

Before breakfast	70–110 mg/dl
Before lunch, supper, and bedtime snack	70–130 mg/dl
One hour after meals	≤180 mg/dl
Two hours after meals	≤150 mg/dl
2:00 AM to 4:00 AM	> 70 mg/dl

B. **Assumptions**

1. The long-acting ultralente insulin provides a background basal dosage of insulin, and its effect is primarily reflected in the results of blood glucose tests during the middle of the night and on arising the next morning.
2. The prebreakfast short-acting regular insulin has major action between breakfast and lunch, and its effect is reflected in the results of blood glucose tests before lunch.
3. The prelunch regular insulin has major action between lunch and supper, and its effect is reflected in the results of blood glucose tests before supper.
4. The presupper regular insulin has major action between supper and bedtime, and its effect is reflected in the results of blood glucose tests at bedtime.

C. **Hyperglycemia (high blood sugar) not explained by unusual diet/exercise/insulin**

1. If the midnight, 2:00–4:00 AM, or prebreakfast blood glucose is greater than 110 mg/dl for 4–5 days in a row, refer to the nocturnal insulin adjustment sheet.
2. If prelunch blood glucose is greater than 130 mg/dl for 2–4 days in a row, increase your prebreakfast regular insulin by 1 or 2 units.
3. If presupper blood glucose is greater than 130 mg/dl for 2–4 days in a row, increase your prelunch regular insulin by 1 or 2 units.
4. If bedtime blood glucose is greater than 130 mg/dl for 2–4 days in a row, increase your presupper regular insulin by 1 or 2 units.

D. **Hypoglycemia (low blood sugar) not explained by unusual diet/exercise/insulin**

1. *Prevent insulin reactions by eating meals and snacks on time.*
2. If midnight, 2:00–4:00 AM, or prebreakfast blood glucose is less than 70 mg/dl, or if there is evidence that hypoglycemic reactions are occurring during the night, refer to the nocturnal insulin adjustment sheet.
3. If prelunch blood glucose is less than 70 mg/dl or if you have a hypoglycemic reaction between breakfast and lunch, reduce your prebreakfast regular insulin by 1 or 2 units.
4. If presupper blood glucose is less than 70 mg/dl or if you have a hypoglycemic reaction between lunch and supper, reduce your prelunch regular insulin by 1 or 2 units.
5. If bedtime blood glucose is less than 70 mg/dl or if you have a hypoglycemic reaction between supper and bedtime, reduce your presupper regular insulin by 1 or 2 units.
6. *Note:* When you change the total ultralente insulin dosage, if you have been taking the ultralente in two injections per day, the two doses should be kept approximately equal unless you are instructed otherwise.

The regiman herein is depicted in Figure 2-5.

insulin administration (lengthening the interval before the meal), increase the insulin dose while adding or increasing an intervening snack, or increase the insulin dose while carefully monitoring the preprandial glucose if it has been in the upper portion of the target range.

Insulin adjustments are of the magnitude of 1 or 2 U of insulin at a time, and increments are made only every 3 or 4 days. Unless the blood glucose level is consistently over 200 mg/dl throughout the day, signifying gross insulin deficiency (and the need to increase all insulin components), we recommend that only one component of the insulin regimen be altered at a time, beginning with the component responsible

Table 2-8. Algorithms for Adjusting Insulin Doses for Patients Using Continuous Subcutaneous Insulin Infusion

A. **Target blood glucose levels**

Before breakfast	70–110 mg/dl
Before lunch, supper, and bedtime snack	70–130 mg/dl
One hour after meals	≤180 mg/dl
Two hours after meals	≤150 mg/dl
2:00 AM to 4:00 AM	> 70 mg/dl

B. **Assumptions**

1. The basal insulin rate provides continuous background amounts of insulin. Its effect is reflected primarily in the results of blood glucose tests during the middle of the night and on arising in the morning.
2. Each premeal bolus of insulin provides for the use and storage of food consumed at that meal. The effect of each bolus is reflected in the results of blood glucose tests after that meal and before the next meal.

C. **Hyperglycemia (high blood sugar) not explained by unusual diet/exercise/insulin**

1. If the midnight, 2:00–4:00 AM, or prebreakfast blood glucose is greater than mg/dl for 2–4 days in a row, refer to the nocturnal insulin adjustment sheet.
2. If prelunch blood glucose is greater than 130 mg/dl for 2–4 days in a row, increase your prebreakfast bolus by 1 or 2 insulin units.
3. If presupper blood glucose is greater than 130 mg/dl for 2–4 days in a row, increase your prelunch bolus by 1 or 2 insulin units.
4. If bedtime blood glucose is greater than 130 mg/dl for 2–4 days in a row, increase your presupper bolus by 1 or 2 insulin units.

D. **Hypoglycemia (low blood sugar) not explained by unusual diet/exercise/insulin**

1. *Prevent insulin reactions by eating meals and snacks on time.*
2. If midnight, 2:00–4:00 AM, or prebreakfast blood glucose is less than 70 mg/dl or if there is evidence that hypoglycemic reactions are occurring during the night, refer to the nocturnal insulin adjustment sheet.
3. If prelunch blood glucose is less than 70 mg/dl or if you have a hypoglycemic reaction between breakfast and lunch, reduce your prebreakfast bolus by 1 or 2 insulin units.
4. If presupper blood glucose is less than 70 mg/dl or if you have a hypoglycemic reaction between lunch and supper, reduce your prelunch bolus by 1 or 2 insulin units.
5. If bedtime blood glucose is less than 70 mg/dl or if you have a hypoglycemic reaction between supper and bedtime, reduce your presupper bolus by 1 or 2 insulin units.

The regimen herein in depicted in Figure 2-6.

for controlling the prebreakfast blood glucose level. When the prebreakfast hyperglycemia is corrected, the patient can sequentially adjust the other insulin components, starting with the prebreakfast regular insulin. Glycemic control is gradually attained in this manner using the algorithms in Tables 2-5 through 2-8.

Hypoglycemia. Whenever possible, hypoglycemic symptoms should be verified by blood glucose determination to ensure that symptoms occurring for some other reason (e.g., anxiety) are not attributed to hypoglycemia. Blood glucose testing also helps patients who have symptoms triggered by counterregulatory hormone release without true hypoglycemia to adapt to lower ambient levels of blood glucose without imposing additional calories. When hypoglycemia is documented, or if blood glucose cannot be determined and hypoglycemic symptoms occur, the patient should consume rapidly absorbed simple sugar (about 10g). Patientss should always carry an acceptable source of sugar for this purpose. If mealtime is more than 1 hr away, additional slowly absorbed food (complex carbohydrate or protein) should be consumed. Hypoglycemic episodes are often readily explainable by known alterations in the food/activity/insulin balance (e.g., a delayed meal or unusual activity). If such is not the case, the relevant insulin component should be reduced by 1 or 2 U the next day, as outlined by the algorithms in Tables 2-5 through 2-8.

Overnight Blood Glucose Levels. Particular care must be taken before there is an alteration in the component of insulin acting overnight. Because CSII and an ultralente-based intensive conventional regimen are designed to provide stable insulinemia without a peak insulin effect, it may be easier to attain overnight control with either of these. Nocturnal adjustments are described in Tables 2-9 and 2-10. It is more difficult to adjust an intermediate-acting insulin regimen overnight because of the peak effect. In such patients there must be even greater vigilance to avert hypoglycemia.

Table 2-9. Nocturnal Adjustment of Insulin by Patients on an Ultralente-Based Insulin Regimen

Ultralente insulin provides a background amount of insulin. Overnight, when no food is consumed, the ultralente insulin ideally results in stable levels of blood glucose. Whether it has this effect may be determined by measuring blood glucose values at midnight, 2:00 AM to 4:00 AM, and before breakfast (7:00 AM to 8:00 AM).

A. **Hyperglycemia (high blood sugar) not explained by unusual diet/exercise/insulin**
   1. If prebreakfast blood glucose is greater than 110 mg/dl for 4–5 days in a row, measure blood glucose at midnight and 2:00–4:00 AM for at least 2–3 days.
   2. If both the midnight and 2:00–4:00 AM blood glucose levels are within the acceptable range (70–110 mg/dl) and the prebreakfast value is higher, increase your dose of ultralente insulin by 1 or 2 units.
   3. If both the midnight and 2:00–4:00 AM blood glucose levels exceed the acceptable range (70–110 mg/dl) but the prebreakfast value is more than 20–25 mg/dl higher, increase your dose of ultralente insulin by 1 or 2 units.
   4. If both the midnight and 2:00–4:00 AM blood glucose levels exceed the acceptable range (70–110 mg/dl) but are approximately equal to the breakfast value (within 20–25 mg/dl), the blood glucose levels are stable overnight and the ultralente insulin dose is adequate. The high midnight level of blood glucose can be corrected either by increasing your presupper (or prebedtime snack) dose of regular insulin or by decreasing your bedtime snack.
   5. If either the midnight or 2:00–4:00 AM blood glucose level is below 70 mg/dl, it must be corrected first, even though the prebreakfast value exceeds the target range. This can be accomplished either by decreasing your presupper (or prebedtime snack) dose of regular insulin or by increasing your bedtime snack.
   6. If you have any uncertainty about interpreting these patterns, consult your physician or a member of the diabetes staff.

B. **Hypoglycemia (low blood sugar) not explained by unusual diet/exercise/insulin**
   1. *Hypoglycemic reactions*
      a. If hypoglycemic reactions occur before 4:00 AM, decrease your presupper (or prebedtime snack) dose of regular insulin or increase your bedtime snack.
      b. If hypoglycemic reactions occur during the morning hours after 4:00 AM, and you do not know if the blood glucose was low earlier in the night as well, decrease your dose of ultralente insulin by 1 or 2 units.
   2. *Low blood sugar*
      a. If prebreakfast blood glucose is less than 70 mg/dl, measure the blood glucose level at midnight and 2:00–4:00 AM for the next 1–2 days.
      b. If the midnight, 2:00–4:00 AM, and prebreakfast blood glucose levels are all below 80 mg/dl but at least one of these is below 70 mg/dl, the blood glucose is relatively stable overnight and the dose of ultralente insulin is adequate. Because the blood glucose level is initially low at midnight, these low levels can be corrected either by decreasing your presupper (or prebedtime snack) dose of regular insulin or by increasing your bedtime snack.
      c. If both the midnight and 2:00–4:00 AM blood glucose levels are above 80 mg/dl, and the prebreakfast value is below 70 mg/dl, decrease your dose of ultralente insulin by 1 or 2 units.

The regimen herein is depicted in Figure 2-5.

Table 2-10. Nocturnal Adjustment of Insulin by Patients on CSII

The basal insulin infusion rate provides a background amount of insulin. Overnight, when no food is consumed, ideally the blood glucose levels are stable. Whether the basal infusion rate has this effect may be determined by measuring blood glucose values at midnight, 2:00–4:00 AM, and before breakfast (7:00–8:00 AM).

A. **Hyperglycemia (high blood sugar) not explained by unusual diet/exercise/insulin**
   1. If prebreakfast blood glucose is greater than 110 mg/dl for 2–4 days in a row, measure blood glucose at midnight and 2:00–4:00 AM for at least 2–3 days.
   2. If both the midnight and 2:00–4:00 AM blood glucose levels are within the acceptable range (70–110 mg/dl) and the prebreakfast value is higher, increase your basal dose by 1 or 2 units.
   3. If both the midnight and 2:00–4:00 AM blood glucose levels exceed the acceptable range (70–110 mg/dl) but the prebreakfast value is more than 20–25 mg/dl higher, increase your basal dose by 1 or 2 units.
   4. If both the midnight and 2:00–4:00 AM blood glucose levels exceed the acceptable range (70–110 mg/dl) but are approximately equal to the breakfast value (within 20–25 mg/dl), the blood glucose levels are stable overnight and the basal dose is adequate. A high blood glucose level at midnight can be corrected either by increasing your presupper (or prebedtime snack) meal bolus or by decreasing your bedtime snack.
   5. If either the midnight or 2:00–4:00 AM blood glucose level is below 70 mg/dl, it must be corrected first, even though the prebreakfast value exceeds the target range. Do this either by decreasing your presupper (or prebedtime snack) meal bolus or by increasing your bedtime snack.
   6. If you can have any uncertainty about interpreting these patterns, consult your physician or a member of the diabetes staff.

B. **Hypoglycemia (low blood sugar) not explained by unusual diet/exercise/insulin**
   1. *Hypoglycemic reactions*
      a. If hypoglycemic reactions occur before 4:00 AM, decrease your presupper (or prebedtime snack) meal bolus or increase your bedtime snack.
      b. If hypoglycemic reactions occur during the morning hours after 4:00 AM and you do not know if the blood glucose was low earlier in the night as well, decrease your basal dose by 1 or 2 units.
   2. *Low blood sugar*
      a. If prebreakfast blood glucose is less than 70 mg/dl, measure the blood glucose level at midnight and 2:00–4:00 AM for the next 1–2 days.
      b. If the midnight, 2:00–4:00 AM, and prebreakfast blood glucose levels are all below 80 mg/dl but at least one of these is below 70 mg/dl, the blood glucose is relatively stable overnight and the basal dose is adequate. Because the blood glucose level is initially low at midnight, these low levels can be corrected either by decreasing your presupper (or prebedtime snack) meal bolus or by increasing your bedtime snack.
      c. If both the midnight and 2:00–4:00 AM blood glucose levels are above 80 mg/dl, and the prebreakfast value is below 70 mg/dl, decrease your basal dose by 1 or 2 units.

The regimen herein is depicted in Figure 2-6.

Physicians and patients should be aware that prebreakfast blood glucose levels may not reflect overnight levels, which may rise during the early morning hours for any one of several reasons, including: (1) waning levels of circulating free insulin; (2) diurnal variation in insulin action (dawn phenomenon); or (3) "rebound" hyperglycemia following hypoglycemia ("Somogyi phenomenon") (Fig. 2-9). The actions required to overcome an early morning rise in glucose level vary, depending on which of these reasons seems to be responsible for the rise. Unfortunately, it is not easy to identify the reason(s) for the early morning rise in glucose level.

After a meal-related subcutaneous injection or bolus of regular insulin, circulating levels of free insulin remain elevated for 4–8 hr. Overnight, circulating insulin consists of the basal insulin infusion (or the overnight component of intermediate- or long-acting insulin) plus a declining contribution from any regular insulin given be-

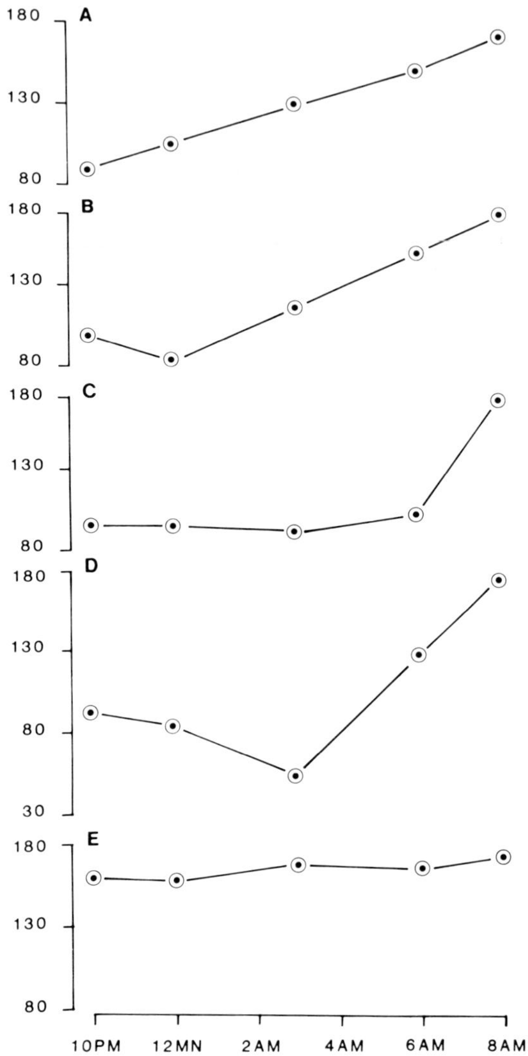

Fig. 2-9 Several patterns of overnight glycemia all resulting in prebreakfast (8:00 AM) glucose values exceeding the target range. In patterns A through D, bedtime values are normal. It can be seen that with only bedtime and prebreakfast glucose values it would be impossible to distinguish these patterns. Patterns A and B indicate deficiency of the overnight insulin component. Pattern C depicts the dawn phenomenon. Pattern D depicts a pattern of rebound hyperglycemia following nocturnal hypoglycemia. Pattern E indicates that the overnight insulin component is adequate to maintain basal glycemia but that the presupper or prebedtime snack insulin is deficient (or the bedtime snack too large). Overnight glycemic patterns should be sought before altering overnight insulin doses.

fore supper or a bedtime snack. Measurements of blood glucose levels at midnight, 3:00–4:00 AM, and 7:00–8:00 AM often reveal a gradually rising trend from a nadir around midnight. If the nadir at midnight is below the acceptable range (or tending toward the lower portion of the acceptable range), the interval between the presupper insulin and supper can be lengthened, and/or the dose decreased, and/or a larger bedtime snack consumed). Once the midnight nadir is in a safe range, the overnight component of insulin can be gradually increased to prevent the early-morning glucose rise.

An abrupt rise in blood sugar during the early morning hours (5:00–8:00 AM) after stable euglycemic values at midnight and 3:00–4:00 AM has been termed the *dawn phenomenon*. Its mechanism is not known, although diurnal variation in sensitivity to insulin (possibly secondary to diurnal fluctation of an anti-insulin hormone), deactivation of insulin-stimulated biological responses, stimulation of the reticular activating system during waking, and other diurnal mechanisms have been proposed. A solution to the dawn phenomenon in patients on CSII is preprogramming of the pump's basal infusion rate to provide incremental insulin availability during the dawn hours. If the phenomenon can be demonstrated in a patient and the other reasons for an early-morning glucose rise can be excluded, this seems a reasonable approach. The preprogramming should be done gradually, with careful surveillance of glycemic response.

The *rebound effect* is a glucose rise following hypoglycemia, presumably triggered by counterregulatory hormones. It is evidenced by documented hypoglycemia at midnight or 3:00–4:00 AM, followed by rising blood sugar into either the euglycemic or hyperglycemic range. The sequence of hypolycemia followed by hyperglycemia is generally a result of excessive circulating insulin levels at the time of the glucose nadir, followed by insufficient insulin levels at the time of the rebound. Rebound is corrected by decreasing the insulin component acting at the time of the hypoglycemia. Additional insulin is needed at the time of any hyperglycemia. Clues to nocturnal hypoglycemia, indicating the need to make additional determinations of blood glucose levels during the night, include nightmares, morning headache or irritability (or both), nocturnal sweating, and morning ketonuria without evidence of insulin deficiency (the ketonuria arising from counterregulatory hormone stimulation of lipolysis and ketogenesis).

The separate nocturnal adjustment sheets for some regimens (Tables 2-9 and 2-10) serve also to emphasize the vigilance that must be exerted to avoid nocturnal hypoglycemia.

Insulin Supplements

Compensatory insulin supplements are used to overcome excessive preprandial hyperglycemia during periods of optimal control as well as periods of acute loss of glycemic control (e.g., with intercurrent illness).

In response to preprandial hyperglycemia, compensatory supplemental insulin is taken, as outlined in Table 2-11. The values given in Table 2-11 are representative and should be adapted for the individual patient based on body size, total daily insulin dosage, and experience with supplements in that patient. Patients vary in their response to a given size of supplement. It is important that the supplement be recorded separately from the basic dose (as in Figure 2-10) because the continuing need for a supplement before a particular meal requires an adjustment in the insulin dose covering the previous meal. For example, if the prelunch level of blood glucose is excessive 3 days in a row, prelunch supplements should be taken to lower the blood glucose level closer to the target range before supper but the prebreakfast basic dose should be adjusted on the fourth day.

During intercurrent illness, larger and more frequent supplements may be needed, perhaps as often as every 3–4 hr. Supplements during illness (Table 2-12) are approximately 1 or 2 units of insulin for every 30–50 mg/dl increment of blood glucose over 120 mg/dl. (As in preprandial supplements, the values given in Table 2-12 are

Table 2-11. Algorithms for Use of Compensatory Insulin Supplements for Premeal Correction of Blood Glucose

1. Once your insulin dose is stable, use the following scheme for premeal supplements of regular insulin. If the blood glucose is:

<70 mg/dl:	reduce the premeal dose by 1 or 2 units
70–110 mg/dl:	take the prescribed premeal dose
110–150 mg/dl:	increase the premeal dose by 1 unit
150–200 mg/dl:	increase the pemeal dose by 2 units
200–250 mg/dl:	increase the premeal dose by 3 units
>300 mg/dl:	increase the premeal dose by 4 units

2. If your blood glucose exceeds 200 mg/dl, you may wish to delay your next meal by an additional 20–30 min.
3. Record the supplement in the ''supplement'' column of your record sheet so that you do not confuse it with your usual premeal dose.
4. In the absence of illness, a need for supplements lasting longer than 2–4 days indicates that you need to adjust your basic insulin dose according to your ''algorithms for adjustment of insulin doses.''

only a general guide and should be modified for the individual patient, as appropriate, based on body size, total daily insulin dosage, food consumption, and previous experience with supplements in that patient.) If glycemic control deteriorates despite the use of supplemental insulin, the size of the supplements should be increased. Again, the supplements should be recorded separately from the basic dose (Fig. 2-10).

As additional preparation for intercurrent illness, an antinauseant (e.g., Emetrol or Coke syrup) and antiemetic suppositories [e.g., trimethobenzamide (Tigan) or

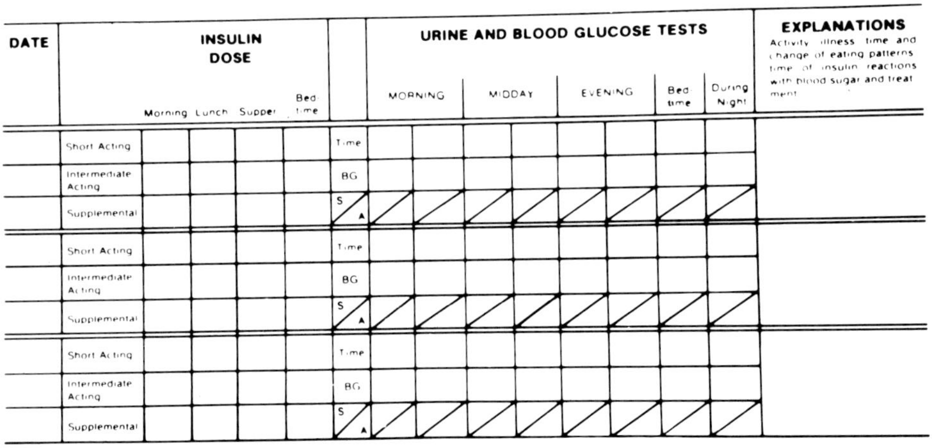

Fig. 2-10 Sample of a diabetes record sheet. This one includes enough space to accomodate any of the insulin regimens described in this chapter. There is also room for recording blood glucose results before and after meals, as well as space for recording insulin supplements (or decrements) separate from the basic dose. This helps prevent ''bookkeeping errors.'' The explanations/comments column is used for clarification of circumstances impacting on glycemia.

Table 2-12. Algorithms for Use of Compensatory Insulin Supplements During Illness

1. Take extra regular insulin according to the following schedule. If the blood glucose is:

110–150 mg/dl	add 1–2 units of insulin
150–200 mg/dl before meals or at bedtime	add 2–3 units of insulin
200–250 mg/dl before meals or at bedtime:	add 3–5 units of insulin
250–300 mg/dl:	add 4–6 units of insulin every 3 or 4 hr.
300–350 mg/dl:	add 6–8 units of insulin every 3 or 4 hr
350–400 mg/dl:	add 8–10 units of insulin every 3 or 4 hr

2. Check urine for ketones at the time of each test of blood glucose. If urine ketones are high and the blood glucose concentration is 300 mg/dl or more, double the amount of insulin to be taken.
3. After taking two or three supplements, contact your physician or nurse if your blood glucose level has not decreased or if you are having any other problem. If you are unable to keep food down or are vomiting, call your physician or nurse immediately.
4. When you are ill, be sure to drink plenty of fluids—more than you think you need. The type of fluid depends on the blood glucose level. If the glucose is higher than 200 mg/dl, the fluids should be free of sugar. If it is lower than 200 mg/dl, the fluids should contain sugar.
5. Record the supplement in the "supplement" columns of your record sheet so that you do not confuse it with your usual premeal dose.

prochlorperazine (Compazine)] may be kept at home for emergency use. Such medication usually should be taken *only* after telephone consultation with the supervising physician or a member of the diabetes health care team. Patients should also be aware that insulin use must be continued during intercurrent illness, and that they should drink plenty of fluids and try to maintain calorie intake; they should learn the carbohydrate values of soft foods and liquids, particularly those that can be tolerated when they are nauseated. During intercurrent illness, close telephone consultation and frequent blood glucose and urine ketone monitoring are necessary.

Anticipatory insulin supplements are used to prevent expected hyperglycemia outside the target range (e.g., when the patient is about to eat a larger-than-usual meal). We usually start with 1–3 U of insulin as an anticipatory supplement for a typical large meal. For patients who have learned the carbohydrate content of food exchanges, the anticipatory supplement may be proportional to the increment in carbohydrates for that meal. Thus if the usual premeal dose is x units per gram of carbohydrate, the anticipatory supplement may parallel the extra carbohydrates by the same proportion. Again, such supplements should be recorded separately from the basic dose (Fig. 2-10). Anticipatory supplements are often arbitrary and are modified on the basis of experience with similar-size meals. Thus if, for example, a 2-U supplement is used for a given meal, and this creates postprandial hypoglycemia, the next time that size meal is anticipated a 1-U supplement might be used. On the other hand, if in response to that meal postprandial glycemia is higher than desired, the next time a similar-size meal is anticipated, a 3-U supplement might be used.

Compensation for Exercise

During activity that is not part of the patient's usual daily routine, we suggest that he or she eat extra food to provide an energy source for the increased energy expended. Initially, this may be 10–15 g of carbohydrates every 30–45 min during activity. Blood glucose should be monitored before, during, and after exercise to determine the effectiveness of this intervention. Anticipatory insulin decrements should be considered in addition to or (in some cases) instead of the dietary supplements. These too should be recorded separately from the basic dose (Fig. 2-10) and as a negative number, e.g., "−2." (In such an example the basic dose of regular insulin may be 8 U, which together with a "supplement" of −2 results in 6 U of regular insulin being administered.)

Exercise-induced hypoglycemia may be less frequent in patients on CSII therapy than on conventional therapy as it can result from the mobilization of insulin from the subcutaneous depots where is has been injected. With CSII there are no insulin depots. Nevertheless, vigorous exercise may result in a lowering of blood glucose, which can be prevented by decreasing the basal infusion rate or by removing the pump during the exercise. Many patients, however, find it unnecessary to decrease or stop the basal insulin infusion during activity.

The monitoring of blood glucose levels before, during, and after exercise helps the patient on CSII make a sensible decision about how to handle the insulin infusion during unusual activity. All patients should have quick-acting, rapidly absorbable carbohydrate available during activity in case of hypoglycemia. If the infusion is maintained, it may be desirable to compensate for unusual activity with extra energy intake, as discussed above.

Patients should realize that moderately intensive exercise may deplete glycogen stores, resulting in a sustained food requirement to replace the glycogen. As a consequence, hypoglycemia may occur well after exercise (e.g., 12 hr after jogging).

Bookkeeping

It is important to separately record insulin supplements and decrements, e.g., when compensating for a low prevailing level of glycemia or in anticipation of either an unusually small meal or increased exercise (Fig. 2-10). This helps prevent "bookkeeping" errors.

Because patients on intensive insulin programs have frequent variations in insulin doses, bookkeeping is crucial for both guiding dosage selections and providing a record for review by the health care team at the time of the next visit. If the supplement is written down as part of the basic dose, it may be inadvertently incorporated into the basic dosage. Rather, supplements and decrements should be recorded separately and thought of as a temporary change in response to prevailing circumstances. Indeed, as noted earlier, a continuing need for a supplement at a particular time (e.g., before lunch) indicates not that the prelunch basic dose of regular insulin should be increased but, rather, that the prebreakfast basic dose of regular insulin should be increased.

It should be noted that at times a patient may be taking a "combined" compensatory and anticipatory supplement. For example, a patient may be anticipating a larger-than-usual meal but also find that the premeal blood glucose level exceeds the target range.

The patient's record is an important tool in guiding daily decisions based on previous experience. In this regard, the "comments" column of the record book is crucial in documenting reasons for particular actions.

The patient's record becomes the focal point of interactions with the physician and health care team. We spend the bulk of our time during office visits reviewing the patient's record, trying to understand the rationale for actions taken, or why actions were not taken despite indications for them (e.g., five consecutive days of prelunch hyperglycemia without supplementation and without a consequent adjustment in prebreakfast regular insulin). Appropriate actions are reinforced by commendation. Inaction or inappropriate actions are discussed in detail. The focus of the discussion is thus how to best use information to take action. In our view, persistent hyperglycemia is not viewed as bad and in need of punishment but as an indicator that different actions need to be taken.

It must be emphasized too that although our algorithms deal with changes in insulin dosage actions to be taken also include changes in food intake and in timing of insulin administration. These are particularly important if there is postprandial hyperglycemia that is restored to the acceptable range prior to the next meal. Insulin should be administered at least 20–30 min and perhaps as long as 45 min before a meal. (The interval might be shortened if premeal blood glucose is *below* the target range or lengthened if premeal blood glucose is much *above* the target range.) Likewise, the site of injection might be altered to avoid exercise-related increases in insulin absorption or to try to create greater day-to-day reproducibility in insulin absorption. Also, a sporadic pattern of glycemia in response to a constant food intake and insulin dosage might indicate variability in absorption from injection sites. For this reason, we recommend rotation of injection sites *within* a given region for each daily injection (e.g., prebreakfast injections in the abdomen, presupper injections in the buttocks) rather than between regions, as is a common practice.

With practice, educated patients learn to appropriately maniuplate an array of variables—food intake, activity, insulin dosage, timing of injections, site of injections—guided by their self-monitored blood glucose and their daily records.

Adapting Algorithms for Special Circumstances

Appropriate algorithms should be designed for each patient's particular circumstances. For example, during pregnancy meticulous glycemic control must be maintained to reduce the risks of fetal morbidity and mortality. Such control is attainable with intensive therapy. The algorthms for pregnant patients are modified so that ideal and target blood glucose levels are identical, and dose increments are generally made at shorter intervals than in nonpregnant patients. Fasting urinary ketones are also carefully monitored to avoid starvation ketosis.

For patients who have difficulty recognizing symptoms of hypoglycemia or who have counterregulatory insufficiency, blood glucose targets should be adjusted upward to lessen the risk of hypoglycemia. A variety of other circumstances may require a change in the target glucose values and appropriate modification of the algorithms.

PATIENT EDUCATION AND MOTIVATION

Patient education and motivation are crucial to the success of any program of intensive therapy of IDDM. Obviously, the most important educational component is that of learning to effectively utilize the algorithms in attainment of the defined glucose targets. Successful implementation of an intensive treatment program requires that the patient pay careful attention to meal planning, activity, and the monitoring of balance between these. To accomplish this, patients should have an overall understanding of their disease and its management. It is our opinion that patient education should be formalized and have defined objectives, e.g., those listed in Table 2-13. The patient's family should be included in the educational program. In particular,

Table 2-13. Objectives of Patient Education

1. *Attitudes:* The patient should:
   a. Appreciate that diabetes is a permanent condition that can be controlled but not cured.
   b. Recognize that self-care is essential to diabetes management and must be routine, although professional support is available whenever needed
   c. Understand that although a few restrictions in life style may be necessary he or she can do almost anything a nondiabetic person can do.
2. *Knowledge:* The patient should be able to:
   a. Discuss the normal relationship between blood glucose and circulating insulin and the absence of circulating insulin response in diabetes
   b. Describe the relationship between the primary factors controlling blood glucose (i.e., food intake, energy expenditure, and insulin)
   c. Discuss the rationale—reducing symptoms and lessening the risk of complications—for careful control of blood glucose
   d. State the goals of therapy (target blood glucose levels) and discuss the importance of routine self-monitoring of blood glucose in attaining and maintaining those goals
   e. Discuss the use of glycosylated hemoglobin as an indicator of glucose control
   f. Describe several possible multiple-component insulin regimens, including the relative advantages and disadvantages of each
   g. Discuss the indications for alterations in insulin dosage
   h. Describe the factors that may predispose a patient to hypoglycemia, how to prevent it, and how to recognize and treat it
   i. Describe the factors that may lead to hyperglycemia and impending ketoacidosis and how to intervene to correct these
   j. Describe the effects of physical illness and emotional stress on blood glucose levels
3. *Self-care:* The patient should be able to demonstrate the following skills and techniques:
   a. Insulin-dose measurements and injection technique
   b. Pump use, including catheter application and needle insertion
   c. Dietary selection and estimation of the calorie or carbohydrate content of meals
   d. Blood glucose monitoring
   e. Urine glucose and ketone monitoring
   f. Recognition and treatment of hypoglycemia
   g. Adjustment of insulin dosage
   h. Use of insulin supplements
   i. Alteration of regimen to accommodate exercise
4. *Responsible others:* The patient's family, friends, or colleagues should be able to recognize hypoglycemia and demonstrate the use of concentrated glucose in the buccal mucosa and the administration of glucagon.

family members should learn how to administer glucagon to treat hypoglycemia. We have also found it helpful to have family members simulate living with diabetes (including taking saline "insulin" injections, blood and urine testing, following a meal plan, etc.). Through simulation, family members gain insights into the disease and the burdens of living with it that generally are not otherwise attained.

Patient motivation is probably the limiting factor in the institution of programs of intensive insulin therapy. Clearly, it is essential to success. We have found that motivation may be enhanced by periodic group meetings of patients. Nevertheless, increasing patient motivation remains a challenge for clinicians.

DOCUMENTATION OF CONTROL—GLYCOSYLATED HEMOGLOBIN

Over the past decade, the measurement of glycosylated hemoglobin has emerged as an important clinical tool useful for assessing average glycemic control over several weeks. Glycosylated hemoglobin is formed by the process of nonenzymatic glycosylation. Nonenzymatic glycosylation of proteins occurs at both N-terminal amino groups and at epsilon amino groups of intrachain amino acids (e.g., lysine). It involves the addition of glucose to protein by a slow continuous reaction that is a function of the duration of contact between the reactants and the integrated glucose concentration during the time of contact. The reaction scheme is depicted in Figure 2-11. The first product is an aldimine (or Schiff base), which then undergoes an internal rearrangement of the double bond (an Amadori rearrangement) to form a ketoamine. The latter reaction is essentially irreversible. Thus although the reaction occurs slowly, the ketoamine is a stable product and reflects integrated glycemic control dur-

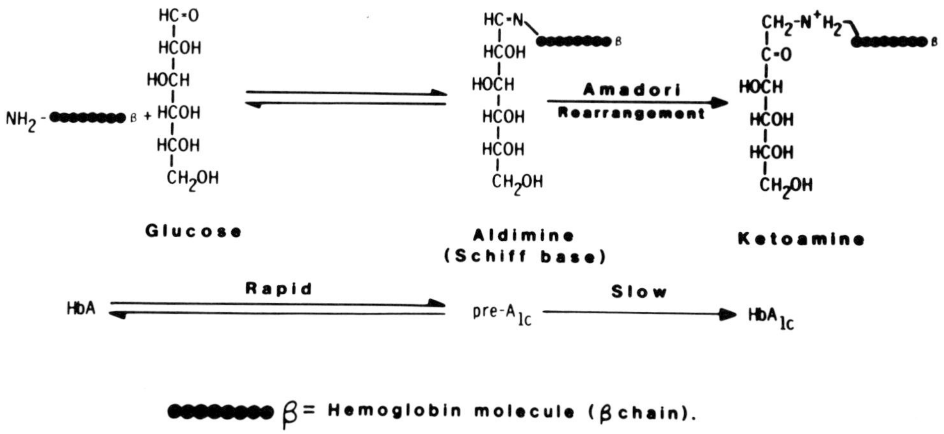

Fig. 2-11 The process of nonenzymatic glycosylation of hemoglobin at the terminal amino group of the hemoglobin beta chain.

ing the life span of the hemoglobin molecule. In contrast, the formation of the aldimine is both relatively rapid and reversible.

The most abundant glycosylated hemoglobin is HbA_{1c}, which is the ketoamine formed by the addition of glucose to the terminal valine groups on the beta chains of hemoglobin HbA. This is also known as "stable HbA_{1c}," whereas "total HbA_{1c}" includes both the stable ketoamine and the labile aldimine, also known as "pre-A_{1c}." Other minor glycosylated hemoglobins include HbA_{1a1}, HbA_{1a2}, and HbA_{1b}, which are formed by the addition of sugar phosphates to the terminal valine of the beta chains of HbA or by a further modification of HbA_{1c}. Collectively, these components involving modification of the terminal valine of the beta chain, have been referred to as HbA_1 which is ($HbA_{1a1+a2+b+c}$). (This too may be stable HbA_1 or total HbA_1 depending on whether the labile pre-A_{1c} has been removed.) In addition, as noted, there are non-HbA_1 glycosylated hemoglobins (HbA-Glc) formed by the addition of glucose either to the N-terminus of alpha chains or to epsilon amino groups on lysine residues. These latter glycosylated components can be measured in chemical assays but not in cation-exchange chromatographic or electrophoretic methods.

Methodologic Considerations

A number of assays have been developed to measure glycosylated hemoglobin. Each has advantages and disadvantages, and each measures different glycosylated hemoglobin components. The most commonly used assays have been chromatographic, based on cation-exchange chromatography in which the negatively charged glycosylated hemoglobins HbA_{1a1}, HbA_{1a2}, HbA_{1b}, and HbA_{1c} elute faster than the predominant HbA. These include: (1) the precise, inexpensive, but time-consuming "macro" column method by which HbA_{1c} can be quantitated; (2) the rapid, inexpensive, but somewhat less precise commercial "mini" column method, which measures HbA_1; and (3) the rapid, highly reproducible but expensive high performance liquid chromatography (HPLC) method, which measures HbA_{1c}. For accurate determinations in all of these methods, the labile pre-A_{1c} fraction should be removed by appropriate sample preparations. This involves incubation of intact erythrocytes in 0.9 percent saline at 37°C for 5 hr. Failure to exclude labile pre-A_{1c} leads to imprecise assessment of glycemic control because the amount of pre-A_{1c} is proportional to the blood glucose at the time of blood sampling.

The chromatographic methods are influenced by a number of circumstances. For example, carbamylated hemoglobin (formed in uremia) and HbA_A (formed by acetaldehyde addition to hemoglobin in alcoholics) coelute with HbA_{1a+b}, whereas fetal hemoglobin (HbF: elevated in pregnancy, thalassemia, and certain hemoglobinopathies) coelutes with HbA_{1c}. These have the potential for creating falsely elevated glycosylated hemoglobin determinations. In contrast, slowly migrating hemoglobins [e.g., sickle hemoglobin (HbS) and HbC], although also glycosylated, cannot be measured by the chromatographic techniques, thus leading to falsely low glycosylated hemoglobin determinations.

Accuracy of the chromatographic methods depend on precise temperature control (± 1°C), pH control (± 0.1 pH units), appropriate sample collection and storage, rapid formation of hemolysate before storage, and careful sample preparation (to remove labile pre-A_{1c}).

Chemically based methods include calorimetric techniques, a fluorometric technique, and affinity chromatography. All of these are specific for the stable ketoamine linkage and do not measure the labile aldimines. They measure total glycosylated hemoglobin, including the glyco moieties at the epsilon amino groups and those at the amino termini of both alpha and beta chains. Colorimetric methods involve the formation of 5-hydroxymethylfurfural (5-HMF) by addition of weak acid to ketoamine linkages and their detection by addition of a color reagent, usually thiobarbituric acid (TBA), with the optical density of the adduct then measured. Because aldimines are not measured, no sample preparation is necessary. The method is relatively inexpensive and has high precision if care is taken with reagent preparation and standardization. The assay time is relatively long, although some modifications have reduced the time from 6 hr to 2 hr. It is most crucial to carefully wash erythrocytes to remove plasma glucose before preparing the hemolysates, as free sugar reacts with TBA.

The fluorometric technique is based on the periodate oxidation of ketoamine groups, which forms formaldehyde. This is measured as the fluorescent 3,5-diacetyl-1,4-dishydrolutidine formed from the condensation of formaldehyde with acetylacetone and ammonia. This is considered an efficient means of determining the true number of total glyco groups. The same general principles apply to the fluorometric technique as to the colorimetric method.

The affinity chromatographic method is based on the interaction of ketoamine groups with a boronate affinity gel (phenylboronic acid immobilized on agarose). The affinity resin reversibly binds *cis*-diol groups of ketoamines, and nonglycosylated hemoglobin is readily eluted from the column. The glycosylated hemoglobins are then eluted with a second buffer, which reverses the binding. Like the colorimetric and fluorometric techniques, the affinity chromatographic method is not influenced by the labile pre-A_{1c} fraction or by other hemoglobins. An advantage over the colorimetric method is that the affinity chromatography method, like ion-exchange chromatography, involves measurement of hemoglobin rather than of a chemically formed product. Careful washing to remove plasma glucose is thus unnecessary.

Electrophoretic methods include isoelectric focusing on polyacrylamide slab gels (a method requiring technical skill and an accurate densitometer) and agar gel electrophoresis (which gives wide separation of hemoglobin components). These methods are quite precise but not widely used.

A radioimmunoassay specific for measurement of HbA_{1c} has also been developed but has had only limited use.

All of the methods should be carefully standardized with appropriate quality control. Clinicians should be familiar with the method used by their local laboratory and its pitfalls. All of the methods show excellent correlation with each other. The absolute numbers obtained by one or another method or between laboratories cannot be directly compared, however.

Clinical Utility

Glycosylated hemoglobin values reflect integrated glycemic control during the life span of the hemoglobin molecule. The correlations are strongest for glycemic control 4–8 weeks before glycosylated hemoglobin determination. Values seem to be more sensitive to deterioration in control than improvement in control, presumably because of the irreversibility of the Amadori rearrangement forming the ketoamine. Measurement of the ketoamine component of glycosylated hemoglobin provides an accurate assessment of the mean level of glycemia over a period of several weeks utilizing a single sample and is only minimally influenced by acute changes in glycemic control.

We utilize glycosylated hemoglobin measurements to document glycemic control and confirm that the patient's blood glucose record is an accurate reflection of events. To this end we determine glycosylated hemoglobin every 1–2 months during stabilization to document progress and approximately every 2–4 months when glycemia seems stable. Our target is normalization or near-mormalization of glycosylated hemoglobin, or the lowest value attainable without inducing an unacceptable frequency of hypoglycemia. Generally, it is possible to achieve levels within 115 percent of the upper limit of normal of the chromatographic methods during a program of intensive therapy of IDDM.

Discrepancies between glycosylated hemoglobin determinations and patient reports of blood glucose measurements indicate a need to review the management program. The patient may not be accurately measuring blood glucose, may be infrequently measuring blood glucose and thus missing wide fluctuations, or may be providing fraudulent results. There are a number of psychological reasons for the latter which we and our colleagues have identified (Table 2-14). These can be sought in a sensitive interview and an action plan developed to deal with them.

Table 2-14. Underlying Mechanisms Responsible for Discrepant Results

Underlying Mechanism	Example: Feeling	Example: Behavioral Response
Seeking perfection	I want to be 100% okay.	Therefore: I put records down 100% okay.
Seeking approval	I want you to be pleased, proud.	Therefore: I give you records that make you pleased, proud.
Seeking independence	I want to be in charge.	Therefore: I give you records that show what I want you to see.
Avoidance of punishment	I don't want you to punish me.	Therefore: I give you records so that you think I don't deserve punishment.
Avoidance of confrontation (criticism)	I don't want you to question or accuse me.	Therefore: I give you records that encourage you to leave me alone.
Avoidance of judgment	I don't want to hear if I'm good or bad.	Therefore: I give you records that you won't have to comment about.
Avoidance of depression	I don't want to pay attention to diabetes and feel sad.	Therefore: I won't test so that I won't have to face sadness.
Expression of denial	I don't have diabetes.	Therefore: I need not test.
Expression of resentment or anger	I hate diabetes, *or* I hate how you make me deal with diabetes.	Therefore: I won't do what you ask me to do.
Expression of guilt	I cheated.	Therefore: I'll hide it.

SELECTION OF PATIENTS FOR INTENSIVE THERAPY

The ideal candidate for an intensive therapeutic program is the patient with IDDM who is otherwise healthy and does not yet have signs of diabetic complications, as there is no evidence for reversibility of complications. It is hoped that metabolic normalization will lessen the frequency and severity of complications or delay their onset, as discussed in the previous chapter. Thus if this proves to be the case, there is a "window of opportunity" between the onset of hyperglycemia and the onset of complications (which usually do not appear before 10 years' duration of diabetes in young people) during which intervention is most likely to be of benefit (Fig. 2-12).

Other criteria which we consider when assessing patients for possible implementation of a program of intensive therapy are summarized in Table 2-15. Patient motivation is crucial and perhaps the determining factor in treatment success or failure.

A preliminary program of counseling, education, and training may be desirable. Because success in achieving near-normalization of glycemia depends on daily self-monitoring of blood glucose and careful adherence to diet, it may be desirable to have most patients begin an intensive therapeutic program with multiple daily injections rather than an infusion device so that they do not attribute their success solely to the device and ignore other important aspects of therapy.

Some authors have recommended psychological screening of patients to ensure that there is no preexisting psychopathology. There should at least be ongoing surveillance to ensure that the patient is able to measure blood glucose levels accurately and adjust insulin doses reliably.

The major risk of intensive therapy of IDDM is unrecognized severe hypogly-

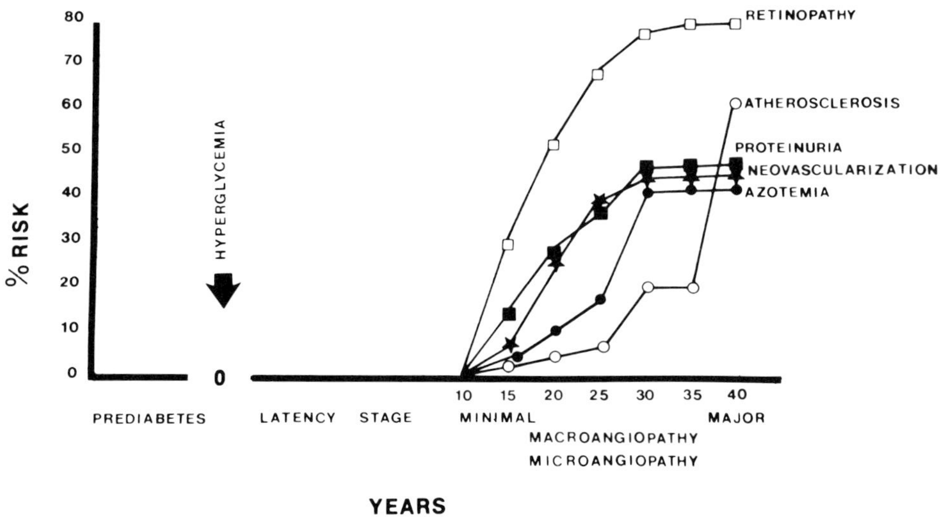

Fig. 2-12 Natural history of type I diabetes and its complications based on epidemiological data. The latency period (in terms of complications) represents the "window of opportunity" for intervention with intensive therapy.

Table 2-15. Criteria for Selection: Intensive Therapy

1. Suboptimal control with conventional therapy
2. Able and willing to use blood glucose self-monitoring
3. Trained and skilled medical staff available to direct treatment and provide increased attention
4. Sufficient education and technical ability to follow a program of intensive therapy
5. Motivation and psychosocial stability adequate to manage intensive therapy

cemia. Hypoglycemia poses a particular danger to patients with coronary or cerebral vascular disease, for whom improved glycemic control is likely to offer little long-term benefit. Thus the presence of coronary or cerebral vascular disease is a contraindication to intensive therapy with a goal of near-normalization of glycemia. Other contraindications include a number of conditions associated with a greater predisposition to hypoglycemia: adrenal or pituitary insufficiency, end-stage liver or kidney disease, autonomic neuropathy, and established or suspected counterregulatory insufficiency. Patients being treated with adrenergic blocking drugs may also be unsuitable.

If a patient manifests recurrent or severe hypoglycemia, the target levels of glycemia should be adjusted to avoid danger.

Health Team Requirements

An American Diabetes Association policy statement concerning infusion devices, in our view, is applicable to all intensive therapy of IDDM:

> The outpatient use of portable insulin infusion devices should be prescribed and managed by diabetologists who are trained and skilled in their use. Initiation of treatment should be in a setting where a trained staff can develop an overall treatment regimen for the patients and provide intense patient education. It is to be emphasized that success of this type of program ultimately depends on cooperation of the patient. Use of continuous insulin delivery in no way allows for discarding diet or the daily scheduling of events necessary for total diabetic management. Before starting treatment the patient must be made aware of the additional demands that will be placed on him/her if satisfactory lowering of blood glucose is to be achieved, as well as the additional expense compared with conventional therapy. The responsible physician must be able to provide 24-hour telephone communication service and emergency room facilities.

Each part of this statement is important. Physicians prescribing intensive therapy should be well versed in diabetes and in the details of such management. Physicians may need specialized advanced training, including practical experience with devices, to master the requisite skills. Such skills are best honed by continuing attention to a group of IDDM patients being treated intensively. The isolated use of one or two pumps by an inexperienced physician may be dangerous.

The trained staff should include a diabetes educator, nurse-clinician, or physician's assistant, as well as a dietitian; access to a psychological support system is desirable. Physicians and staff involved in diabetes management should recognize that it requires an unusual amount of their time and resources, including a great deal of telephone contact.

In many treatment centers, patient group meetings seem to contribute to patient morale and facilitate compliance with the intensive therapy program. Involvement of a patient's family members has also been found helpful.

EMERGING FORMS OF THERAPY: THEIR CLINICAL USE

Mechanical Devices

The delivery of insulin by mechanical infusion pump, as described above, without an automated modulating feedback signal (e.g., continuous glucose measurement) has been referred to as "open-loop" insulin delivery. In contrast, "closed-loop" insulin delivery involves glucose-sensor-controlled automated insulin delivery. The latter devices have been labeled "artificial endocrine pancreas."

A number of investigators have fabricated closed-loop systems, and one is commercially available, the Biostator GCIIS, manufactured by the Life Sciences Instruments Division of Miles Laboratories. This device, which sells for over $50,000, is the size of a large television set on a rolling cart. Its use entails tethering the patient to the device via at least two intravenous lines. The fragility of the sampling line is such that it rarely remains patent more than 24–48 hr. An operator must be continually available to calibrate and control the device. Although of potential clinical utility for the control of diabetes during ketoacidosis, labor and delivery, or surgical procedures, or to establish insulin requirements, the practicality of the Biostator GCIIS is such that its use is largely confined to specific research protocols.

In theory, it should be possible to develop a miniaturized implantable closed-loop insulin delivery system. The limiting factor in the technological development of such systems has been the absence of an appropriate glucose sensor. Recently, however, progress has been made toward the development of a miniaturized potentially implantable glucose sensor. Such sensors, coupled with either external or implanted insulin delivery systems, will likely come to clinical testing within the next 2–3 years.

Open-loop insulin delivery systems currently exist in both external and implantable forms. These provide insulin delivery by a variety of routes: subcutaneous, intravenous, and intraperitoneal. Many investigators testing implantable systems have favored the peritoneal route, as a portion of the insulin seems to be absorbed via the hepatic portal circulation. Although implantable systems, controlled via telemetry, have been tested in experimental animals and human beings, two technical problems remain. These are: (1) finding an appropriate "pump" insulin that does not aggregate in the pump reservoir (where it is at 37°C), particularly because such aggregated insulin may result in amyloidosis in experimental animals; and (2) verifying that the pump reservoir cannot leak, potentially leading to profound hypoglycemia. The latter problem is being solved by titanium-encased reservoirs that are virtually leakproof ot that are maintained at negative pressure so that in the event of damage tissue fluid leaks in, rather than insulin leaking out. A number of "pump" insulins are currently being tested, and that problem should also be solved. Our personal bias is that implantable pumps will become a mainstay in the management of IDDM during the course of the next decade.

External open-loop insulin pumps are undergoing rapid evolution and miniaturization. External pumps are now smaller than a package of cigarettes and are fully programmable for maximum flexibility in design of an appropriate insulin delivery profile. Such pumps are more palatable and less cumbersome to patients than previously available versions. However, open-loop systems are not a panacea to diabetes control, and comparable results can be obtained in many patients with intensified multiple-injection therapy. Thus the limiting factor in the use of these systems is patient acceptability.

Pancreatic Transplantation

Transplantation of pancreatic islet tissue, either as isolated islets or pancreatic segments, has successfully reversed experimentally induced diabetes in animals and has prevented and reversed early diabetic microvascular complications involving the eyes and kidneys or recipient animals. As of 31 December 1983, the world experience with pancreas transplantation has included at least 404 transplants in 380 patients, of which at least 37 were from living related donors. As of that date, only 14 percent were functioning, and only 8 percent had been functioning for 12 months or more. The largest experience has been at the University of Minnesota where the current (since 1 July 1977) series has included 86 segmental transplants in 75 patients. Of these, there have been 10 deaths (13 percent of patients), 22 technical failures (26 percent of grafts), and 30 nontechnical (? rejection) failures (35 percent of grafts). There are 24 functioning grafts (26 percent of grafts), of which 13 have functioned for 12 months or more, the longest nearly 6 years. These patients seem to be ameliorated of diabetes. Interestingly, in the Minnesota series the frequency of functioning grafts is much greater in patients receiving grafts from living related donors (43 percent) than from cadaver donors (18 percent).

In addition, there have been a number of islet allotransplant procedures attempted in diabetic patients, almost all of which have failed. (Of four alleged successes, insufficient details have been reported to permit critical analysis.) Morbidity and mortality have been minimal. In addition, there have been over 100 autotransplants following pancreatectomy. Of these, 40–50 percent of patients have remained free of the need for insulin therapy. However, the completeness of pancreatectomy may be questioned in some of these cases. Also, fatalities have been reported in recipients of intraportal autografts.

Thus it is evident that pancreatic transplantation is a highly experimental procedure. In addition to the obvious problems of technical difficulties and rejection, other problems include tissue acquisition and tissue preservation. Moreover, the possibility exists that there may be recurrence of diabetes in the graft. (This has occurred in at least three instances in which a graft was received from an identical twin and no immunosuppressive therapy was used.)

Nevertheless, all of these problems appear solvable. Current emphasis has favored the development of islet transplantation. Progress has been made in a number of areas. One of the major problems in islet transplantation has been the relatively low yields obtained in islet isolation procedures from adult pancreases. (In rodents, this does not represent a major obstacle, since one can obtain sufficient islets to reverse diabetes by using islets from several donors for each recipient). Recently, newer techniques for islet isolation have markedly improved the yields such that sufficient islets may be obtained from a single canine pancreas to reverse diabetes in that species. The same methods have been used to obtain similar yields from human pancreases, but human implantation studies have not yet been undertaken. Thus, it remains to be established whether islet cell isolation and preservation procedures will be suitable for human studies. Moreover, the source of donor tissue (fetal versus adult, allografts versus xenografts) remains an area where more investigation is needed.

Another problem has been the purity of islet preparations. Preparations containing acinar tissue, and the proteolytic enzymes contained therein, have resulted in such problems as disseminated intravascular coagulation and systemic hypotension. Current purification strategies thus are designed to eliminate acinar tissue.

One potential prospect of islet implantation is that of immunomodulation of donor tissue. Thus, it might be possible to eliminate from the donor tissue those signals mediating the rejection response. This primarily involves the Ia or class II antigens, which are a crucial signal in the sequence of events that accompany graft rejection. Thus, strategies include modifying or eliminating Ia antigen bearing cells, or depleting the donor preparation of such Ia antigens. The latter approach is feasible because it appears that Ia antigen is not expressed on pancreatic islet beta cells, but rather on a number of other cell types in pancreatic tissue, including vascular endothelium, passenger leucocytes, and dendritic cells. A number of laboratories have been pursuing various experimental approaches that are designed to implement one or another of these strategies to alter islet immunogenicity.

In addition, in an attempt to lessen rejection studies will address a multitude of other questions. One such issue is improved tissue typing and immune monitoring. Another is the development of newer modalities to prevent both rejection and reactivation of the autoimmune immunodestructive processes that initially created type I diabetes. This includes the use of various immunosuppressive agents, both nonspecific and potentially specific immunosuppressive strategies targeted for pancreatic islet tissues. Also in need of study are the techniques to be used for islet implantation, including the site of such implantation. Finally, to be answered is the ultimate question of whether the use of any pancreatic transplantation procedure will influence the rate of progression and/or the extent of microvascular or neurological complications of diabetes.

Over the next decade it is likely that further progress in these areas will result in the clinical application of pancreatic transplantation at least in a selected subset of diabetic patients. In the interim, carefully designed clinical research protocols will continue to answer the remaining questions.

Human Insulin

Until recently most commercial insulin preparations have been derived from bovine and porcine pancreas. There are known differences in amino acid sequence between these animal insulins and human insulin (Table 2-16). These differences in primary structure, as well as impurities in commercial insulin preparations, have been held responsible for the appearance of antiinsulin antibodies in patients treated with insulin. The immunogenicity of commercial insulin also may lead to local or systemic insulin allergy, immunological insulin resistence (IIR), and lipoatrophy at injection sites. The use of insulin of homologous sequence to native human insulin might be expected to obviate some of the immunogenicity of commercial preparations.

Human insulin, i.e., insulin homologous in sequence to native insulin produced by human beings, can be prepared in four ways. One potential source is extraction from pancreases of human cadavers. Although some insulin has been produced in this manner, there are two problems: obtaining human pancreases and postmortem autodigestion by enzymes derived from the exocrine pancreas. Although the latter problem could be resolved by obtaining pancreases from "heart-beating" cadavers (i.e., individuals who have sustained brain death but are maintained on life-support systems), the numbers of such pancreases are limited and would best be directed to basic research or for potential use in transplantation.

A second potential source is by full chemical synthesis, as insulin is a relatively small protein. Although some insulin has been produced in this manner, the yield is relatively low owing to the production of a number of error peptides. As a consequence, this is a very expensive process not suitable for widescale clinical application.

A third source is the enzymatic conversion of porcine insulin to human insulin. Porcine insulin differs from human insulin only by a single amino acid difference at the carboxy terminal of the beta chain. Therefore, it has been possible to develop enzymatic methods that remove the alanine residue at that position in porcine insulin and replace it with a threonine residue, with a resultant semisynthetic human insulin. This method is suitable for commercial preparation and is being used for such by several manufacturers.

A fourth source is the production of human insulin by recombinant DNA technology. In fact, human insulin of recombinant DNA origin is the first product of this technology to come to potential usefulness. Production of human insulin in this manner ensures unlimited insulin availability in the future, thus obviating any potential shortages of insulin, which have been projected for the future.

The commercially available human insulins (those produced by enzymatic conversion of porcine insulin and by recombinant DNA technology) have been found to

Table 2-16. Differences in the Amino Acid Structure of Insulin Species

Species	A-chain A 8	A-chain A 10	B-chain B 30
Bovine	Alanine	Valine	Alanine
Porcine	Threonine	Isoleucine	Alanine
Human	Threonine	Isoleucine	Threonine

be chemically, physically, immunologically, and biologically equivalent to pancreatic human insulin.

Some formulations of intermediate and long-acting human insulins seem to have a more rapid onset and shorter duration of action than their animal insulin counterparts. This sometimes has an impact on the design of intensive therapy regimens. For example, human insulin may be less effective than animal insulin in the split-and-mixed program in which intermediate-acting insulin is given before supper. Given at that time, it may not last through the night. With these exceptions, human insulin may be used in the same way as animal insulins.

In theory, human insulin might be expected to be less immunogenic than beef or pork insulin. Although this has proved to be the case, human insulin is not non-immunogenic. On the other hand, antiinsulin antibody levels seem to decrease when patients are transferred from animal insulins to human insulin. Studies of patients with immunological complications of insulin therapy (immunological insulin resistance, insulin allergy, lipoatrophy) are too few to permit a conclusion as to the efficacy of human insulin in these circumstances. On a theoretical basis, these patients might be considered particularly desirable candidates for therapy with human insulin.

In comparison with purified pork insulin, human insulin may offer no unique advantages. On the other hand, in comparison with beef insulin or mixed beef-pork insulin, human insulin is less immunogenic and less antigenic in that levels of pre-formed antiinsulin antibodies decrease on transfer to human insulin.

Because of their favorable immunogenicity, human insulin or purified pork insulin seem preferable to beef insulin or mixed beef-pork insulin in patients being exposed to insulin for the first time or in whom insulin use is anticipated to be temporary (e.g., type II patients undergoing surgery or those with gestational diabetes).

There are no obvious circumstances in which human insulin seems to be contraindicated. On the other hand, there are no clear indications for switching patients with established diabetes to human insulin, except in the presence of immunological complications of insulin therapy, as noted above.

SUMMARY

We have attempted to provide details of our approach to implementation of a program of intensive insulin therapy of type I diabetes. Although not for all patients with type I diabetes, this approach permits improved glycemic control in patients willing and able to embark on this course of therapy. The results are quite gratifying. We trust that the reader too will find that to be the case.

ACKNOWLEDGMENTS

This work was supported by funds from the Diabetes Research Institute Foundation, Miami, Florida, and by the University of Miami/Southeastern Florida Regional Diabetes Program, funded by the Health Program Office, Department of Health and Rehabilitative Services, State of Florida.

BIBLIOGRAPHY

This bibliography includes general references for each section, and focuses largely on review articles. It is by no means comprehensive.

General

Schade DS, Santiago JV, Skyler JS, Rizza R: Intensive Insulin Therapy. Excerpta Medica, Princeton, NJ, 1983

Insulin Secretion and the Design of Insulin Regimens

Berger M, Cuppers HJ, Hegner H, et al: Absorption kinetics and biologic effects of subcutaneously injected insulin preparations. Diabetes Care 5:77, 1982

Binder C: Absorption of injected insulin: a clinical-pharmacological study. Acta Pharmacol Toxicol 27:[Suppl. 2] 1, 1969

Clarke W, Haymond MW, Santiago J: Overnight basal insulin requirements in fasting insulin-dependent diabetics. Diabetics 29:78, 1980

Danowski TS, Sunder JH: Jet injection of insulin during self-monitoring of blood glucose. Diabetes Care 1:27, 1978

Eaton RP, Allen RC, Schade DS, Standefer JC: Normal insulin secretion: the goal of artificial insulin delivery systems? Diabetes Care 3:270, 1980

Galloway JA, Spradlin CT, Nelson RL, et al: Factors influencing the absorption, serum insulin concentration, and blood glucose responses after injections of regular insulin and various insulin mixtures. Diabetes Care 4:366, 1981

Holman RR, Turner RC, Diabetes: The quest for basal normoglycemia. Lancet 1:469, 1977

Kitabchi AE, Fisher JN, Matteri R, Murphy MB: The use of continuous insulin delivery systems in treatment of diabetes mellitus. Adv Intern Med 28:449, 1983

Philips M, Simpson RW, Holman RR, Turner RC: A simple and rational twice daily insulin regime: distinction between basal and meal insulin requirements. Q J Med 48:493, 1979

Reeves ML, Seigler DE, Ryan EA, Skyler JS: Glycemic control in insulin-dependent diabetes mellitus: compariosn of outpatient intensified conventional therapy with continuous subcutaneous insulin infusion. Am J Med 72:673, 1982

Rizza RA, Gerich JE, Haymond MW, et al: Control of blood sugar in insulin-dependent diabetes: comparisons of an artificial endocrine pancreas, continuous subcutaneous insulin infusion, and intensified conventional insulin therapy. N Engl J Med 303:1313, 1980

Schiffrin A, Belmonte MM: Comparison between continuous subcutaneous insulin infusion and multiple injections of insulin: a one year prospective study. Diabetes 31:255, 1982

Schmidt MI, Nadji-Georgopoulos A, Rendell M, et al: The dawn phenomenon, an early morning glucose rise: implications for diabetic instability. Diabetes Care 4:579, 1981

Skyler JS: Type I diabetes: regimens, targets and caveats. Diabetes Care 5:547, 1982

Skyler JS, Reeves ML, Seigler DE: Intensive Insulin Therapy. In Sakamoto N, Hotta N (ed): Proceedings of the Second Japan-Korea Symposium on Diabetes Mellitus. International Congress Series. Excerpta Medica, Amsterdam, 1984 (in press)

Skyler JS, Seigler DE, Reeves M,: A compariosn of insulin regimens in insulin-dependent diabetes mellitus. Diabetes Care 5:suppl. 1, 11, 1982

Initial Insulin Doses and Distribution

Jovanovic L, Peterson CM: Optimal insulin delivery for the pregnant diabetic patient. Diabetes Care 5:suppl. 1, 24, 1982

Schiffrin A: Treatment of insulin-dependent diabetes with multiple subcutaneous insulin injections. Med Clin North Am 66:1251, 1982

Skyler JS, Seigler DE, Reeves ML: Optimizing pumped insulin delivery. Diabetes Care 5:135, 1982

Skyler JS, Skyler DL, Seigler DE, O'Sullivan MJ: Algorithms for adjustment of insulin dosage by patients who monitor blood glucose. Diabetes Care 4:311, 1981

Food Intake and Activity Planning

American Diabetes Association Special Report: Principles of nutrition and dietary recommendations for individuals with diabetes mellitus. Diabetes 28:1027, 1979; and Diabetes Care 2:520, 1979

Richter E, Ruderman N, Schneider S: Diabetes and exercise. Am J Med 70:201, 1981

Skyler JS: Diabetes and exercise: clinical implications. Diabetes Care 2:307, 1979

Skyler, JS: Dietary management of diabetes mellitus. In: Peterson CM (ed): Diabetes Management in the 80's: The Role of Home Blood Glucose Monitoring and New Insulin Delivery Systems. pp. 126–151. Praeger Scientific, New York, 1982

Skyler JS: Dietary planning in insulin dependent diabetes mellitus. Pediatr Ann 12:652, 1983

Skyler JS: Nutritional management of diabetes mellitus. In: Katzen HM, Mahler RJ (eds): Advances in Modern Nutrition. Vol. 2, pp. 645–698. Hemisphere Publishing, Washington DC, 1978

Vranic M, Berger M: Exercise and diabetes mellitus. Diabetes 28:147, 1979

Self-Monitoring of Blood Glucose

American Diabetes Association: Policy statement: indications for use of continuous insulin delivery systems and self-measurement of blood glucose. Diabetes Care. 5:140, 1982

Peacock I, Tattersall R: Methods of self-monitoring of diabetic control. Clin Endocrinol Metab 11:485, 1982

Schiffrin A, Belmonte M: Multiple daily self-glucose monitoring: its essential role in long-term glucose control in insulin-dependent diabetic patients treated with pump and multiple subcutaneous injections. Diabetes Care 5:479, 1982

Skyler JS: Patient self-monitoring of blood glucose. Clin Diabetes 1:4:12, 1983

Skyler JS: Patient self-monitoring of blood glucose. Med Clin North Am 66:1227, 1982

Tattersall RB: Home blood glucose monitoring. Diabetologia 16:71, 1979

Tattersall RB, Gale E: Patient self-monitoring of blood glucose and refinements of conventional insulin treatment. Am J Med 70:177, 1981

Attainment of Excellent Glucose Control

Jovanovic L, Peterson CM: Optimal insulin delivery for the pregnant diabetic patient. Diabetes Care, 5:suppl. 1, 24, 1982

Schiffrin A: Treatment of insulin-dependent diabetes with multiple subcutaneous insulin injections. Med Clin North Am 66:1251, 1982

Schiffrin A, Belmonte MM: Compariosn between continuous subcutaneous insulin infusion and multiple injections of insulin: a one year prospective study. Diabetes 31:255, 1982

Skyler JS, Seigler DE, Reeves ML: Optimizing pumped insulin delivery. Diabetes Care 5:135, 1982

Skyler JS, Skyler DL, Seigler DE, O'Sullivan MJ: Algorithms for adjustment of insulin dosage by patients who monitor blood glucose. Diabetes Care 4:311, 1981

Patient Education and Motivation

Citrin WS, Kleiman GA, Skyler JS: Emotions: a critical factor in diabetic control. In Davidson MB (ed): Diabetes Mellitus: Diagnosis and Treatment. pp. 400–419. Wiley, New York, 1981

Citrin WS, Zigo MA, LaGreca AM, Skyler JS: Diabetes in adolescence: effects of multi-family group therapy and parent simulation of diabetes. Diabetes, 31:suppl. 2, 13A, 1982

Citrin WS, Zigo MA, LaGreca AM, Skyler JS: Group strategies for diabetes in adolescence. Pediatr Adolescent Endocrinol 10:219, 1982

Strowig S: Patient education: a model for autonomous decision-making and deliberate action in diabetes self-management. Med Clin North Am 66:1293, 1982

Welborn TA, Duncan N: Diabetic staff simulation of insulin dependent diabetic life. Diabetes Care 3:679, 1980

Documentation of Control—Glycosylated Hemoglobin

Bunn HF: Evaluation of glycosylated hemoglobin in diabetic patients. Diabetes 30:613, 1981

Citrin WS, Ellis GJ, Skyler JS: Glycosylated hemoglobin: a tool in identifying psychological problems? Diabetes Care 3:563, 1980

Fluckinger R, Woodtli T, Berger W: Quantitation of glycosylated hemoglobin by boronate affinity chromatography. Diabetes 33:73, 1984

Goldstein DE, Parker KM, England JD, et al: Clinical application of glycosylated hemoglobin measurements. Diabetes, 31:suppl. 3, 70, 1982

Jovanovic L, Peterson CM: Clinical utility of glycosylated hemoglobin. Am J Med 70:331, 1981

Selection of Patients for Intensive Therapy

American Diabetes Association: Policy statement: indications for use of continuous insulin delivery systems and self-measurement of blood glucose. Diabetes Care 5:140, 1982

Mecklenberg R, Benson J, Becker N, et al: Clinical use of the insulin infusion pump in 100 patients with type I diabetes. N Engl J Med 307:513, 1982

Unger R: Meticulous control of diabetes: benefits, risks, and precautions. Diabetes 31:479, 1982

White NH, Skor DA, Cryer PE, et al: Identification of type I diabetic patients at increased risk for hypoglycemia during intensive therapy. N Engl J Med 308:485, 1983

Emerging Forms of Therapy: Their Clinical Use

Mechanical Devices

Eaton RP (ed): Symposium on insulin delivery systems. Diabetes Care 3:253, 1980

Irsigler K, Kritz H, Hagmuller G, et al: Long-term continuous intraperitoneal insulin infusion with an implanted remote-controlled insulin infusion device. Diabetes 30:1072, 1981

Kitabchi AE, Fisher JN, Matteri R, Murphy MB: The use of continuous insulin delivery systems in treatment of diabetes mellitus. Adv Intern Med 28:449, 1983

Santiago JV, Clemens AH, Clarke WL, Kipnis DM: Closed-loop and open-loop devices for blood glucose control in normal and diabetic subjects. Diabetes 28:71, 1979

Schade DS, Eaton RP, Carlson GA, et al: Future therapy of the insulin-dependent diabetic patient—the implantable insulin delivery system. Diabetes Care 4:319, 1981

Shichiri M, Kawamori R: Feasibility of a needle-type glucose sensor and a wearable artificial pancreas system in human diabetic subjects. In Irsigler K, Kritz H, Lovett R (eds): Diabetes Treatment with Implantable Insulin Infusion Systems. pp. 224–230. Urban & Schwarzenberg, Munich, 1983

Soeldner JS: Treatment of diabetes mellitus by devices. Am J Med 70:183, 1981

Soeldner JS (ed): Symposium on potentially implantable glucose sensors. Diabeties Care 5:147, 1982

Pancreatic Transplantation

Lacy, PE, Davie JM, Finke EH: Transplantation of insulin-producing tissue. Am J Med 70:589, 1981

Sutherland DER: Pancreas and islet transplantation. I. Experimental studies. Diabetologia 20:161, 1981

Sutherland DER: Pancreas and islet transplantation. II. Clinical trials. Diabetologia 20:435, 1981

Sutherland DER, Goetz FC, Najarian JS: Pancreas transplantation. Clin Endocrinol Metab 11:549, 1982

Human Insulin

Heding LG: Human insulin: facts and perspectives. Acta Med Scand [suppl] 671:107, 1983

Home PD, Alberti KGMM: Human insulin. Clin Endocrinol Metab 11:453, 1982

Karam JH, Etzwiler DD (eds): International symposium in human insulin. Diabetes Care, 6:suppl. 1, 1, 1983

Skyler JS: Human insulin of recombinant DNA origin: clinical potential. Diabetes Care, 5:suppl. 2, 181, 1982

Skyler, JS (edr): Symposium on human insulin of recombinant DNA origin. Diabetes Care 5:suppl. 2, 1, 1982

Skyler JS, Raptis S (eds): Symposium on biosynthetic human insulin. Diabetes Care 4:139, 1981

3 Metabolic Risks of Insulin Therapy

Robert A. Rizza

Blood glucose concentrations are generally maintained between 60 and 150 mg/dl in nondiabetic man in both the fasting and the postprandial state. This is accomplished by a careful integration of insulin secretion and secretion of a variety of "antiinsulin" or "counterregulatory" hormones including glucagon, epinephrine, norepinephrine, cortisol, and growth hormone. It is believed by many (and hoped by even more) physicians that maintenance of plasma glucose concentrations in diabetic patients within the range observed in nondiabetic man prevents or, if already present, slows the progression of the chronic microvascular and macrovascular diabetic complications.

Because to date this belief remains an unproved hypothesis, the risks of pursuing these goals must be carefully assessed. This chapter attempts to summarize our current understanding of the potential metabolic risks of intensive insulin therapy. Because hypoglycemia is the major known risk of intensive insulin therapy, mechanisms responsible for defense against, and recovery from, hypoglycemia are extensively reviewed. Counterregulatory defects that place certain diabetic patients at increased risk of hypoglycemia are emphasized. In addition, other potential risks of intensive insulin therapy, e.g., an increased frequency of diabetic ketoacidosis, alterations in insulin action, acceleration of atherosclerosis, and changes in vascular permeability, are discussed.

GLUCOSE COUNTERREGULATION IN NONDIABETIC MAN

Effects of Insulin and the Counterinsulin Hormones on Glucose Metabolism

In nondiabetic man[1] the postabsorptive blood glucose concentration (i.e., 6–14 hr after meal ingestion) is kept between 70 and 100 mg/dl by a closely linked balance between the amount of glucose released by the liver and the amount utilized by extrahepatic tissues. The glucose production and utilization average approximates 2 mg·kg^{-1}·min^{-1} in the postabsorptive state. If the rate of glucose production decreases without a concomitant decrease in the rate of glucose utilization or, conversely, if the rate of glucose utilization increases without an equivalent increase in glucose production, blood glucose concentration decreases until the rates of glucose production and utilization are equal once again. In the postabsorptive state, approximately 75 percent of the glucose released by the liver is derived from glycogenolysis (i.e., breakdown of glycogen) and 25 percent from gluconeogenesis (new glucose synthesis).

A variety of factors regulate the rate of hepatic glucose release[1] (Table 3-1). Insulin suppresses glucose production by inhibiting both glycogenolysis and gluconeogenesis. The liver is exquisitely sensitive to small changes in insulin concentrations. Under euglycemic conditions an increase in circulating insulin concentrations from 10 μU/ml (a typical fasting insulin concentration in normal subjects) to approximately 25–30 μU/ml results in half-maximal suppression of glucose production[2] (Fig. 3-1). Maximal suppression occurs at insulin concentrations in excess of 50–60 μ U-ml. Thus small changes in the circulating insulin concentrations may have a major effect on blood glucose concentration.

Glucagon, catecholamines, and cortisol all increase hepatic glucose release. The effects of changes in glucagon and catecholamine concentrations are almost instantaneous, whereas several hours are required for an increase in cortisol to stimulate glucose production. Epinephrine stimulates glucose production primarily through a beta-adrenergic mechanism. In addition to its acute effects, cortisol plays a key role in chronic regulation of hepatic glucose production, as "permissive" concentrations must be present for normal glycogen synthesis and for glucagon and catecholamine to stimulate glycogenolysis and gluconeogenesis. Although growth hormone has only minimal direct effects on hepatic glucose metabolism, changes in growth hormone concentrations may alter hepatic sensitivity to insulin.[1]

As with glucose production, insulin and the counterinsulin hormones also have opposite effects on glucose utilization[1] (Table 3-1) with insulin increasing and the counterinsulin hormones decreasing glucose utilization. Aside from glucagon, which has negligible effects on glucose utilization, the other counterinsulin hormones are able to decrease glucose uptake by nonhepatic tissues. Half-maximal stimulation of glucose utilization occurs at insulin concentrations of 50–60 μU/ml and maximal stimulation at insulin concentrations in excess of 200–500 μU/ml in nondiabetic subjects studied under euglycemic conditions.[2] Thus whereas a 15–20 μU/ml is neces-

Table 3-1. Effects of Insulin and Counterregulatory Hormones

Hormone	Glucose Uptake	Gluconeogenesis	Glycogenolysis	Lipolysis	Ketogenesis
Insulin	↑	↓	↓	↓	↓
Glucagon	↓ ?	↑	↑	↑	↑
Catecholamines	↓	↑	↑	↑	↑
Cortisol	↓	↑	↑	↑	↑
Growth hormone	↓	↑ ?	↑ ?	↑	↑

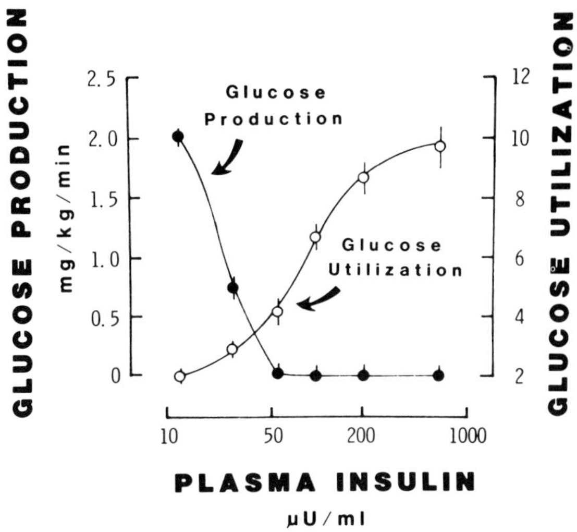

Fig. 3-1 Insulin dose-response curve for suppression of glucose production and stimulation of glucose utilization. (Adapted with permission from Rizza R, Mandarino L, Gerich J: Dose-response characteristics for effects of insulin on production and utilization of glucose in man. Am J Physiol 240:E630, 1981.)

sary for half-maximal suppression of hepatic glucose release, an increment of 40–50 μU/ml is necessary for a half-maximal effect on glucose utilization. Therefore small increases in circulating insulin concentration have a proportionately greater effect on hepatic glucose release than on tissue glucose utilization. Glucose utilization is also influenced by the circulating glucose concentration due to "mass action," with utilization increasing as the glucose concentration increases and decreasing as the glucose concentration decreases.

Catecholamines, cortisol, and growth hormone all antagonize the ability of insulin to increase glucose utilization.[1] These hormones seem to act at a postbinding site, with variable effects on insulin binding having been reported. Catecholamines act primarily through a beta-adrenergic mechanism. These agents also may indirectly inhibit glucose utilization by increasing circulating free fatty acid concentrations through the "glucose-fatty acid cycle."

Glucose Counterregulation After Insulin-Induced Hypoglycemia

Hypoglycemia is associated with an increase in the circulating concentrations of each of the counterregulatory hormones[3] (Fig. 3-2). The timing of the changes in the concentration of these hormones provides insight as to the potential role of each of these hormones in the counterregulation process. After intravenous injection of insulin, the blood glucose concentration initially decreases because of suppression of glucose production and stimulation of glucose utilization. Counterregulation begins when glucose production begins to increase and/or glucose utilization begins to decrease. The plasma glucose concentration ceases falling when the rates of glucose production and utilization become equal, and it increases when the rate of glucose production exceeds the rate of glucose utilization. Because the blood glucose concentration begins to increase at a time when the rate of glucose utilization remains above

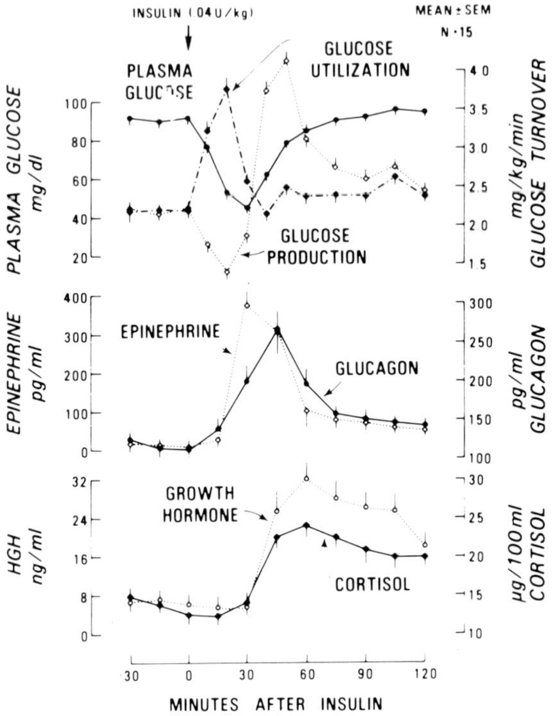

Fig. 3-2 Temporal relationships between changes in plasma glucose, glucose flux rates, and counterregulatory hormone concentrations in normal man during insulin-induced hypoglycemia. (Adapted from Gerich J, Cryer P, Rizza R: Hormone mechanisms on acute counterregulation: the relative roles of glucagon, epinephrine, norepinephrine and cortisol. Metabolism 29:1165, 1980.)

baseline (Fig. 3-2), the primary counterregulatory event is a compensatory increase in glucose production rather than a decrease in glucose utilization.

Although the circulating concentrations of all the counterregulatory hormones increase during hypoglycemia, only the concentrations of glucagon and epinephrine are elevated at the initiation of the compensatory increase in glucose production. Because glucagon is secreted into the portal vein, the increase in portal venous glucagon concentrations presumably occurs even earlier. The delay in the increase in the plasma concentrations and the delay in onset of action makes it unlikely that cortisol and growth hormone contribute significantly to the compensatory increase in glucose production. These conclusions, derived from the temporal pattern of secretion, are supported by the effects of selective deficiency of each of these hormones on glucose counterregulation.

Glucagon deficiency, which can be produced by infusion of somatostatin (a hormone that inhibits both glucagon and growth hormone secretion) along with infusion of sufficient growth hormone to mimic the normal posthypoglycemic plasma concentrations, markedly impairs glucose counterregulation[4] (Fig. 3-3). Glucagon deficiency blunts the normal hypoglycemic-induced compensatory increase in glucose production. Glucose utilization is not altered. In contrast, so long as an adequate increment in plasma glucagon is maintained, neither acute growth hormone deficiency (produced by infusion of somatostatin and sufficient glucagon to mimic posthypoglycemic glucagon concentrations) nor complete adrenergic blockage (produced by in-

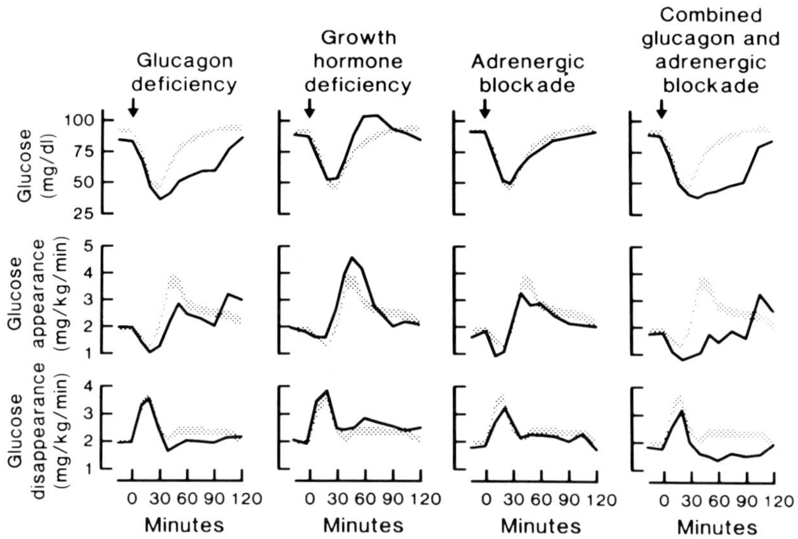

Fig. 3-3 Effects of glucagon deficiency, growth hormone deficiency, and adrenergic blockage on glucose counterregulation in normal man. (Adapted with permission from Rizza R, Cryer P, Gerich J: Role of glucagon, catecholamines, and growth hormone in human glucose counter regulation: effect of somatostatin and combined α and β adrenergic blockade on plasma glucose recovery and glucose flux rates after insulin-induced hypoglycemia. J Clin Invest 64:62, 1979.)

fusion of propranolol and phentolamine) impairs counterregulation.[3] These experiments strongly suggest that glucagon is the primary counterregulatory hormone and that the hypoglycemic-induced increases in catecholamines, growth hormone, and cortisol are not essential for normal restoration of euglycemia after moderate hypoglycemia. The lack of a primary role of catecholamines, although somewhat surprising, is supported by the observation that glucose counterregulation is normal in adrenalectomized patients receiving maintenance corticosteroid replacement (i.e., epinephrine-deficient, cortisol secretion absent)[5] and in patients with functional sympathectomy due to high cervical cord transsection (i.e., epinephrine- and norephinephrine-deficient).[6]

Catecholamines, however, do have an important role in glucose counterregulation. Counterregulation persists albeit impaired in the presence of glucagon deficiency. This residual counterregulation is primarily mediated by catecholamines. Although adrenergic blockade in itself has no effect on counterregulation when adrenergic blockade is produced along with glucagon deficiency, the residual compensatory increase in glucose production is virtually abolished, resulting in persistent hypoglycemia[4] (Fig. 3-3). Similarly, counterregulation is also virtually abolished when glucagon deficiency is produced in adrenalectomized patients by a somatostatin infusion.[5]

Thus glucagon seems to be the primary hormone responsible for the restoration of euglycemia following the induction of hypoglycemia. So long as glucagon secretion is intact, catecholamine secretion is not required for normal counterregulation. However, in the absence of glucagon secretion or when counterregulatory mechanisms are stressed, e.g., following severe hypoglycemia (nadir plasma glucose concentrations of 20–30 mg/dl), catecholamines become essential.[7,8]

Glucose Counterregulation after a Carbohydrate Meal

After ingesting a carbohydrate meal, glucose and insulin concentrations increase and glucagon concentrations decrease. These alterations in substrate and hormone concentrations result in suppression of endogenous hepatic glucose release and stimulation of hepatic and extrahepatic glucose uptake. Glucose concentrations increase until the compensatory processes exceed the rate of glucose absorption from the intestine; thereafter the blood glucose concentration returns toward, and transiently drops slightly below, preprandial glucose concentrations. The decrease in glucose concentration is accompanied by an increase in glucagon, catecholamine, cortisol, and growth hormone release. The process that prevents hypoglycemia is referred to as postprandial counterregulation.

Postprandial glucose counterregulation is also dependent on glucagon.[9] Symptomatic hypoglycemia rarely if ever occurs in normal man. On the other hand, when

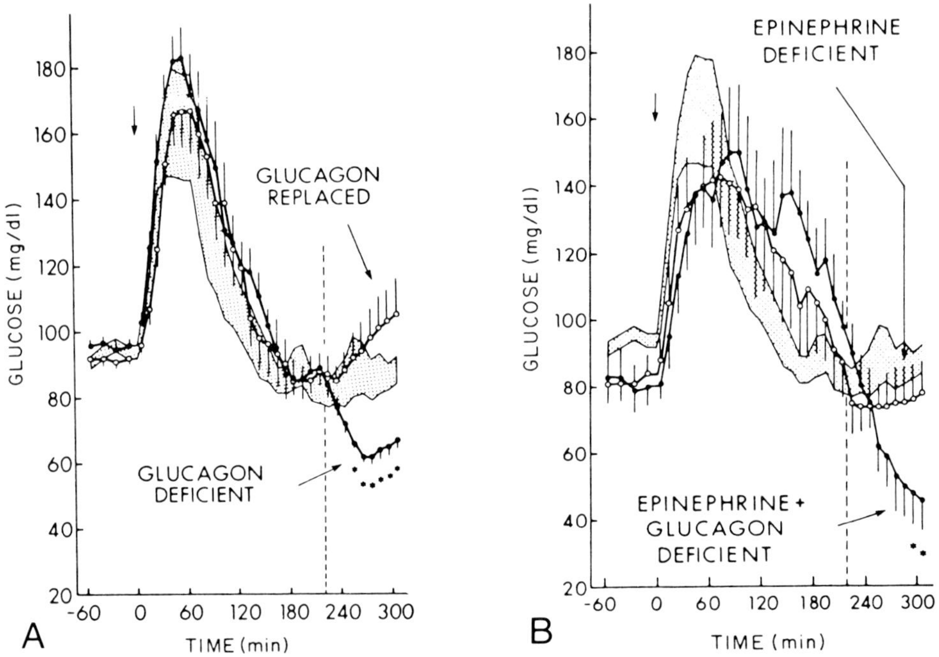

Fig. 3-4 Effects of glucagon deficiency (A), epinephrine deficiency (B), and combined glucagon and epinephrine deficiency on postprandial counterregulation. Shaded area represents the normal response to ingestion of an oral glucose challenge. Glucagon deficiency was produced by infusion of somatostatin. Epinephrine deficiency represents studies in adrenalectomized patients. (Adapted with permission from Tse T, Clutter W, Shah S, Cryer P: Mechanisms of postprandial glucose counterregulation in man. J Clin Invest 72:278, 1983.)

glucagon secretion is absent (e.g., during an infusion of somatostatin), counterregulation is impaired and glucose concentrations decrease below preprandial levels (Fig. 3-4A). Postprandial hypoglycemia is not observed in either adrenalectomized patients (epinephrine-deficient) or patients receiving adrenergic blocking agents (combined epinephrine and norepinephrine deficiency) so long as glucagon secretion is intact. However, when subjects are made both glucagon- and epinephrine-deficient, postprandial counterregulation is virtually abolished (Fig. 3-4B).

GLUCOSE COUNTERREGULATION IN DIABETIC MAN

Hypoglycemia, if not the major metabolic risk in diabetic patients treated with insulin, is certainly one of them. Diabetic patients receiving exogenous insulin are not only more vulnerable to the development of hypoglycemia than nondiabetic subjects but also have a decreased ability to counterregulate once hypoglycemia has occurred.

Vulnerability to Hypoglycemia

The loss of feedback regulation between plasma glucose and insulin secretion makes the diabetic patient more vulnerable to hypoglycemia. Although both patient and physician carefully attempt to define the "appropriate" amount of insulin to be injected subcutaneously, even under optimum conditions the resultant circulating insulin concentrations vary widely in the same individual both throughout the day and between days.[10] Differences in depth of injection, site of injection, preparation of insulin, and physical activity may enhance this variation. Even when these parameters are controlled, coefficients of variation in daily insulin absorption of 40–50 percent may be observed in the same individual, resulting in marked and unexpected changes in circulating insulin concentrations. The presence of insulin antibodies may further alter the kinetics of circulating insulin concentrations.[10] Because in the postabsorptive state minimal increments in circulating insulin concentrations can markedly suppress the rate of hepatic glucose release, diabetic patients frequently have periods of negative glucose balance with glucose utilization exceeding glucose production. This results in a progressive decline in blood glucose concentration. In the absence of effective counterregulation, the time required to produce hypoglycemia depends on the duration of the excessive insulin concentrations and the initial blood glucose concentration.

Patients with diabetes mellitus also may be more vulnerable to hypoglycemia following meal ingestion even when "appropriate" amounts of insulin are given. As discussed in the previous section, prevention of postprandial hyposlycemia is dependent on glucagon secretion. Patients with diabetes mellitus commonly seem to lack this response.[11] When glucose concentrations are rapidly lowered from hyperglycemic to euglycemic levels under conditions when circulating insulin concentrations are maintained constant, both diabetic and nondiabetic subjects secrete growth hormone, cortisol, epinephrine, and norepinephrine.[12,13] In contrast, whereas glucagon concentrations increase in nondiabetic subjects, they do not increase in patients with diabetes mellitus.[12,13] This lack of glucagon secretion in response to changing glucose concentrations may partially explain why hypoglycemia is commonly observed several hours after a meal with intensive therapy programs that attempt to normalize postprandial glucose excursions.

Impaired Recovery From Hypoglycemia

Recovery from insulin-induced hypoglycemia is frequently impaired in patients with diabetes mellitus.[14,15] As in nondiabetic subjects, the ability to counterregulate is determined by the balance between the relative activities of insulin and the antiinsulin hormones. Unfortunately, patients with insulin-dependent diabetes mellitus (IDDM) commonly do not release glucagon during hypoglycemia. This defect is not due to absolute glucagon deficiency as these same individuals release excessive amounts of glucagon in response to other stimuli, e.g., glucose or amino acids.[11] The impairment in hypoglycemia-induced glucagon release seems to be an acquired defect.[14] Newly diagnosed diabetic patients have normal glucagon secretion during hypoglycemia which progressively decreases with increasing duration of diabetes mellitus (Fig. 3-5). The loss of hypoglycemia-induced glucagon release does not seem to represent a genetic abnormality coincident with diabetes mellitus as it is also observed in animals following drug-induced diabetes mellitus.[16] Although beta cell function also decreases with increasing duration of diabetes, there is no relationship between glucagon release and residual insulin secretion.[17] The defect in glucagon release is not reversed with improved diabetic control.[18] Glucagon response to hypoglycemia is more impaired in patients who have autonomic neuropathy than those who do not.[19] This seems to be due to an association of both processes with increasing duration of diabetes rather than a causal relationship, as hypoglycemia-induced glucagon release is not dependent on the autonomic nervous system.

The ability of diabetic subjects to counterregulate parallels their ability to secrete glucagon in response to hypoglycemia.[14] In the experiments shown in Fig. 3-5, Bolli et al. have examined glucose counterregulation in patients with insulin-dependent diabetes of duration ranging from less than 1 month to 30 years. Counterregulation in the patients with new-onset diabetes (Fig. 3-, column A) did not differ from nondiabetic subjects. Glucagon, epinephrine, norepinephrine, cortisol, and growth hormone secretion was normal. In contrast, the rate of recovery from hypoglycemia was impaired in patients (Group B) who had diabetes of 1–5 years' duration. This could be ascribed to decreased glucagon release, as secretion of the other counterregulatory hormones was either normal or increased. Counterregulation was still further impaired in patients with longer duration of diabetes mellitus (group C). These patients had a more marked deficit in glucagon release in addition to a decrease in epinephrine release compared to patients in group B. Although glucose counterregulation has not been as extensively examined in patients with noninsulin-dependent diabetes mellitus (NIDDM) as in patients with IDDM, patients with NIDDM generally have intact hypoglycemia-induced glucagon release and normal glucose counterregulation.[20]

The lack of adequate glucagon response to hypoglycemia makes epinephrine the primary counterregulatory hormone in patients with IDDM. Adrenergic blockade severely impairs the ability of these individuals to recover from insulin-induced hypo-

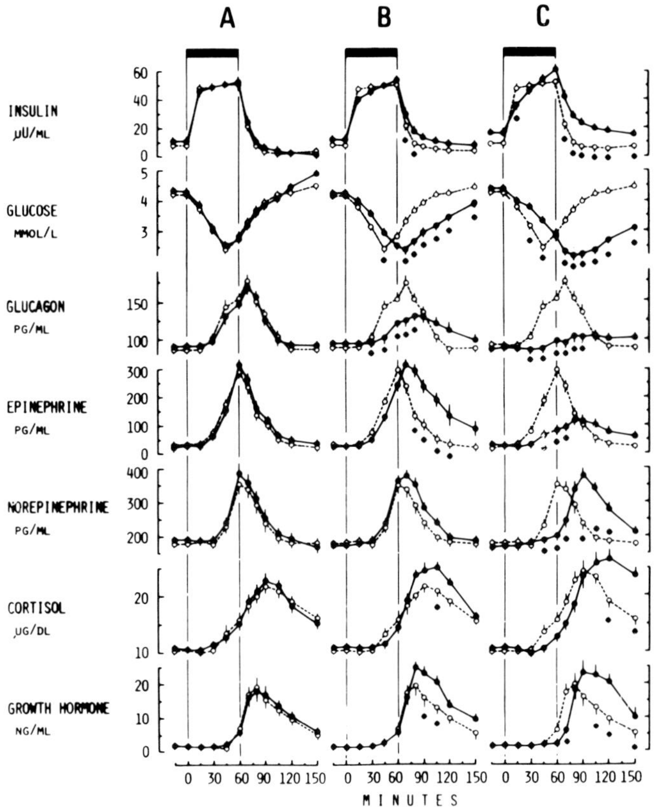

Fig. 3-5 Plasma glucose and counterregulatory hormone responses during insulin-induced hypolycemia in diabetic patients. (A) Patients with diabetes of duration less than 1 month. (B) Diabetes duration 1–5 years. (C) Diabetes duration 14–31 years. (Adapted with permission from Bolli G, Pierpaolo D, Compagnucci P, et al: Abnormal glucose counterregulation in insulin-dependent diabetes mellitus. Diabetes 32:134, 1983)

glycemia.[15,21] The degree of dependence on epinephrine seems to be an inverse function of their capacity to secrete glucagon.[21] It is of interest that although beta-adrenergic block impairs recovery from hypoglycemia it also attenuates the posthypoglycemic hyperglycemic rebound that may be observed in diabetic patients with limited insulin secretory capacity.[15] The lack of epinephrine release during hypoglycemia thus not only makes it difficult for patients with diabetic autonomic neuropathy to recognize hypoglycemia but also places them at risk for severe and prolonged hypoglycemia.

Antiinsulin antibodies may influence glucose counterregulation by altering the kinetics of blood free (unbound) insulin concentrations.[18] After administration of insulin, insulin antibodies initially may decrease the rate of fall of blood glucose by slowing the increase in blood free insulin concentrations. Subsequently, insulin antibodies may impair counterregulation by releasing insulin into the circulation, thereby maintaining blood free insulin concentrations at higher levels for longer intervals than would be observed in the absence of antibodies. This is illustrated by the experiments shown in Figure 3-6. Despite comparable circulating counterinsulin hormone concentrations, the rate of recovery from hypoglycemia is slower in the patients with insulin antibodies because of the persistence of higher circulating free insulin concentrations. The development of insulin antibodies, and therefore their adverse effects on counterregulation, presumably can be minimized by the exclusive use in the treatment of diabetes of the purest possible preparations of an insulin whose structure is the same as, or closely resembles, human insulin. The use of such insulin preparations may be particularly important in the therapy of patients with newly diagnosed diabetes because once antibody production is stimulated it may continue even when patients are switched to purified "human" insulin preparations.[22]

Counterregulation, although impaired, may still occur in diabetic patients in the absence of counterregulatory hormone secretion due to "autoregulation." This term refers to the ability of hypoglycemia per se to directly increase glucose production and decrease glucose utilization (the latter presumably through a mass action effect). This mechanism may become important when the rate of fall of glucose is sufficiently

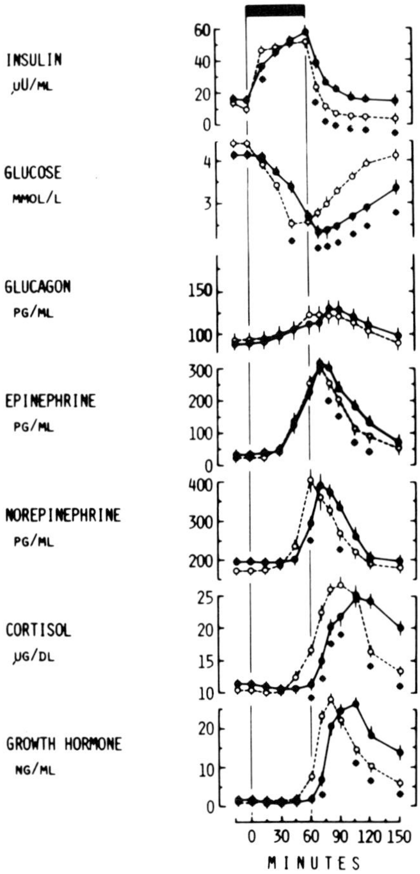

Fig. 3-6 Effects in insulin antibodies on glucose counterregulation in diabetic patients. ○—○ Diabetic patients without antibodies. ●—● Diabetic patients with antibodies. (Adapted with permission from Bolli G, Pierpaolo D, Compagnucci P, et al: Abnormal glucose counterregulation in insulin-dependent diabetes mellitus. Diabetes 32:134, 1983)

slow that minimal if any counterregulatory hormone secretion occurs. In nondiabetic man, blood glucose seems to be stabilized during a low-dose insulin infusion primarily by an increase in glucose production. In contrast, the autoregulatory process seems to differ in diabetic patients in whom glucose concentrations are stablized during a low-dose insulin infusion by a decrease in glucose utilization rather than an increase in glucose production.[23] It is not known if this abnormal pattern of autoregulation improves after long-term intensive insulin therapy.

Clinical Considerations

Two clinical considerations commonly face the physician caring for patients with diabetes mellitus: (1) Can patients at increased risk for hypoglycemia during either conventional or intensified insulin therapy be prospectively identified? (2) Can insulin-requiring patients safely be treated with selective or nonselective beta-adrenergic blocking agents? The answers to these questions remain controversial.

Several groups of investigators have measured patient response during controlled induction of hypoglycemia produced by intravenous infusion of insulin in an effort to predict which subjects are at increased risk for hypoglycemia during subcutaneous insulin therapy.[24,25] Polonsky et al., using an insulin infusion test, were unable to distinguish patients who in the preceding 6 months had two or more episodes of hypoglycemia that were severe enough to produce unconsciousness from patients who by history had no clinical evidence of serious episodes of hypoglycemia.[24] The presence or absence of normal heart rate variation with deep breathing (a measure of sympathetic innervation of the heart), the rate of fall of glucose during insulin infusion, or hypoglycemia-induced changes in epinephrine, norepinephrine, cortisol, and growth hormone did not differ between groups.

In contrast, White et al. were able to prospectively identify diabetic patients who were at increased risk for hypoglycemia during subsequent intensive insulin therapy.[25] Eight of the nine patients classified as having inadequate counterregulation during the insulin infusion test had recurrent severe hypoglycemia during the succeeding 6–36 months of therapy. In contrast, only one of the 13 patients classified as having adequate glucose counterregulation during the insulin infusion test had recurrent severe hypoglycemia over the same interval. Whereas all diabetic patients had decreased glucagon release during the test induction of hypoglycemia, patients with inadequate counterregulation also had impaired epinephrine release.

The differences between these two studies and the ability to predict risk for hypoglycemia may be explained in part by the higher insulin infusion rate (1.7 $mu{\cdot}kg^{-1}{\cdot}min^{-1}$) utilized by Polonsky et al. relative to that used by White et al. (1.0 $mu{\cdot}kg^{-1}{\cdot}min^{-1}$). The resultant plasma insulin concentrations may have been sufficiently high in the study of Polonsky et al. that any differences in counterregulatory responses may have been masked. In any case, the clinical usefulness of these tests, although promising, awaits further verification.

Another commonly encountered problem is assessment of the risks of using beta-adrenergic blocking agents in insulin-dependent diabetic patients. Diabetic patients frequently either require or potentially could benefit from administration of beta-adrenergic blocking agents for the treatment of concurrent disease processes, e.g., cardiac arrhythmias, angina pectoris, and hypertension. On the other hand, because many diabetic patients depend primarily on catecholamines for glucose counterregulation, use of adrenergic blocking agents could place these individuals at substantial risk for hypoglycemia. A variety of factors—including the degree of adrenergic blockade achieved, the amount of residual glucagon secretion present, and the proximity of the glycemic goals to the euglycemic range—are likely to influence the magnitude of the risk. It is of interest that in a prospective trial Barnett et al. reported that neither the frequency nor the severity of hypoglycemia differed in 50 "routinely" insulin-treated diabetic subjects taking beta-adrenergic blocking agents compared to a control group of diabetic subjects managed otherwise identically except they were not taking adrenergic blocking agents.[26] Although the diabetic subjects were not classified as to whether they were IDDM or NIDDM, because the mean age of the subjects was approximately 50–55 years with a mean duration of diabetes of approximately 20 years it is likely that patients with both types of diabetes were included in the study. No efforts were made to optimize glycemic control, and levels of glycemic control were not reported. Thus although this study suggests that cautious use of moderate doses of adrenergic blocking agents is not associated with a disproportionate incidence of hypoglycemia, in the author's opinion it is prudent to avoid using adrenergic blocking agents in insulin-treated diabetic patients whenever possible. When the goals of diabetic therapy are maintenance of euglycemia, which in itself may place the patient at increased risk of hypoglycemia, their use should be assiduously avoided.

A corollary question is: If beta-adrenergic blocking agents are strongly indicated, can their adverse effects on glucose counterregulation be minimized by the use of drugs that have "selective" rather than nonselective effects? The answer seems to be maybe. Because catecholamines influence glucose metabolism through both $beta_1$- and $beta_2$-adrenergic mechanisms, several investigators have compared glucose counterregulation during nonselective adrenergic blockade (propranolol, oxprenolol) to that observed during selective $beta_1$-adrenergic blockade (metoprolol, atenolol) (Table 3-2).[27–35] $Beta_1$-adrenergic blocking agents were chosen because this class of drugs can replace propranolol for most cardiovascular indications.

These studies suggest that when severe hypoglycemia is induced in nondiabetic man (i.e., when catecholamines play a significant role in counterregulation) nonselective blocking agents modestly impair glucose counterregulation. In contrast, in approximately half of the reported studies,[27–31] selective blocking agents did not impair counterregulation. Nonselective blocking agents slow the rate of recovery from hypoglycemia in diabetic patients unless they are explicitly screened for intact glucagon secretion.[32–35] $Beta_1$ selective blocking agents have been reported to either not,[34] minimally,[33–35] or significantly impair glucose counterregulation in diabetic patients.[33] Part of the explanation for these discrepant results may relate to differences in the severity of hypoglycemia examined. The studies in which the most severe hypoglycemia was produced (i.e., when catecholamines are most important) were those in which the selective $beta_1$ blocking agents had the greatest adverse effect on glucose counterregulation. Taken together, the data available to date suggest that $beta_1$ selective blocking agents may have a slightly less deleterious effect on glucose counterregulation than nonselective agents. It thus seems reasonable to utilize selective rather than nonselective agents when adrenergic blockade is absolutely indicated in diabetic patients receiving exogenous insulin.

Table 3-2. Effects of Selective and Nonselective Adrenergic Blocking Agents on Glucose Counterregulation in Normal and Diabetic Man

Ref.	Insulin Dose (U/kg)	Type of Blocking Agent		Glucose Nadir (mg/dl)			Impairment or Glucose Recovery		Significant Differences
		Nonselective	β_1 Selective	Saline	Nonselective	β_1 Selective	Nonselective	Selective	Nonselective
Nondiabetic									
27	0.15	Propranolol	Metoprolol	~35	~35	~35	No	No	No
28	0.15	Propranolol	Metoprolol	~18	~18	~18	Yes	No	Yes
29	0.15	Propranolol	Atenolol	~20	~20	~20	Yes	Yes	No
30	0.10	Propranolol	Betaxolol	24	22	24	Yes	No	Yes
31	~0.1	Oxprenolol	Metoprolol	~22	~27	~22	Yes	Yes	No
Diabetic									
Type I									
32	~0.1	Oxprenolol	Metoprolol	18	18	18	Yes	Yes	No
33	0.15–0.25	Propranolol	Metoprolol	28	23	29	Yes	+/–	No
34									
Glucagon intact	~0.05	Propranolol	Metoprolol	~45	45	45	No	No	No
Glucagon deficient,	~0.05	Propanolol	Metoprolol	~42	34	45	Yes	No	Yes
Type II									
35	0.2–0.35	Propranolol	Atenolol	~41	~41	41	Yes	+/–	No

RISK OF DIABETIC KETOACIDOSIS DURING CSII

In addition to being at risk for hypoglycemia, diabetic patients are also at risk for hyperglycemia and ketoacidosis. Ketoacidosis may develop in patients with either NIDDM or IDDM. The propensity to develop ketoacidosis depends on the relative balance between insulin deficiency (either absolute due to lack of insulin or relative due to lack of insulin action) and antiinsulin hormone excess. Diabetic ketoacidosis is less common in patients with NIDDM because they generally have significant residual beta cell function. Insulin-dependent diabetic subjects, who by definition are totally dependent on exogenous insulin therapy, have little if any endogenous insulin release. Any therapeutic program that may be associated with rapid onset of insulin deficiency therefore places these individuals at risk for the rapid onset for ketonemia and acidosis.

Continuous subcutaneous insulin infusion (CSII) represents such a program. The chief advantage of this form of therapy, i.e., the presence of only a small subcutaneous reservoir of insulin subject to the vagaries of subcutaneous blood flow, is also one of its chief potential disadvantages. Interruption of the insulin infusion for whatever reason is accompanied by rapid onset of insulin deficiency with a prompt increase in both blood glucose and ketone body concentrations ensuing[36] (Fig. 3-7). If the interruption occurs during the night, the patient may have significant hyperglycemia and ketonemia by the following morning. Because ketonemia and acidosis may occur in the presence of only modest elevations in the blood glucose concentration (200–300 mg/dl), a patient who is customarily monitoring blood but not urine glu-

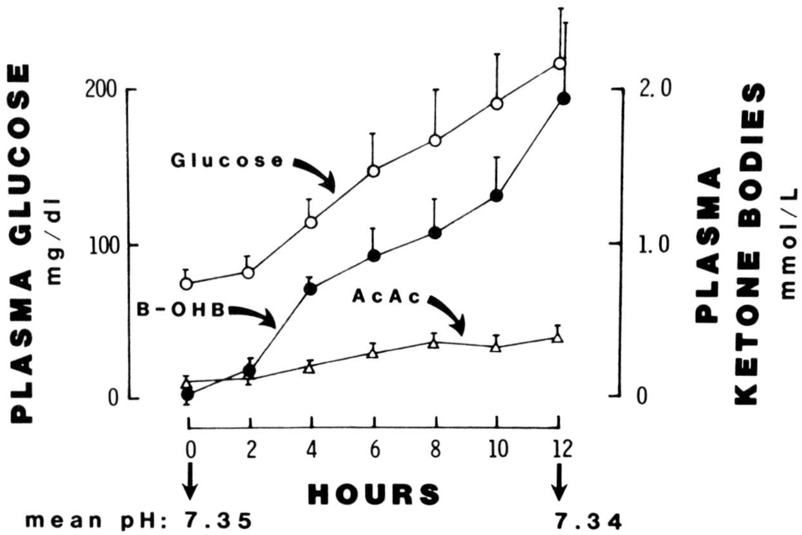

Fig. 3-7 Changes in plasma glucose, beta-hydroxybutyrate (B-OHB), and acetoacetate (ACAC) in diabetic patients after discontinuation of a CSII (Adapted with permission from Champion M, Shepherd G, Rodger N, Dupre J: Continuous subcutaneous infusion of insulin in the management of diabetes mellitus. Diabetes 29:206, 1980.)

cose concentrations (and therefore unlikely to measure urine ketone body concentrations) may not appreciate the impending danger. Furthermore, if the interruption of the insulin infusion is due to cathether obstruction, leakage, or pump malfunction, the patient may become progressively ketotic if he attempts to utilize the pump to treat what he perceives as only mild hyperglycemia.

Although many newer pumps are designed to alarm when an obstruction occurs, these alarms are relatively insensitive, with many hours being required before the obstruction is sensed. Furthermore, the pumps cannot detect leakage which may amount to only 0.01 cc/hr in the basal state.[1]

All patients utilizing insulin infusion pumps therefore should be instructed to check their urine for ketone bodies and to carefully inspect their pump and infusion site whenever unexplained hyperglycemia occurs. If ketone bodies are present, the subcutaneous needle should be removed, the insulin infusion tubing replaced, and the catheter inserted in a new subcutaneous site. Supplemental insulin should be given and blood glucose concentrations and urine ketone body concentrations monitored at frequent intervals until euglycemia is reestablished and the ketone bodies are cleared from the urine. If hyperglycemia and ketonuria do not promptly resolve, the patients should be instructed to remove their pump, contact their physician, and give themselves an injection of short-acting insulin using a syringe. Because intensive insulin programs using multiple daily injections of insulin utilize an intermediate- or long-acting insulin preparation to maintain adequate nocturnal blood insulin concentrations, a substantial reservoir of subcutaneous insulin is present, making rapid-onset insulin deficiency unlikely.

POTENTIAL ADVERSE EFFECTS OF HYPERINSULINEMIA

Although it is well recognized that untreated patients with IDDM are severely insulin-deficient, it is less well appreciated that these individuals have circulating insulin concentrations that are greater than those in nondiabetic subjects during treatment with exogenous insulin.[37] This presumably is due to the need to achieve a portal venous insulin concentration comparable to that in nondiabetic subjects. Because the liver extracts approximately 50 percent of the insulin secreted by the pancreas, in nondiabetic man portal venous insulin concentrations are generally two-fold higher than peripheral venous insulin concentrations in the postabsorptive state and several-fold higher in the fed state.[38] In contrast, because patients with IDDM receive virtually all of their insulin by absorption of exogenously administered subcutaneous insulin, peripheral venous and portal venous insulin concentrations are equal. Therefore when sufficient exogenous insulin is given to achieve portal venous insulin concentrations comparable to those present in nondiabetic individuals, peripheral hyperinsulinemia ensues. Other factors—e.g., the lack of a cephalic phase of insulin release, a mismatch between changes in glucose and insulin concentrations, and the presence of insulin resistance—may all contribute to hyperinsulinemia by increasing insulin requirements.

Chronic hyperinsulinemia may be undesirable for several reasons. Insulin seems to be able to regulate its own action by modulating the number and activity of its tissue receptors and by altering intercellular responsiveness.[39] Hyperinsulinemia per se, whatever the etiology therefore may either cause or exacerbate insulin resistance, leading to further hyperinsulinemia.

Peripheral hyperinsulinemia may also alter the pattern of glucose disposal. After meal ingestion, hepatic and extrahepatic tissues contribute to glucose and other substrate clearance. The lack of a normal portal-peripheral venous insulin gradient and the presence of peripheral hyperinsulinemia may result in altered sites of glucose metabolism despite "normal" plasma glucose concentrations. The demonstration that insulin can stimulate incorporation of glucose into aortic lipid may provide an explanation for the reported correlations between circulating insulin concentration and the development of atherosclerosis.[40] Although much of the data relating hyperinsulinemia to atherosclerotic risk is either indirect or preliminary in nature, it seems prudent until further information is available to pursue therapeutic strategies designed to minimize peripheral hyperinsulinemia.

OTHER METABOLIC COMPLICATIONS OF INSULIN THERAPY

In addition to regulating glucose, fat, and protein metabolism, insulin has a variety of other actions. Administration of insulin has been reported to be associated with a decrease in vascular volume, an increase in vascular permeability, distal nephron sodium absorption, and circulating catecholamine concentrations.[41–43] The insulin-induced changes in vascular permeability may also contribute to the development of "insulin edema" and the rapid progression of diabetic proliferative retinopathy that allegedly has been observed when insulin therapy is either initiated or intensified in diabetic patients who previously have been in poor diabetic control.[44,45]

Development of insulin antibodies is also a complication of exogenous insulin therapy. Insulin antibodies develop after injection of currently available formulations of both nonhuman and human insulin, although the titers tend to be lower with human insulin.[22] Insulin antibodies may result in insulin resistance, insulin allergy, and alterations in the kinetics of insulin clearance. Although no definitive role has been established, a contribution of circulating antigen-antibody complexes to the microvascular complications of diabetes remains a worrisome possibility. Injection of insulin may also be associated with local cutaneous changes, e.g., lipoatrophy and lipohypertrophy. Use of purified preparations of porcine (and presumably human) insulin has decreased the incidence of lipoatrophy. Lipohypertrophy, however, can still occur with these preparations. Lipohypertrophy particularly may be a problem during continuous subcutaneous insulin therapy or injection of long-acting insulin preparations, e.g., ultralente, when adequate attention is not paid to site rotation.

SUMMARY

Hypoglycemia represents the chief complication of both conventional and intensive insulin therapy. The more stringent the goals of glycemic control, the greater is the potential for hypoglycemia. An understanding of the mechanisms responsible for the production of and recovery from hypoglycemia hopefully will provide a framework for minimizing the incidence and severity of this complication. Insulin therapy programs should be designed to match changes in insulin and glucose concentrations.

Patients who have intact glucagon release in response to hypoglycemia (NIDDM and recent-onset IDDM) and normal glucose counterregulation are likely able to tolerate transient mismatches between insulin need and circulating insulin concentrations without severe hypoglycemia. Patients with a longer duration of diabetes who have absent glucagon release but intact epinephrine secretion, although not able to counterregulate normally, are still capable of defending against hypoglycemia. Patients with autonomic neuropathy, or patients who have defective glucagon secretion and are given beta-adrenergic blocking agents have markedly impaired glucose counterregulation and are poor candidates for intensive insulin therapy programs. If a beta-adrenergic blocking agent is strongly indicated in a diabetic patient being treated with insulin, selective $beta^1$ blockers may have fewer adverse effects on glucose counterregulations than do nonselective agents.

Intensive insulin therapy programs as well as all other insulin programs should be designed to minimize insulin antibody formation (i.e., use pure "human-like" insulin preparations) and peripheral hyperinsulinemia (i.e., remove treatable causes of insulin resistance, e.g., obesity). Hopefully, normalization of patterns of glucose disposal as well as portal and peripheral venous insulin concentrations by development of more physiological methods of insulin delivery will either prevent or slow the progression of the chronic microvascular and macrovascular complications of diabetes.

REFERENCES

1. Substrate and hormonal alterations in diabetes mellitus. In Schade D, Santiago J, Skyler J, Rizza R (eds): Intensive Insulin Therapy. Excerpta Medica, Princeton, NJ, 1983
2. Rizza R, Mandarino L, Gerich J: Dose-response characteristics for effects of insulin on production and utilization of glucose in man. Am J Physiol 240:E630, 1981
3. Gerich J, Cryer P, Rizza R: Hormonal mechanisms in acute glucose counterregulation: the relative roles of glucagon, epinephrine, norepinephrine, growth hormone, and cortisol. Metabolism 29:1165, 1980
4. Rizza R, Cryer P, Gerich J: Role of glucagon, catecholamines, and growth hormone in human glucose counter regulation: effect of somatostatin and combined α and β adrenergic blockade on plasma glucose recovery and glucose flux rates after insulin-induced hypoglycemia. J Clin Invest 64:62, 1979
5. Gerich J, Davis J, Lorenz M, et al: Hormone mechanisms of recovery from hypoglycemia in man. Am J Physiol 236:380, 1979
6. Palmer JP, Henry DP, Benson JW, et al: The glucagon response to hypoglycemia in sympathecotomized man. J Clin Invest 57:522, 1976
7. Lilavivat U, Brodows R, Campbell R: Adrenergic influence on glucocounterregulation in man. Diabetologia 20:482, 1981
8. Cryer P: Glucose counterregulation in man. Diabetes 30:261, 1981
9. Tse T, Clutter W, Shah S, Cryer P: Mechanisms of postprandial glucose counterregulation in man: physiologic roles of glucagon and epinephrine vis-à-vis insulin in the prevention of hypoglycemia late after glucose ingestion. J Clin Invest 72:278, 1983
10. Binder C, Lauritzen T, Faber O, Pramming S: Insulin pharmacokinetics. Diabetes Care 7: 1984.

11. Gerich J, Langlois M, Noacco C, et al: Lack of a glucagon response to hypoglycemia in diabetes: evidence for an intrinsic pancreatic alpha cell defect. Science 182:171, 1973.
12. Santiago J, Clarke W, Shah S, Cryer P: Epinephrine, norepinephrine, glucagon, and growth hormone release in association with physiological decrements in the plasma glucose concentration in normal and diabetic man. J Clin Endocrinol Metab 51:877, 1980
13. DeFronzo R, Hendler R, Christensen N: Stimulation of counterregulatory hormonal responses in diabetic man by a fall in glucose concentration. Diabetes 29:125, 1980
14. Bolli G, Pierpaolo D, Compagnucci P, et al: Abnormal glucose counterregulation in insulin-dependent diabetes mellitus. Diabetes 32:134, 1983
15. Popp D, Shah S, Cryer P: Role of epinephrine mediated adrenergic mechanisms in hypoglycemic glucose counterregulation and posthypolycemic hyperglycemia in insulin-dependent diabetes mellitus. J Clin Invest 69:315, 1982
16. Patel D: Lack of glucagon response to hypoglycemia in long-term experimental diabetic rats. Diabetes 32:55, 1983
17. Madsbad S, Hilsted J, Krarup T, et al: Hormonal metabolic and cardiovascular responses to hypoglycaemia in type I (insulin dependent) diabetes with and without residual β cell function. Diabetologia 23:499, 1982
18. Bolli G, Calabrese G, DeFeo P, et al: Lack of glucagon response in glucose counterregulation in type I (insulin dependent) diabetes: absence of recovery after prolonged optimal insulin therapy. Diabetologia 22:100, 1982
19. Hilsted J, Madsbad S, Krarup T, et al: Hormonal metabolic and cardiovascular response to hypoglycemia in diabetic autonomic neuropathy. Diabetes 30:626, 1981
20. Boden G, Soriano M, Hoeldke R, Owen O: Counterregulatory hormone release and glucose recovery after hypoglycemia in noninsulin dependent diabetic patients. Diabetes 32:1055, 1983
21. Bolli G, DeFeo P, Compagnucci P, et al: Important role of adrenergic mechanisms in acute hypoglycemia in type I diabetes: evidence for an effect mediated by beta-adrenoreceptors. Diabetes 31:641, 1982
22. Fineberg S, Galloway J, Fineberg N, Rathbun M: Immunologic improvement resulting from the transfer of animal insulin-treated diabetic subjects to human insulin (recombinant DNA). Diabetes Care, suppl. 2, 5:107, 1982
23. Sacca L, Sherwin R, Hendler R, Felig P: Influence of continuous physiologic hyperinsulinemia on glucose kinetics and counterregulatory hormones in normal and diabetic humans. J Clin Invest 63:849, 1979
24. Polonsky K, Bergenstal R, Pons G, et al: Relation of counterregulatory responses to hypoglycemia in type I diabetics. N Engl J Med 307:1106, 1982
25. White N, Skor D, Cryer P, et al: Identification of type I diabetic patients at increased risk for hypoglycemia during intensive therapy. N Engl J Med 308:485, 1983
26. Barnett A, Leslie D, Watkins P: Can insulin-treated diabetics be given beta-adrenergic blocking drugs. Br Med J 1:976, 1980
27. Nilsson O, Anderberg B, Karlberg B, Kagedal B: Crotisol, growth hormone, and prolactin responses to insulin-induced hypoglycemia in hyperthyroid patients before and during β-adrenoreceptor blockade. Clin Endocrinol 12:581, 1980
28. Corrall R, Frier B, Davidson N, French E: Hormonal and substrate responses during recovery from hypoglycemia in man during $beta_1$ selective and nonselective beta-adrenergic blockade. Eur J Clin Invest 11:279, 1981
29. Lauridsen U, Christensen N, Lyngsoe J: Effects of nonselective and β-1-selective blockade on glucose metabolism and hormone responses during insulin-induced hypoglycemia in normal man. J Clin Endocrinol Metab 56:876, 1983
30. Saunders J, Prestwich S, Avery A, et al: The effect on nonselective and selective beta-1-

blockade on the plasma potassium response to hypoglycemia. Diabetes Meta 7:239, 1981
31. Viberti G, Keen H, Bloom S: Beta blockade and diabetes mellitus: effect of oxprenolol and metoprolol on the metabolic, cardiovascular, and hormone response to insulin-induced hypoglycemia in normal subjects. Metabolism 29:866, 1980
32. Viberti G, Keen H, Bloom S: Beta blockade and diabetes mellitus: effect of oxprenolol and metoprolol on the metabolic, cardiovascular, and hormonal response to insulin-induced hypoglycemia in insulin dependent diabetics. Metabolism 29:873, 1980
33. Lager I, Blohme G, Smith U: Effect of cardioselective and nonselective β-blockade on the hypoglycemic response in insulin dependent diabetics. Lancet 1:458, 1979
34. DeFeo P, Bolli G, Perriello G, et al: The adrenergic contribution to glucose counterregulation: dependency on A-cell function and mediation through $beta_2$adrenergic receptors. Diabetes 32:887, 1983
35. Deacon S, Karunanayake A, Barnett D: Acebutolol, atenolol, and propranolol and metabolic responses to acute hypoglycemia in diabetics. Br Med J 2:1255, 1977
36. Champion M, Shepherd G, Rodger N, Dupre J: Continuous subcutaneous infusion of insulin in the management of diabetes mellitus. Diabetes 29:206, 1980
37. Rizza R, Gerich J, Haymond M, et al: Control of blood sugar in insulin dependent diabetes: comparison of an artificial endocrine pancreas, continuous subcutaneous insulin infusion and intensified conventional insulin therapy. N Engl J Med 303:1313, 1980
38. Horwitz D, Starr J, Mako M, et al: Proinsulin, insulin, and c-peptide concentrations in human portal and peripheral blood. J Clin Invest 55:1278, 1975
39. Olefsky J: The insulin receptor: its role in insulin resistance of obesity and diabetes. Diabetes 25:1154, 1976
40. Stout R: The role of insulin in atherosclerosis in diabetics and nondiabetics: a review. Diabetes, suppl. 2, 30:54, 1981
41. Osterby, R, Gundersen H, Christensen N: The acute effect of insulin on capillary endothelial cells. Diabetes 27:745, 1978
42. DeFronzo R: The effect of insulin on renal sodium metabolism. Diabetologia 21:165, 1981
43. Gundersen H, Christensen N: Intravenous insulin causing loss of intravascular water and albumin and increased adrenergic activity in diabetics. Diabetes 26:551, 1977
44. Shaper A: The insulin edema syndrome in African diabetic subjects. Trans Soc Trop Med Hyg 60:519, 1966
45. Daneman D, Drash A, Lobes L, et al: Progressive retinopathy with improved control in diabetic dwarfism (Maurine's syndrome). Diabetes Care 4:360, 1984

4 Retinopathy and Other Ocular Complications in Diabetes

Ronald Klein

Diabetic retinopathy is a leading cause of visual impairment in the United States.[1] Although its natural history has been described, its pathogenesis is not known.[2] Available data suggest that identification of the presence of retinopathy is important because intervention with photocoagulation may prevent or delay the development of severe visual loss.[3] This chapter describes current concepts about the natural history, pathogenesis, diagnosis, and management of retinopathy as well as other ocular complications of diabetes that may result in visual loss.

DIABETIC RETINOPATHY

Retinal Anatomy

The retina[4] is a thin, transparent neural tissue lining the inner part of the eye. It is in contact with the clear vitreous gel internally and the choroid externally. The retina varies in thickness from 0.1 mm at the fovea and far periphery to 0.55 mm at the macula. There are 10 well-defined retinal layers consisting of the nuclei of three sequential neurons, their axons and synaptic connections, and glial supporting cells with little extracellular space. A central retinal artery derived from the ophthalmic artery branches into arterioles at the optic nerve head and supplies blood to the internal two-thirds of the retina; the choriocapillaris of the choroid supplies nutrition to the external one-third. A blood-retinal barrier comprised of tight junctions of the en-

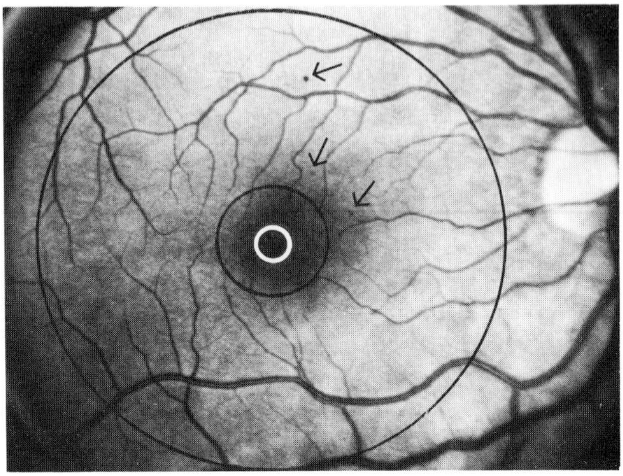

Fig. 4-1 Fundus photograph of right eye. The macular area corresponds approximately to the largest, the fovea to the middle, and the foveola to the smallest black circle. Three retinal microaneurysms (dark arrows) appear as small dark spots with sharp margins.

dothelial cells of the retinal blood vessels and the retinal pigment epithelial cells prevents penetration of all but a few important metabolic products into the retina.

The macular area measures approximately 4 mm in diameter and is centered 4mm temporal to the optic disc (Fig. 4-1). The fovea, a depression in the inner retinal surface of the macula, is 1.5 mm in diameter. A retinal capillary free zone of 450–600 μm exists in its center, where the retinal tissue is fed by the choriocapillaris of the choroidal circulation. The central portion of the fovea (or foveola) contains only cone photoreceptors, which are important for the best visual acuity (finest spatial resolution) and highest quality trichromatic color vision.

Natural History

The earliest clinically apparent manifestations of diabetic retinopathy are classified as nonproliferative. During this phase a number of pathophysiological changes associated with diabetes occur in the microvasculature; these include occlusion, dilation, and increased permeability of the small retinal blood vessels.[5,6] Early retinal vascular change may be detected using fluorescein angiography. Yamana et al.[7] reported abnormal dye leakage followed by localized capillary dilation, focal filling defects in capillaries, and spot-like dilations analogous to retinal microaneurysms. Histological changes that occur early in the course of the disease are degeneration of retinal capillary pericytes (mural cells) and thickening of the capillary basement membrane.[5,6]

Usually the first changes seen with the ophthalmoscope are retinal microaneurysms, small outpouchings of the retinal capillaries (Fig. 4-1). They appear as small circular red dots, varying in size from about 20 to 200 μm. Retinal microaneurysms typically arise in areas of capillary closure (Fig. 4-2) and on histopathological sections have an endothelial lining and a basement membrane of variable thickness. These lesions demonstrate abnormal permeability of the endothelial cell wall to fluorescein and possibly to lipoproteins (Fig. 4-2). With time, the walls may thicken with deposition of periodic acid-Schiff (PAS)-positive and lipid material, and stagnant blood may be trapped in the lumen. If there is further thickening of the wall and obliteration of the lumen, the microaneurysm may then appear yellow or white on clinical examination. Occlusion of the feeding capillary or complete hyalinization of the lumen may be responsible for the microaneurysm's ultimate disappearance.[5]

Microaneurysms have been reported to have variable survival rates, and their average disappearance rate has been estimated at 3.3 percent/month.[8] Baudoin et al.[9] developed a standarized reproducible method for quantitating the number of retinal microaneurysms using fluorescein angiograms. This technique may prove useful for study of the early natural history of diabetic retinopathy and as an endpoint in clinical trials to evaluate the effects of treatment or intervention.

Retinal microaneurysms generally do not make their appearance until at least 3 years after diagnosis of diabetes.[10–12] They are found in about 69 percent of people with a history of 10 years of insulin-dependent diabetes.[12] In adults with noninsulin-dependent diabetes, retinal microaneurysms are present in 55 percent of the population who have had diabetes for 10 years.[13] They can occur in nondiabetic patients with other conditions associated with retinal ischemia, e.g., branch retinal vein occlusion and carotid artery disease.

Retinal microaneurysms by themselves are usually not a threat to vision. However, as the disease progresses, retinal blot hemorrhages and hard exudates appear. Retinal blot hemorrhages are round with blurred edges and result from an extravasation of blood from retinal capillaries or microaneurysms into the inner nuclear layer of the retina (Figs. 4-3 and 4-4). They are not fluorescent on angiography and usually disappear within 3–4 months.

Retinal hard exudates are variable in size, sharply defined, and yellow; they may be scattered, aggregated, or "ring-like" in their distributions (Fig. 4-4). Hard exudates result from leakage of lipoprotein material from retinal capillaries or microaneurysms into the outer retinal layer; and they may last from months to years.[14] The exudate forms preferentially in the posterior retina, especially temporal to the macula, and may extend into the macula, reducing visual acuity. On ophthalmoscopy retinal hard exudates are sometimes confused with drusen, which are deposits of PAS-positive material located between the retinal pigment epithelium and Bruch's membrane. Drusen are not characteristic of diabetes but occur frequently in older individuals. Differentiation between hard exudates and drusen may be difficult in some cases if the examination is done without stereopsis; drusen are usually rounder, more regular, and less yellow than hard exudates.

In the more advanced stages of nonproliferative retinopathy, closure of the retinal capillaries and arterioles occurs, causing decreased nutrition to the inner layers of the retina. These changes cause whitish or grayish swellings in the nerve fiber layer of the retina, termed "cotton-wool spots" or "soft exudates," which are infarcts of the nerve fiber layer (Fig. 4-5). They remain only a few weeks to months. After their disappearance, the retina may appear normal on ophthalmoscopy, but nonperfusion

(Text continues on page 108.)

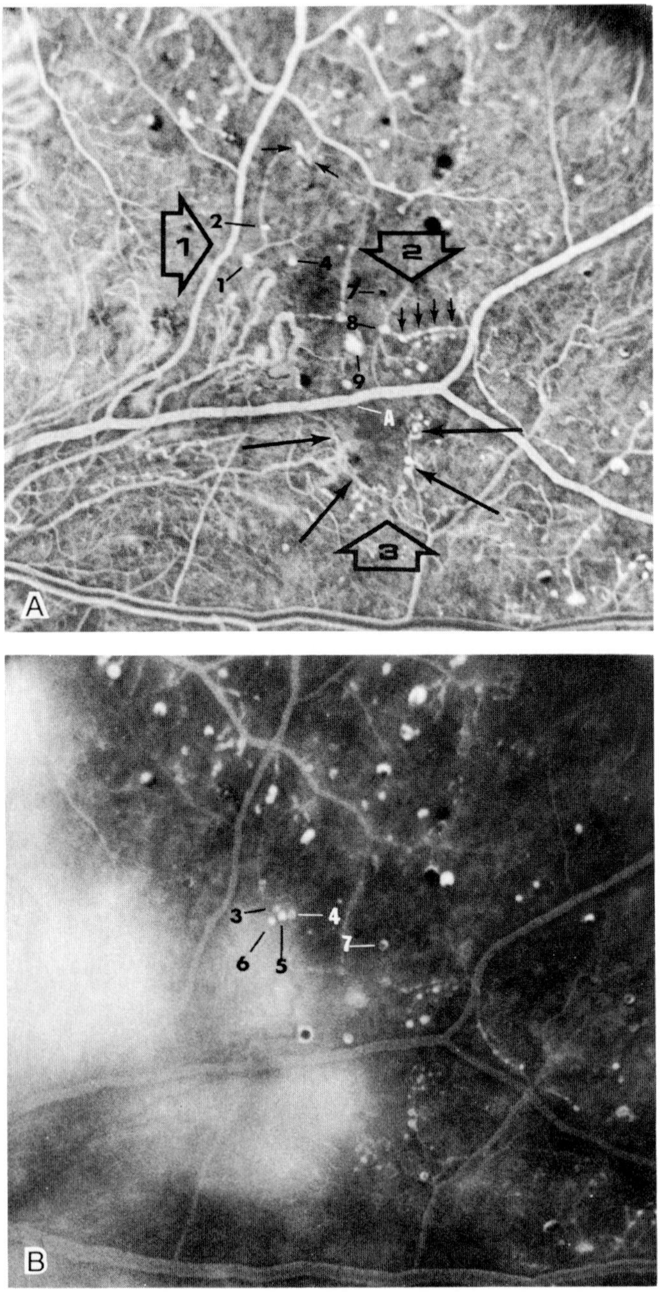

Fig. 4-2 Retinal microaneurysms are demonstrated on fluorescein angiograms and trypsin digest preparation of the retina to illustrate clinicopathological correlations. (A) Fluorescein angiogram: capillary phase. Areas are denoted by large open arrows and specific lesions by unenclosed numbers. (B) Fluorescein angiogram: late venous phase [same field as in (A)]. Note intense fluorescein leakage from preretinal new vessel system (left).

Fig. 4-2 (cont.) (C) Trypsin digest specimen of area 1 [compare to (A) and (B)]. PAS stain. ×10. Note the following correlations: Fluorescent spot 1 is hyalinized microaneurysm H1. Fluorescent spot 2 is hyalinized microaneurysm H2. Fluorescent spot 4 is microaneurysm M4. Fluorescent spots 3, 5, and 6 did not fill until the late venous phase (B); they correlate with hyalinized microaneurysms M5 and M6. Arrows point to dilated hypercellular capillary channels that are prominent in angiogram (A). (D) Trypsin digest specimen of area 2. PAS stain. ×10. Spot 7 has a dark center and a fluorescent cap (A), and it develops a full fluorescent halo in the late venous phase (B); this spot correlates with hyalinized microaneurysm H7. Fluorescent spot 9 correlates with a hyalinized microaneurysm with a large irregular pouch, P9. Arrows point to a dilated hypercellular vessel that demonstrates an interrupted fluorescent column (A).

(Figure continues on next page.)

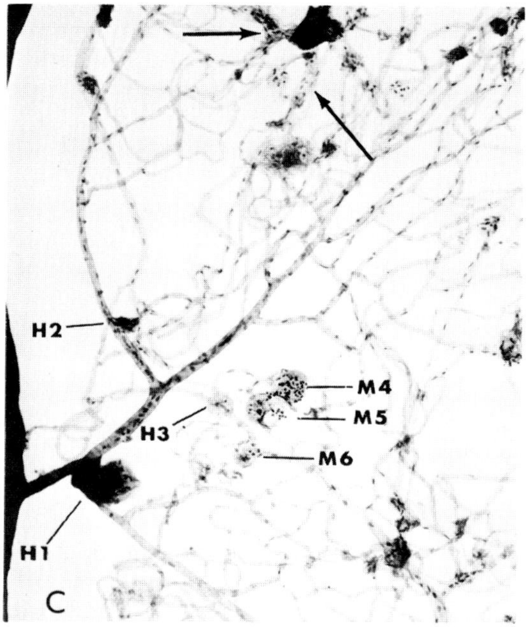

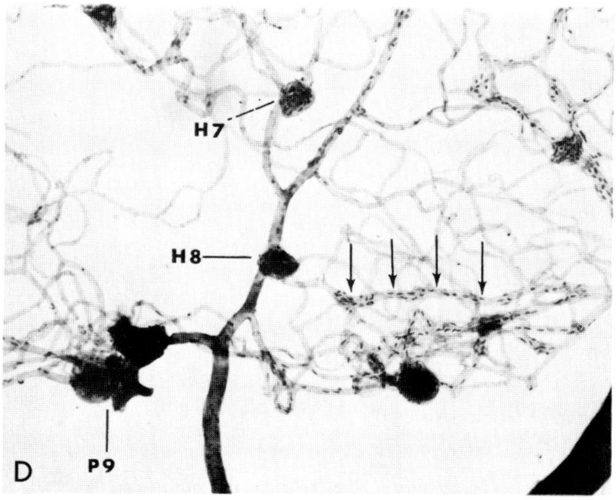

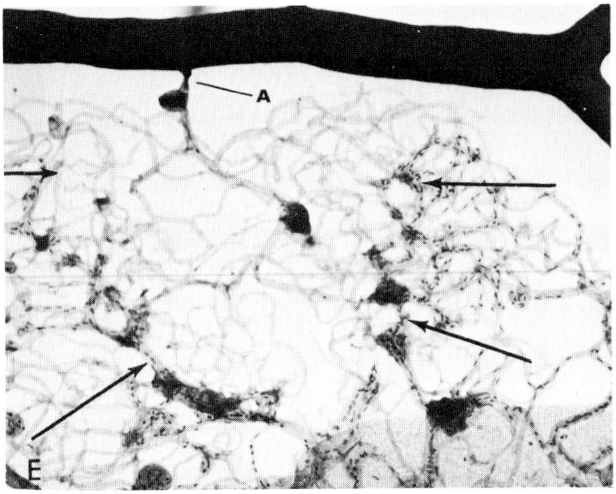

Fig. 4-2 (cont.) (E) Trypsin digest specimen of area 3. PAS stain. ×10. Note that the acellular capillaries correspond to an apparently nonperfused area in fluorescein angiogram (A). Note the absence of a normal reticular appearance in this portion of the angiogram. Arrows point to dilated hypercellular capillary channels and microaneurysms that surround an acellular zone. (Reprinted with permission from Bresnick GH: Diabetic retinopathy. In Peyman G, Sanders DR, Goldberg MR (eds): Principles and Practice of Ophthalmology. Saunders, Philadelphia, 1980.)

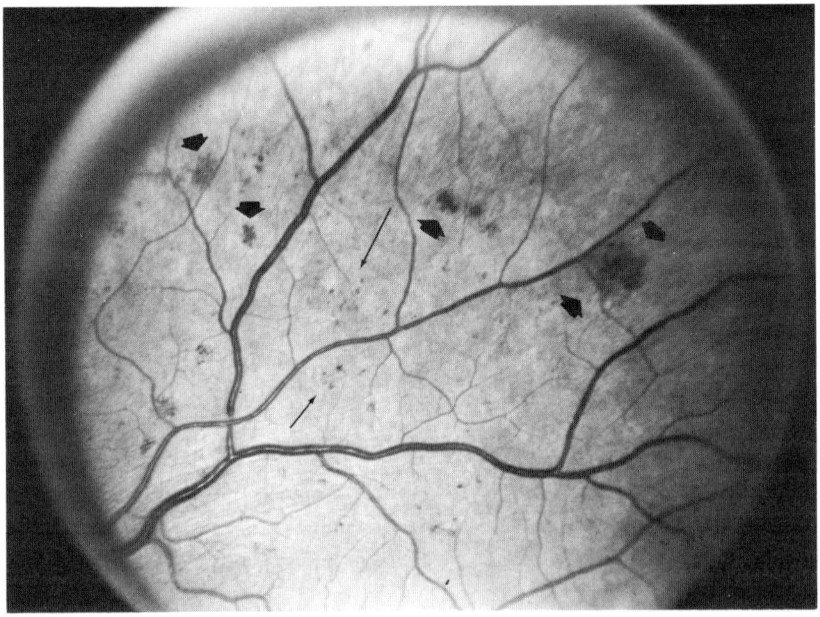

Fig. 4-3 Fundus photograph of the left eye. A number of retinal microaneurysms (long dark arrows) appear as small dark spots with sharp margins, and retinal blot hemorrhages (short thick arrows) appear as spots of varying size with irregular margins and uneven densities. (Reprinted with permission from Klein R: Management of eye disease in the insulin-dependent diabetic patient. In MacDonald M (ed): Managing Diabetes Mellitus in Children and Adolescents. Saunders, Philadelphia, 1983.)

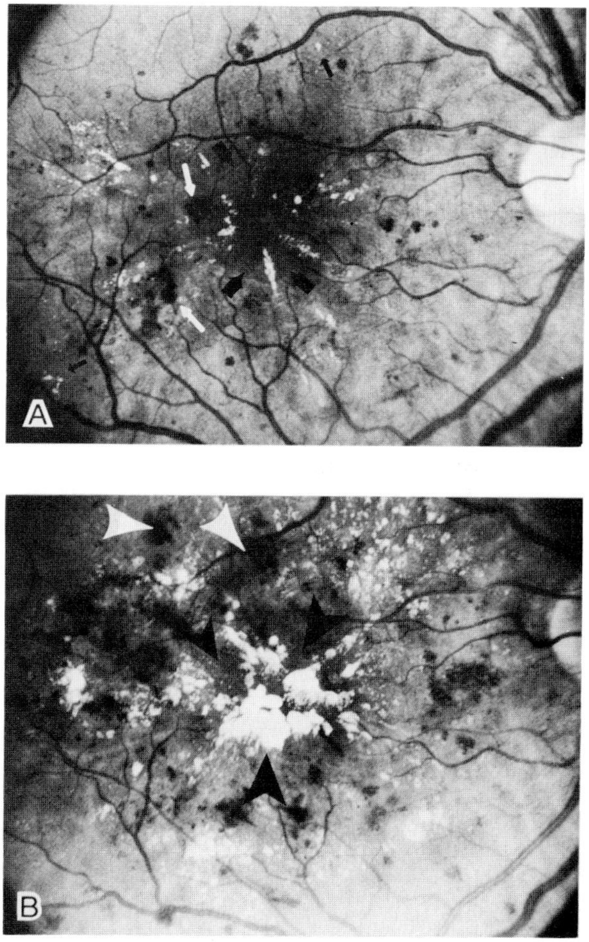

Fig. 4-4 Fundus photographs of the macular area of the right eye demonstrating retinal hard exudates that appear as white deposits with sharp margins either scattered (short thin black arrows), "ring-like" (short thick black arrows), or aggregated in their distributions (large black arrowheads). Retinal blot hemorrhages (small white arrows) and dark intraretinal hemorrhages (large white arrowheads) are present. At the time photograph (A) was taken, the visual acuity was 20/15; 1 year later, when photograph (B) was taken, the visual acuity had dropped to 20/50.

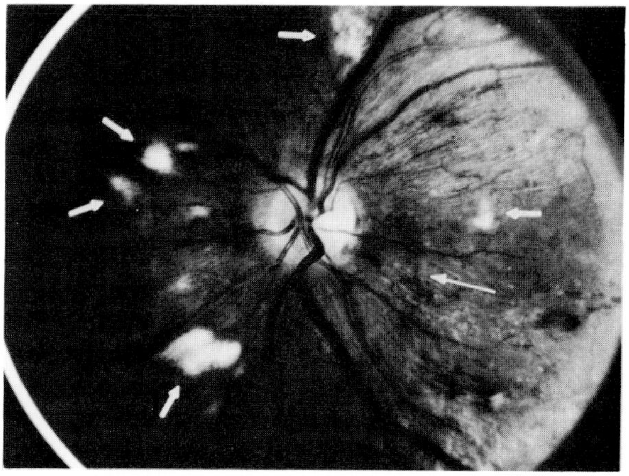

Fig. 4-5 Fundus photograph of the left eye with "preproliferative" retinopathy. Cotton-wool spots or soft exudates appear as grayish white areas with ill-defined edges (small thick white arrows); intraretinal microvascular abnormalities (thin white arrow), venous dilation, and retinal hemorrhages are present

of retinal arterioles may be seen in fluorescein angiography. In some patients with severe ischemia, occlusion of larger arterioles results in larger areas of irreversible retinal nonperfusion, especially in the retinal midperiphery. Late in the course of the disease, severe ischemia may manifest by thin sheathed sclerotic (white "thread-like") arterioles (Figs. 4-6 and 4-7).

Shimizu et al.[15] suggested that the midperipheral retina is more susceptible than the macular area to the vasoobliterative process that occurs in the diabetic microcirculation. Using wide-angle fluorescein angiography, they demonstrated that the main change in the diabetic retinal midperiphery was capillary nonperfusion, whereas in the macular area the most common changes were "vasodilation, capillary microaneurysm formation, hyperpermeability," and occasional capillary nonperfusion.

Another manifestation of focal retinal ischemia is the presence of dilated capillaries [intraretinal microvascular abnormalities (IRMAs)] (Figs. 4-5 and 4-6). IRMAs are found in areas of capillary nonperfusion and may be abnormally permeable to plasma proteins; they are considered by some to be a compensatory response to hy-

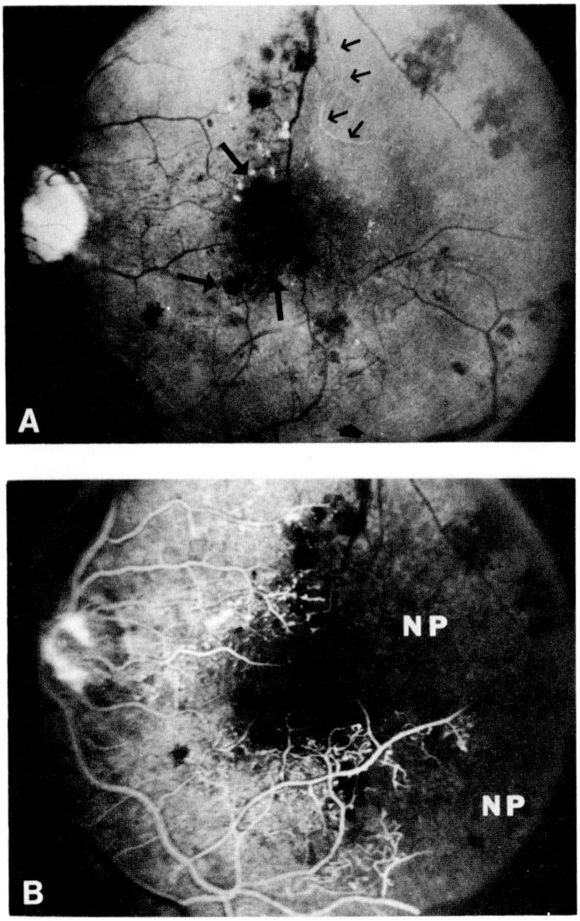

Fig. 4-6 (A) Fundus photograph, left eye. Closure of a large retinal arteriole appears white (short arrows). Dark intraretinal hemorrhages (large black arrows) and intraretinal microvascular abnormalities (black arrowhead) are present. (B) Fluorescein angiogram, capillary phase, left eye. This photograph, taken at the same time as the fundus photograph, demonstrates several nonperfused zones (NP) of the retina on the right. Visual acuity was 20/40.

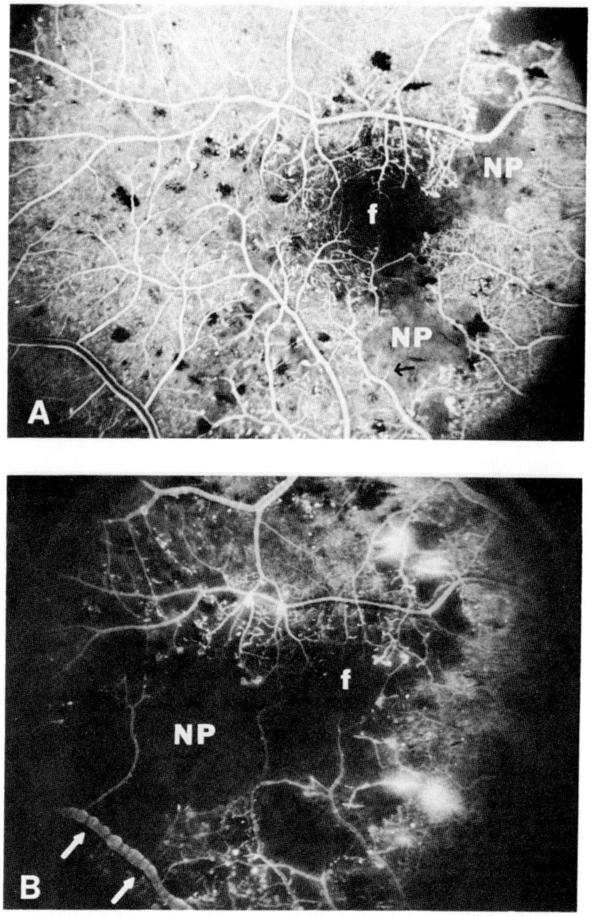

Fig. 4-7 Progression of ischemic process is shown in fluorescein angiograms taken 18 months apart. (A) Note the several nonperfused zones (NP). The stump of one small arteriolar branch supplying the ischemic zone is marked by a black arrow. There is capillary drop-out to the right of the foveal area (f). Visual acuity is 20/30. (B) Eighteen months later there has been a pronounced progression of ischemic process with new large areas of nonperfused retina (NP) at the left as well as at the right of the foveal area (f). Venous beading (white arrows) is present. Visual acuity is 20/40.

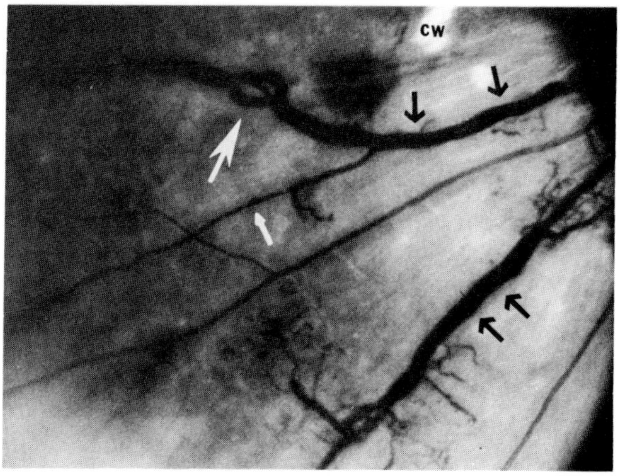

Fig. 4-8 Fundus photograph of the left eye. Retinal venous dilation and beading (black arrows) and an area of reduplication are present (large white arrow). Slow flow is manifested by ''box-carring'' in the small retinal branch vein (small white arrow). Intraretinal microvascular abnormalities and a cotton-wool spot (CW) are present in this very ischemic retina.

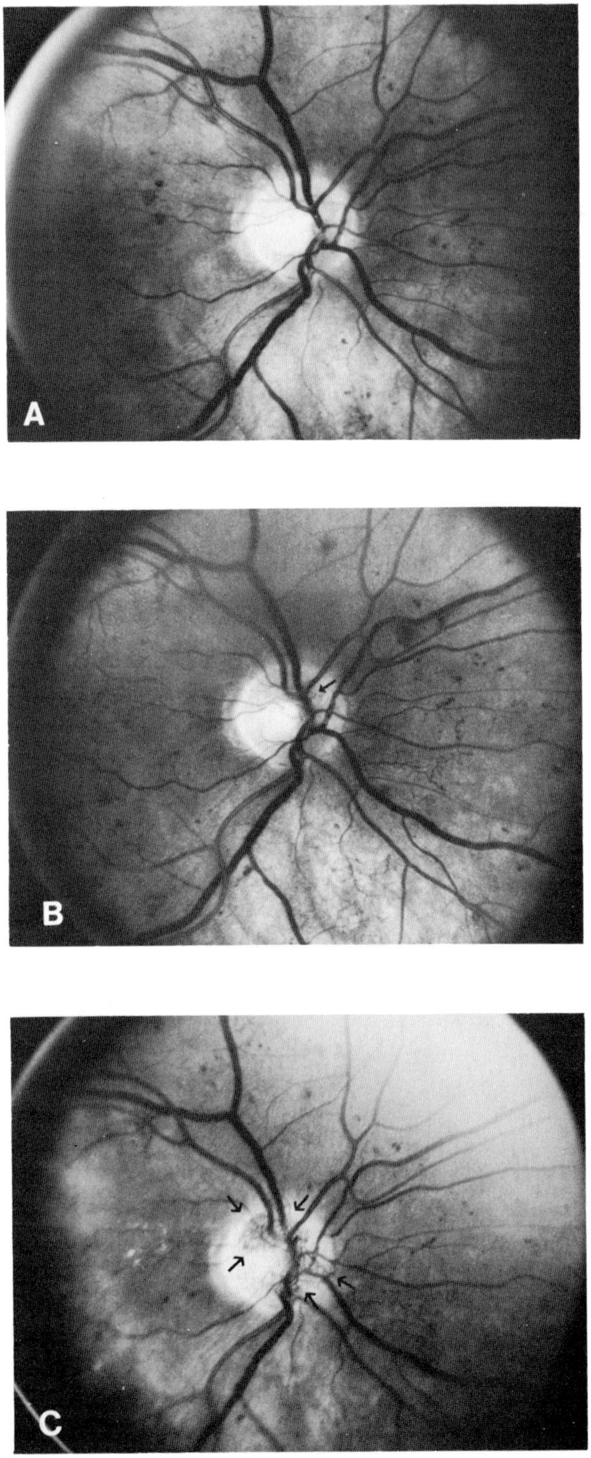

Fig. 4-9 Fundus photograph of the right eye. This sequence of photographs demonstrates progression from the nonproliferative stage (A, 7/74) to early proliferative retinopathy manifested initially as fine tufts of retinal new vessels on the optic disc (B, 2/75) (black arrows).

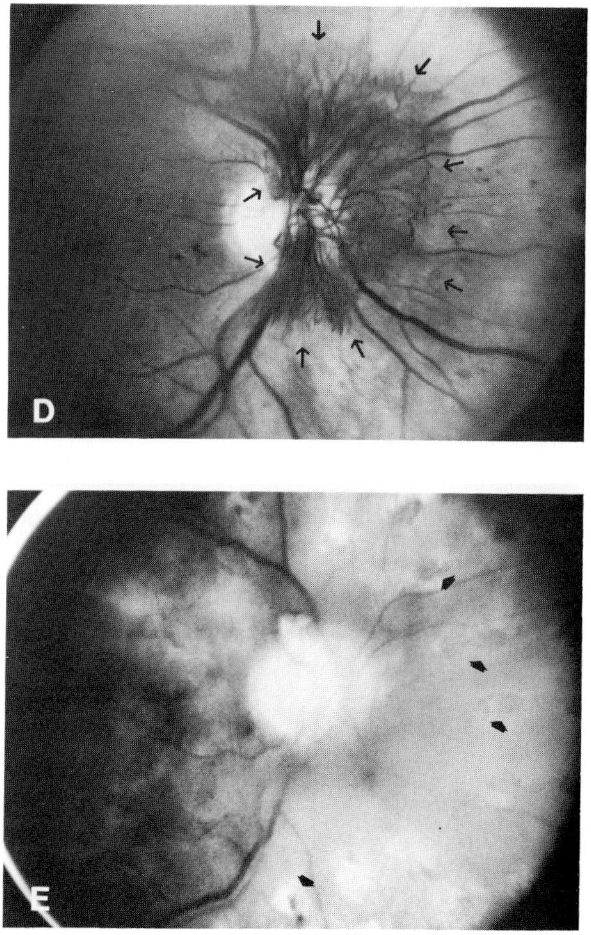

Fig. 4-9 (cont.) There was further growth of retinal new vessels (C, 8/75 and D 4/76) with regression after photocoagulation treatment (E, 8/76). Pigmented photocoagulation scars are present (black arrowheads).

poxia.[6] Venous beading, duplication, and kinks also occur in response to hypoxia in areas of focal ischemia (Figs. 4-7 and 4-8). Many large, dark intraretinal hemorrhages may also appear secondary to retinal ischemia and are thought to represent hemorrhagic infarcts (Figs. 4-4 through 4-6).[5]

The presence of cotton-wool spots, venous irregularities, IRMAs, and dark intraretinal hemorrhages constitutes what has been called the "preproliferative phase"; eyes with these changes have an increased risk of developing proliferative retinopathy.[5] Therefore the appearance of cotton-wool spots and other manifestations of retinal ischemia are considered a warning sign of impending growth of new retinal vessels.

Proliferative diabetic retinopathy is characterized by growth of abnormal blood vessels and fibrous tissue from the optic nerve head (Fig. 4-9) or from the inner retinal surface (usually near or from retinal veins) (Fig. 4-10). The vessels, which appear initially as fine tufts on the surface of the retina, subsequently grow into the

(Text continues on page 115.)

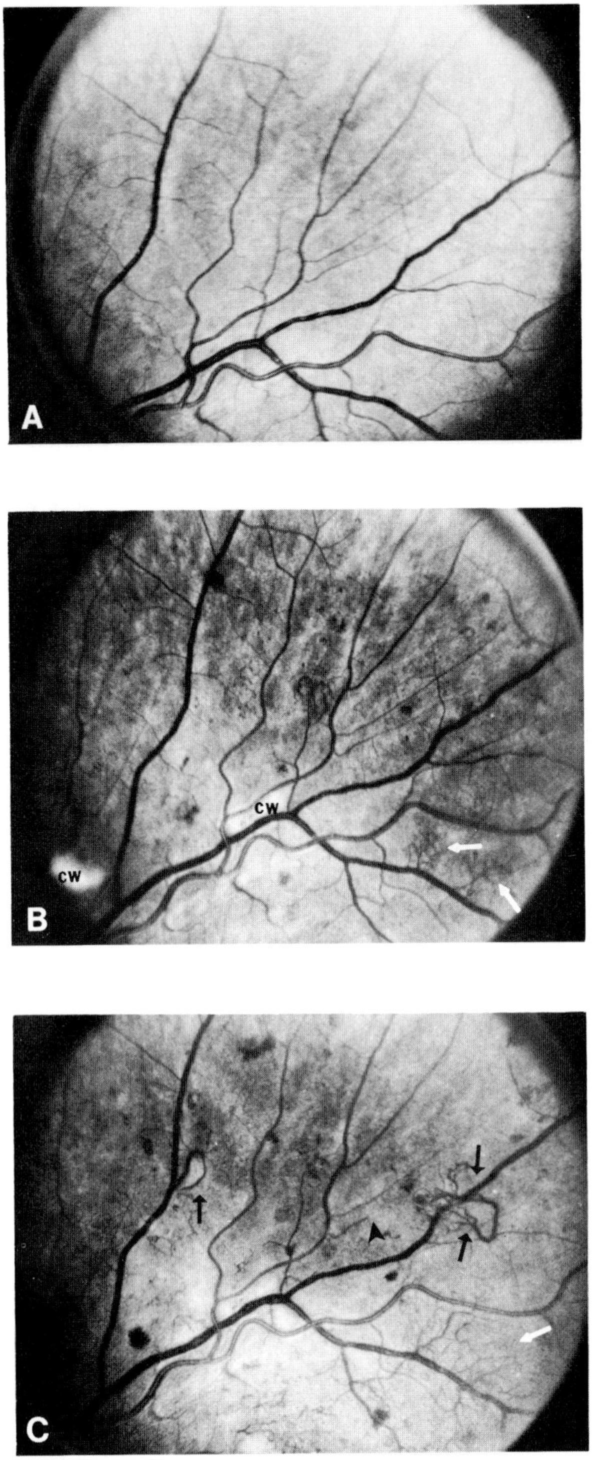

Fig. 4-10 Fundus photograph of the left eye showing progression from nonproliferative to proliferative diabetic retinopathy in an area superior and temporal to the macula. (A) When the patient was seen in 11/72 she was 25 years old and had a 14-year history of insulin-dependent diabetic retinopathy. A few dilated capillaries and retinal microaneurysms are present here, and cotton-wool spots and blot hemorrhages were present in the macular area (not in photograph). The visual acuity was 20/15. (B) One year later (12/73) a number of intraretinal microvascular abnormalities (white arrows), cotton-wool spots (CW), and blot hemorrhages are present, indicating a progression of the ischemic process. (C) In 3/76 flat retinal new vessels (small black arrows) are present. An abrupt termination of a branch arteriole (black arrowhead), intraretinal microvascular abnormalities (white arrow), and venous beading are present.

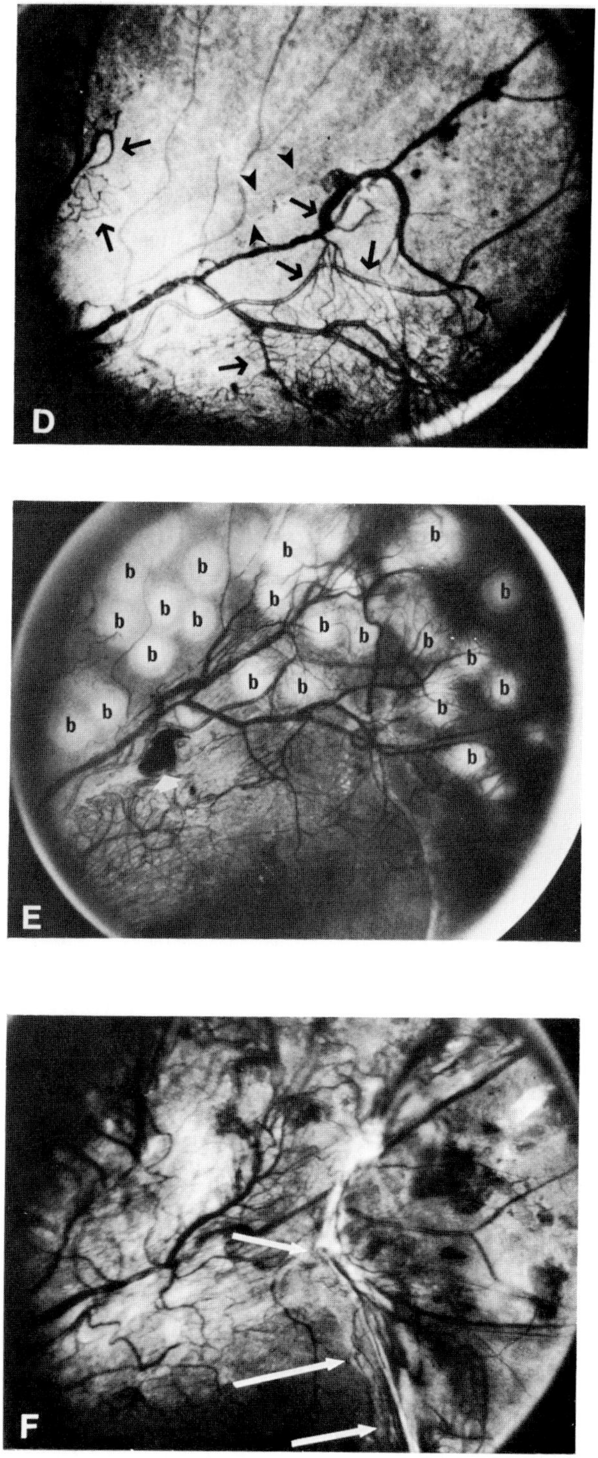

Fig. 4-10 (cont.) (D) By 10/76, there is an increase in the size of the retinal new vessels (black arrows) and the "feeder" vessel from the vein. The small arterioles above the vein are sheathed and appear white (small black arrowheads). (E) This picture was taken in 2/77, 2 hr after laser treatment; the photocoagulation burns appear white (b). A small preretinal hemorrhage, appearing black, is present (white arrowhead). (F,G) In 6/73 the visual acuity was 20/30. An area of fibrovascular proliferation with traction on the retina superior and temporal to the macula was present (white arrows).

(Figure continues on next page.)

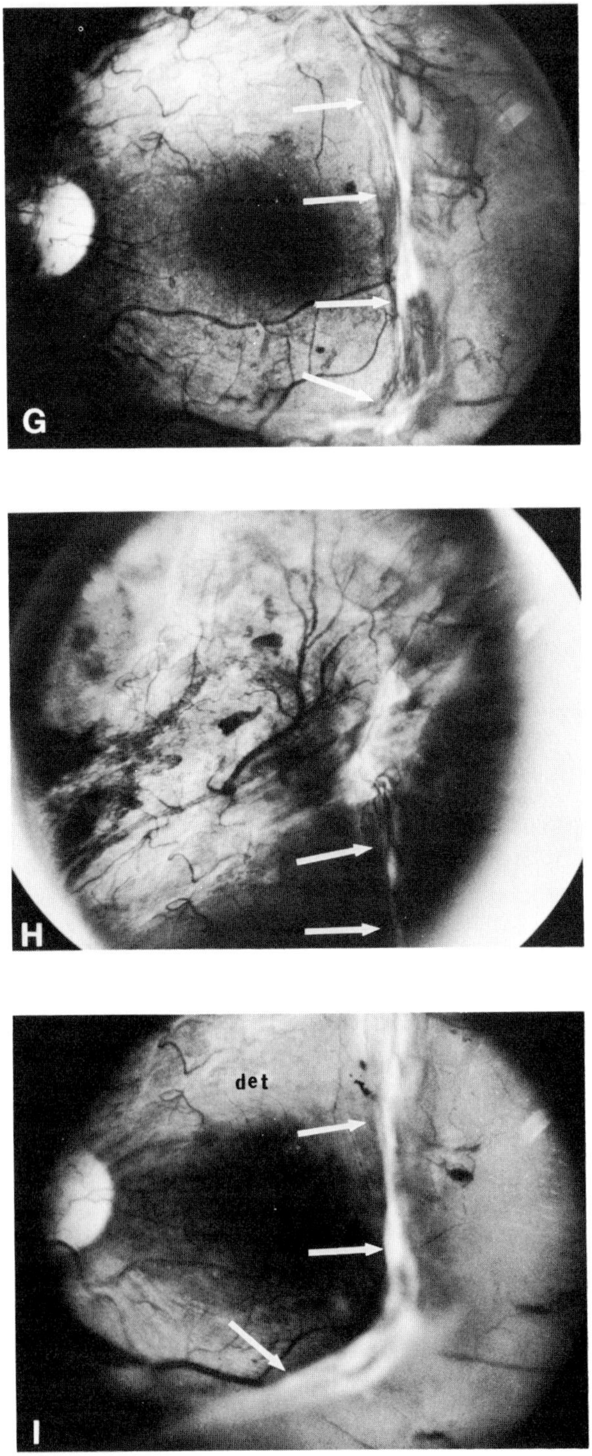

Fig. 4-10 (cont.) (H,I) On 7/15/77 further elevation of fibroproliferative tissue (white arrows) led to increased traction with detachment (det) of the area above the macula. The visual acuity had dropped to 20/70.

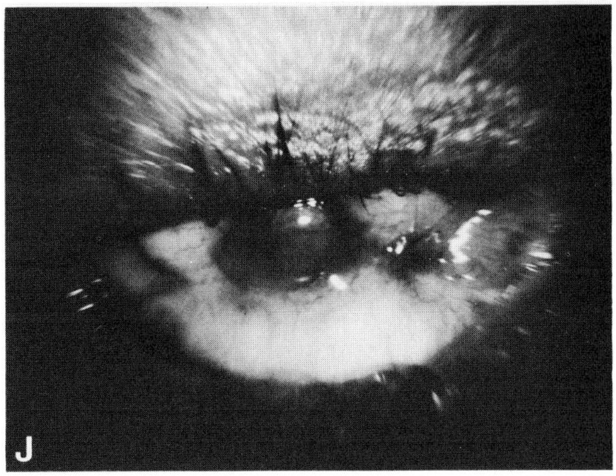

Fig. 4-10 (cont.) (J) The macular area became detached, and she underwent a vitrectomy and scleral buckle on 7/28/77. Corneal edema and blood in the anterior chamber developed after surgery. Later the eye became phthisical, and she had no light perception when this photograph was taken in 10/78. Her other eye had been enucleated in 4/77 as a result of pain from rubeotic glaucoma, secondary to traction retinal detachment and vitreous hemorrhage. (Courtesy of Dr. G. Bresnick, University of Wisconsin.)

outermost layer of the vitreous. Initially they consist of fine "naked" vessels which are permeable to fluorescein. These vessels may hemorrhage into the vitreous.

The mesenchymal cells responsible for the development of new blood vessels may also form fibrous tissue. Contraction of fibrovascular tissue may result in traction detachment of the retina. Fibrous tissue predominates and may remain as the only evidence of proliferative retinopathy if regression of new vessels occurs later in the course of the disease.

Diabetic Maculopathy

Occlusion or increased permeability of the retinal microvasculature that results in abnormal structure or function of the macular area has been called a "primary" or "intraretinal" maculopathy. Traction or dragging of the sensory retina due to shrinkage of fibrovascular vitreoretinal membranes causing altered macular function has been called "secondary" or "vitreoretinal" maculopathy.[5]

Intraretinal maculopathies associated with increased permeability are more common in patients with noninsulin-dependent diabetes and nonproliferative disease. Kohner[16] reported that 75 percent of patients with noninsulin-dependent diabetes seen in an ophthalmological clinic had intraretinal maculopathies. On the other hand, intraretinal maculopathies are less common in insulin-dependent diabetes and, when they occur, are more likely to be ischemic due to occlusion of the retinal blood vessels.

Increased permeability of retinal capillaries and retinal microaneurysms may result in accumulation of extracellular fluid and thickening of the normally compact retinal tissue. Initially, there may be a slight loss of the normal transparency of the retina, and the edema may be missed easily by direct ophthalmoscopy. The leakage and resulting edema may be focal around retinal microaneurysms or be diffuse and in some cases lead to the appearance of cystoid spaces in the outer retina. Focal leakage is usually associated with the deposition of hard exudative material, either in small clumps, rings, or large deposits (Fig. 4-4). The rings of hard exudate usually surround edematous centers, leaking retinal vessels and microaneurysms, and they demarcate the border of nonedematous and edematous retina. The accumulation of hard exudate in the macular area is usually gradual, and spontaneous resolution of the exudate may occur in time.[14]

Macular edema appearing as diffuse thickening of the posterior retina is associated with retinal ischemia, and hard exudate is seldom present. The diffuse leakage of retinal blood vessels is a result of an extensive breakdown of the normally impermeable blood-retinal barrier of the capillary endothelial cells. Patients with diffuse edema have widespread extravasation of fluorescein dye from the capillaries to the retinal tissue during angiography.

Reduced oncotic pressure due to decreased serum albumin levels, increased intravascular fluid load, increased arterial perfusion pressure, and tissue hypoxia have been postulated to cause macular edema by exacerbating breakdown of the blood-retinal barrier.[17] However, studies in patients with macular edema often fail to reveal a specific medical abnormality systematically associated with such edema. Bresnick,[17] summarizing recent data from fluorophotometric, histopathological, and photocoagulation studies, suggested that a diseased retinal pigment epithelium may contribute to the presence of macular edema. He suggested that the mechanism responsible for macular edema may be decreased transport of fluid out of the sensory retina and increased flow in.

Occlusion of retinal vessels may or may not be associated with increased vascular permeability. Using serial fluorescein angiograms, enlargement of the normal 450–600 μm diameter foveal avascular zone due to perifoveal capillary occlusion can be demonstrated.[5] If there is closure of the precapillary arterioles, larger areas of macular nonperfusion result (Fig. 4-7) and visual acuity may diminish. Severe ischemic maculopathy is associated with the appearance of cotton-wool spots, sheathing of the retinal arterioles, and proliferative retinopathy.

The vitreoretinal maculopathies all involve traction on the macular area, vary in severity, and result from a number of processes. A grayish or translucent glistening epiretinal glial membrane may be seen on the inner retinal surface, and contraction of this membrane may lead to a ''wrinkling'' effect. These membranes are also found in older nondiabetic patients, in diabetic patients with nonproliferative disease, and after panretinal photocoagulation, but they are more common in patients with proliferative retinopathy.[18]

In patients with proliferative retinopathy, shrinkage of fibrovascular tissue and detachment of the posterior vitreous surface may lead to an elevation or displacement of the sensory retina at the macula (Fig. 4-11).[19] A macular detachment may result from traction leading to a retinal tear with fluid accumulation beneath the retina including the macular area (Fig. 4-10).

Classification

Various classification schemes for diabetic retinopathy have been used beginning with that of Hirschberg in 1890.[20–24] Most schemes have been based on the natural history of the disease.

The modified Airlie House Classification of diabetic retinopathy[23,24] has been used in a number of clinical and epidemiological studies.[3,12] This system allows spec-

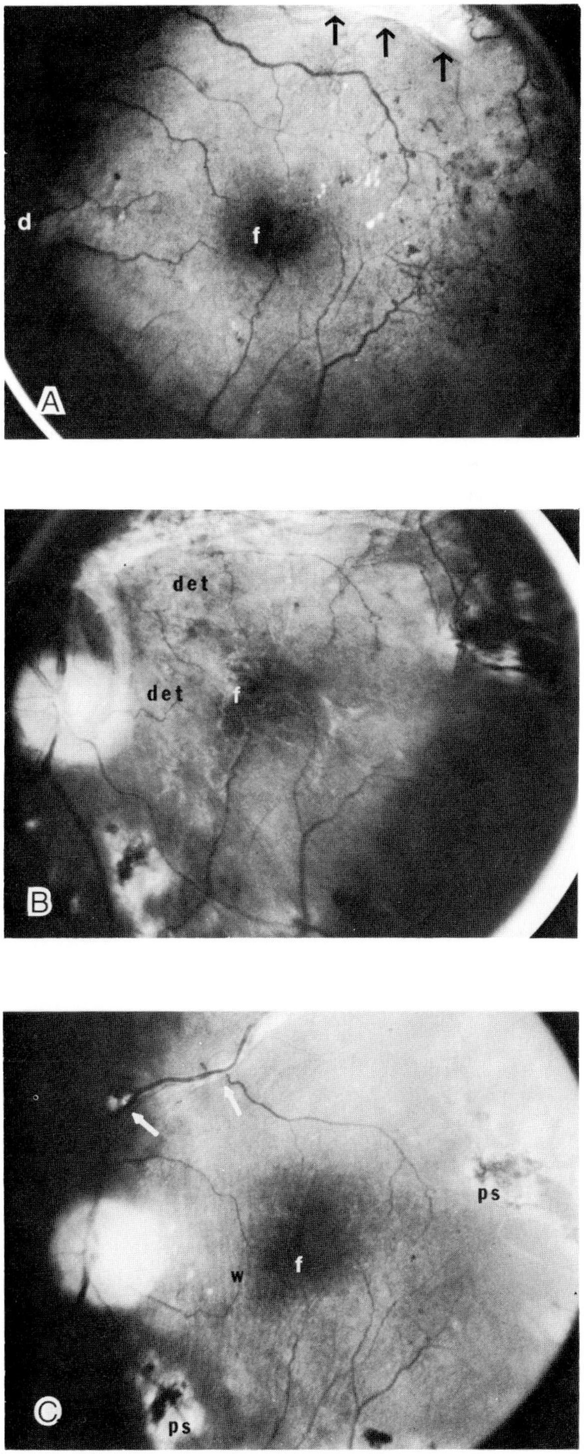

Fig. 4-11 (A) Fundus photograph of the left eye of a 45-year-old man with a 17-year history of insulin-dependent diabetes. Proliferative diabetic retinopathy with fibrovascular tissue is present superior to the macular area (black arrows). f = foveal area. d = optic disc. Hard exudates, intraretinal microvascular abnormalities, and blot hemorrhages and microaneurysms are present temporal to the macula. The visual acuity was 20/40 at the time this photograph was taken in 7/80. (B) After argon laser photocoagulation treatment in 10/80 and 11/80, some displacement of the macula was present with progressive reduction of visual acuity to 5/200 when this photograph was taken in 3/82. A low traction retinal detachment (det) temporal to the optic disc and cystoid changes were present at the foveal area in (A) and (B). (C) Photograph of the same area, taken 9/83, 7 months after vitrectomy. Visual acuity had improved to 8/200. The fibrovascular tissue superior and temporal to the disc had been cut (white arrows), and the foveal area (f) had moved slightly temporal to its position in (B). Wrinkling of the retina (W) is present. Pigmented photocoagulation scars (ps) are present. (Courtesy of Dr. T. Stevens, University of Wisconsin.)

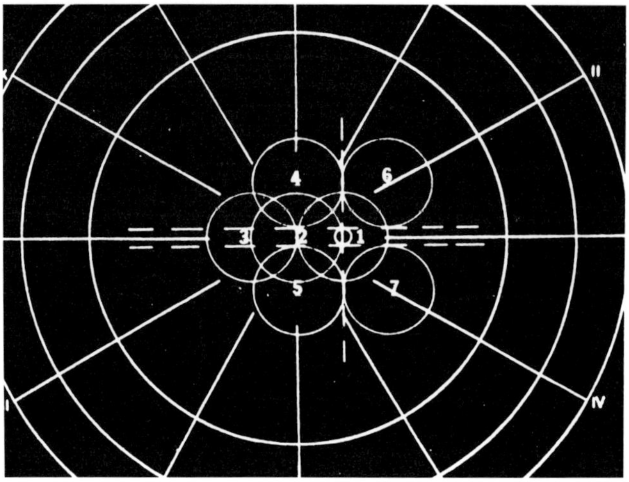

Fig. 4-12 Posterior pole area of the retina of the right eye demonstrating seven standard photographic fields. Field 1 is taken centered on the disc; field 2 is centered on the foveal area; field 3 is centered temporal to the foveal area with its nasal edge passing through the foveal area; field 4 is superior temporal and field 6 is superior nasal to the optic disc; field 5 is inferior temporal and field 7 is inferior nasal to the optic disc.

ification of the presence or absence, as well as the severity, of each of 17 major lesions characteristic of diabetic retinopathy. These lesions are identified by grading stereoscopic color fundus photographs of seven standard 30° fields of the posterior retina (Fig. 4-12). The graders determine the severity of the specific lesions using photographic color standards for comparison.[24]

A number of modified schemes have been developed to provide an indication of overall severity of retinopathy for a given eye or patient as the modified Airlie House Classification scheme does not do this.[12,25] In reporting a study of the natural history of diabetic retinopathy in 191 insulin-dependent patients, Klein et al.[25] developed one such scheme based on increasing severity of the disease. This "191" classification system is presented in Table 4-1. Using this system various degrees of severity from simple presence or absence to 45 hierarchical levels of retinopathy may be defined depending on the specific needs of the study.

Photographic documentation of retinopathy and use of photographic standards for grading severity of retinal lesions allows detection of early changes, minimizes observer bias by masking the graders with respect to patient characteristics and treatments, provides monitoring of quality control of the documentation, and permits comparisons over time. Palmberg et al.[11] reported that grading stereoscopic fundus photographs was 57 percent more sensitive than ophthalmoscopy in detecting retinopathy at all levels of severity.

Pathogenesis

Although many pathophysiological changes have been found in association with diabetic retinopathy, the exact pathogenesis is unknown. It is frequently assumed that retinopathy is a consequence of hyperglycemia. This is supported by: (1) the strong association of retinopathy with increasing duration of disease[2,12,13]; (2) the finding of retinopathy in secondary diabetes[26]; and (3) the production of retinopathy in experimental diabetes in animal models.[27–29] However, the actual mechanism by which high

Table 4-1. Classification of Diabetic Retinopathy

Level	Description
1	No retinopathy
2	Microaneurysms only
3	Microaneurysms and mild hemorrhages and/or mild hard exudates without other lesions, e.g., soft exudates, early venous beading, intraretinal microvascular abnormalities (IRMAs), new vessels, vitreous hemorrhage
4	Microaneurysms plus more severe hemorrhages or more severe hard exudates and/or presence of mild soft exudates, venous beading, or IRMAs without new vessels or vitreous hemorrhage
5	Preproliferative retinopathy with more soft exudates or IRMAs or venous beading present
6	Proliferative retinopathy in the absence of DRS high-risk characteristics for visual loss
7	DRS high-risk characteristics—one or more of the following: new vessels elsewhere greater than one-half disc area and preretinal hemorrhage or vitreous hemorrhage; new vessels on or within 1 DD of the disc graded less than one-third disc area with preretinal or vitreous hemorrhage; new vessels on or within 1 DD of disc graded ≥ one-third disc area with or without preretinal or vitreous hemorrhage
8	Eyes which could not be graded for retinopathy level because of vitreous hemorrhages obscuring the retina, phthisis bulbi, or enucleation secondary to a complication of diabetic retinopathy

blood glucose levels lead to retinopathy is not known. There are several hypothesized but unproved pathogenetic explanations. One explanation is an increase in sorbitol as a result of sugar metabolism through the polyol pathway.[30] According to this theory, aldose reductase-initiated accumulation of sorbitol may lead to selective degeneration of mural cells. A second role of the polyol pathway in diabetic retinopathy may be its relationship to the development of abnormal basement membrane thickening,[23,31] which has been hypothesized to cause closure of retinal capillary vessels. This thickening can be prevented by aldose reductase inhibitors in galactosemic rats.[31,32]

A second proposed mechanism is abnormal release of growth hormone associated with impaired glucose metabolism.[33] Increased growth hormone in turn is thought to result in plasma protein abnormalities (increases in alpha-$_2$-globulins, fibrinogen, haptoglobins, and C-reactive proteins) which may be associated with increased plasma viscosity and decreased retinal blood flow.

The relationship of nonenzymatic or enzymatic glycosylation of proteins which occurs in diabetes to the pathogenesis of retinopathy remains obscure.

Whatever the cause, most proposed pathogenetic mechanisms are based on the assumption that retinal hypoxia is present early in the development of retinopathy.[2,5,33–36] Retinal hypoxia has been hypothesized to result from decreased oxygen release from hemoglobin, as has been reported by Ditzel in diabetic patients.[36] This has been attributed to decreased red blood cell 2,3-diphosphoglycerate, increased hemoglobin A_1, and increased blood lipids.[33–36]

Another explanation for the development of hypoxia is that abnormalities in oxygen delivery result from altered retinal blood flow.[6,33,35] Abnormalities in retinal blood flow have been found even before the development of ophthalmoscopically visible diabetic retinopathy.[37–39] Kohner et al.[37,38] measured retinal blood flow based on an indicator dilution technique adapted to retinal blood vessels. They reported a decreased transit time of fluorescein dye and an increased volume flow in diabetic patients with no or early retinopathy compared to normal controls. Increased blood flow has also been found in the renal, cerebral, and peripheral circulations in persons with diabetes.[40]

In contrast, Yoshida et al.[41] reported decreased segmental blood flow in retinal vessels in diabetic patients without retinopathy compared to normal control subjects using laser doppler velocitometry, which measures flow velocity of the red blood cells. The discrepancies in blood flow changes early in the disease that are reported by the various studies[37,38,40] may result from the alternative techniques used to examine flow.

Later in the course of the disease, with the appearance of nonproliferative retinopathy, retinal blood flow has been reported to be decreased.[41,42] Reduction in retinal blood flow in diabetes has been hypothesized to result from abnormalities in plasma viscosity, platelet and red blood cell function, blood vessel wall structure and permeability, and autoregulatory mechanisms.[5,33–36]

Reduction in blood flow has been attributed to increased blood viscosity.[33] Abnormalities in blood viscosity have been found by some investigators.[33,43–45] Little demonstrated increased plasma viscosity in diabetic patients without retinopathy compared to nondiabetic control patients.[33] Others have shown a strong correlation between increased plasma viscosity and increased severity of retinopathy.[45] Increased red blood cell aggregation found in diabetic patients may also cause an increase in plasma viscosity.[46] However, this same investigator[46] as well as others[47] found no difference in plasma viscosity of persons with short duration of diabetes and no retinopathy compared to a group of nondiabetic persons.

A second possible cause of reduced blood flow in diabetic patients may be platelet abnormalities. In a recent review Colwell et al.[48] described a number of studies in which increased platelet aggregation was present before the appearance of retinopathy and further increased in patients with severe microvascular disease. Aggregated platelets *in vitro* were more stable and less likely to disaggregate in diabetic patients than in control subjects. Increased platelet aggregation may be a result of increased production of aggregatory thromboxane A_2, decreased antiaggregatory prostacyclin synthesis, and elevated von Willebrand factor, all of which are found in diabetic patients in contrast to nondiabetic patients.[48]

A third possible cause of decreased retinal blood flow may be narrowing of blood vessel lumens due to encroachment of thickened retinal capillary wall. Thickening may result if there is an increased permeability of the endothelial cells to plasma proteins. Normally, the capillary endothelial cells are impermeable to plasma proteins.[49] However, cell membrane damage may occur as suggested by increased permeability of fluorescein early in the course of diabetes.[2,5,6] Possible causes of such damage include increased retinal capillary rigidity, decreased deformability of the red blood cells, increased blood viscosity, and increased hydrostatic pressure.[33] It may be that the increased capillary rigidity makes the endothelial cell lining more susceptible to damage from the effects of high blood pressure and from the shearing force of the red blood cells.[33,50]

Autoregulation of retinal blood flow, which is normally controlled by local factors, e.g., pCO_2, pH,$p0_2$, may respond insufficiently to the reduced oxygen caused by the aforementioned mechanisms, resulting in further tissue hypoxia. Hickam and Sieker[51] reported a reduction in the normal retinal vasoconstriction response to 100 percent oxygen in diabetic patients. This abnormality became worse with the development of diabetic retinopathy.[52] Using a blue-field entoptic technique, Sinclair et al.[53] reported abnormalities in autoregulation of macular blood flow in response to changes in the intraocular pressure in diabetic patients.

The pathophysiological findings described above suggest that abnormalities in the diabetic microvasculature may play a primary role in diabetic retinopathy. Metabolic and physiological alterations in the neuronal retina may also precede or accompany the circulatory changes. This is suggested by retinal function abnormalities in diabetic patients without ophthalmoscopically detectable vascular retinopathy. Examples are the reduction in the amplitude of the oscillatory potentials of the electroretinograms and the decrease in the electrooculogram light-peak/dark-trough ratio in the diabetic patients with no retinopathy[54] and abnormalities in spectral sensitivity.[55] Tritan (blue-yellow) color vision defects with red and blue cone sensitivity have been reported to occur before the appearance of retinopathy.[55] Delay in the visual evoked cortical response, suggesting the possibility of physiological abnormalities in the optic nerve or higher visual pathway has been reported in 62 percent of 16 diabetic subjects without evidence of retinopathy or multiple sclerosis.[56]

Why the microvasculature is differentially affected in different organs is still an unanswered question. Although the brain and retina are both neural tissue, it is rare to find microvascular abnormalities in the brains of diabetic patients.[57] Studies are needed to assess the role of early retinal neuronal abnormalities as an initiating cause of the retinopathy.

Description of the pathogenesis of retinopathy will require the development of improved classification schemes of early retinopathy, new animal models (the BB Wistar rat[58]), improved physiological methods of measuring retinal blood flow (doppler measurements[59]) and oxygenation of retinal tissue (retinal oximetry[60]), and cellular biological techniques to describe early abnormalities on the cellular level (endothelial and pericyte tissue culture[61,62]).

Little is known about the processes responsible for the formation of new retinal blood vessels. Retinal ischemia and resultant hypoxia are hypothesized to liberate retinal angiogenic substances.[63,64] A number of angiogenic substances have been identified as being present in retinal tissue, but their role in the development of retinal new vessels remains unclear.[65] Also unclear is the role of the vitreous gel in inhibiting angiogenesis.

Risk Factors

Knowledge of various demographic, genetic, systemic, and ocular factors that are associated with increased risk of incidence or progression of retinopathy is of great importance in: (1) efforts to prevent or modify the course of retinopathy; (2) characterization of the "high-risk" patient; and (3) prediction of health service needs.[66,67] Data about risk factors for retinopathy have been obtained largely from specialty clinics[10,11,68–73] and from geographically defined populations.[12,13,74–79] A number of methodological problems due to the size or the selection of the population studied,[68–73] failure to use standardized examination protocols,[68–71] and use of arbitrary classification schemes or definitions[2,68–71] have resulted in difficulty in interpretation and lack of comparability of the data collected. For example, the presence and severity of retinopathy was determined by a retrospective chart review of routine examinations by internists through undilated pupils in one study,[73] whereas in other studies fluorescein angiography was used.[10,11] Such discrepancies may be responsible for findings from various studies of significant positive or no associations between risk factors (e.g., blood pressure, metabolic control) and retinopathy.[70,71,74,75,80]

Duration of Diabetes

Insulin-Dependent Diabetes. The frequency and severity of diabetic retinopathy increases with increasing duration of diabetes.[2,10–13,74–77] In the Wisconsin Epidemiologic Study of Diabetic Retinopathy (WESDR), a large geographically defined population of diabetic patients was examined.[81] Objective recording of retinopathy by use of stereoscopic fundus photography and use of a standardized protocol for grading the retinopathy were employed.[12] In the 995 insulin-taking diabetic participants diagnosed before 30 years of age examined in this study, the rates of retinopathy rose from 17 percent in persons who had diabetes for less than 5 years to 97.5 percent in those who had had diabetes for 15 years or more (Fig. 4-13).[12] Similarly, in a population-based study in Poole, England, Houston[76] reported a rise in the prevalence of diabetic retinopathy in insulin-taking persons from 5 percent during the first 5 years to 80 percent in persons with 25–30 years of diabetes.

In two clinic-based studies, Frank et al.[10] and Palmberg et al.,[11] using fundus photographs and fluorescein angiograms, reported low rates of retinopathy during the

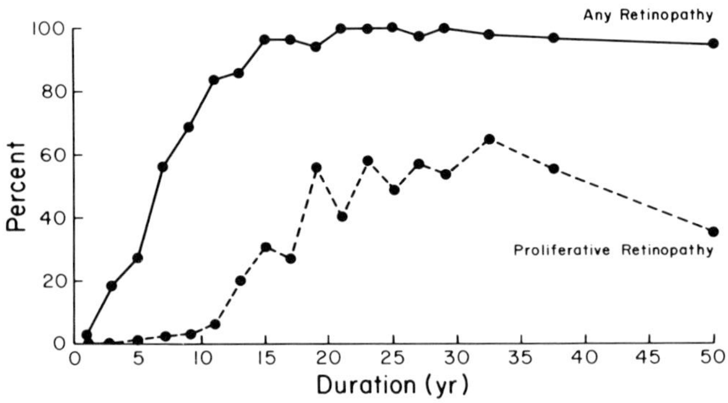

Fig. 4-13 The frequency of retinopathy or proliferative retinopathy by duration of diabetes (years) in 995 insulin-taking persons diagnosed to have diabetes before 30 years of age who participated in the WESDR. (Reprinted with permission from Klein R, Klein BEK, Moss SE, et al: The Wisconsin epidemiologic study of diabetic retinopathy. 2. Prevalence and risk of diabetic retinopathy when age at diagnosis is less than 30 years. Arch Ophthalmol, 102:520, 1984.)

first 5 years of insulin-dependent diabetes (less than 20 percent), rising to 29 or 63 percent, respectively, after 9 years. All of the above findings differ from three studies[82–84] in which a high prevalence of retinopathy (appearance of retinal microaneurysms on fluorescein angiograms but not on color photographs) was reported in insulin-dependent diabetic children shortly after diagnosis. It is probable that hyperfluorescence of retinal drusen and other retinal pigment epithelial abnormalities were mistaken for retinal microaneurysms in these studies.

One exception to the relationship between retinopathy and duration of diabetes is found in children. It is rare to find diabetic retinopathy during the first decade of life, regardless of the duration of the disease.[10–12,85,86] In the WESDR, insulin-taking patients diagnosed at age 14 years were found to be three times as likely to have retinopathy at 22 years of age as patients diagnosed at 4 years of age when they are 12.[12] In a follow-up study of 60 insulin-dependent diabetic children, Frost-Larsen and Starup[87] found the incidence of retinopathy to be higher after puberty than before independent of duration, metabolic control of diabetes, or type of treatment. A number of studies suggest that possible hormonal changes (i.e., growth hormone, somatomedin C) associated with puberty may play a role in the development of retinopathy.[29,88,89]

However, aside from the young children, the severity of retinopathy tends to increase with increasing duration. In the WESDR, the prevalence of proliferative retinopathy rose from 0 percent before 5 years to 4 percent at 9–10 years, 26 percent at 15–16 years, and 56 percent at 20 years or greater duration of diabetes (Fig. 4-13).[12] These rates are similar to those reported by White for the Joslin Clinic[90] but higher than those reported by others.[2,11,74,75]

In the WESDR, 9.5 percent of persons with onset of insulin-requiring diabetes before age 30 had macular edema.[91] The prevalence of macular edema rose from 0 percent in persons with diabetes of 5 years to 21 percent in persons with diabetes duration of more than 20 years.

There have been few studies which have examined the incidence of new retinopathy and rates of progression of existing retinopathy in insulin-dependent diabetes.[68–71] In one retrospective study, Burditt et al.[68] reported the incidence and progression of retinopathy in patients diagnosed before 30 years of age who underwent routine ophthalmoscopic examination in the Radcliffe Diabetes Clinic. They reported that the 5-year incidence of new retinopathy or progression of existing retinopathy was approximately 40 percent. In another study of insulin-dependent patients with 5 years or more of diabetes (the Wisconsin "191" Study), 39 percent of persons with no retinopathy when first seen developed nonproliferative retinopathy in 2 years, and 86 percent developed it in 6 years.[25] In persons who had retinopathy at the first examination, progression was observed in 19 percent 2 years later and in 58 percent 6 years after their baseline examination. In patients with moderate to severe nonproliferative retinopathy in each eye at the baseline visit, 72 percent had progressed to proliferative retinopathy in at least one eye in 6 years. Progression of retinopathy was a function of the duration of the diabetes as well as the severity of the retinopathy when the patients were first seen.

Diabetic retinopathy regresses infrequently. Five-year rates of regression in persons with early nonproliferative retinopathy (consisting of retinal microaneurysms) have been reported to vary from 7 percent to 36 percent.[2] Spontaneous regression with disappearance of any sign of proliferative retinopathy is relatively infrequent.

Noninsulin-Dependent Diabetes. Less information is available about prevalence of retinopathy in persons with noninsulin-dependent diabetes.[2,13,68–71,73–79] Many of the published reports have defined this condition by age at diagnosis of diabetes (at or after 30 or 40 years of age) but have not described hypoglycemic medication status, body weight, or history of ketosis[2,68–71,73,76]; therefore it is likely that insulin-dependent patients are included in these reports.

Diabetic retinopathy has been reported at the time of diagnosis in a small percentage of older-onset patients.[2,76,92] In most reports rates of retinopathy are higher in noninsulin-taking patients diagnosed after 30 years of age than for insulin-taking younger-onset patients during the first few years after diagnosis (Figs. 4-13 and 4-14).[2,12,13,68,76] In the Poole population, the rate of retinopathy in noninsulin-treated patients was 17 percent during the first year of diabetes.[76] In the WESDR the prevalence of retinopathy during the first 3 years of diabetes was 24 percent in noninsulin-taking persons diagnosed to have diabetes at or after 30 years of age compared to 2 percent in insulin-taking persons diagnosed before 30 years of age (Figs. 4-13 and 4-14).[12,13] The finding of higher rates of retinopathy shortly after diagnosis in noninsulin-dependent diabetic patients may represent a detection bias; that is, persons diagnosed after 30 years of age are less likely to be diagnosed at the time of onset of their disease; they may have been diabetic for years before the actual date of diagnosis. Alternatively, the microvasculature in the older-onset diabetic persons may be more sensitive to factors responsible for the development of retinopathy.

With increasing duration of diabetes, rates of retinopathy in noninsulin-taking patients fail to reach levels reported in insulin-taking patients. In the WESDR popu-

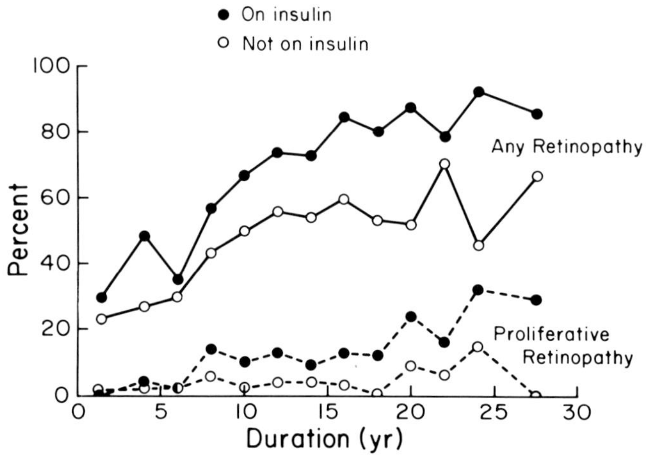

Fig. 4-14 The frequency of retinopathy or proliferative retinopathy by duration of diabetes (years) in 673 insulin-taking and 697 noninsulin-taking persons diagnosed to have diabetes after 29 years of age who participated in the WESDR. (Reprinted with permission from Klein R, Klein BEK, Moss SE, et al.: The Wisconsin epidemiologic study of diabetic retinopathy. 3. Prevalence and risk of diabetic retinopathy when age at diagnosis is 30 or more years. Arch Ophthalmol, 102:527, 1984.)

lation, retinopathy developed in approximately 60 percent of noninsulin-taking older-onset persons (diagnosis after 29 years of age) but in 84 percent of insulin-taking older-onset and in 97.5 percent of insulin-taking younger-onset persons (Figs. 4-13 and 4-14).[12,13] Forty-two percent of noninsulin-treated diabetic persons in Poole, England, were found to have retinopathy after 15–20 years of diabetes.[76]

The severity of retinopathy increases with increasing disease duration in noninsulin-taking patients, as in the insulin-taking patients. In the WESDR, rates of proliferative retinopathy in noninsulin-taking older-onset patients rose from 1 percent during the first 3 years of the disease to about 10 percent after 20 years of diabetes (Fig. 4-14).[13] Comparable rates have been reported by Burditt et al.[68] in older-onset patients (30–59 years of age, medication status unspecified) and in Poole, England.[76]

Less information is available about the incidence or progression of retinopathy in persons with noninsulin-dependent diabetes than in insulin-dependent persons. Burditt et al.[68] reported a 5-year incidence of retinopathy of 45 percent and a rate of progression of 60 percent in diabetic persons whose age at diagnosis was 30–59 years. If these patients had mild or moderately severe nonproliferative retinopathy and 5–9 years of diabetes when they were first seen, they had a 20 percent 5-year risk of developing proliferative retinopathy. Lower rates of progression were found in persons diagnosed to have diabetes after 60 years of age.

In the noninsulin-taking Pima Indian population, Knowler et al.[93] reported the 6-year incidence of retinopathy to be 24 percent. Increased incidence was associated with longer duration of diabetes.

Macular edema is reported to be more common in older-onset patients than in younger-onset patients.[94,95] In the WESDR, rates of macular edema also increase with increasing duration of diabetes, ranging from 3 percent at 5 years to 13 percent at 15 years or more in noninsulin-taking patients.[91] In a referral practice at the Joslin Clinic, macular edema was found to be more common (45 percent) in noninsulin-dependent patients diagnosed after 40 years of age than in insulin-dependent patients (17 percent) who were diagnosed before 30 years of age.[94]

Sex

Most studies have shown no sex difference in the prevalence of retinopathy[2]; this was not true in the WESDR, where a higher rate of proliferative disease (with Diabetic Retinopathy Study high-risk characteristics for visual loss) or actual loss of vision due to retinopathy was reported in younger-onset insulin-taking males (11 percent) than in females (6 percent).[12,96] In a case-control study, Bodansky et al.[97] also reported a higher proportion of males (68 percent) in the group with proliferative retinopathy than in the group with minimal or no retinopathy (45 percent). The reason for the sex difference is unknown.

Race

There are no population-based data comparing the prevalence or severity of diabetic retinopathy between blacks and whites in the United States. Jackson et al.[98] found no differences between the frequency of retinopathy in white or black diabetic patients studied in Cape Town, South Africa.

Genetic Factors

There is considerable disagreement regarding the relationship between the prevalence of retinopathy and genetic factors.[99–113] In favor of a relationship is the finding that retinopathy occurs more often among concordant (both have diabetes) identical twin pairs.[99–101] In addition, the time of appearance of retinopathy, as well as its severity are similar among concordant identical twins, suggesting that the tendency to develop diabetic retinopathy and possibly its progression are influenced by genetic factors. Furthermore, a positive association between the severity of diabetic retinopathy and the presence of HLA-B8 or HLA-B15 and DR-4 antigens in insulin-dependent diabetes mellitus has been reported in several studies.[102–106] In one study the odds ratio for retinopathy among patients with HLA-DR4 was 2.0; patients with both DR4 and poor control of blood sugar were at greatly increased risk of retinopathy. In contrast, Rand[107] reported a relative protective effect with respect to retinopathy when DR3 and DR4 were both present (in Joslin Clinic patients studied in a case-control investigation).[107] However, several studies report no association between HLA antigens or antigens of the BF locus, also located on chromosome 6, and retinopathy.[108–113] The reasons for discrepancies among studies may be due to the limited size or the select nature of the groups studied, failure to use standardized protocols, absence of objective recording of retinopathy, and inadequate statistical control of confounding risk variables.[102–113] Accurate data concerning the relationship between genetic markers and the incidence and progression of diabetic retinopathy are of interest and importance in describing patients at increased risk and in developing better understanding of possible causal relationships.

Control of Hyperglycemia

Review of the existing experimental literature using animal models leaves little doubt as to the strong relationship between good metabolic control and less retinopathy.[27,114] In a prospective trial of "good" and "poor" control in alloxan-induced diabetes in dogs, Engerman et al.[114] demonstrated fewer and less severe retinal microangiopathic changes (microaneurysms, capillary dropout, etc.) in "well" controlled than in "poorly" controlled animals.

It has not been easy to determine the relationship between metabolic control and retinopathy in diabetic patients. Despite the numerous clinical and epidemiological studies suggesting a beneficial effect of good metabolic control on retinopathy, a number of limitations exist in the interpretation of these data.[2,12,13,68,70–72,75,77,78,115,116] There have been problems in defining and achieving "good" metabolic control, as well as in measuring it. There has been little information available in these studies on the role of patient compliance. The question of underlying severity of the diabetes, leading to poorer control and possibly to more severe retinopathy, has not been answerable in the absence of a randomized therapeutic trial of metabolic control.

The Univeristy Group Diabetes Program (UGDP) initiated in 1960 was a long-term prospective clinical trial designed to evaluate the effects of four methods of treatment (oral hypoglycemic agents, insulin in fixed or variable doses, and diet only) on mortality and vascular complications in noninsulin-dependent diabetes.[117] No significant differences were found in the incidence or progression of retinopathy in the groups studied at 5 years or at 12 years (for the insulin and diet groups) despite differences in levels of control as measured by fasting blood glucose values.

With the advent of continuous subcutaneous insulin infusion (CSII) systems, the wider acceptance of multidose (three or four doses per day) treatment regimens, the development of newer means of determining control using home glucose monitoring and glycosylated hemoglobin, randomized therapeutic trials comparing differences in metabolic control in insulin-dependent diabetes became feasible. Data from three such trials have recently been reported.[118–120]

A prospective randomized study comparing CSII to conventional treatment (CT) in achieving metabolic control and reducing the progression of retinopathy in 30 insulin-dependent diabetic patients was done at the Steno Memorial Hospital in Denmark.[118] Significantly lower mean blood sugars and glycosylated hemoglobin levels were reported in the CSII group compared to the CT groups after 3 months and were maintained up to 24 months after the start of the study. Measures of retinal function (electroretinographic oscillatory potential, macular recovery time, and posterior vitreous fluorophotometry) improved in the CSII group and deteriorated in the CT group at 6 and 12 months of this study. However, in both groups there was significant progression of the retinopathy. At 1 year, progression of retinopathy was found in 67 percent of CSII patients and 33 percent of CT patients. After 2 years, progression of retinopathy was similar between the CSII and CT groups. In most cases, progression of retinopathy was associated with the appearance of cotton-wool spots or retinal hemorrhages. Similarly, in the Kroc study, a multicentered therapeutic trial involving 69 insulin-dependent patients who were randomly assigned to either CSII or CT, progression of retinopathy was reported for both groups over an 8-month period, despite significant improvement in metabolic control in the CSII group.[119] The CSII group tended to show slightly faster progression of retinopathy (between-group differences were of borderline significance). Progression in the CSII group was associated with the appearance of cotton-wool spots. Similar findings have been reported from a small trial in Oslo.[120] The appearance of cotton-wool spots in the well-controlled experimental group in all three studies have been hypothesized to have resulted directly from the abruptly decreased supply of glucose and changes in retinal blood perfusion or indirectly from elevations in other factors (e.g., somatomedin C) which have been associated with progression of retinopathy.[121] Hypoglycemia which has been reported to cause enhanced intravascular platelet aggregation, and intravascular coagulation may have contributed to development of cotton-wool spots.[122]

Conclusions drawn from these studies are limited because of the small sample sizes and the short period of time the patients were studied.[118–120] These studies included no patients without retinopathy, and thus the question of preventing the development of retinopathy by metabolic control has not been answered. The 7- to 10-year Diabetes Control and Complications Trial was designed to assess the relationship between metabolic control and the development or progression of early retinopathy in persons with insulin-dependent diabetes mellitus.[123] It is currently in its feasibility stage.

Blood Pressure

Because high blood pressure per se can cause many of the lesions associated with diabetic retinopathy (e.g., cotton-wool spots, retinal hemorrhages, and microaneurysms), it was not unexpected that a positive association between blood pressure and severity of retinopathy has been reported by a number of investigators.[12,13,74,75,79,93,97] The relative risk for the presence of retinopathy during the first 10 years of diabetes for the WESDR younger-onset insulin-taking persons with diastolic blood pressure in the highest quartile compared to those in the lowest quartile was about two; for persons with 10 years or more of diabetes, the relative risk of proliferative retinopathy in persons whose diastolic blood pressure was in the highest quartile compared to those whose diastolic blood pressure was in the lowest quartile was also about 2.[12] Similarly, the highest risk for retinopathy was reported for persons with highest blood pressure in the older-onset insulin- or noninsulin-taking persons.[13]

Macular edema has also been reported to be associated with increased blood pressure. Deutsch et al. found that patients with macular edema in one clinic in the Early Treatment Diabetic Retinopathy Study (ETDRS) had higher mean blood pressure than patients without edema.[124] Similar findings have been reported in the WESDR for insulin- or noninsulin-taking persons.[91]

Whether the relationship between blood pressure and retinopathy is etiological or both are the result of the effect of diabetes on the microvascular system is difficult to assess from prevalence studies. To date there has been only one longitudinal study examining this relationship.[93] In a 5-year follow-up of a population of noninuslin-dependent Pima Indians, Knowler et al.[93] reported twice the incidence of retinal hard exudates in persons with elevated blood pressure. However, the failure to find a similar relationship of elevated blood pressure with other retinal lesions and the possibility that retinal drusen may have been confused with hard exudates in that study leave the nature of this relationship obscure. Because hypertension is a known risk factor for cardiovascular disease,[125] even though its relationship to retinopathy is unclear, it is reasonable for blood pressure to be controlled.

Smoking

Smoking, a known risk factor for cardiovascular disease, has been implicated in some studies as being causally related to retinopathy.[126,127] One might anticipate such an association because smoking may cause tissue hypoxia by increasing blood carbon monoxide levels.[128] Additionally, smoking may lead to increased platelet adhesiveness.[129] Paetkau et al.[126] first reported a positive association between smoking and proliferative diabetic retinopathy in 181 patients referred to a fluorescein angiography unit. Nielsen and Hjollund[127] also found a relationship between severity of retinopathy and cigarette smoking in male, but not in female, insulin-dependent diabetic patients. Five subsequent studies have failed to demonstrate an association between the risk of retinopathy and a smoking history.[77,130–133] However, results of cross-sectional studies may be limited if selective mortality is occurring; that is, if smokers with severe retinopathy die, the relationship of smoking and retinopathy in survivors may be minimal.

Body Mass (Obesity)

The severity of retinopathy has been reported to be associated inversely with body mass index in noninsulin-taking persons.[13,75,77] This finding is compatible with the concept that obese older-onset noninsulin-taking patients have a milder form of the disease. No association has been reported for insulin-taking younger- or older-onset patients.[12,13]

Pregnancy

In a review of the literature, Rodman et al.[134] found that only 17 (8 percent) of 201 cases of pregnant diabetic patients with no or early nonproliferative retinopathy at the onset of their pregnancy progressed; only 4 of these 17 developed proliferative diabetic retinopathy. In 127 cases of women known to have proliferative retinopathy at the onset of their pregnancy, 32 (25 percent) experienced progression during the pregnancy. In a review of the Joslin Clinic data by Beetham[135] in 1950 and in a study by Carstensen et al.,[136] duration of diabetes before pregnancy was found to be the most important determinant of the progression of retinopathy.

Larinkari et al.,[137] in an uncontrolled follow-up series of patients, observed progression of retinopathy in 8 of 42 pregnant diabetic patients. Progression of retinopathy was related to increased duration of diabetes, increased severity of retinopathy at the onset of disease, poor control of blood glucose during the first trimester, and higher serum progesterone concentrations.

In a prospective study, Moloney and Drury[138] reported a 40 percent incidence of retinopathy in patients who were free of retinopathy at the beginning of the pregnancy. There was a 0 percent incidence of retinopathy in 120 nonpregnant insulin-dependent control subjects. In patients with background retinopathy at the onset of their pregnancies, progression, manifested by streak or blot hemorrhages, occurred in 53 percent, and cotton-wool spots occurred in 29 percent. In comparison, streak or blot hemorrhages occurred in only 8 percent and soft exudates in 0 percent of the diabetic nonpregnant control group. Only one of the pregnant women with nonproliferative retinopathy progressed to proliferative disease. In the pregnant group ophthalmoscopic manifestations of retinopathy disappeared in 12 (22.6 percent) patients after delivery. Development of streak and blot hemorrhages was associated with increased insulin requirement, higher fasting blood glucose, and hemoglobin A_1 levels early in pregnancy. Soft exudates were associated with lower fasting blood glucose levels late in pregnancy but not with hypertension or preeclamptic toxemia.

With the development of photocoagulation there has been much change in the management of female diabetic patients since 1950, when Beetham recommended "in their own best interests, patients presenting a large amount of retinal hemorrhage, or proliferating retinopathy, should not be permitted to undertake pregnancy."[135] Current management recommendations include evaluation by an ophthalmologist of all insulin-dependent diabetic patients considering pregnancy or those who have become pregnant. Those women with no or mild retinopathy, although at low risk of progression, should be followed by an ophthalmologist and seen more frequently than usual during gestation (perhaps every 2–3 months), especially if they develop complications, e.g., toxemia or progression of retinopathy. Because panretinal photocoagulation has been shown to cause significant regression of retinal new blood vessels and prevent serious reduction of vision, women with severe preproliferative or proliferative retinopathy should be referred for possible treatment.[3,139,140]

Education, Occupation

There are few data available assessing the relationships between socioeconomic factors and severity of retinopathy. Roy et al.[141] reported a significant association between proliferative retinopathy and occupational status (working class) or a lower income in a case-control study of 49 insulin-dependent diabetic patients. West et al.[77] failed to find a relationship of retinopathy with education level in a population of diabetic Oklahoma Indians.

Renal Disease

The prevalence and severity of diabetic retinopathy is associated with the presence of diabetic nephropathy. Diabetic retinopathy is usually seen before clinical detection of nephropathy [measured by proteinuria, increased blood urea nitrogen (BUN), or serum creatinine] although physiological manifestations of early renal dysfunction, e.g., increased glomerular filtration rate, may be detected early in the course of the disease.[142]

Although most patients develop diabetic retinopathy of varying severity during the course of their disease, only approximately 50 percent of insulin-dependent patients develop clinically manifest diabetic nephropathy.[142] In the WESDR, proteinuria (30 mg% or greater) was present in 27 percent of insulin-taking persons diagnosed before 30 years of age who had retinopathy; for persons diagnosed at or after 30 years who were not taking insulin, proteinuria was present in 19 percent of those with retinopathy.[12,13] In a study of a population of diabetic Oklahoma Indians, West et al.[77] reported that 58 percent of persons with severe retinopathy had heavy proteinuria.

In the younger-onset persons with 10 years or more of diabetes who participated in the WESDR, proliferative retinopathy was found three times as often in persons with proteinuria as in those without proteinuria; similarly, in noninsulin-taking older-onset persons, proliferative retinopathy was 2.7 times as frequent in the presence of proteinuria as in its absence.[12,13]

Most diabetic persons who develop end-stage renal disease that requires dialysis or transplantation have proliferative retinopathy. Ramsey et al.[143] reported that 75 percent of eyes of diabetic patients who were undergoing renal transplantation or dialysis had proliferative retinopathy, and 32 percent had visual acuity of 20/160 or worse in the better eye.

Retinopathy, nephropathy, and neuropathy have long been thought to be manifestations of diabetic microvascular disease. Why 97.5 percent of diabetic patients (insulin-dependent) develop retinopathy whereas only about 50 percent develop clinically apparent renal disease is not known. Differing underlying pathogenetic or anatomical factors have been postulated to explain such differences.[40,142] The higher frequency of retinopathy may also be secondary to its easier detection via ophthalmoscopy.

Aiello et al.[144] described a "renal retinopathy" in diabetic patients consisting of a "hypertensive and renal component." A high frequency of flame-shaped hemorrhages, arteriolar narrowing and irregularity, cotton-wool spots, and diffuse retinal and disc edema were described in diabetic patients in renal failure seen at the Joslin Clinic. These patients were also said to be less responsive to photocoagulation; successful treatment of renal failure was suggested as a means of reducing the macular edema.

Patients on dialysis or following renal transplantation usually have a stabilization of visual function.[143] In one study, 54 percent (165/308) of eyes of diabetic patients had visual acuity of 20/50 or better at the time of their renal transplant for diabetic end-stage renal disease. With a mean follow-up time of 3–5 years, 51 percent (157/308) of eyes had retained this visual acuity level. Progression of retinopathy was reported (no comparison group) in 38 percent (30/78) of eyes which had nonproliferative disease before transplantation. However, of eyes that had active proliferative retinopathy at the time of transplantation, 71 percent (43/61) became inactive and were at lower risk of visual loss after the transplantation. Similar findings were reported for patients on dialysis.

Patients undergoing transplantation are at risk of developing decreased visual acuity due to cataract formation, secondary to systemic corticosteroids, or due to cytomegalic virus retinitis (secondary to immunosuppression).[144]

Patients undergoing hemodialysis have been thought to be at greater risk of vitreous hemorrhage due to heparinization or to rapid metabolic and blood pressure changes.[144] However, Ramsey et al.[143] reported no difference in visual prognosis (if metabolic and blood pressure control is brought about gradually) in diabetic patients managed by peritoneal dialysis compared to chronic hemodialysis. Patients undergoing hemodialysis are also at risk of developing increased intraocular pressure.[144] The mechanism for this is unknown. Monitoring of intraocular pressures of such patients is indicated.

Blindness is not a contraindication to chronic ambulatory peritoneal dialysis. Flynn[145] reported the lowest rate of peritonitis in blind diabetic patients (one in every 66 patient-weeks) who have been trained in this procedure.

Retinopathy and Prognosis for Survival

The probability for survival decreases with increasing severity of retinopathy. In a group of 709 diabetic persons with proliferative diabetic retinopathy, the observed 5-year survival rate was 56 percent compared to 98 percent in persons without retinopathy.[146] Men with proliferative diabetic retinopathy had a poorer 5-year survival rate than women. In another case series, Caird et al.[2] found that the 5-year survival rates for 128 diabetic patients were 92 percent for patients without retinopathy, 90 percent for patients with microaneurysms only, 63 percent for patients with more severe nonproliferative retinopathy, and 55 percent for those with proliferative retinopathy.

Sharma et al.,[147] studying 907 patients at a referral practice at an ophthalmic clinic for diabetic patients, found a 5-year survival rate of 100 percent in patients without retinopathy and one of 86 percent for females and 79 percent for males with proliferative diabetic retinopathy. Death was associated with coronary artery disease in 50 percent of cases. Unfortunately, no comparisons for age-specific rates for a nondiabetic population were provided in this study.

The higher prevalence of systemic conditions, e.g., uremia, coronary heart disease, and hypertension, in patients with severe retinopathy is responsible for the increased risk of death.[77,147] Oklahoma Indians with diabetic retinopathy were found to have a higher prevalence of coronary disease.[77] The percentage of patients with electrocardiographic major Q waves was 9 percent in those without retinopathy, 15 percent with retinopathy, and 21 percent with severe retinopathy in this group. These data suggest that diabetic patients with retinopathy should be under closer medical surveillance for diagnosis and treatment of cardiovascular disease.

Medical Therapy

No drugs have been found to prevent or decrease the progression of diabetic retinopathy.[2,66] Treatment regimens involving androgenic and nonandrogenic anabolic steroids, lipid-lowering agents, rutnin, vitamins B_{12}, C, E, and K, calcium debosilate, calcium phosphate, cyclandelate, anticoagulants, and fructose have been proposed, tried, or have not proved to be of therapeutic or preventive value in altering the course of diabetic retinopathy.[2,66]

Aspirin is being studied in a multicentered therapeutic trial, the ETDRS, to determine if it retards the progression of retinopathy.[148] The rationale for using aspirin is that it may interrupt the process of abnormal platelet aggregation, which is presumed to play a role in the retinal capillary closure.

In another multicentered therapeutic trial, sorbinil, an aldose reductase inhibitor, is being studied to see if it prevents or slows the progression of retinopathy.[149]

The role of reducing hyperglycemia and/or blood pressure in preventing or reducing the progression of retinopathy is discussed above.

Surgical Therapy

Photocoagulation. The rationale for the use of panretinal photocoagulation resulted from the observation that the eyes of diabetic patients with disseminated chorioretinal scars due to trauma or infection had lower rates of retinopathy than the fellow eye without such changes.[2] As a result of these observations, high-energy light sources (xenon arc; ruby, argon, and krypton lasers) have been developed to produce burns leading to scars in the outer layer of the retina.

Despite a number of clinical studies, five of which used concurrent controls, the efficacy of photocoagulation in preventing severe visual loss due to proliferative retinopathy was not widely accepted prior to the onset of the Diabetic Retinopathy Study (DRS) in 1972.[150] That therapeutic trial was sponsored by the National Eye Institute and was conducted between 1972 and 1979.[3] A total of 1,758 patients were involved. To be eligible for participation, patients had to have visual acuity of 20/100 or better in each eye, no previous photocoagulation, and proliferative retinopathy in at least one eye or severe nonproliferative or proliferative retinopathy in both eyes. There was random assignment of one eye of each patient to photocoagulation (either xenon arc or argon laser) and the other to follow-up without photocoagulation. The photocoagulation technique involved ''scatter'' panretinal photocoagulation of retinal new vessels (Fig. 4-15).

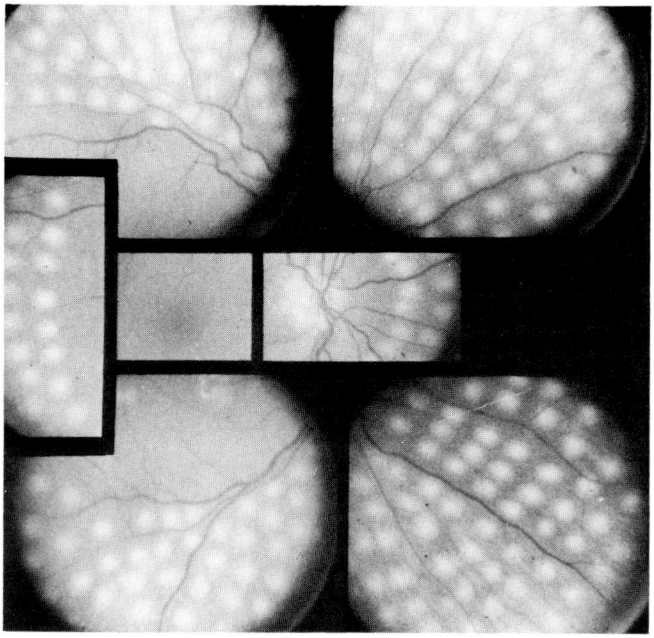

Fig. 4-15 Fundus photograph of the right eye demonstrating fresh panretinal argon laser photocoagulation burns which have been delivered in a grid-like fashion sparing the macular area. (Reprinted with permission from Klein R: Management of eye diseases in the insulin-dependent diabetic patient. In MacDonald M (ed): Managing Diabetes Mellitus in Children and Adolescents. Saunders, Philadelphia, 1983.)

The major endpoint in the DRS was "severe visual loss," defined as a visual acuity of less than 5/200 in two consecutive follow-up visits 4 months apart. The major finding of the DRS was that the risk of severe visual loss in treated eyes was less than one-half that in untreated control eyes (Fig. 4-16).[3] The 6-year cumulative event rate for severe visual loss was 38 percent for untreated and 16 percent for treated eyes. High-risk retinopathy characteristics for severe visual loss in untreated eyes in the DRS included new vessels at the optic disc equalling or exceeding one-third the disc area in extent (Fig. 4-17), new vessels at the disc less than one-third the disc area in extent with preretinal or vitreous hemorrhage, and new vessels more than one disc diameter away from the optic disc greater than one-half the disc area in size associated with preretinal or vitreous hemorrhage. The conclusion reached by the DRS was that in eyes with such high-risk characteristics the risk of severe visual loss without treatment was 25 percent at 2 years and in eyes with treatment it was 12 percent (Fig. 4-18); this beneficial effect outweighed the risk of harmful treatment effects.[3]

The British Multicentre Photocoagulation Trial,[151] a randomized trial of xenon arc photocoagulation for patients with symmetrical proliferative diabetic retinopathy, also reported findings consistent with those of the DRS.

Before undergoing treatment, the patient is told that photocoagulation may re-

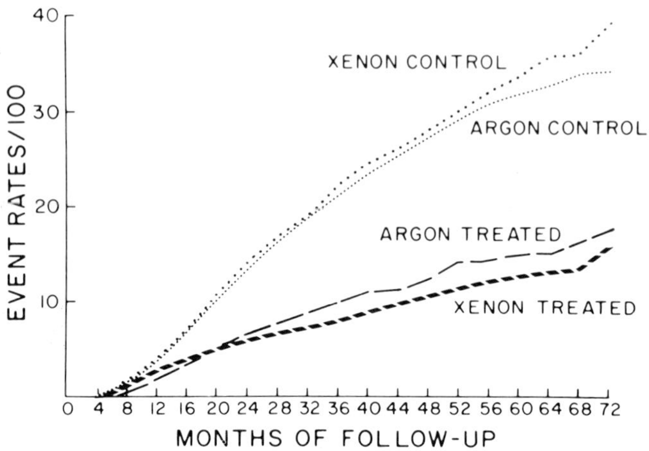

Fig. 4-16 Cumulative rates of severe visual loss (5/200 or less) in the DRS. (Reprinted with permission from Diabetic Retinopathy Study Group: Photocoagulation treatment of proliferative diabetic retinopathy. Ophthalmology 88:583, 1981.)

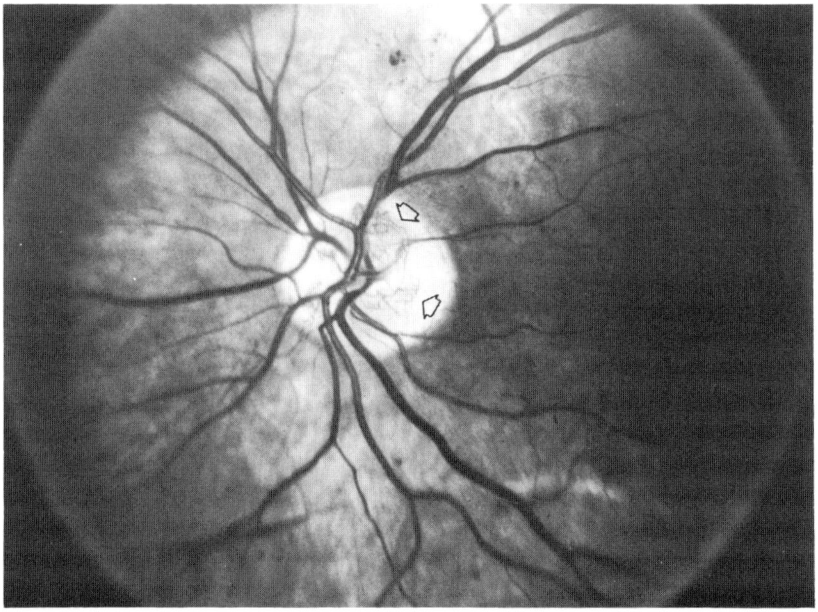

Fig. 4-17 Fundus photograph of the left eye showing stringy new vessels equalling one-third the disc area in front of the optic disc (arrows). This patient, who is asymptomatic and has normal visual acuity, is at high risk of developing severe visual loss if not treated with panretinal photocoagulation. (Reprinted with permission from Klein R: Management of eye disease in the insulin-dependent diabetic patient. In MacDonald M (ed): Managing Diabetes Mellitus in Children and Adolescents. Saunders, Philadelphia, 1983.)

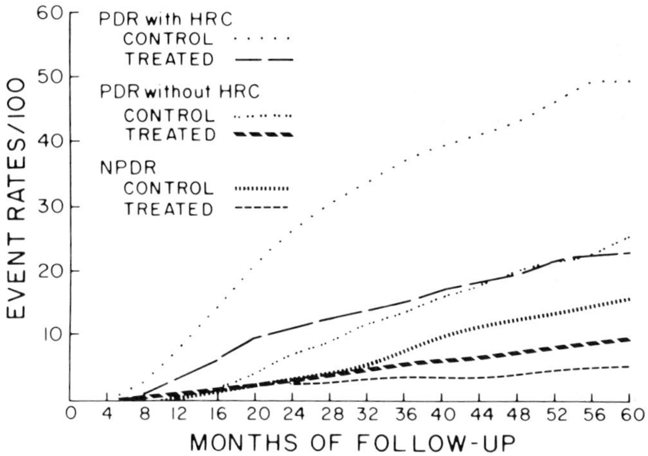

Fig. 4-18 Cumulative rates of severe visual loss for eyes classified by the presence of proliferative retinopathy (PDR) and high-risk characteristics (HRC) in baseline fundus photographs, argon and xenon groups combined. NPDR = nonproliferative diabetic retinopathy. (Reprinted with permission from Diabetic Retinopathy Study Group: Photocoagulation treatment of proliferative diabetic retinopathy. Ophthalmology 88:583, 1981.)

duce the chances of severe loss of vision (to less than 5/200) but that it does not completely eliminate its possibility. The patient is also told that photocoagulation may cause moderate reduction of visual function as an unavoidable side effect, but that this reduction usually is of minor consequence. Such reduction includes mild loss of central vision (e.g., if the visual acuity was 20/20 before treatment, it might be reduced to 20/25 to 20/30 after panretinal argon laser treatment in 10 percent of patients), mild constriction of peripheral visual fields (5 percent of cases with argon laser), impaired night vision, and decreased accommodation.[3,152] The patient is also informed about the rare more-severe side effects, e.g., severe constriction of visual fields and severe loss of central vision due to development of vitreous hemorrhage, traction retinal detachment after treatment, or an inadvertent foveal burn.

Panretinal photocoagulation is usually done as an outpatient procedure. To achieve anesthesia, proparacaine drops are applied to the cornea or a retrobulbar injection of lidocaine is used. The pupil is dilated, and a contact lens is applied to the cornea. Under direct visualization of the retina, 800–1,800 burns, usually of 500 μm diameter in size, are delivered in a grid-like pattern (sparing the central retina) in one or more treatment sessions (Fig. 4-15). A successful treatment usually leads to partial or complete regression of abnormal new preretinal and optic disc blood vessels (Fig. 4-19), in most cases within 4 weeks.[153] If the high-risk characteristics remain, further treatments are usually scheduled. Underlying reasons for failure to respond to laser treatment were not defined in the DRS.

The mechanisms of action of panretinal photocoagulation are not known. A number of theories of how photocoagulation works have been suggested. They include destruction of hypoxic retinal tissue resulting in decreased production of a hypothetical

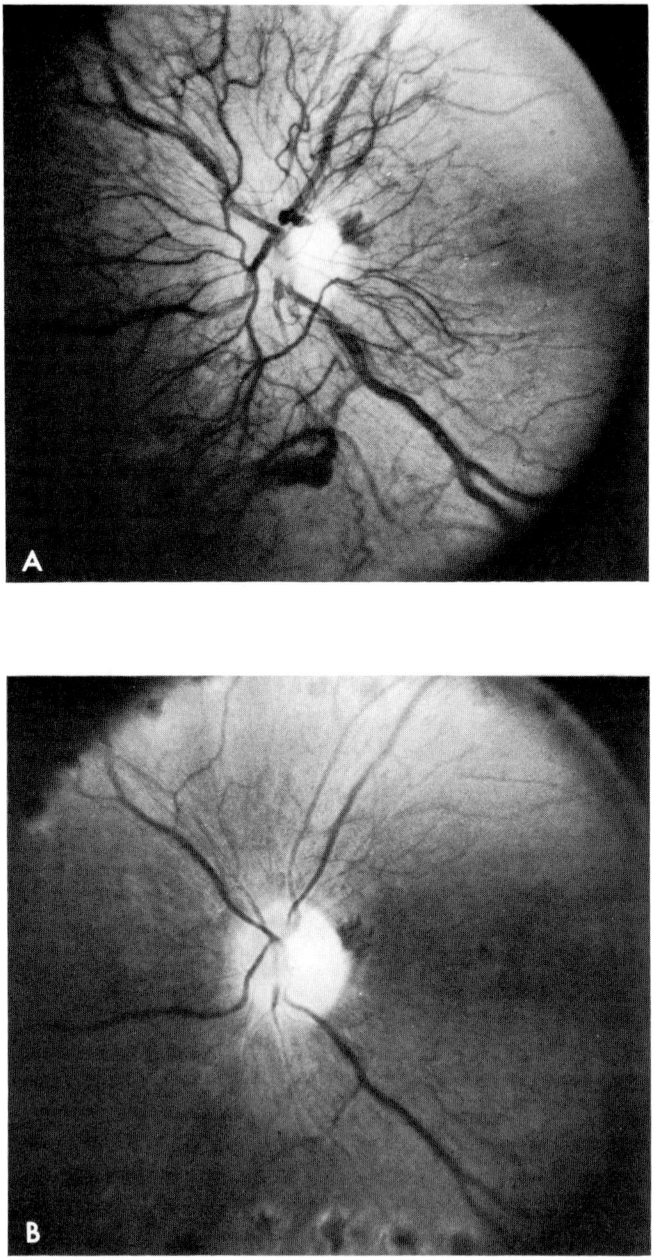

Fig. 4-19 (A) Fundus photograph of the left eye demonstrating extensive retinal new vessels in front of the disc and preretinal hemorrhage. (B) Four weeks after panretinal argon laser photocoagulation there has been a dramatic regression of retinal new vessels. Pigmented photocoagulation scars are present in the periphery of the picture. (Reprinted with permission from Klein R: Management of eye disease in the insulin-dependent diabetic patient. In MacDonald M (ed): Managing Diabetes Mellitus in Children and Adolescents. Saunders, Philadelphia, 1983.)

vasoproliferative factor, increased oxygenation of untreated retinal tissue leading to vasoconstriction and regression of proliferative tissue, and increased passage of metabolites through the blood-retinal barrier at the level of the retinal pigment epithelium.[5,6]

The question of whether use of argon laser panretinal photocoagulation at an earlier stage (before the development of high-risk characteristics) would reduce the development of severe visual loss even further is being examined in the ETDRS.[148] In the DRS, the 1-year risk of progression of retinopathy from the severe nonproliferative stage to the proliferative phase was 15.3 percent in the untreated compared to 8.8 percent in the treated; for eyes with proliferative retinopathy but without high-risk characteristics (HRCs) initially, the progression of HRCs or visual acuity of 5/200 or poorer was 34.6 percent in the untreated and 14.3 percent in the treated.[3,148] Thus these data demonstrate an approximate 50 percent reduction in progression of retinopathy by treating at an earlier stage. However, because the risk of severe visual loss is less than in eyes with HRCs [8 percent at 2 years for untreated eyes with nonproliferative retinopathy (Fig. 4-18)], it is not clear from the DRS whether the benefits of earlier treatment outweigh the risk of complications. This question as well as the efficacy of less extensive scatter treatment than that done in the DRS are being examined in the ETDRS.[148]

A number of prospective studies have examined the role of photocoagulation in the treatment of macular edema.[154–159] Most of these studies have shown better vision at follow-up in treated than untreated eyes. However, many of these studies have had methodological problems limiting interpretation of the data. The problems include failure to allocate eyes randomly to treatment, to specify the type of maculopathy, and to mask the person determining visual acuity as to which eye was treated.

The British Multicentre Study was a randomized controlled clinical trial using xenon arc photocoagulation to treat diabetic maculopathy.[159] In that study, 99 patients with similar severity of diabetic maculopathy had one eye chosen by a random procedure. Treatment to the center of hard exudate rings (except when they were at the fovea), focal treatment of retinal microaneurysms and IRMAs, or scatter treatment to lesions outside the superior and inferior temporal vessels was done. In persons with either 20/20–20/30 or 20/40–20/80 visual acuity at entry or circinate retinopathy (Fig. 4-4), treated eyes had significantly less deterioration in visual acuity than untreated eyes over 5 years of follow-up. Eyes with visual acuity of 20/120 or worse or eyes with diffuse edema or ischemia seemed to do worse than eyes with focal areas of edema or hard exudates. This study[159] and others[157,158] suggest that patients with minimal loss of vision secondary to macular edema, or those who have threatened loss of vision secondary to encroachment of the foveal area by hard exudates, may benefit from focal laser photocoagulation. The ETDRS is currently assessing the role of argon laser photocoagulation in treating various types of intraretinal diabetic maculopathy.[148]

During treatment for macular edema, a fluorescein angiogram projected on a wall or in a special viewer is used to demonstrate abnormal leakage from retinal blood vessels which may be responsible for macular edema, as well as for areas of ischemia (closure of retinal capillaries) (Fig. 4-7). Retrobulbar anesthesia is used only if akinesia is desired (for treatment around the foveal area); otherwise topical anesthesia

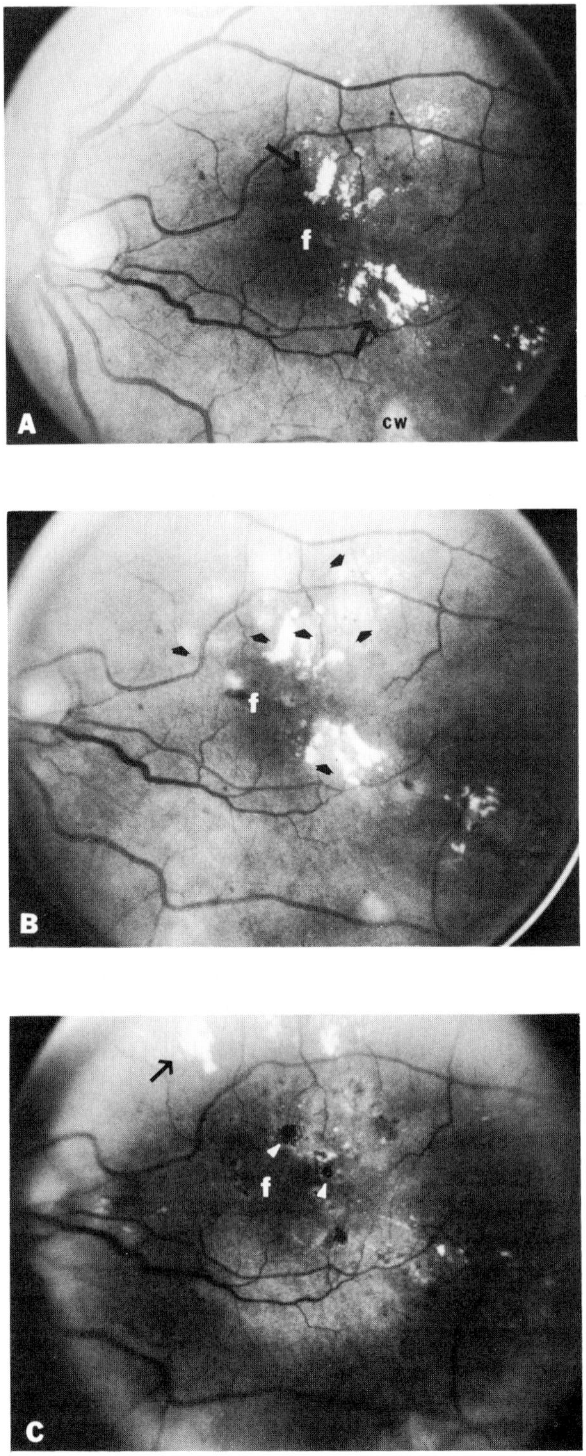

Fig. 4-20 Fundus photograph of the left eye. (A) Hard exudates (black arrows), retinal microaneurysms, and a cotton-wool spot (CW) are present. Macular edema is present temporal to the foveal area (f). Visual acuity is 20/40. (B) Photograph on 8/10/79 shows fresh photocoagulation burns (black arrowheads) around retinal microaneurysms which leaked on fluorescein angiography. (C) In this photograph, taken 5/22/80, the macular area is no longer edematous and the visual acuity is 20/30. Photocoagulation scars appear black (white arrows), and there is a minimal amount of scattered retinal hard exudate material present in the macula. However, new areas of hard exudate are present above the superior temporal arteriole (black arrow).

with proparacaine drops is routinely used. Photocoagulation burns 0.05–0.1 sec duration and 100–200 μm in size are directed at leaking retinal microaneurysms as identified on the fluorescein angiograms (Fig. 4-20). Burns of 50 μm may be added to get further whitening of the retinal microaneurysms. Nonperfused areas may also be treated to destroy ischemic retina. Follow-up examination is done within 3 months; if the edema persists, the angiogram is repeated and any remaining leaks are treated.

The rationale for photocoagulation for macular edema includes ablation of leaking microaneurysms. Wallow[160] and Bresnick[17] have suggested that a "débridement" of abnormal retinal pigment epithelial cells with replacement by normal cells may reestablish the blood-retinal barrier, facilitating absorption of retinal edema fluid.

Vitrectomy. Vitrectomy, in widespread use for the past 12 years, is done to remove vitreous hemorrhage or to cut fibrous bands that cause tractional detachments of the retina due to proliferative disease. Prior to the development of vitrectomy, the only treatment for vitreous hemorrhage was patching of both eyes and elevation of the head. Currently, if a significant vitreous hemorrhage obscures visualization of the retina, bilateral patching and elevation of the head for 24–28 hr is sometimes recommended. The fundus is examined, and if there has been enough settling of the vitreous hemorrhage panretinal photocoagulation is done if indicated and feasible.

Vitrectomy may be recommended if there has been no clearing of the vitreous hemorrhage after 6–12 months or sooner if there is ultrasound or other evidence of a traction retinal detachment threatening or involving the macular area. The major objectives of vitreous surgery are to clear the optical axis of opacities and to release mechanical traction on the retina. Vitrectomy may also act to increase the oxygenation of the inner retina. Stafansson et al.[161] found constriction of retinal blood vessels after vitrectomy and suggested that, after removal of vitreous, the aqueous humor, which has a higher oxygen tension than the vitreous, may provide the retina with more oxygen.

Vitrectomy is a procedure which requires hospitalization and is usually performed under general anesthesia; the average duration of the operation is 2–4 hr. Because the surgery is generally performed on an elective basis, preoperative evaluation includes a thorough examination to diagnose and control numerous medical problems often found in the diabetic patient undergoing vitrectomy. Cardiovascular, renal, and metabolic problems must be managed during and after surgery.

The vitrectomy device and fiberoptic illuminators are introduced into the eye through small openings made in the sclera overlying the pars plana (flat portion) of the ciliary body (Fig. 4-21). Usually the lens is left undisturbed; however, if a cataract is present and prohibits visualization for vitrectomy, the lens may be removed before or during surgery. Under direct observation, the vitrectomy instrument is used to cut and remove fibrous tissues and blood from the vitreous cavity, and vitreous volume is restored with a balanced salt solution (Fig. 4-22). Using special intraocular scissors, the surgeon may cut fibroproliferative tissue and epiretinal membranes which are responsible for traction on the retina (Figs. 4-23 and 4-24).

In cases where a prior retinal tear is present or a tear occurs during the procedure, choroidoretinal adhesion is produced around the tear with cryopexy to prevent detachment of the retina. Additionally, air with or without expanding gas mixtures (e.g., sulfur hexafluoride) may be exchanged for the fluid in the vitreous cavity to

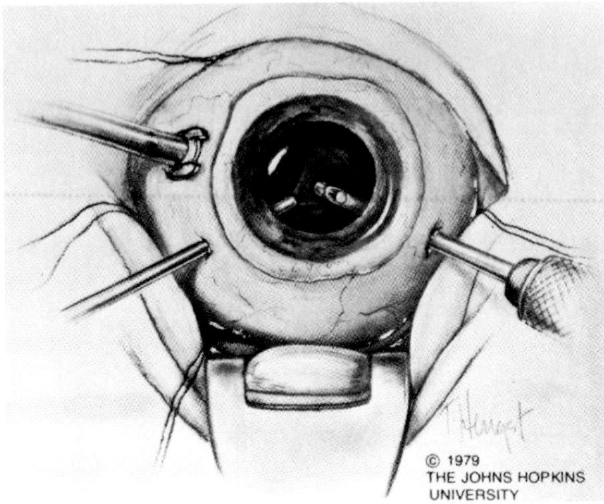

Fig. 4-21 Divided-system instrumentation for pars plana vitrectomy using the O'Malley ocutome system. Separate scleral incisions are made for introduction of: (1) an inferior cannula, sutured to the sclera; (2) a vitrectomy cutting probe; and (3) a fiberoptic illuminator. (Reprinted with permission from Michels RG: Vitreous surgery for visual loss from proliferative diabetic retinopathy. In Freidman EA, L'Esperance FA (eds): Diabetic Renal-Retinal Syndrome: Prevention and Management. The Johns Hopkins University Press, New York, 1982.)

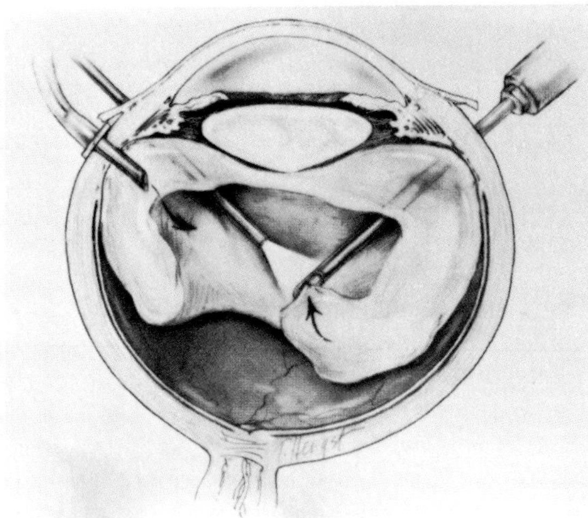

Fig. 4-22 Intraocular illuminator provides reflex free illumination as opaque vitreous gel is cut and removed via a vitrectomy cutting probe. A separate infusion cannula replaces the intraocular volume loss as opaque tissue is removed. (Reprinted with permission from Michels RG: Vitreous surgery for visual loss from proliferative diabetic retinopathy. In Friedman EA, L'Esperance FA (eds): Diabetic Renal-Retinal Syndrome: Prevention and Management. The Johns Hopkins University Press, New York, 1982.)

tamponade the retinal tear, and the subretinal fluid may be drained during the operation. Scleral buckling (with hard episcleral silicone or sponges) may also be used to indent the sclera, reduce traction further, and thus seal the tear.

Before the development of vitrectomy, when vitreous hemorrhage resulted in a reduction of vision of 20/200 or worse, only 8 percent of eyes in one study had spontaneous improvement of vision to better than 20/200 in a 1-year interval.[150] In recent series of patients undergoing vitrectomy, visual improvement to better than 20/200 was reported in 50 percent of operated cases.[162] Michaels[163] described a series of 596

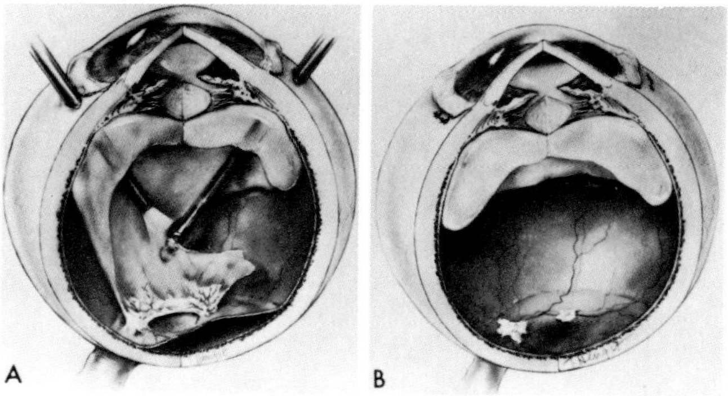

Fig. 4-23 Excision of vitreous gel in a diabetic eye with posterior traction retinal detachment. (A) The central vitreous gel is excised, and the posterior vitreous surface is then cut to relieve traction between the vitreous base anteriorly and zones of fibrovascular proliferation posteriorly. (B) Release of anteroposterior vitreous surgery for visual loss from proliferative diabetic retinopathy. In Friedman EA, L'Esperance FA (eds): Diabetic Renal-Retinal Syndrome: Prevention and Management. The Johns Hopkins University Press, New York, 1982.

consecutive eyes with severe loss of visual acuity and reported a successful result (visual acuity of 5/200 or better and stable anatomical findings) in 384 (66 percent) of 579 eyes. Successful results after vitrectomy are more likely in eyes with vitreous hemorrhage alone than in eyes with traction retinal detachment involving the macular area. In the latter, the effects of preexisting anatomical damage to the macular area are more likely to limit visual improvement postoperatively.

Vitrectomy carries with it a high overall complication rate (about 25 percent). These complications include iatrogenic retinal tears resulting in retinal detachment, recurrent vitreous hemorrhage, corneal edema, cataract (up to 20 percent of eyes at 1 year), the development of neovascularization of the iris (up to 22 percent of eyes), and rubeotic glaucoma (up to 12 percent of eyes).[164]

Rubeotic glaucoma (secondary to neovascularization of the anterior chamber angle), when it occurs, usually develops within 6 months of vitrectomy and is more likely to arise in eyes with severe retinal ischemia, retinal detachment, or removal of the lens. Panretinal photocoagulation during (using an endophotocoagulator) or after the procedure may reduce the incidence of this serious complication.[165]

The Diabetic Retinopathy Vitrectomy Study (DRVS) was funded in 1975 by the National Eye Institute to assess indications, risks, and benefits for early (shortly after the development of vitreous hemorrhage) versus late (a year) vitrectomy.[166] The rationale for early vitrectomy include avoiding prolonged visual disability and possibly avoiding the presumed deleterious effects of longstanding intraocular hemorrhage (possible acceleration of growth of fiboproliferans, exacerbation of retinal vascular occlusive process, and a possible toxic effect of blood on the retina). The rationale for late vitrectomy (at 1 year after the initial vitreous hemorrhage) included the possibility of spontaneous resolution of hemorrhage and that with time the retinopathy would be stabilized and there would be fewer vision-threatening complications of sur-

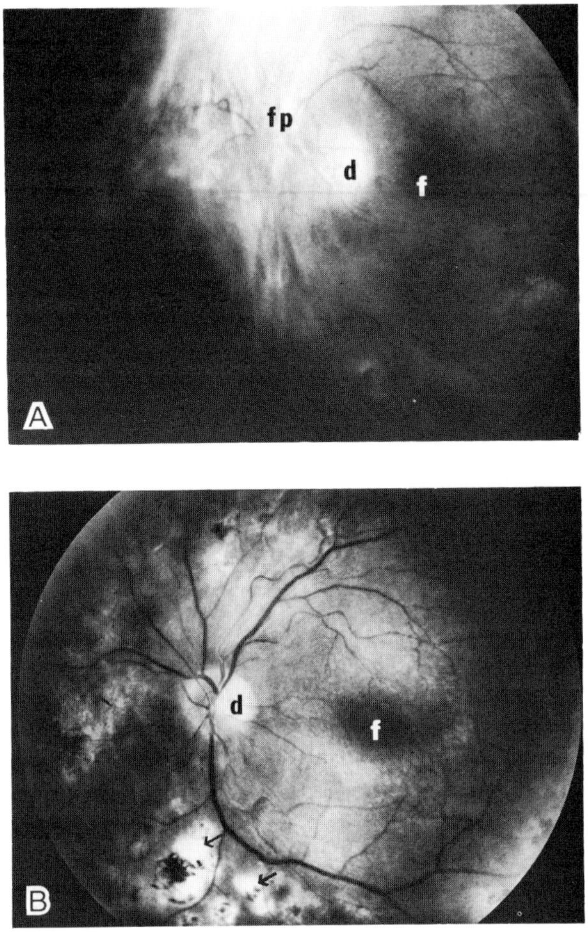

Fig. 4-24 Fundus photograph of the left eye of a 35-year-old woman with a 14-year history of insulin-dependent diabetic retinopathy. (A) Fibroproliferative tissue (fp) at the optic disc (d) has contracted and caused displacement of the foveal area (f) closer to the optic disc (d), resulting in visual acuity of 20/200 on 3/3/83. (B) A pars plana vitrectomy with excision of an epiretinal membrane responsible for displacement of the fovea was performed on 3/28/83. When this photograph was taken on 8/19/83 [at a lower magnification than (A)] visual acuity had returned to 20/70 and the foveal area had moved back to its normal position. Photocoagulation scars (black arrows) are present, and fibroproliferative tissue is no longer seen at the optic disc (d). (Courtesy of Dr. T. Stevens, University of Wisconsin.)

gery, e.g., neovascular glaucoma. The study is also assessing whether early vitrectomy or conventional clinical management (photocoagulation) is indicated in eyes with severe proliferative retinopathy before vitreous hemorrhage or macular detachment occurs. Data monitoring in the DRVS has yet to reveal a significant difference in early versus delayed vitrectomy in the two parts of the study. Results from one uncontrolled study in which vitrectomy was done in 140 eyes with visual acuity of 20/200 or better suggest that removal of epiretinal or preretinal fibrovascular proliferative tissue and cutting or circumcision of epiretinal membranes might reduce the risk of vitreous hemorrhage or retinal detachment and preserve useful visual acuity.[167]

Pituitary Ablation. Prior to the widespread use of panretinal photocoagulation, pituitary ablation was used to prevent blindness in individuals with rapidly progressive severe retinopathy.[150] A number of studies (most without adequate control groups) demonstrated regression of retinopathy and preservation of vision in some cases, presumably as a result of the hormonal changes associated with hypopituitarism.[150] Pituitary ablation is rarely used today because it is believed that the numerous

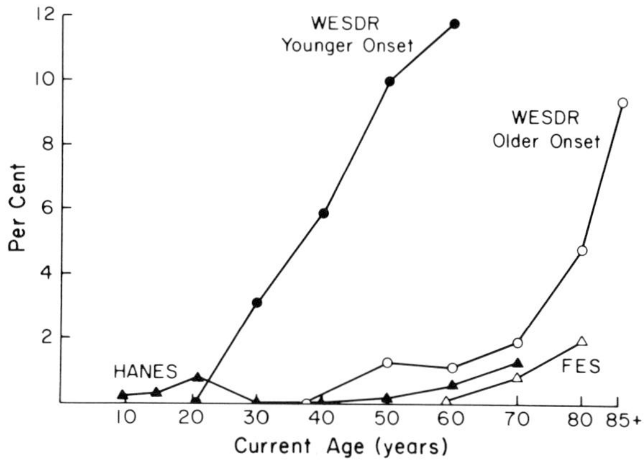

Fig. 4-25 Percent of persons with visual acuity of 20/200 or worse in the better eye in the WESDR, the Health and Nutrition Examination Survey (HANES),[172] and the Framingham Eye Study (FES),[171] by current age. (Reprinted with permission from Klein R, Klein BEK, Moss SE: Visual impairment in diabetes. Ophthalmology, 91:1, 1984.)

side effects from panhypopituitarism outweigh the benefits of preservation of vision, and most patients may be treated with photocoagulation or vitrectomy surgery instead.

VISUAL IMPAIRMENT

Diabetes is estimated to account for 5,000 new cases of legal blindness (visual acuity of 20/200 or worse in the better eye) in the United States each year.[1,168] Caird and Garrett[169] estimated that for an insulin-taking diabetic patient diagnosed at 20 years of age the risk of blindness was 0.1 percent after 10 years, 1.6 percent after 20 years, and 3.5 percent after 30 years of diabetes. For persons diagnosed at 60 years of age, the risk of blindness was 1.8 percent after 10 years and 5.5 percent after 20 years.

Blindness is 20 times more common in diabetic than in nondiabetic persons (Fig. 4-25).[96,170–172] Approximately 8 percent of people who were legally blind reported diabetes as the etiology of their blindness.[173] The prevalence of blindness in diabetic persons is related to current age and the duration of the diabetes.[96] In the WESDR, legal blindness was found to be substantially more frequent in persons who had diabetes for 15 years or more.[96] In that study, in younger-onset insulin-requiring persons after 30 years of diabetes, 21 percent of the population had some degree of visual impairment (visual acuity of 20/40 or worse in the better eye), and 12 percent were legally blind (Fig. 4-26).

In older-onset persons, a greater frequency of legal blindness was found earlier but was less frequent in those with longer duration of diabetes than in younger-onset persons with comparable disease duration (Figs. 4-26 and 4-27).[96]

Retinopathy

Retinopathy is an important cause of visual impairment in diabetes. Eyes with more severe retinopathy have been found to be at higher risk of blindness. The cumulative 5-year rate of blindness (visual acuity of 20/200 or worse) for eyes with

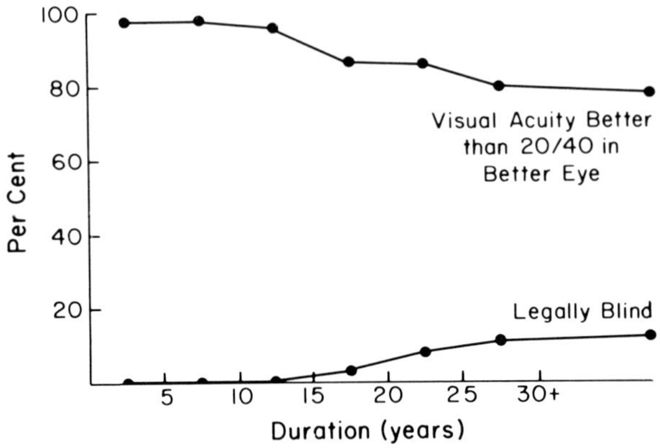

Fig. 4-26 Percent of insulin-taking persons diagnosed to have diabetes before 30 years of age who participated in the WESDR with visual acuity of 20/40 or better, and of those with legal blindness, by duration of diabetes. (Reprinted with permission from Klein R, Klein BEK, Moss SE: Visual impairment in diabetes. Ophthalmology, 91:1, 1984.)

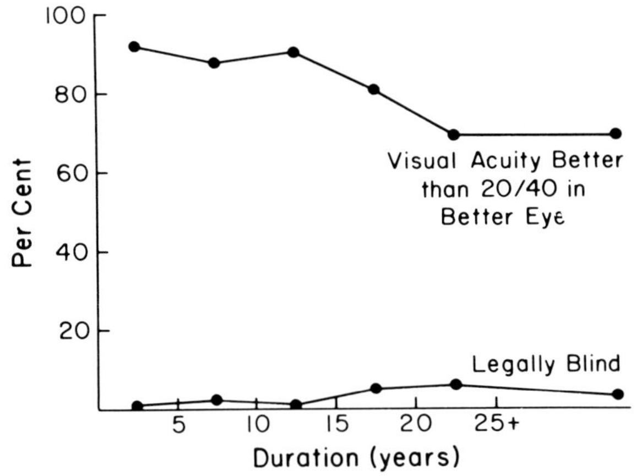

Fig. 4-27 Percent of persons diagnosed to have diabetes after 29 years of age who participated in the WESDR with visual acuity of 20/40 or better and of those with legal blindness, by duration of diabetes. (Reprinted with permission from Klein R, Klein BEK, Moss SE: Visual impairment in diabetes. Ophthalmology, 91:1, 1984.)

good vision (20/60 or better) at the beginning of one study was 1.6 percent if retinopathy was not present and 14.8 percent if retinal blot hemorrhages and/or exudates were present.[169] Untreated eyes in the DRS had a cumulative event rate of severe visual loss (less than 5/200) of 14 percent at 2 years, 27 percent at 4 years, and 38 percent at 6 years (Fig. 4-16).[3] In the WESDR, diabetic retinopathy was partially or totally responsible for 86 percent of cases of visual loss (acuity of 20/200 or worse) in eyes of younger-onset insulin-taking patients and 30 percent in eyes of older-onset persons.[96]

In insulin-dependent younger-onset persons, reduction of vision to 20/200 or worse is more likely to be due to proliferative retinopathy resulting in vitreous hemorrhage or retinal traction detachment involving the macular area.[6] In older-onset persons, similar visual loss in patients with retinopathy is often associated with macular edema.[6,96] In both groups, macular ischemia due to closure of retinal capillaries in the foveal area may also result in a decrease of vision.[5,6]

If proliferative diabetic retinopathy is present, vitreous hemorrhage from fragile abnormal new preretinal blood vessels may result in an acute decrease in vision. In such cases the sudden appearance of a number of small dark floaters, a large spot obscuring vision, or "complete" loss of vision is described. Contraction of fibrous proliferative tissue leading to traction on the macular area may cause distortion in vision. Traction on the retina may also result in retinal detachment; if the macula is involved, severe blurry vision and darkening of vision may result. In some diabetic patients there may be marked fluctuations in vision due to clearing and recurrence of vitreous hemorrhage or macular edema.

In older diabetic patients with macular edema, the visual disturbance may go unnoticed until both eyes are involved. The patient may complain of a blur or distortion in central vision, especially when reading. In the absence of proliferative retinopathy, patients with diabetic maculopathy and loss of central vision are usually left with peripheral vision which is sufficient to navigate, unless glaucoma or severe cataracts are present.

Diabetic patients as a group have poorer color vision than nondiabetic persons (G. H. Bresnick, R. Condit, K. Korth, et al., personal communication).[55,174] Even before the development of retinopathy, disturbances in yellow-blue hue discrimination may be detected.[55] With progression of maculopathy, manifested by edema or hard exudate, further deterioration in color vision is found.[174] This has therapeutic significance as many patients using either home blood glucose monitoring or urine glucose testing may have difficulty correctly interpreting results of glucose testing. Bresnick et al.[175] recommended testing color vision of diabetic patients who do home urinary glucose monitoring, especially those with proliferative retinopathy or macular edema. If an impairment exists, enhancement of lighting conditions when testing glucose and use of alternate devices (e.g., meters with digital display of glucose concentration) should be considered. Further studies to determine the effect of this color vision defect on blood glucose monitoring are needed.

Other Causes

A frequent cause for sudden change in vision, especially in children and adolescents with diabetes, is related to a change in the refractive media.[2] In adults this may be one of the presenting symptoms at the time of diagnosis. The patient may complain of blurriness in vision which can usually be corrected to 20/20 or better with appropriate glasses. Reversible osmotic swelling of the lens due to rapid alterations in blood sugar has been postulated to be responsible for this phenomenon.[176] With better control of the blood sugar, the refraction and acuity return to previous levels.

Cataract. Cataractous lens changes often cause a decrease in vision.[2] This affects a small percentage of young type I diabetic patients but occurs more frequently than in age-matched nondiabetic persons. Cataracts in young diabetic patients have been described as vacuolar or snowflake in appearance, involving the cortical or posterior subcapsular area of the lens. In the young, rapidly progressive cataracts have been associated with poor control.[2] It has been suggested that high glucose concentrations in the aqueous humor surrounding the lens enters lens cells and is converted to sorbitol in the polyol pathway.[177,178] Sorbitol cannot leave the lens cells and so accumulates, leading to osmotic swelling and destruction of cells. The use of aldose reductase inhibitors has been found to inhibit such cataract formation in poorly controlled diabetic animals.[179]

Prevalence rates of cataract have been reported to increase with increasing age and are higher for diabetic than nondiabetic persons for each age.[2,180] The association between cataracts and diabetes is stronger at younger ages.[180]

Burditt and Caird[181] found a relationship between metabolic control of blood sugar and the frequency of lens opacity for middle-aged men. Potential environmental exposures may also affect rates of cataracts. Cotlier et al.[182,183] reported an inverse association between aspirin usage and frequency of cataract in diabetic persons. Seigel et al.[184] failed to find a similar relationship in all participants in the Framingham Eye Study.

If a cataract causes significant visual impairment, the patient may no longer be able to read. Cataract extraction, if successfully performed, usually results in good vision with the use of glasses or contact lenses, assuming that concomitant retinopathy has not affected central vision.

Results of recent clinical surveys suggest that intraocular lens implants may be used without excess morbidity to the eye in some diabetic patients with no or early nonproliferative retinopathy.[185,186] Straatsma et al.[185] reported no difference in complications or final postoperative visual acuity level between diabetic and nondiabetic patients. They recommended use of an intraocular lens only in diabetic patients 60 years of age or older with a cataract-related decrease in vision that interfered with the patient's activities and if proliferative diabetic retinopathy or rubeosis was not present.

Glaucoma. Glaucoma is a disease in which there is loss of vision or visual field from damage to the optic nerve fibers due to absolute or relative elevations in intraocular pressure. Two types of glaucoma, open-angle and rubeotic, are reported to be more common in persons with diabetes.[2,165,187,188]

There is conflicting information about the relationship between diabetes and open-angle glaucoma.[2,187–190] Most reports describe a higher prevalence of ocular hypertension and open-angle glaucoma in diabetic than in nondiabetic persons.[187,188,191] Additionally, patients with open-angle glaucoma or ocular hypertension are reported to have a higher prevalence of diabetes. Persons in the Framingham Eye Study with an intraocular pressure greater than 20 mm Hg were two to three times as likely to have diabetes as others,[192] although other investigators have failed to find this relationship.[189,190]

It has been hypothesized that diabetic patients are at increased risk of optic nerve damage due to vascular factors.[192] Because diabetic patients may be at increased risk of glaucoma, measurement of the intraocular pressure and ophthalmoscopic examination for changes of the cup to disc configuration and size is an important part of the ophthalmological management of these patients. In patients who develop glaucoma, medical intervention is usually successful in preventing or retarding further field and visual loss.

Eyes with severe ischemic retinopathy or detachment of the retina, or eyes that have undergone vitrectomy, are at increased risk of developing rubeotic glaucoma.[2,5,165] In this condition, abnormal new vessels on the iris and in the anterior

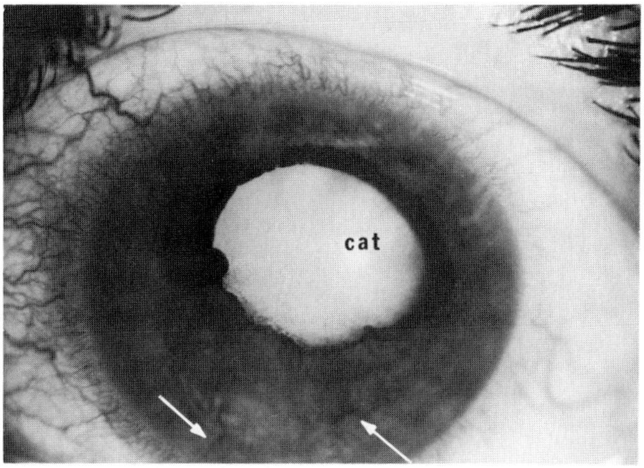

Fig. 4-28 Left eye of a patient with new vessels on the iris (white arrows) and the cataractous lens (cat). This patient had a traction retinal detachment secondary to proliferative diabetic retinopathy, no light perception, and severe pain.

chamber angle of the eye (Fig. 4-28) may lead to elevations of the intraocular pressure, severe optic nerve damage, and blindness with possible enucleation of the eye if it is painful. In some cases, panretinal photocoagulation may result in regression of the rubeotic vessels and control of the intraocular pressure.[165] Other surgical (cyclocryotherapy and valve implants) or medical intervention (antiglaucoma medications, topical corticosteroids, and mydriatic cycloplegics) for rubeotic glaucoma are rarely successful in preserving vision.[165]

OPHTHALMOLOGICAL MANAGEMENT

Because it is possible in many cases to prevent severe visual loss with photocoagulation, and because proliferative retinopathy may be present before it affects vision, it is important to identify those diabetic persons in need of ophthalmological evaluation.[3] The need for careful examination by ophthalmologists has been documented by Sussman et al.[193] They found that internists, diabetologists, and senior medical residents correctly diagnosed the presence of proliferative retinopathy in only 49 percent of patients they examined (under optimal conditions), whereas ophthalmologists and retinal specialists correctly diagnosed its presence in 96 percent of cases.

It is suggested that all diabetic patients be informed of the possible ocular complications and of the role of the ophthalmologist in the management (detection and prevention) of these complications. It is rare for young (pre-pubertal) insulin-dependent patients to develop serious vision-threatening retinopathy during the first 5–10 years of diabetes[10–12]; furthermore, because no known measures are available to prevent development of early retinopathy, frequent examinations by an ophthalmologist need not begin until 5–10 years after diagnosis of diabetes. For older-onset individuals, because the age of onset of diabetes is frequently uncertain and there is a higher frequency of vision-threatening retinopathy at the time of diagnosis,[76,92] regular periodic examinations by an ophthalmologist should begin shortly after diagnosis. Pa-

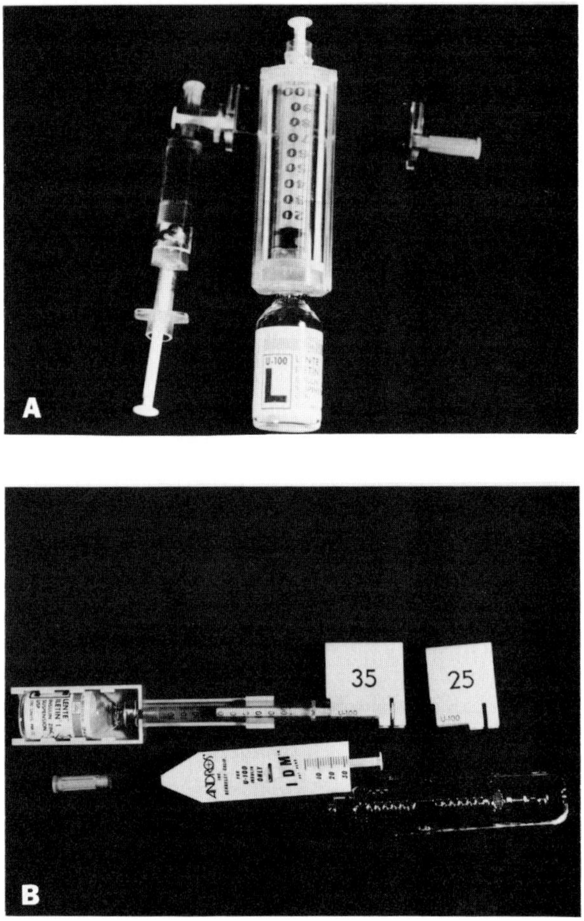

Fig. 4-29 Devices which aid the visually impaired diabetic patient draw up insulin in the correct dosage.

tients who are pregnant or who have proteinuria should be examined by ophthalmologists as they may be at higher risk for progression of retinopathy.

At each visit the ophthalmological examination may include refraction and measurement of the visual acuity, measurement of the intraocular pressure, dilation of the pupil, and examination of the lens by slit lamp biomicroscopy. The vitreous and retina are examined using direct and indirect ophthalmoscopy. Retinal edema is more easily detected using slit lamp biomicroscopy and a corneal contact lens to provide a magnified stereoscopic view of the retina.

Sketches of the retina and/or color stereoscopic fundus photographs should be obtained to document the presence and severity of the retinopathy. Photographs are used to document accurately the progression of retinal disease. Fluorescein angiography is used when focal photocoagulation treatment is considered and when the extent of retinal ischemia needs to be assessed. The angiograms demonstrate abnormal leakage from retinal blood vessels which may be responsible for macular edema and may also demonstrate closure of small capillaries or arterioles. More highly specialized procedures, e.g., vitreous fluorophotometry,[194] macular recovery time measured with nyctometry,[195] and electrophysiological testing,[54,195] are being evaluated experimentally as tools to indicate retinal functional or physiological abnormalities due to diabetes before the appearance of retinopathy.

REHABILITATION

The visual impairment in diabetes may range from minimal changes in color vision to total blindness and may include periods of rapid or slow progression with fluctuations in vision due to recurrent vitreous hemorrhage or macular edema. The unique problems confronted by visually impaired insulin-taking diabetic patients include identification of the type of insulin, determination of the amount of insulin in the vial, measurement of dose, and location of injection sites. Monitoring glucose levels using urine or blood test strips and foot care become more difficult or impossible for the visually impaired diabetic patient. A number of low-vision aids, devices for insulin administration, and aids in glucose monitoring are available for the visually impaired diabetic patient (Fig. 4-29).[196] Depending on the degree of visual impairment, supportive rehabilitation services, including low-vision clinics, state vocational rehabilitation centers, and schools for the blind, are available. Social workers, psychologists, orientation and mobility instructors, and rehabilitation teachers working as a team are needed to develop successful programs. They must help in handling the anxiety, anger, guilt, loss of self-esteem, and difficulties in social adjustment suffered by diabetic patients with visual loss.[197] Other current or potential systemic problems must be taken into account when planning the program. Helping the patient accept the partial or complete visual loss is an essential step in planning living arrangements and in developing coping strategies.

ACKNOWLEDGMENTS

The author acknowledges the support of grant EY03083 from the National Eye Institute. He thanks Drs. Barbara E. K. Klein, George H. Bresnick, and Edward Ehrlich, Mr. Scot Moss, and Ms. Jean Espenshade for reviewing the manuscript; Gene Knutson and Michael Neider for preparing the photographs; and Kathy Kaap, Lorraine Boyle, and Bernadette Bull for secretarial assistance.

REFERENCES

1. Palmberg PF: Diabetic retinopathy. Diabetes 26:703, 1977
2. Caird FI, Pirie A, Ramsell TG: Diabetes and the Eye. Blackwell, Oxford, 1969
3. Diabetic Retinopathy Study Group: Photocoagulation treatment of proliferative diabetic retinopathy: clinical application of Diabetic Retinopathy Study (DRS) findings, DRS report number 8. Ophthalmology 88:583, 1981
4. Hogan MJ, Alvarado JA, Weddell JE: Histology of the Human Eye: An Atlas and Textbook. Saunders, Philadelphia, 1971

5. Bresnick GH: Diabetic retinopathy. In Peyman GA, Sanders DR, Goldberg MF (eds): Principles and Practice of Ophthalmology. Saunders, Philadelphia, 1977
6. Kohner EM, McLeod D, Marshall J: Diabetic eye disease. In Keen H, Jarrett J (eds): Complications of Diabetes. 2nd Ed. Arnold, London, 1982
7. Yamana Y, Ohnishi Y, Taniguchi Y et al: Early signs of diabetic retinopathy by fluorescein angiography. Jpn J Ophthalmol 27:218, 1983
8. Kohner EM, Dollery CT: The rate of formation and disappearance of microaneurysms in diabetic retinopathy. Europ J Clin Invest 1:167, 1970
9. Baudoin C, Maneschi F, Quentel G, et al: Quantitative evaluation of fluorescein angiograms: microaneurysm counts. Diabetes suppl. 2, 32:1, 1983
10. Frank RN, Hoffman WH, Podgor MJ, et al: Retinopathy in juvenile-onset diabetes of short duration. Ophthalmology 87:1, 1980
11. Palmberg P, Smith M, Waltman S, et al: The natural history of retinopathy in insulin-dependent juvenile-onset diabetes. Ophthalmology 88:613, 1981
12. Klein R, Klein BEK, Moss SE, et al: The Wisconsin epidemiologic study of diabetic retinopathy. 2. Prevalence and risk of diabetic retinopathy when age at diagnosis is less than 30 years. Arch Ophthalmol 102:520, 1984
13. Klein R, Klein BEK, Moss SE, et al: The Wisconsin epidemiologic study of diabetic retinopathy. 3. Prevalence and risk of diabetic retinopathy when age at diagnosis is 30 or more years. Arch Ophthalmol 102:527, 1984
14. Dobree JH: Simple diabetic retinopathy. Evolution of the lesions and therapeutic considerations. Br J Ophthalmol 54:1, 1970
15. Shimizu K, Kobayashi Y, Muraoka K: Midperipheral fundus involvement in diabetic retinopathy. Ophthalmology 88:601, 1981
16. Kohner EM: The evolution and natural history of diabetic retinopathy. Int Ophthalmol Clin 18:1, 1978
17. Bresnick GH, Diabetic maculopathy: a critical review highlighting diffuse macular edema. Ophthalmology 90:1301, 1983
18. Gass JDM: Stereoscopic Atlas of Macular Diseases. Mosby, St. Louis, 1977
19. Bresnick GH, Haight B, de Venecia G: Retinal wrinkling and macular heterotopia in diabetic retinopathy. Arch Ophthalmol 97:1890, 1979
20. Hirschberg J: Über diabetische Netzhautenzündung. Dtsch Med Wochenschr 16:1181, 1890
21. Ballantyne AJ: The state of the retina in diabetes mellitus. Trans Ophthamol Soc UK 66:503, 1946
22. Oakley NW, Joplin GF, Kohner EM, et al: Practical experience with a method for grading diabetic retinopathy. In Goldberg MF, Fine SL (eds): Treatment of Diabetic Retinopathy. Service Publication 1890. Government Printing Office, Washington, DC, 1968
23. Davis MD, Norton EWD, Myers FL: The Airlie classification of diabetic retinopathy. In Goldberg MF, Fine SL (eds): Treatment of Diabetic Retinopathy. Public Service Publication 1890. Government Printing Office, Washington, DC, 1968
24. Diabetic Retinopathy Study: Report 7. A modification of the Airlie House classification of diabetic retinopathy. Invest Ophthalmol 7:210, 1981
25. Klein BEK, Davis MD, Segal P, et al: Diabetic retinopathy: assessment of severity and progression. Ophthalmology 91:10, 1984
26. Verdonk CA, Palumbo PJ, Gharib H, et al: Diabetic microangiopathy in patients with pancreatitic diabetes mellitus. Diabetologia 11:395, 1975
27. Engerman RL: Animal models of diabetic retinopathy. Trans Am Acad Ophthalmol Otol 81:710, 1976
28. Engerman RL, Davis MD, Bloodworth JMB: Retinopathy in experimental diabetes: its relevance to diabetic retinopathy in man. In: Proceedings of the VII Congress of the In-

ternational Diabetes Federation. International Congress 231. Excerpta Medica, Amsterdam, 1971
29. Engerman RL, Kern TS: Experimental galactosemia produces diabetic-like retinopathy. Diabetes 33:97, 1984
30. National Diabetes Advisory Board: Eye Complications in Progress and promise in diabetes research. Report of the Second National Conference on Diabetes, Reston, Virginia, National Institutes of Health NIH Publication No. 84–661, 1984
31. Robison WG Jr, Kador PF, Kinoshita JH: Retinal capillaries: basement membrane thickening prevented with aldose reductase inhibitor. Science 221:1177, 1983
32. Frank RN, Keirn RJ, Kennedy A, et al: Galactose-induced retinal capillary basement membrane thickening: prevention by sorbinil. Invest Ophthalmol Vis Sci 24:1519, 1983
33. Little HL: The role of abnormal hemorrheodynamics in the pathogenesis of diabetic retinopathy. Trans Am Ophthalmol Soc 74:574, 1976
34. Ditzel J: Functional microangiopathy in diabetes mellitus. Diabetes 17:388, 1968
35. Ditzel J, Standl E: The problem of tissue oxygenation in diabetes mellitus. 1. Its relation to the early functional changes in the microcirculation of diabetic subjects. August Krogh Memorial Symposium, 1974, p. 49
36. Ditzel J: Impaired oxygen release caused by alterations of the metabolism in the erythrocytes in diabetes. Lancet 1:721, 1972
37. Kohner EM, Hamilton AM, Saunders SJ, et al: The retinal blood flow in diabetes. Diabetologia 11:27, 1975
38. Kohner EM: The problems of retinal blood flow in diabetes. Diabetes, suppl. 2, 25:839, 1976
39. Soeldner JS, Christacopoulos PD, Gleason RE: Mean retinal circulation time as determined by fluorescein angiography in normal, prediabetic, and chemical-diabetic subjects. Diabetes, suppl. 2, 25:903, 1976
40. Parving HH, Viberti GC, Keen H, et al: Hemodynamic factors in the genesis of diabetic microangiopathy. Metabolism 32:943, 1983
41. Yoshida A, Feke GT, Morales-Stoppello T, et al: Retinal blood flow alterations during progression of diabetic retinopathy. Arch Ophthalmol 101:225, 1983
42. Blair NP, Feke GT, Morales-Stoppello J, et al: Prolongation of the retinal mean circulation time in diabetes. Arch Ophthalmol 100:764, 1983
43. Skovborg F, Nielsen AV, Schlichtkrull J, et al: Blood viscosity in diabetic patients. Lancet 1:129, 1966
44. McMillan DE: Disturbance of serum viscosity in diabetes mellitus. J Clin Invest 53:1071, 1983
45. Lowe GDO, Lowe JM, Drummond MM, et al: Blood viscosity in young male diabetics with and without retinopathy. Diabetologia 18:359, 1980
46. Ditzel J: Whole-blood viscosity and related components in diabetes mellitus. Dan Med Bull 15:49, 1968
47. Cogan G, Merola L, Laibson PR: Blood viscosity, serum hexosamine and diabetic retinopathy. Diabetes 10:393, 1961
48. Colwell JA, Winscour PD, Halushka PV: Do platelets have anything to do with diabetic microvascular disease? Diabetes, suppl. 2, 32:14, 1982
49. Cunha-Vaz JG, Shakeb M, Ashton N: Studies on the permeability of the blood-retinal barrier. I. On the existence, development, and site of a blood-retinal barrier. Br J Ophthalmol 50:441, 1966
50. McMillan DE: The effect of diabetes on blood flow properties. Diabetes, suppl. 2, 32:56, 1982

51. Hickam JB, Sieker HO: Retinal vascular reactivity in patients with diabetes mellitus and with atherosclerosis. Circulation 22:243, 1960
52. Hickam JB, Frayser R: Studies of the retinal circulation in man: Observations on vessel diameter, arterio-venous oxygen difference, and mean circulation time. Circulation 33:302, 1966
53. Sinclair SH, Grunwald JE, Riva CE, et al: Retinal vascular autoregulation in diabetes mellitus. Ophthalmology 89:748, 1982
54. Yonemura D, Kawasaki K: New approaches to ophthalmic electrodiagnosis by retinal oscillatory potentials, drug-induced responses from retinal pigment epithelium and cone potential. Doc Ophthalmol 48:163, 1979
55. Kinnear P, Aspinall P, Lakowski R: The diabetic eye and colour vision. Trans Ophthalmol Soc UK 92:69, 1972
56. Puvanendran K, Devathasan G, Wong PK: Visual evoked responses in diabetes. J Neurol Neurosurg Psychiatry 46:643, 1983
57. DeOliveira J: Pericytes in diabetic retinopathy. Br J Ophthalmol 50:134, 1966
58. Sima AAF, Garcia-Salinas R, Basu PK: The BB Wistar rat: an experimental model for the study of diabetic retinopathy. Metabolism, suppl. 1, 32:136, 1983
59. Riva CE, Grunwald TE, Sinclair SH: Laser doppler velocimetry study of the effect on pure oxygen breathing on retinal blood flow. Invest Ophthalmol Vis Sci 24:47, 1983
60. Delori FC, Weiter JJ, Mainster MA, et al: Oxygen saturation measurements in retinal vessels. Invest Ophthalmol Vis Sci, suppl., 24:13, 1983
61. Buzney SM, Frank RN, Robison WG Jr: Retinal capillaries: proliferation of mural cells in vitro. Science 190:985, 1975
62. Buzney SM, Massicotte SJ: Retinal vessels: proliferation of endothelium in vitro. Invest Ophthalmol Vis Sci 18:1191, 1979
63. Michaelson IC: The mode of development of the retinal vessels and some observations of its significance in certain retinal diseases. Trans Ophthalmol Soc UK 68:137, 1948
64. Wise GN: Retinal neovascularization. Trans Am Ophthalmol Soc 54:729, 1956
65. Glaser BM, D'Amore PA, Michels RG, et al: Demonstration of vasoproliferative activity from mammalian retina. J Cell Biol 84:298, 1980
66. Rand LJ: Recent advances in diabetic retinopathy. Am J Med 70:595, 1982
67. Hamman RF: Data assessment and problem identification—reviewing the experience. In: Proceedings, Diabetic Control Conference, 1982, p. 32
68. Burditt AF, Caird FI, Draper GJ: The natural history of diabetic retinopathy. Q J Med 37:303, 1968
69. Miki E, Fukuda M, Kuzuya T, et al: Relation of the course of retinopathy to control of diabetes, age, and therapeutic agents in diabetic Japanese patients. Diabetes 18:773, 1969
70. Pirart J: Diabetes mellitus and its degenerative complications: a prospective study of 4,400 patients observed between 1947 and 1973. Diabetes Care 1:168, 1978
71. Pirart J, Diabetes mellitus and its degenerative complications: a prospective study of 4,400 patients observed between 1947 and 1973. Diabetes Care 1:252, 1978
72. Jackson RL, Ide CH, Guthrie RA, et al: Retinopathy in adolescents and young adults with onset of insulin-dependent diabetes in childhood. Ophthalmology 89:7, 1982
73. Kahn HA, Bradley RF: Prevalence of diabetic retinopathy, age, sex, and duration of diabetes. Br J Ophthalmol 59:345, 1975
74. Kornerup T: Studies in diabetic retinopathy: an investigation of 1,000 cases of diabetes. Acta Med Scand 153:81, 1955
75. Nilsson SE, Nilsson JE, Frostberg N, et al: The Kristianstad Survey II studies in a representative adult diabetic population with special reference to comparison with an adequate control group. Acta Med Scand 469:1, 1967

76. Houston A: Retinopathy in the Poole area: an epidemiological inquiry. In Eschwege E (ed): Advances in Diabetes Epidemiology. INSERM Symposium No. 22. Elsevier, Oxford, 1982
77. West KM, Erdreich LJ, Stober JA: A detailed study of risk factors for retinopathy and nephropathy in diabetes. Diabetes 29:501, 1980
78. Dorf A, Ballintine EJ, Bennett PH, et al: Retinopathy in Pima Indians: relationships to glucose level, duration of diabetes, age at diagnosis of diabetes, and age at examination in a population with a high prevalence of diabetes mellitus. Diabetes 25:554, 1976
79. King H, Balkau B, Zimmet P, et al: Diabetic retinopathy in Nauruans. Am J Epidemiol 117:659, 1983
80. Harrold BP: Diabetic retinopathy and hypertension. Br J Ophthalmol 55:225, 1971
81. Klein R, Klein BEK, Moss SE, et al: Prevalence of diabetes in southern Wisconsin. Am J Epidemiol 119:54, 1984
82. Barta L, Brooser G, Molnar M: Diagnostic importance of fluorescein angiography in infantile diabetes. Acta Diabetol Lat 9:290, 1972
83. Brooser G, Barta L, Anda L, et al: Frühdiagnose der mikroangiopathie bei kindlichem diabetes. Klin Monatsbl Augenheilkd 166:233, 1975
84. Malone JI, Van Cader TC, Edwards WC: Diabetic vascular changes in children. Diabetes 26:673, 1977
85. Dorchy H, Toussaint D, Vanderschueren-Lodeweyckx M, et al: Leakage of fluorescein: first sign of juvenile diabetic retinopathy; role of diabetic control and duration of diabetes. Acta Paediatr Scand 277:48, 1979
86. Starup K, Larsen HW, Enk B, et al: Fluorescein angiography in diabetic children. Acta Ophthalmol (Copenh) 58:347, 1980
87. Frost-Larsen K, Starup K: Fluorescein angiography in diabetic children: a follow-up. Acta Ophthalmol (Copenh) 58:355, 1980
88. Merimee TJ: Comparative metabolic and clinical studies of sexual ateliotic dwarfs and diabetics. In Camerini-Davalos RA, Cole HS (eds): Vascular and Neurological Changes in Early Diabetes. Academic Press, New York, 1973
89. Merimee TJ, Zapf J, Froesch ER: Insulin-like growth factors. N Engl J Med 309:527, 1983
90. White P: Childhood diabetes. Diabetes 9:345, 1960
91. Klein R, Klein BEK, Davis MD, et al: Risk factors for macular edema in diabetes. Invest Ophthalmol Vis Sci, suppl., 25:127. 1984
92. Lundbaek K: Diabetic retinopathy in newly diagnosed diabetes mellitus. Acta Med Scand 152:33, 1955
93. Knowler WC, Bennett PH, Ballintine EJ: Increased incidence of retinopathy in diabetics with elevated blood pressure: a six-year follow-up study in Pima Indians. N Engl J Med 302:645, 1980
94. Aiello LM, Rand LI, Briones JC, et al: Diabetic retinopathy in Joslin Clinic patients with adult-onset diabetes. Ophthalmology 88:619, 1981
95. Patz A, Berkow JW: Visual and systemic prognosis in diabetic retinopathy. Trans Am Acad Ophthalmol Otol 72:253, 1968
96. Klein R, Klein BEK, Moss SE: Visual impairment in diabetes. Ophthalmology 91:1, 1984
97. Bodansky HJ, Cudworth AG, Drury PL, et al: Risk factors associated with severe proliferative retinopathy in insulin-dependent diabetes mellitus. Diabetes Care 5:97, 1982
98. Jackson WPU, Goldin C, Marine N: Diabetics-interracial comparisons SA Med J 40:206, 1966
99. Tattersall RB, Pyke DA: Diabetes in identical twins. Lancet 2:1120, 1972
100. Pyke DA, Tattersall RB: Diabetic retinopathy in identical twins. Diabetes 22:613, 1973

101. Leslie RDG, Pyke DA: Diabetic retinopathy in identical twins. Diabetes 31:21, 1982
102. Larkins RG, Martin FIR, Tait BD: HLA patterns and diabetic retinopathy. Br Med J 1:1111, 1978
103. Anderson O, Vejtorp L, Christy M, et al: HLA factors in insulin-dependent diabetes mellitus: clinical significance. Diabetologia 11:329, 1975
104. Standl E: HLA-antigens and diabetic retinopathy: a different view warranted. Diabetologia 18:79, 1980
105. Barbosa J, Ramsay RC, Knobloch WH, et al: Histocompatibility antigen frequencies in diabetic retinopathy. Am J Ophthalmol 90:148, 1980
106. Dornan TL, Ting A, McPerson CK, et al: Genetic susceptibility to the development of retinopathy in insulin-dependent diabetics. Diabetes 31:226, 1982
107. Rand LI: HLA DR loci and diabetic retinopathy. Invest Ophthalmol Vis Sci, suppl., 24:80, 1983
108. Becker B, Shin DH, Burgess D, et al: Histocompatibility antigens and diabetic retinopathy. Diabetes 26:997, 1977
109. Moller E, Persson B, Sterky G: HLA phenotypes and diabetic retinopathy. Diabetologia 14:155, 1978
110. Jervell J, Solheim B: HLA-antigens in long standing insulin dependent diabetics with terminal nephropathy and retinopathy with and without loss of vision. Diabetologia 17:391, 1979
111. Cove DH: Are HLA types or BF alleles markers for diabetic retinopathy? Diabetologia 19:402, 1980
112. Bodansky HJ, Cudworth AG, Whitelocke RAF, et al: Diabetic retinopathy and its relation to type of diabetes: review of a retinal clinic population. Br J Ophthalmol 66:496, 1982
113. Bodansky JH, Wolf E, Cudworth AG, et al: Genetic and immunologic factors in microvascular disease in type I insulin-dependent diabetes. Diabetes 31:70, 1982
114. Engerman R, Bloodworth JMB, Nelson S: Relationship of microvascular disease in diabetes to metabolic control. Diabetes 26:760, 1977
115. Job D, Eschwege E, Guyotargenton C, et al: Effect of multiple daily insulin injections on the course of diabetic retinopathy. Diabetes 25:463, 1976
116. Tchobroutsky G: Relation of diabetic control to development of microvascular complications. Diabetologia 15:143, 1978
117. University Group Diabetes Program: A study of the effects of hypoglycemic agents on vascular complications in patients with adult-onset diabetes. VI. Supplementary report on nonfatal events in patients treated with tolbutamide. Diabetes 25:1129, 1976
118. Lauritzen T, Frost-Larsen K, Larsen HW, et al: Effect of 1 year of near-normal blood glucose levels on retinopathy in insulin-dependent diabetics. Lancet 1:200, 1983
119. The KROC Collaborative Study Group: Blood glucose control and the evolution of diabetic retinopathy and albuminuria. A preliminary multicenter trial. N Engl J Med 311:365, 1984
120. Dahl-Jorgensen K, Hanssen KF, Smelland E, et al: Long-term strict control in type 1 (insulin-dependent) diabetes mellitus: effect on late diabetic complications. Diabetologia 25:149, 1984
121. Lorenzi M, Goldbaum MH, Spencer EM: Improved diabetic control and retinopathy. N Engl J Med 308:1600, 1983
122. Hilsted J, Nielsen JD, Sestaft L, et al: Hypoglycemia may cause intravascular coagulation in juvenile diabetics. Diabetes, suppl. 2, 29:23, 1980
123. National Institute of Arthritis, Metabolism and Digestive Diseases: Request for research cooperative agreement applications: clinical centers for a collaborative clinical trial on

the relationship between blood glucose control and vascular complications on insulin-dependent diabetes mellitus. RFA NIAMDD 81–01. Government Printing Office, Washington, DC

124. Deutsch TA, O'Riordan JF, Ernest JT, et al: Systemic blood pressure and diabetic macular edema. Invest Ophthalmol Vis Sci, suppl., 24:80, 1983
125. Garcia MJ, McNamara PM, Gordon T, et al: Morbidity and mortality in diabetics in the Framingham population: sixteen year follow-up study. Diabetes 23:105, 1974
126. Paetkau ME, Boyd TAS, Winship B, et al: Cigarette smoking and diabetic retinopathy. Diabetes 26:46, 1977
127. Nielsen MM, Hjollund E: Smoking and diabetic microangiopathy. Lancet 2:533, 1978
128. Ball K, Turner R: Smoking and the heart. Lancet 2:822, 1974
129. Hawkins RL: Smoking, platelets and thrombosis. Nature 236:450, 1972
130. Christiansen JS, Nerup J: Smoking and diabetic nephropathy. Lancet 1:605, 1978
131. Madsbad S, McNair P, Christensen MS, et al: Influence of smoking on insulin requirement and metabolic status in diabetes mellitus. Diabetes Care 1:146, 1978
132. Rand LI, Perrin ED, Soeldner JS: Case-control study of diabetic retinopathy. Invest Ophthalmol Vis Sci, suppl., 20:59, 1981
133. Klein R, Klein BEK, Davis MD: Is cigarette smoking associated with diabetic retinopathy? Am J Epidemiol 118:228, 1983
134. Rodman HM, Singerman LJ, Aiello LM, et al: Diabetic retinopathy and its relationship to pregnancy. In Merkatz KR, Adams PAJ (eds): The Diabetic Pregnancy: A Perinatal Perspective. Grune & Stratton, New York, 1979
135. Beetham WP: Diabetic retinopathy in pregnancy. Trans Am Ophthalmol Soc 48:205, 1950
136. Carstensen LL, Frost-Larsen K, Fugleberg S, et al: Does pregnancy influence the prognosis of uncomplicated insulin-dependent diabetes mellitus? Diabetes Care 5:1, 1982
137. Larinkari J, Laatikainen L, Mooronen P, et al: Metabolic control and serum hormone levels in relation to retinopathy in diabetic retinopathy. Diabetologia 22:327, 1982
138. Moloney JBM, Drury MI: The effect of pregnancy on the natural course of diabetic retinopathy. Am J Ophthalmol 93:745, 1982
139. Hercules BL, Wozencroft M, Gayed II, et al: Peripheral retinal ablation in the treatment of proliferative diabetic retinopathy during pregnancy. Br J Ophthalmol 64:87, 1980
140. Johnston GP: Pregnancy and diabetic retinopathy. Am J Ophthalmol 90:519, 1980
141. Roy M, Hanna AK, Zimman B, et al: Risk factors for proliferative diabetic retinopathy. Invest Ophthalmol Vis Sci, suppl., 24:80, 1983
142. Feldman JN, Hirsh SR, Beyer MM, et al: Prevalence of diabetic nephropathy at time of treatment for diabetic retinopathy. In Friedman EA, L'Esperance FA (eds): Diabetic Renal-Retinal Syndrome: Prevention and Management. Vol. 2. Grune & Stratton, New York, 1982
143. Ramsey RC, Knobloch WH, Cantrill HL, et al: Visual status in transplanted and dialyzed diabetic patients. In Friedman EA, L'Esperance FA (eds): Diabetic Renal-Retinal Syndrome: Prevention and Management. Vol 2. Grune & Stratton, New York, 1982
144. Aiello LM, Rand LI, Brines JC, et al: Nonocular clinical risk factors in the progression of diabetic retinopathy. In Little HL, Jack RL, Patz A, et al (eds): Diabetic Retinopathy. Thieme-Stratton, New York, 1983
145. Flynn CT: The diabetics on CAPD. In Friedman EA, L'Esperance FA (eds): Diabetic Renal-Retinal Syndrome: Prevention and Management. Vol. 2. Grune & Stratton, New York, 1982
146. Davis MD, Hiller R, Magli YL, et al: Prognosis for life in patients with diabetes: relation to severity of retinopathy. Trans Am Ophthalmol Soc 77:144, 1979

147. Sharma NK, Archer DB, Hadden DR, et al: Morbidity and mortality in patients with diabetic retinopathy. Trans Am Ophthal Soc UK 100:83, 1980
148. Early Treatment Diabetic Retinopathy Study Coordinating Center: Manual of Operation. Chapters 1, 2, and 4. Diabetic Retinopathy Coordinating Center, Baltimore, 1980
149. Sorbinil Retinopathy Trial Coordinating Center: The Sorbinil Retinopathy Trial. A Brief Summary, Data Coordinating Center, Brookline Mass. 1983
150. Goldberg MF, Fine SL (eds): Treatment of Diabetic Retinopathy. Public Health Service Publication 1890. Government Printing Office, Washington, DC, 1968
151. British Multicentre Photocoagulation Trial: Proliferative diabetic retinopathy: treatment with xenon-arch photocoagulation; interim report of multicentre randomized controlled trial. Br Med J 1:739, 1977
152. Little HL: Complications of argon laser photocoagulation in the treatment of diabetic retinopathy. In Little HL, Jack RL, Patz A, et al (eds): Diabetic Retinopathy. Thieme-Stratton, New York, 1983
153. Doft BN, Blankenship GW: Early retinopathy risk factor regression after laser panretinal photocoagulation in proliferative diabetic retinopathy. Ophthalmology, suppl., 90:52, 1982
154. Patz A, Shatz H, Berkow JW, et al: Macular edema—an overlooked complication of diabetic retinopathy. Trans Am Acad Ophthalmol Otolaryngol 77:34, 1973
155. Rubinstein K, Myska V: Pathogenesis and treatment of diabetic maculopathy. Br J Ophthalmol 58:76, 1974
156. Marcus DF, Aaberg TM: Argon laser photocoagulation treatment of diabetic cystoid maculopathy. Ann Ophthalmol 9:365, 1977
157. Wyznia RA: Photocoagulation of nonproliferative exudative diabetic retinopathy. Am J Ophthalmol 88:22, 1979
158. Blankenship GW: Diabetic macular edema and laser photocoagulation. Ophthalmology 86:69, 1979
159. British Multicentre Study Group: Photocoagulation for diabetic maculopathy: a randomized controlled clinical trial using the xenon arc. Diabetes 32:1010, 1983
160. Wallow IH: Repair of the pigment epithelial barrier following photocoagulation. Arch Ophthalmol 102:126, 1984
161. Stefansson E, Landers MB III, Wolbarsht ML: The role of oxygen and vasodilation in diabetic retinopathy. In Friedman EA, L'Esperance FA (eds): Diabetic Renal-Retinal Syndrome: Prevention and Management. Vol. 2. Grune & Stratton, New York, 1982
162. Michaels RG, Rice TA, Rice EF: Vitrectomy for diabetic vitreous hemorrhage. Am J Ophthalmol 95:12, 1983
163. Michaels RG: Vitreous surgery for visual loss from proliferative diabetic retinopathy. In Friedman EA, L'Esperance FA (eds): Diabetic Renal-Retinal Syndrome: Prevention and Management. Vol. 2. Grune & Stratton, New York, 1982
164. Rice TA, Michaels RG: Complications of vitrectomy. In Little HL, Jack RL, Patz A, et al (eds): Diabetic Retinopathy. Thieme-Stratton, New York, 1983
165. Rosenthal RA: The diagnosis and management of rubeosis iridis. In Little HL, Jack RL, Patz A, et al (eds): Diabetic Retinopathy. Thieme-Stratton, New York, 1983
166. Diabetic Retinopathy Vitrectomy Study Coordinating Center: Manual of Operations. Diabetic Retinopathy Vitrectomy Coordinating Center, Minneapolis, 1976
167. Shea M: Early vitrectomy in proliferative diabetic retinopathy. Arch Ophthalmol 101:1204, 1983
168. Kahn HA, Hiller R: Blindness caused by diabetic retinopathy. Am J Ophthalmol 78:58, 1974
169. Caird FI, Garrett CJ: Prognosis for vision in diabetic retinopathy. Diabetes 12:389, 1963

170. Vision Problems in the U.S. Data Analysis. National Society to Prevent Blindness, New York, 1980
171. Leibowitz HM, Krueger DE, Maunder LR, et al: The Framingham eye study monograph. Surv Ophthalmol 24:335, 1980
172. Roberts J: Monocular visual acuity of persons 4–74 years, United States, 1971–1972. Vital and Health Statistics: Series 11, Data from National Health Survey, Data from the Health Examination Survey, No. 201, 1977
173. Howe LJ, Drury JT: Current estimates from the Health Interview Survey, United States, 1977. Vital and Health Statistics Series 10, No. 126, 1978
174. Begg IS, Lakowski R: A comparison of colour vision with other methods of clinical assessment in diabetics with macular edema. In Verriest G, Brist G (eds): Colour Vision Deficiencies, Vol. 3. Adam Hilger, Bristol, England, 1980
175. Bresnick GH, Crawford J, Groo A: Urine testing inaccuracies among diabetic patients with color vision deficiency. Symposium on Color Vision. Adam Hilger, Bristol, England, (in press)
176. Riordan P, Pascoe PT, Vaughan DG: Refractive change in hyperglycaemia: hyperopia, not myopia. Br J Ophthalmol 66:500, 1982
177. Kinoshita JH, Fukushi S, Kador P, et al: Aldose reductase in diabetic complications of the eye. Metabolism 28:462, 1979
178. Kinoshita JH: Mechanisms initiating cataract formation. Invest Ophthalmol Vis Sci 13:713, 1974
179. Fukushi S, Merola LO, Kinoshita JH: Altering the course of cataracts in diabetic rats. Invest Ophthalmol Vis Sci 19:313, 1980
180. Ederer F, Hiller R, Taylor HR: Senile lens changes and diabetes in two population studies. Am J Ophthalmol 91:381, 1981
181. Burditt AF, Caird FI: The natural history of lens opacities in diabetics. Br J Ophthalmol 52:433, 1968
182. Cotlier E, Fagadau W, Cicchetti DV: Methods for evaluation of medical therapy of senile and diabetic cataracts. Trans Ophthalmol Soc UK 102:416, 1982
183. Cotlier E: Senile cataracts: evidence for acceleration by diabetes and deceleration by salicylate. Can J Ophthalmol 16:113, 1981
184. Seigel D, Sperduto RD, Ferris FL: Aspirin and cataracts. Ophthalmology 89:47, 1982
185. Straatsma BR, Pettit TH, Wheeler N, et al: Diabetes mellitus and intraocular lens implantation. Ophthalmology 90:336, 1983
186. Clayman HM, Jaffe NS, Light DS: Lens implantation and diabetes mellitus. Am J Ophthalmol 88:990, 1979
187. Becker B: Diabetes mellitus and primary open angle glaucoma. Am J Ophthalmol 70:1, 1971
188. Vacharat N: Risk factors in glaucoma. Int Ophthalmol Clin 19:157, 1979
189. Bankes JLK: Ocular tension and diabetes mellitus. Br J Ophthalmol 51:557, 1967
190. Armaly MF, Baloglu PJ: Diabetes mellitus and the eye. I. Intraocular pressure and aqueous outflow facility. Arch Ophthalmol 77:493, 1967
191. Kahn HA, Leibowitz HM, Ganley JP, et al: The Framingham eye study. II. Association of ophthalmic pathology with single variables previously measured in the Framingham heart study. Am J Epidemiol 106:33, 1977
192. Leske MC: The epidemiology of open-angle glaucoma: a review. Am J Epidemiol 118:166, 1983
193. Sussman EJ, Tsiaras WG, Soper K: Diagnosis of diabetic eye disease. JAMA 247:3231, 1982

194. Waltman SR: Vitreous fluorophotometry. In Little HL, Jack RL, Patz A, et al (eds): Diabetic Retinopathy. Thieme-Stratton, New York, 1983
195. Frost-Larsen K, Larsen HW, Simonsen SE: Oscillatory potential and nyctometry in insulin-dependent diabetics. Acta Ophthalmol (Copenh) 58:879, 1980
196. The Carroll Center for the Blind: Diabetic control: equipment for use with vision loss. Aids Appliances Rev 6:1, 1982
197. Bluhm HP, Stone JB: Diabetic retinopathy patients: characteristics and rehabilitation implications. J Rehabil 49:50, 1983

5 Diabetes and the Kidney: An Update

Ralph A. DeFronzo

It has been estimated that 2–5 percent of the population of the United States has diabetes mellitus.[1,2] During the preinsulin era the mean life expectancy from the time of diagnosis was only 5 years. With the advent of insulin therapy the mean life expectancy has progressively increased and is now more than 20 years. With this increase in longevity the frequency of deaths from renal disease has also risen, from 3 percent to over 10 percent.[3–6] Further breakdown of this increase in renal mortality, based on data published from the Joslin Clinic and the Steno Memorial Hospital, reveals that it is primarily the young insulin-dependent (type I—IDD) diabetic, who develops his disease during the first two decades of life, who is affected. In this younger population end-stage renal failure accounts for slightly over 50 percent of the mortality.[3–6] In contrast, in patients whose onset of diabetes is after the age of 40, the primary cause of mortality is related to accelerated atherosclerosis and manifests in the form of myocardial infarction and stroke. This older group comprises 80–90 percent of the total diabetic population, and the great majority are noninsulin-dependent (type II—NIDD). In this NIDD group, advanced renal insufficiency is relatively uncommon compared to that in the young IDD.[7]

DIABETIC NEPHROPATHY

Kimmelstiel and Wilson in 1936 were the first to draw attention to the prominent renal histopathological changes in juvenile-onset diabetes.[8] In eight patients studied at autopsy there was diffuse intercapillary glomerulosclerosis in association with nodule formation. Clinically these patients manifested hypertension, edema, heavy albuminuria, and varying degrees of renal insufficiency. Since this initial description,

Table 5-1. Diabetic Nephropathy: Histological Changes

Glomerulosclerosis
Diffuse intercapillary glomerulosclerosis
Nodular glomerulosclerosis
Glomerular basement membrane thickening
Vascular disease: arteriosclerosis and arteriolosclerosis
Tubulointerstitial disease

numerous studies have reported on the changes in renal histology.[9–22] The major histopathological changes observed in the diabetic kidney are outlined in Table 5-1 and are summarized below. For a more detailed description the reader is referred to references 9–22.

Glomerulosclerosis

Three distinctive glomerular lesions have been described: diffuse intercapillary gluomerulosclerosis, nodular glomerulosclerosis, and glomerular basement membrane (GBM) thickening (Fig. 5-1). Two other lesions, which have been reported less commonly, are the capsular-drop lesion and the exudative, or fibrin-cap, lesion.

Diffuse and Nodular Lesions. The diffuse form of intercapillary glomerulosclerosis is the most frequently encountered and is characterized by increased amounts of periodic acid-Schiff (PAS)-positive, eosinophilic material within the mesangial region (Fig. 5-1A). The process is diffuse, involving the entire glomerulus, and is generalized, affecting all glomeruli throughout the kidney. The first changes involve a widening of the normally delicate strands of mesangial matrix with little or no increase in the number of mesangial cells. With time this mesangial material coalesces, expanding the mesangial region and encroaching on adjacent capillary lumens. As this process progresses entire glomeruli may become hyalinized. As the mesangial matrix increases, it sometimes forms large acellular nodules at the center of peripheral glomerular lobules (Fig. 5-1B). This nodular lesion occurs in 40–50 percent of all patients with glomerular involvement. It is invariably seen in association with the diffuse lesion and is highly *pathognomonic* of diabetes mellitus. Although it is the most specific lesion observed in diabetics, it correlates poorly with the severity of clinical renal disease. The best predictor of the severity of renal insufficiency is the diffuse lesion.[8,13,23–25] Thus, it is very common to see advanced diabetic nephropathy [glomerular filtration rate (GFR) $<$ 20 ml/min] without Kimmelstiel-Wilson nodules; conversely, it is not uncommon to see nodules in diabetic individuals with relatively well preserved renal function. In essentially all diabetic patients with advanced renal insufficiency, diffuse intracapillary glomerulosclerosis is present.

Two other glomerular lesions may be observed with diabetic renal involvement. The exudative, or fibrin-cap, lesion is an eosinophilic, lipid-containing mass found within the lumen of a peripheral capillary loop. This histological abnormality is not specific for diabetes and may be seen in a variety of disorders including glomerulonephritis and arteriolosclerosis. Its presence correlates best with the severity of vascular disease. The last lesion characteristic of diabetic glomerulosclerosis is the capsular-drop lesion. This appears as a small, rounded, homogeneous, eosinophilic mass

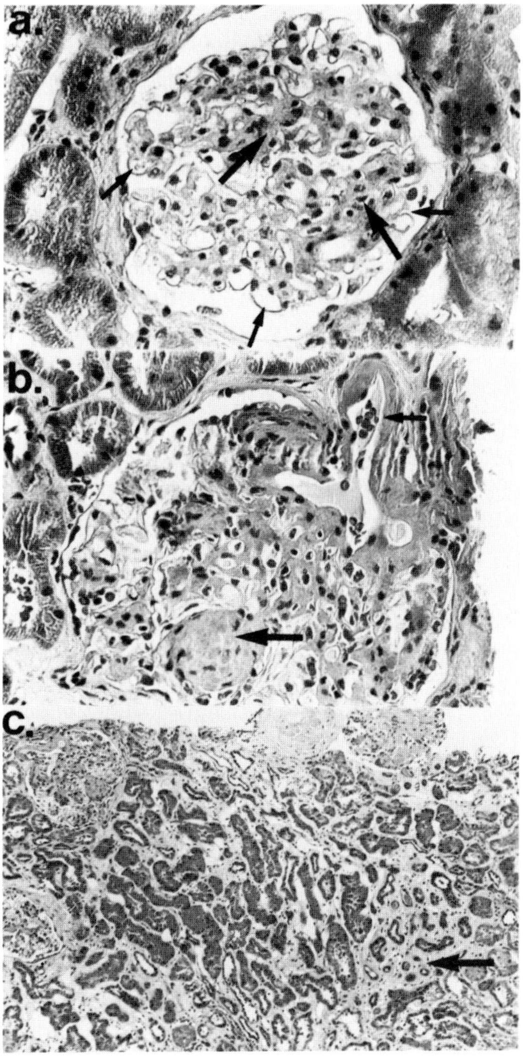

Fig. 5-1 (a) Diffuse diabetic glomerulosclerosis with marked mesangial matrix hyperplasia (thick arrows) and thickened glomerular basement membranes (thin arrows). No hypercellularity is evident. (b) Nodules (thick arrows) are usually observed in the peripheral capillary loops and are almost never seen in the absence of the diffuse lesion. Note the prominent arteriolosclerosis in the efferent and afferent arterioles with ischemic injury (thin arrows). (c) Interstitial fibrosis and tubular atrophy (thick arrows). Evidence of both diffuse and nodular glomerulosclerosis is also present.

situated between the capillary basement membrane and the overlying parietal epithelium of Bowman's capsule. It is unusual to observe the fibrin-cap or capsular-drop lesion in the absence of diffuse diabetic glomerulosclerosis.

Immunofluorescent examination has revealed a diffuse linear deposition of immunoglobulin G (IgG) along the glomerular basement membrane to be the most frequent finding.[8,18] Other immunoglobulins and complement have not been demonstrated. Although this linear pattern of immunoglobulin deposition is reminiscent of anti-GBM nephritis, IgG eluted from the glomerulus has been shown to have no affinity for glomerular basement membrane. It is likely, therefore, that the presence of IgG represents nonspecific trapping of filtered proteins and is not an important mediator of the renal disease. Although an increase in the mesangial matrix is characteristic of diabetes, immunoglobulin deposition in this area is quite rare.

Basement Membrane Thickening. The third lesion which characterizes diabetic glomerulosclerosis is thickening of the glomerular basement membrane (Fig. 5-1A). Studies by Osterby et al.[12,17,22] have documented that basement membrane thickening is absent in newly diagnosed insulin-dependent (type I) diabetics. She also failed to demonstrate any abnormalities in mesangial morphology at the time of initial diagnosis. Within 3–5 years, however, significant basement membrane thickening as well as expansion of the mesangial region was observed. These observations have been confirmed by others.[26,27] Initially, the basement membrane changes are detectable only by electron microscopic examination, but with time the thickening is easily visible by light microscopy. The absence of basement membrane and mesangial abnormalities early in the course of clinical diabetes provides evidence that alterations in the metabolic environment rather than genetic abnormalities are responsible, at least in part, for the development of the renal disease. We return to this issue in subsequent sections. It should be emphasized that thickening of the capillary basement membrane is not limited to the glomerulus but can be observed in all capillaries throughout the body, including muscle, skin, and retina.

Like other basement membranes in the body, the glomerular capillary basement membrane has been shown to be a collagen-like protein[11,28–31] that is synthesized by visceral epithelium of the glomerulus. Studies in rats have shown that the turnover of the normal glomerular basement membrane is quite slow,[32,33] with continuous addition of new membrane material from the epithelial aspect and simultaneous removal from the endothelial side, where it is phagocytosed by the mesangial cells. It has been estimated that the half-life of the glomerular basement membrane may be as long as 100 days. Studies[24,34–38] have indicated that both increased epithelial synthesis as well as impaired removal contribute to the basement membrane thickening observed in IDDM. Failure of the mesangial cell to normally phagocytose and remove old basement membrane[32] leads to the accumulation of basement membrane-like material within the mesangium.

Biochemical analysis of the glomerular basement membrane has demonstrated significant differences in the collagen and protein content compared to basement membranes from nonrenal tissues[29,30]: Unlike other collagen, most of the proline is hydroxylated into hydroxyproline; there is a high content of hydroxylysine; and cysteine, which is absent in ordinary collagen, is present in significant amounts. The carbohydrate content is also much higher than in other collagen, approaching 10 percent. Approximately half of the carbohydrate is present as a disaccharide, glucose-galactose-hydroxylysine, and the other half as a heterogeneous polysaccharide, containing variable amounts of sialic acid, galactose, hexosamine, and frucose bound to asparagine. These differences in chemical composition somehow are responsible for the very high glomerular filtration coefficient, which permits a water flux that is 50- to 100-fold greater than in other capillaries, yet totally restricts the passage of serum proteins. The ability to selectively restrict proteins seems to be related to the strong negative charge provided by heparin sulfate and sialic acid residues within the glomerular basement membrane.[39–41]

Considerable controversy exists concerning biochemical alterations in the composition of the glomerular basement membrane in diabetic nephropathy. Studies by Beisswenger and Spiro have demonstrated an abnormal composition of the glycoprotein comprising the basement membrane isolated from diabetics with advanced renal disease.[42] Hydroxylysine and glycine content are increased, whereas valine and tyrosine are diminished. In addition, the glucosylgalactose disaccharide, which is linked via a beta-glycositic bond to the hydroxyl group of hydroxylysine, is also increased. Subsequent studies in alloxan diabetic rats demonstrated increased activity of glucosyltransferase, which is involved in the assembly of hydroxylysine-linked carbohydrate units.[35] Tight regulation of the plasma glucose concentration with insulin returned the activity of this enzyme to normal.[35] These results suggest that the thickened glomerular capillary basement membrane may result from accelerated synthesis of hydroxylysine-glucose-galactose subunits, which are the biochemical representation of the metabolic derangement stemming from insulin deficiency. However, other groups have been unable to demonstrate a significant alteration in amino acid or glucosylgalactose content in glomerular basement membranes isolated from diabetic individuals.[43–46] These apparently discrepant results may be related to methodological differences and have been discussed in detail.[47] Falk et al,[48] demonstrated a polyantigenic expansion, involving all of the intrinsic components of the glomerular basement membrane and mesangium. This suggests an overall increase in the synthetic rate of "normal" basement membrane and/or a decrease in the rate of degradation. There seems to be agreement that in glomeruli isolated from diabetics with advanced nephropathy the sialic acid content of the basement membrane is diminished.[44,49] This may contribute to the increased clearance of negatively charged macromolecules, e.g., albumin, in these diabetic patients.

Lastly, it should be emphasized that *in vitro* studies employing isolated glomeruli have shown that glucose per se, independent of insulin, is capable of stimulating its own incorporation into capillary basement membrane in a dose-dependent fashion in both man[50] and rats.[51,52] Furthermore, hyperglycemia has been shown to be responsible for other structural protein abnormalities *in vivo,* including abnormal circulating levels of glycosylated hemoglobin. The functional significance of excessive glucosylation of glomerular basement membranes is presently unclear, but it has been suggested that glucosylated collagen may be more resistant to degradation.

Vascular Involvement

Both renal arteriosclerosis and arteriolosclerosis are quite common and more severe in diabetic than in nondiabetic individuals (Fig. 5-1B). In the larger arteries atheromatous changes, characterized by lipid deposition and intimal fibrosis, are often advanced and may contribute to renal failure by secondarily leading to ischemic parenchymal atrophy. The degenerative process in the smaller renal arterioles is different from that involving the larger vessels. Here arteriolosclerosis is characterized by pronounced hyaline thickening, in which both the afferent and efferent vessels are involved. Hyaline appears as an acidophilic, finely granular material containing fibrinogen, globulins, lipids, and other protein. It is first deposited in the intima of the renal arterioles and gradually invades the media, resulting in loss of muscle cells. Although both arteriosclerosis and arteriolosclerosis may be quite extensive in diabetic subjects, neither process seems to correlate with the severity of glomerular change. Although several authors have suggested that narrowing of large and small renal vessels may contribute to the frequent occurrence of hypertension in diabetics with advanced renal involvement, recent studies have shown that plasma renin levels are often low, making a renovascular etiology unlikely[53,54] in the majority of diabetic hypertensive patients. Paradoxically, however, it has been our impression that in patients with documented renal artery stenosis diabetes mellitus is a common occurrence. In keeping with this, Shapiro et al.[55] reported that 29 of 55 patients with renal artery stenosis were diabetic.

Tubulointerstitial Disease

Although not commonly appreciated, tubulointerstitial changes (Fig. 5-1C) are quite common in the diabetic kidney, and in advanced cases there is marked tubular atrophy and interstitial fibrosis.[9,10] Such changes are commonly observed with renal ischemia, but in the diabetic the tubular changes often correlate poorly with the degree of vascular involvement and may even be seen in their absence. The involved tubules often show thickening of the tubular basement membrane, and immunofluorescence studies have demonstrated deposition of IgG along the tubular basement membrane.[9,56] The interstitial area surrounding the involved tubules is fibrotic and often contains a cellular infiltrate of lymphocytes and plasma cells. These changes progress with increasing duration of the diabetes.[9,57] Many investigators have attributed such changes to pyelonephritis, but it should be pointed out that such an interstitial reaction does not necessarily imply infection. It is true that asymptomatic bacteriuria and pyelonephritis are twice as common in diabetics, particularly women, as in nondiabetics.[58] This propensity to urinary tract infection probably results from a variety of factors including impaired renal blood flow, bladder dysfunction, interstitial scarring, impaired polymorphonuclear leukocyte function, defective leukocyte chemotaxis, and glucosuria, which enhances bacterial growth. However, it has been difficult to demonstrate any relationship between either the frequency or severity of interstitial changes and the presence of urinary tract infection. In fact, Batalla et al.[59] failed to detect any deterioration of renal function in 104 diabetic patients with urinary tract infection over a 4-year period. Furthermore, patients whose bacteriuria was not eradicated fared no worse than those in whom the bacteriuria was cured. As stated above, the interstitial changes correlate poorly with vascular disease and ischemic injury, raising the possibility that they are a direct representation of the diabetic state per se. The only tubular lesion which is characteristic of the diabetic state is the Aramanni-Ebstein lesion. This is characterized by vacuolation of the proximal tubular cells of the pars recta. These vacuoles have been shown to contain glycogen and are most often observed in poorly controlled diabetics. Today this lesion is uncommon.

A special type of interstitial lesion, papillary necrosis, may be observed in diabetics. In all large series reported to date[60–62] diabetes mellitus has accounted for over 50 percent of the cases. This is the result of ischemic damage to the inner medulla with eventual infarction and sloughing of part of or the whole papilla. Such patients may present with an acute fulminant illness with fever, shock, flank pain, gross hematuria, pyuria, oliguria, and renal failure, or they may have a more subacute form characterized by microscopic hematuria, pyuria, and indolent renal failure. After diabetes mellitus, urinary tract obstruction and pyelonephritis represent the two next most common causes of renal papillary necrosis. Because these two conditions commonly complicate the diabetic state, it is not surprising that the incidence of papillary necrosis is so high in diabetic patients. Because phenacetin has commonly been associated with papillary necrosis, this analgesic should be avoided in the diabetic population.

PATHOGENESIS OF DIABETIC GLOMERULOSCLEROSIS

Two theories have been proposed to explain the development of diabetic nephropathy (Table 5-2). The first states that the renal changes are secondary to alterations in the metabolic milieu that results from insulin deficiency. The second argues that genetic factors are responsible for the changes in renal histology and function.

Metabolic Theory

Several strong arguments favor the theory that diabetic nephropathy is acquired. First, renal involvement is absent in diabetics who are biopsied at the time their disease is first diagnosed. Basement membrane thickening and mesangial and vascular changes do not become manifest until at least 2–3 years later.[12,17,21,22,26,27,63] Second, the typical changes of diabetic nephropathy have been observed in pancreatic diabetes resulting from hemochromatosis, chronic pancreatitis, and pancreatectomy for cancer.[27,64,65] Basement membrane thickening, diffuse mesangial cell matrix hyperplasia, and even nodules (which are thought to be highly specific for diabetes) have been observed, and the renal involvement may progress to clinically significant renal insufficiency.

Third, lesions similar to those of diabetic nephropathy have been observed in a variety of animal models including the rat,[66–81] mouse,[82–85] dog,[86–89] and monkey[90] irrespective of the means by which diabetes was induced, i.e., pancreatectomy, alloxan, streptozotocin, spontaneous, genetic. In animals tightly regulated with insulin, diabetic renal lesions did not develop.[71–73,91] Also, transplantation of pancreatic islets into diabetic rats has prevented the development of renal lesions or led to the resolution of established diabetic nephropathy.[67,92–97] Furthermore, if kidneys of diabetic rats are transplanted into nondiabetic rats, the renal lesions resolve.[98] Conversely, if normal kidneys are transplanted into diabetic rats, diabetic nephropathy ensues.[69] The development of retinal lesions, including microaneurysms, have also been described in dogs made diabetic with alloxan.[99]

Fourth, kidneys from nondiabetic individuals transplanted into diabetics have developed histological changes suggestive of diabetic nephropathy.[16,98,100–102] Although the transplanted kidneys have been in place for less than 2–5 years, prominent hyalinosis of the afferent and efferent arterioles, basement membrane thickening, diffuse glomerulosclerosis, and linear staining of IgG along the glomerular basement membrane have developed in most grafts, and in some cases nodular glomeruloscle-

Table 5-2. Etiology of Diabetic Nephropathy: Metabolic and Genetic Theories

A. **Metabolic (acquired) theory**
   1. Renal involvement is absent in diabetics biopsied when their disease is first diagnosed. Basement membrane and mesangial changes do not become manifest until at least 2–3 years later.
   2. Typical changes of diabetic nephropathy have been observed in pancreatic diabetes, resulting from hemochromatosis, chronic pancreatitis, pancreatectomy, and cystic fibrosis.
   3. Animal models—In the dog, monkey, rat, and mouse, lesions similar to those observed in human diabetic nephropathy have been documented following the induction of diabetes.
      a. Tight regulation with insulin prevents the development of renal lesions in the above models, even if insulin therapy is initiated several months after the renal lesion has become demonstrable.
      b. Transplantation of kidneys from diabetic into normal rats cures the renal disease. Conversely, transplantation of normal kidneys into diabetic rats leads to diabetic changes within 2–4 months.
   4. Human diabetes—In man, normal kidneys transplanted into diabetic individuals develop changes of diabetic nephropathy within 2–5 years. Transplantation of diabetic kidneys into nondiabetic humans leads to a resolution of the diabetic renal lesion.

B. **Genetic theory**
   1. There is poor correlation between diabetic glomerulosclerosis and the degree of diabetic control as judged by blood glucose levels. The literature is replete with studies that claim to "conclusively document" that good control "prevents" the development of diabetic nephropathy. However, an equal number of studies claim the opposite.
   2. Artificial pancreas—Excellent glucose control with the insulin pump for upward of 1–2 years has failed to reverse proteinuria. Some diabetics have experienced progressive proteinuria and azotemia (no renal biopsies).
   3. Only a minority of individuals with pancreatic diabetes develop glomerulosclerosis.
   4. Occasional cases of diabetic nephropathy have been reported early in the course of diabetes, in the "prediabetic" state, and in individuals with normal glucose tolerance.
   5. Siperstein stated that muscle basement membrane thickening is present when diabetes mellitus is first diagnosed and occurs in approximately half of individuals with "prediabetes" (i.e., offspring of two diabetic parents) at a time when glucose tolerance is entirely normal. These findings have been challenged by others (see text for a more detailed discussion).

rosis also has been observed. The later lesion is highly specific for diabetic nephropathy. In a recent study Abouna et al.[103] performed two cadaveric renal transplants from a donor with a 17-year history of IDDM with established proteinuria and biopsy-proved diabetic nephropathy. After transplantation into two nondiabetic patients, the kidneys demonstrated excellent function. After 7 months both recipients were free of proteinuria, and renal biopsy showed resolution of the diffuse diabetic glomerulosclerosis. Sutherland et al.[104] also reported the regression of diabetic nephropathy in diabetic patients after pancreatic transplantation.

Taken in toto, the preceding evidence provides strong support for the concept that the development of diabetic nephropathy is, in large part, determined by the deranged metabolic milieu in which the kidney is bathed.

Genetic Theory

In favor of the genetic theory (Table 5-2), it has been stated that there is a poor correlation between diabetic glomerulosclerosis and the degree of diabetic control as judged from blood glucose levels. Numerous extensive reviews have addressed this issue,[105–109] and the reader is referred to an excellent updated discussion by Tchobroutsky.[110] The literature is replete with studies that claim to ''conclusively document'' that good metabolic control ''prevents'' or ''does not prevent'' the development of diabetic nephropathy. Depending on one's particular bias, one can find evidence that either supports or negates the role of metabolic control in the pathogenesis of diabetic complications. We agree with the analysis of Kaplan and Feinstein,[111] who concluded that major flaws in study design, inability to achieve and document good metabolic control over a prolonged period of time, imprecise data analysis, etc. make it difficult to draw any firm conclusions concerning the effect of diabetic control on the development of microvascular complications.

It was hoped that clinical trials comparing tight versus poor control with the artificial pancreas might help to resolve the issue of ''what is inherited, what is acquired.'' However, in short-term studies with follow-up of 1–2 years, the achievement of good metabolic control (normal fasting plasma glucose concentration; normalization of glycosylated hemoglobin levels) has failed to reverse or ameliorate established nephropathy (proteinuria, azotemia) or prevent the emergence of new cases of diabetic renal disease.[112–114] The genetic proponents have used this information to argue against the metabolic theory and in favor of inheritance as the primary determinant of diabetic nephropathy as well as other microvascular complications. It is important, however, to point out the limitation of these published studies.[112–114] First, the follow-up period was quite short, in the order of several years, and it is likely that a much longer time is necessary to fully evaluate the true impact of tight metabolic control on microvascular complications. Second, none of the published studies were designed to examine whether good metabolic control can slow (as opposed to reverse) the progression of diabetic nephropathy. Third, and in our opinion most important, insulin pump therapy was not instituted until after patients had had their diabetes for many years. There are now abundant data (see subsequent discussion) to indicate that major renal hemodynamic and structural changes occur within the first several months to years after the development of fasting hyperglycemia. If these changes are not reversed with tight control within the first 1–2 years after the development of diabetes, they may lead to fixed, irreversible alterations that, of themselves, are responsible for the relentless progression to renal insufficiency (see discussion later in the chapter on the hyperfiltration process).

Additional arguments that have been used to support the genetic theory include: the development of diabetic glomerulosclerosis in only a minority of patients with secondary diabetes,[27,64,65] occasional cases of diabetic nephropathy early in the course of diabetes or in the ''prediabetic'' state,[8,115,116] and the development of typical diabetic glomerulosclerosis in individuals without glucose intolerance.[117–123]

Studies by Siperstein et al.[124–126] also provide support for the genetic theory. These authors observed significant muscle capillary basement membrane thickening in adult IDDs from the moment the diagnosis of diabetes was first made. In contrast, basement membrane thickening was not observed in patients whose diabetes was secondary to an acquired pancreatic disease. They also found muscle capillary basement thickening in over half of "prediabetic" individuals, i.e., the offspring of two diabetic parents. In contrast, Williamson and colleagues[127–129] found normal basement membrane thickness at the onset of diabetes and an increase in width that paralleled the duration of diabetes. Furthermore, they found significant muscle capillary basement membrane thickening in patients with secondary or acquired diabetes mellitus. As reviewed by Williamson and Kilo,[130,131] the difference between their results and those of Siperstein et al.[124–126] most likely is explained by differences in fixation techniques. Other investigators have repeated these studies, and there seems to be agreement that at the onset of diabetes the muscle capillary basement membranes are not thickened but increase in thickness with the length of diabetes.[132–136] In addition, Ireland et al.[27] provided evidence that the capillary basement membrane is thickened in patients with secondary diabetes. The study by Raskin et al.[136] is of particular interest. They found that thickened skeletal muscle basement membranes could be restored to normal width by continuous subcutaneous insulin pump therapy in some patients. When considered together, these studies seem to indicate that muscle capillary basement thickening is not present at the onset of diabetes, develops in relationship to poor metabolic control, and can be reversed with normalization of the metabolic milieu.

In summary, it seems that metabolic disturbances contribute, in large part, to the development of diabetic nephropathy. However, it is likely that these metabolic derangements operate on a genetic background that predisposes the kidney to the development of diabetic glomerulosclerosis.

CLINICAL COURSE

Studies from the Joslin Clinic[2,3,137,138] and other diabetes centers[5,6,11,139–143] have documented that fewer than half of all IDDs who have had their disease for 20–30 years or longer will develop clinically significant renal disease. At the time of initial presentation there seem to be no clinical or laboratory findings that predict which individuals will eventually progress to end-stage renal failure. Although diabetic glomerulosclerosis is more common in juvenile-onset (insulin-dependent) than in maturity-onset (noninsulin-dependent) diabetics, it is not clear whether this difference in prevalence is the result of basic differences in the etiology of the diabetes, the longer duration of diabetes in the juvenile-onset diabetics, or poorer control in the younger group.

Early Changes in Renal Function

Early in the course of diabetes the GFR is characteristically increased,[20–22,144–153] and this correlates with increased kidney weight and size [11,20–22,144,153–155])Fig. 5-2). Morphometric studies have shown this increase to result from an increase in mean glomerular volume and increased capillary luminal area per glomerulus.[12,17,21,22,63,144,156] Neither increased cellularity, mesangial matrix, nor basement membrane thickening are present at this stage. Tubular size is also in-

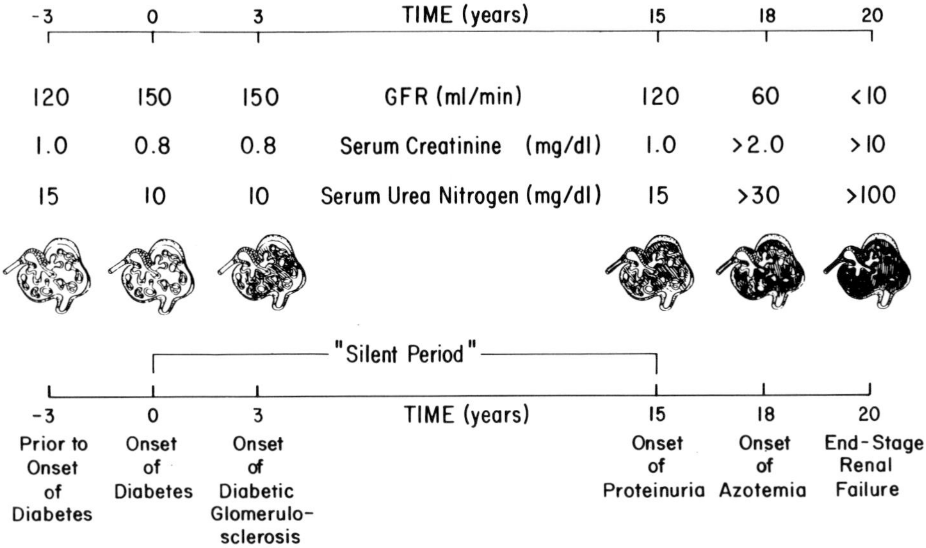

Fig. 5-2 Natural course of diabetic nephropathy. At the time of initial diagnosis, renal function and glomerular histology are normal. Within 2–3 years, increased mesangial matrix and basement membrane thickening are observed. Renal function remains normal until 15 years when proteinuria first develops. This is an ominous sign and usually indicates advanced diabetic glomerulosclerosis. Within 3 years after the onset of proteinuria, elevation of the serum urea nitrogen and creatinine levels are observed, and within 2 years after the development of azotemia half of the patients have advanced to end-stage renal insufficiency.

creased during this early diabetic state.[22] In man the increase in GFR is closely correlated with these structural changes, especially the filtration surface area.[157] Insulin therapy for as little as 2–3 months is capable of returning kidney size and GFR to normal.[154,158]

Introduction of experimental diabetes in the rat also is associated with a marked increase in renal weight within 48–72 hr. As in man, the total glomerular capillary length, basement membrane surface area, glomerular volume, and proximal tubular length and diameter are markedly increased without any thickening of the glomerular basement membrane[159,163–165] Insulin treatment[159,160,170] or islet cell transplantation,[171] if started at the onset of hyperglycemia, prevents the increase in kidney size and GFR. As discussed by Seyer-Hansen,[159] these changes in kidney size and function seem to be independent of changes in glucagon, growth hormone, catecholamines, or prostaglandins; some combination of hyperglycemia and/or insulin lack seems to be essential for these early renal changes to occur. We return to this issue when we discuss the possible role of renal hemodynamic alterations in the progressive decline in renal function observed in patients with established diabetic nephropathy.

In early diabetes in man changes in renal plasma flow (RPF) have been less consistently observed than GFR changes. Although RPF has been reported to be increased by some authors,[172] most investigators have found a normal[20,21,144,146] or even decreased[148–150] renal plasma flow. In all studies the filtration fraction (GFR/RPF) was found to be increased.

Late Changes in Renal Function

In those 30–40 percent of diabetics who are destined to develop renal disease, a very predictable sequence of events ensues (Fig. 5-2 and 5-3). There is a silent period of approximately 15–18 years, during which time there is no laboratory evidence of renal dysfunction.[17,20,21,22,25,143–146,173,174] During this period, however, renal biopsy demonstrates a progressive and widespread increase in eosinophilic PAS-positive material within the mesangial region, thickening of the capillary basement membrane, interstitial fibrosis, and arteriolosclerosis. Amazingly, the GFR remains elevated during this silent period[20,21,143,174,175] and may even persist into the proteinuric stage.[176] The only abnormality that can be demonstrated during this silent period is an excessive increase in exercise-induced albuminuria.[144,177–179] Although some investigators have suggested that identification of patients with exercise-induced proteinuria may provide a helpful means of identifying those who are at risk to develop progressive renal disease, in our opinion there is little evidence to support this concept. In fact, in the only study in which diabetic patients have been reexamined after the original exercise test, no laboratory evidence of renal disease was found.[20] However, the follow-up period was relatively short, 5 years, and it could be argued that a longer period of observation is needed to define the true predictive value of the exercise test.

The earliest manifestation of diabetic glomerulosclerosis is proteinuria (Fig. 5-2 and 5-3), which begins approximately 15–18 years after the diagnosis of diabetes.[17,20–22,25,143–146,173,174] At this time the GFR may still be normal or even elevated, but within a mean of 3 years after the onset of proteinuria an impairment in GFR can

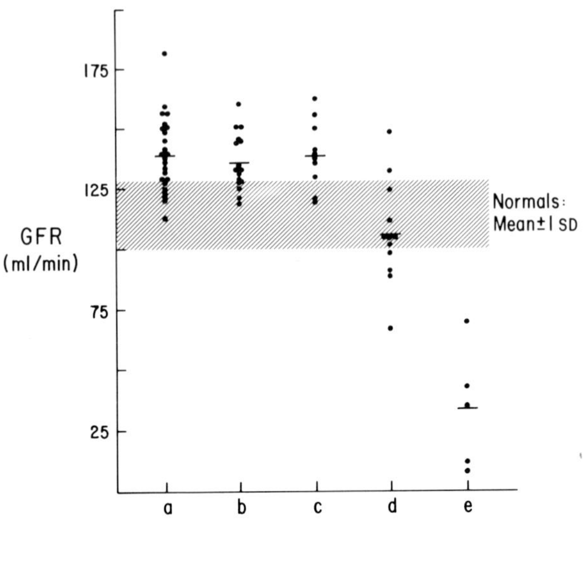

Fig. 5-3 GFR in (a) short-term diabetics (diabetes duration 1–12 years), (b) long-term diabetics without proteinuria (diabetes duration > 15 years), (c) long-term diabetics with intermittent proteinuria, (d) constant and pronounced proteinuria but normal serum creatinine, and (e) severe retinopathy and increased serum creatinine and proteinuria. (Redrawn from Mogensen CE: Abnormal physiological processes in the kidney. In Brownlee M (ed): Handbook of Diabetes Mellitus. Vol. 4. pp. 23–85. Garland STPM Press, New York, 1981.)

be demonstrated as evidenced by an increase in the serum urea nitrogen and creatinine concentrations. Within 2–3 years after the first elevation in serum creatinine concentration, half of the patients progress to end-stage renal insufficiency. Unlike other causes of progressive renal failure, significant proteinuria persists despite the marked decline in renal function. As stated earlier, proteinuria (>200–300 mg/day) is the earliest laboratory manifestation of renal involvement and provides the best correlate with the degree of renal involvement. Massive proteinuria (more than 3 g/day) and the nephrotic syndrome are common, occurring in over half of those individuals who progress to end-stage renal failure. It should be noted that the course described above may be quite different in maturity-onset diabetics. Such patients not uncommonly have significant but low-grade proteinuria (200–500 mg/day), yet renal function remains stable and serial kidney biopsies fail to demonstrate progressive renal disease.[7,14]

LABORATORY ABNORMALITIES

Proteinuria

The mechanism of proteinuria in the diabetic patient has been extensively studied. In normal individuals the rate of urinary albumin excretion does not exceed 10–20 μg/min (15–30 mg/day). In poorly controlled diabetic patients urinary albumin excretion rates above this are common,[20,148,158,180–182] and albumin excretion rates often exceed 100 μg/min. This is the level at which the Albustix reaction becomes positive (i.e., 75–125 μg/min, or about 100 mg/dl). However, tight control with insulin corrects this abnormality in protein excretion.[20,144,158,180–182] It is important, therefore, to take into account the degree of metabolic control when evaluating the clinical significance of albuminuria. As discussed earlier, diabetics also manifest increased rates of urinary albumin excretion in response to exercise or stress.[20,144,177–181] When collecting urine for protein determination, the patient should be instructed to avoid heavy exercise or other stressful situations.

In recent years much attention has been focused on the concept of microalbuminuria. This is defined as a baseline urinary albumin excretion greater than 15–20 μg/min but less than 300 μg/min. Viberti et al. suggested that such microalbuminuria is a predictor of clinical nephropathy in IDDs.[183] However, before accepting their suggestion, it is important to examine closely the data on which their statement has been based. In 1966–1967 they had the opportunity to obtain quantitative urinary ablumin excretion rates on 87 IDDs among whom follow-up information was obtained in 63 patients in 1980–1981. Of 55 IDDs with albumin excretion rates less than 30 μg/min, only two had become clinically proteinuric as defined by a positive Albustix. In contrast, seven of eight with albumin excretion rates above 30 μg/min on initial screening had developed "clinical proteinuria." However, there was a large difference in the duration of diabetes between the two groups. In the IDDs with albumin excretion rates in excess of 30 μg/min, the mean duration of diabetes on initial screening was 14 years. It is quite likely that these diabetics had overt diabetic nephropathy at the time of initial screening and the "microalbuminuria" simply represented the tip of the iceberg. Unfortunately, data on serum creatinine concentrations were not given and creatinine clearances were not obtained. This information would have been of help in establishing whether GFR was already diminished at the time of initial screening.

Furthermore, even if microalbuminuria were a predictor of eventual renal involvement, data from the same group,[113] as well as others,[112,114] have demonstrated that the institution of tight metabolic control in patients who have had their diabetes for more than 5–10 years has little if any effect on altering the course of established diabetic nephropathy. Therefore it is unlikely that the detection of "microalbuminuria" 14 years after the onset of diabetes[113] is likely to have major therapeutic implications. As will be discussed, it is probable that after 5 years (or even less) of poorly controlled diabetes there are fixed structural and hemodynamic changes that largely determine the course of diabetic renal involvement. Mogensen et al.[20] reported on seven IDDs with microalbuminuria (15–300 μg/min) who were followed for 6 years. In three there was a small increase in albuminuria, and in four there was no change. More importantly, the mean GFR was unchanged (142 versus 139 ml/min) in the seven subjects. Obviously, many more IDDs will have to be studied with much longer periods of follow-up before the true significance of microalbuminuria can be established. One further consideration needs to be kept in mind when interpreting the significance of microalbuminuria. Circulating albumin is to a large extent retained by the normal glomerular capillaries. Of that which is filtered, over 90 percent is reabsorbed by the proximal renal tubular cells. Thus, a defect in tubular reabsorption of albumin could account for the presence of "microalbuminuria." In an attempt to examine this question, several groups have looked at the excretion of beta$_2$-microglobulin, a small-molecular-weight protein that is freely filterable but completely reabsorbed by the proximal tubular cells.[144,179,182] The failure to find beta$_2$-microglobulin in the urine of diabetic patients with "microalbuminuria" has been used as an argument against a tubular origin for the albumin. This presumes, however, that albumin and beta$_2$-microglobulin are handled in identical fashion by the diabetic kidney, and this has not been established.

Using fractional dextran clearances and urinary albumin/IgG excretion, several groups have attempted to examine the mechanism(s) responsible for the proteinuria observed in IDDs.[20,144,183–189] Three primary factors control the transglomerular flux of proteins: (1) the transglomerular ultrafiltration pressure gradient; (2) pore size and pore number; and (3) the molecular charge of the glomerular barrier.[190,191] Myers and colleagues performed the most definitive studies in IDDs with macroproteinuria [184–186]; the data from their 1982 report are shown in Fig. 5-4. Neutral dextrans of differing molecular radii were infused into diabetic and control subjects, and the clearance of dextran was related to the clearance of inulin. A value of 1.0 indicates that the dextran molecule is completely permeable, whereas a value of 0 implies that the dextran is completely restricted from passage through the glomerular barrier. The Einstein-Stokes radius of albumin is 36Å. As can be seen in Figure 5-4, at molecular radii less than this the fractional clearance of dextran is significantly decreased compared to controls, indicating that the albuminuria cannot be explained by a generalized increase in pore size. In contrast, there is an increased clearance of neutral dextrans with Einstein-Stokes radii greater than 50–55 Å. Using pore theory analysis, Myers

	Diabetics	Controls
Number	20	15
Age (years)	48	49
Duration (years)	19	–
GFR (ml/min/1.73 m²)	19*	100
RPF (ml/min/1.73 m²)	89*	481
FF	0.21	0.21
Albuminuria (µg/min)	3560*	3
IgG Excretion (µg/min)	494*	0

*p < 0.001 vs controls

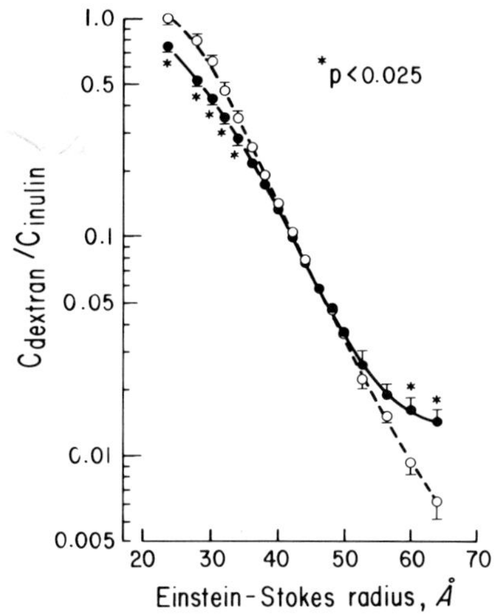

Fig. 5-4 Mechanism of proteinuria in insulin-dependent diabetics with advanced diabetic nephropathy. The patient and laboratory characteristics are summarized in the left panel. The fractional clearance of dextran is plotted as a function of the Einstein-Stokes radius in the right panel. The molecular radius of albumin is 36 Å. In diabetic patients (closed circles) the excretion of dextrans with molecular weights less than 50 Å was not increased compared to controls (open circles), indicating that the albuminuria was not the result of a generalized increase in pore size (see text for a more detailed discussion). (*) = a p value of < 0.025. (Data from Winetz JA, Golbetz HV, Spencer RJ et al: Glomerular function in advanced human diabetic nephropathy. Kidney Int 21:750, 1982.)

and colleagues interpreted these results to indicate the presence of two populations of pore sizes within the glomerular basement membrane. The main component is responsible for the major portion of the glomerular filtrate and is a "small pore" ultrafilter that is responsible for the restriction barrier to neutral dextrans with small radii (less than 40 Å). The minor component represents a "large pore" ultrafilter through which large, as well as small, macromocules can pass. This would explain the leakage of large, neutrally charged proteins such as IgG, which has a molecular radius of 55 Å. However, because the total number of these "large pore" ultrafilters is small, they cannot account for the very high excretion rates of albumin. It is now well established that the negative charge of the glomerular basement membrane provides a highly selective electrostatic barrier to the passage of albumin, which is also negatively charged.[190,191] Therefore it has been postulated that the increased transglomerular passage of circulating polyanions, including albumin, results from defective electrostatic barrier function.[184–186] Similar findings and conclusions have been reported by Viberti et al.[187] and Parving et al.[188,189] Such a hypothesis is consistent with cytochemical studies which have demonstrated the loss of polyanions from glomerular basement membranes isolated from patients with diabetic nephropathy.[44,49] In a recent study Viberti et al.[187] reported on 29 IDDs with normal renal function and "microalbuminuria" (10–150 mg/day). They found a proportional rise in the clearance of both albumin and IgG. Taken in concert with the data of Mogensen,[145] who found that the fractional dextran clearance was not altered in early insulin-dependent diabetes, it seems likely that the increased fractional clearance of albumin and IgG[187] results from an increased transglomerular capillary pressure gradient that drives both albumin and IgG across the glomerular barrier in unchanged proportions. Such a hypothesis is consistent with micropuncture studies that have documented an elevated transglomerular pressure gradient in diabetic rats.[170] If this explanation is correct, the pathophysiological mechanisms responsible for early ''microalbuminuria'' and late ''microalbuminuria'' would be quite distinct and it would be very surprising if ''microalbuminuria'' turned out to be a reliable predictor of clinically significant diabetic nephropathy.

Lastly, a few comments about basement membrane changes and how they relate to proteinuria are indicated. In early diabetes basement membrane thickening is not present, yet albuminuria may be observed, especially during periods of poor control or after exercise or stress. Conversely, after 10–15 years of diabetes marked basement membrane thickening is uniformly observed, yet proteinuria is often absent. Such findings argue against a significant role for basement membrane changes in the pathogenesis of proteinuria. In a theoretical analysis of their dextran clearance data, Winetz et al.[185] came to the same conclusion.

Glomerular Filtration Rate

In order to detect the presence of impaired renal function, follow the progression of renal disease, and evaluate the impact of therapeutic interventions, it is important to have reliable indices of the GFR in diabetic individuals. The most widely employed laboratory tests are the serum creatinine and serum urea nitrogen concentrations. However, both of these chemical determinations have their limitations. The serum urea nitrogen and, to a lesser extent serum creatinine, are influenced by both prerenal (i.e., extracellular fluid volume depletion) and postrenal (i.e., urinary tract obstruction) factors. More importantly, the GFR may decline as much as 40–50 percent before either test becomes elevated into the abnormal range. Furthermore, the plasma creatinine concentration is highly dependent on the muscle mass and protein intake, and both of these may be diminished in the diabetic patient, particularly if renal insufficiency is present. Many authors have advocated following the creatinine clearance. Assuming that a complete 24-hr urine specimen can be collected, this represents the most practical and reliable means of assessing renal function in diabetic patients with normal or near-normal renal function. In advanced glomerular disease, however, the tubular secretion of creatinine increases and glomerular function may be overestimated. Both inulin and ^{54}Cr-EDTA have proved reliable in following changes in renal function in the diabetic[144,192]; however, neither of these tests can be practically performed by most physicians. Use of the reciprocal of the serum creatinine concentration has proved useful in following the progression of renal disease in patients with renal failure of diverse etiology. First advocated by Mitch et al. and Walser et al.,[193,194] subsequent studies proved its usefulness in diabetic individuals as well.[144,195,196] If one plots 1/serum creatinine (1/Cr) as a function of time in diabetics with impaired renal function, a straight line is obtained (Fig. 5-5). Extrapolation of

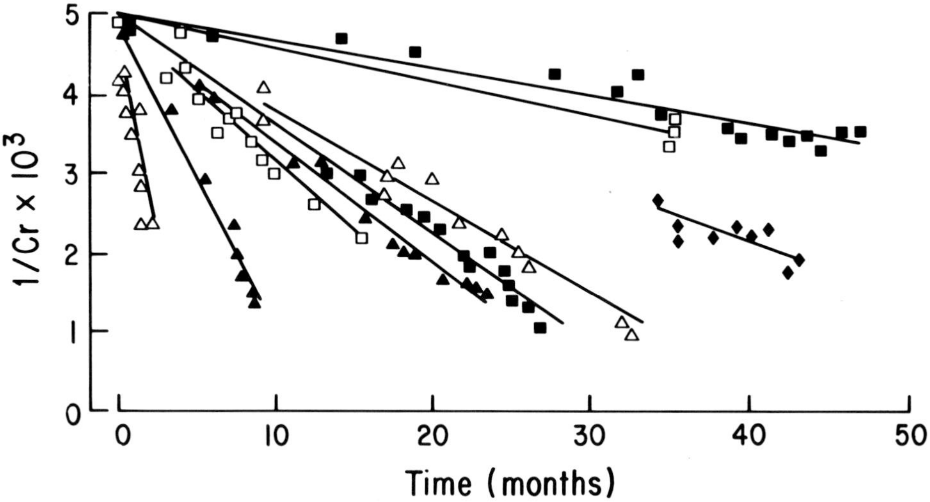

Fig. 5-5 Plot of the inverse of serum creatinine against time in nine insulin-dependent diabetic patients with renal insufficiency. (Reprinted with permission from Jones RH, Hayakawa M, Mackay JD, et al: Progression of diabetic nephropathy Lancet 1:1105, 1979.)

this line to the abscissa allows one to predict when intervention with dialysis will be necessary. In addition, if therapeutic intervention has a beneficial effect on renal function, an abrupt break in the slope of the line is evident. From a purely pragmatic standpoint, we advocate following the creatinine clearance in diabetic patients with normal serum creatinine levels. Once the serum creatinine concentration becomes elevated, either the reciprocal of the serum creatinine or the creatinine clearance can be followed. Studies by Viberti et al.[192] suggest that 1/Cr is the more reliable of the two methods.

Glucosuria

In normal subjects the maximum tubular reabsorptive capacity for glucose (Tm_G) varies with the GFR. This also holds true for recent-onset IDDs in whom the elevated GFR is paralleled by an increase in Tm_G.[144,200] However, in longstanding diabetics with reduced GFR and diabetic glomerulosclerosis, the Tm_G is raised[11,201,202] and the presence or absence of glucose in the urine becomes an unreliable means of monitoring the adequacy of diabetic control.

Hyperkalemia

In normal man the maintenance of normal potassium homeostasis is dependent on both renal[203] and extrarenal[203,204] mechanisms. The total amount of potassium in the body is about 50 mEq/kg, or 3500 mEq for a 70-kg man. Of this, only 2 percent is located within the extracellular fluid. It is important to note that gain from the extracellular space of an amount of potassium equal to only 1 percent of the total body potassium content (35 mEq) can cause a 50 percent increase in the plasma potassium concentration and lead to profound disturbances in neuromuscular and cardiac function. The maintenance of this high intracellular/extracellular potassium concentration ratio is dependent not only on the Na-K-ATPase pump but also on a number of other factors, including hydrogen ion balance, plasma tonicity, and the plasma concentrations of insulin, epinephrine, and aldosterone.[203,204]

Approximately 100 mEq of potassium is ingested per day, and essentially all of this is absorbed from the stomach and upper gastrointestinal tract. About 10 mEq of potassium per day is excreted in stool. Although the epithelial cells of the colon are clearly capable of potassium secretion, their capacity is limited, and the *kidney* is the major organ responsible for the maintenance of *chronic* potassium balance. In contrast, *acute* potassium homeostasis is, in large part, regulated by *extrarenal tissues.* During the first, 4–6 hr after oral and intravenous potassium administration, only half of the potassium load appears in the urine.[203–205] If all of the infused or ingested potassium that was not excreted were retained in the extracellular fluid compartment, the increase in plasma potassium concentration would produce life-threatening hyperkalemia. This does not occur because nearly 80 percent of the retained potassium load is translocated into cells.

Based on this brief review of normal potassium homeostasis, it should be obvious that the diabetic individual is particularly prone to the development of hyperkalemia (Table 5-3). Basal hyperkalemia is common for two reasons: (1) the normal distribution of potassium between intracellular and extracellular compartments in altered; and (2) there may be an increase in total body potassium content secondary to a decrease in renal excretion.

The primary hormone that regulates the distribution of potassium between intracellular and extracellular compartments is insulin. Because type I diabetics are both insulin-deficient and insulin-resistant, they are particularly predisposed to develop hyperkalemia. Furthermore, as the plasma glucose concentration rises, the increased tonicity causes an osmotic shift of fluid and electolytes, primarily potassium, out of cells. The two other hormones, aldosterone and epinephrine, that play an important role in extrarenal potassium homeostasis [206,207] are also frequently diminished in insulin-dependent diabetics. As discussed below, the syndrome of hyporeninemic hypoaldosteronism is very common in diabetic individuals, as is autonomic insuffi-

Table 5-3. Causes of Hyperkalemia in the Diabetic

Extrarenal mechanisms (muscle, liver, gut)
Insulin lack
Aldosterone lack
Epinephrine lack
Hyperosmolality
Acidemia—metabolic
Drugs (beta-adrenergic antagonists)
Renal mechanisms
Reduced GFR
Renal disease—interstitial nephritis
Hypoaldosteronism (hyporeninemia)
Drugs (prostaglandin inhibitors, aldactone, beta-adrenergic antagonists)

ciency. The combination of insulinopenia and adrenal hormone deficiency is particularly worrisome, as it has an additive effect in the development of hyperkalemia.[208] Metabolic acidemia, which is common in the diabetic patient (see subsequent discussion), also predisposes to the development of hyperkalemia. Approximately half of a hydrogen ion load is buffered within cells, and this occurs in exchange for potassium ions.[203,204]

Renal mechanisms also contribute to the development of hyperkalemia in the diabetic patient (Table 5-3). Because the majority of potassium that appears in the final urine represents potassium that is secreted by the mid-late distal and collecting tubular cells, decreases in GFR are an uncommon cause of hyperkalemia. However, if the GFR falls to values less than 15–20 ml/min, the ability to excrete potassium may be impaired.[203] Therefore in patients with advanced diabetic nephropathy, reduced renal mass per se may contribute to the defect in potassium excretion. As discussed earlier, many patients with IDDM demonstrate a very marked interstitial process characterized by fibrosis, tubular atrophy, and tubular basement membrane thickening. Because the majority of urinary potassium is derived from distal and collecting tubular cell secretion, it is not surprising that this interstitial process should contribute to the renal defect in potassium excretion.

The syndrome of hypoaldosteronism is very common in diabetics, particularly in those with evidence of impaired renal function.[209,210] During the last 10 years a number of patients with hyperkalemia in association with hyporeninemia and hypoaldosteronism have been reported. When this subject was initially reviewed in 1980 by DeFronzo,[209] 81 cases of this syndrome had been reported. Since then many more cases have been described, primarily in diabetic subjects.[210–216] The clinical presentation is quite typical (Table 5-4). Most patients are old (mean age 65 ± 7 years), and this may be an important underlying substrate as both renin and aldosterone secretion are known to decrease with advancing age. The majority of patients (approximately 75 percent) have no clinical symptoms and are diagnosed on routine laboratory screening or during evaluation for some other unassociated illness. Only 25 percent of patients

Table 5-4. Clinical and Laboratory Characteristics in 81 Patients with Selective Hypoaldosteronism

1. Mean age = 65 years (range 32–82 years)
2. Findings at presentation
   a. Asymptomatic hyperkalemia (75%)
   b. Muscle weakness (25%)
   c. Cardiac arrhythmia (25%)
   d. Hyperchloremic acidosis (~50%)
   e. Salt wasting (unusual)
3. Normal glucocorticoid function
4. Mild to moderate renal insufficiency, 57/81 (70%)
5. Diabetes mellitus, 40/81 (49%)
6. Low or low-normal baseline plasma aldosterone levels: all patients had a subnormal increase following volume contraction, 81/81 (100%)
7. Normal baseline and/or stimulated plasma renin levels, 13/74 (18%)
8. Normal aldosterone response to angiotensin II infusion, 4/27 (15%)
9. Normal aldosterone response to ACTH administration, 7/34 (21%)

Data from DeFronzo RA: Hyperkalemia and hyporeninemic hypoaldosteronism. Kidney Int 17:118, 1980.

present with symptoms referable to the hyperkalemia, i.e., muscle weakness and cardiac arrhythmias. A hyperchloremic metabolic acidosis (see subsequent section) is common, being present in over half of the cases. Salt wasting is distinctly uncommon. Most of these patients have a partial defect in aldosterone secretion, but the low circulating aldosterone levels are sufficient to maintain normal sodium balance. Baseline plasma cortisol levels and the cortisol response to ACTH are by definition normal in all patients. The majority of patients (approximately 70–80 percent) have some degree of chronic renal insufficiency. Diabetic glomerulosclerosis is the most common renal disease and is followed by a variety of interstitial renal processes including gouty nephropathy, nephrolithiasis, analgesic nephropathy, obstructive uropathy, and sickle cell disease.

Baseline plasma aldosterone concentrations are low or low normal, and after volume contraction a subnormal increase has been observed in all reported cases (Table 5-4). Although patients may demonstrate some rise in plasma aldosterone concentration after volume depletion, the absolute increase is always much less than expected in normal subjects. Renin, acting through angiotensin II, is an important physiological regulator of aldosterone synthesis, and in the great majority of patients with selective hypoaldosteronism the low circulating plasma aldosterone levels can be explained in large part by the hyporeninemia.[203,209] Schambelan et al.[211] provided evidence that the decrease in plasma aldosterone concentration is usually proportional to the decrease in plasma renin activity. However, normal basal renin values have been reported in several series.[203,209,210] Moreover, patients with the syndrome of hyporeninemic hypoaldosteronism all have clinically significant hyperkalemia, and hyperkalemia is the most potent stimulus to aldosterone secretion. Therefore it is surprising to observe a low plasma aldosterone concentration in diabetic patients with "hyporeninemic" hypoaldosteronism. This suggests that, in addition to hyporeninemia, a primary adrenal defect may contribute to the hypoaldosteronism. Several additional pieces of evidence suggest that, at least in a significant minority of patients, factors other than impaired renin secretion may play a role in the development of the hypoaldosteronism. First, baseline and/or stimulated renin levels have been reported to be normal in 13 of 74 (18 percent) patients in whom they were measured (Table 5-4). Similar observations were reported by Schambelan et al.[211] Among 23 hyperkalemic patients with hypoaldosteronism, plasma renin activity was normal in four, or 21 percent. This is very similar to that found by DeFronzo[209] (18 percent) in his review of the literature. Second, the response to intravenous angiotensin II infusion was normal in only 4 of 27 (15 percent) patients (Table 5-4). Because angiotensin II directly stimulates aldosterone release by the zona glomerulosa, one would anticipate a normal response if the adrenal gland were intact. Likewise, the aldosterone response to ACTH, another agent which directly stimulates adrenal production of aldosterone, was normal in only 7 of 34 (21 percent) patients (Table 5-4). In summary, these studies show that a variety of physiological stimuli (ACTH, angiotensin II infusion, hyperkalemia) are capable of stimulating aldosterone secretion in patients with selective hypoaldosteronism, but in absolute terms the aldosterone response is almost universally impaired. Whether this represents a primary defect in aldosterone secretion or represents adrenal atrophy secondary to prolonged hyporeninemia remains to be determined.

In the diabetic individual it is possible that the defect in aldosterone biosynthesis is related to insulin lack per se or some cellular function that is mediated by insulin (Fig. 5-6). It is well established that insulin stimulates potassium uptake by a variety of tissues, including muscle and liver.[203,204,216] In addition, basal insulin levels have been shown to serve an important regulatory role in potassium homeostasis.[205] If insulin also regulates potassium uptake by the adrenal gland, a state of intracellular potassium depletion might develop in diabetic patients. Previous studies[217,218] have shown that the ability of ACTH and angiotensin II to stimulate aldosterone secretion by cultured zona glomerulosa cells is decreased in the presence of low potassium concentrations. Thus, intracellular hypokalemia per se may contribute to the defect in aldosterone biosynthesis in diabetic patients with "hyporeninemic" hypoaldosteronism.

Although many hypotheses have been put forward to explain the defect in renin secretion, no single explanation can satisfactorily account for the pathogenesis of the hyporeninemia. Selective damage to the juxtaglomerulosa apparatus is most frequently cited to explain the hyporeninemia. However, there is very little evidence to support this pathogenetic sequence. Several investigators have identified the presence of high concentrations of the biologically inactive renin precursor, "big renin," in

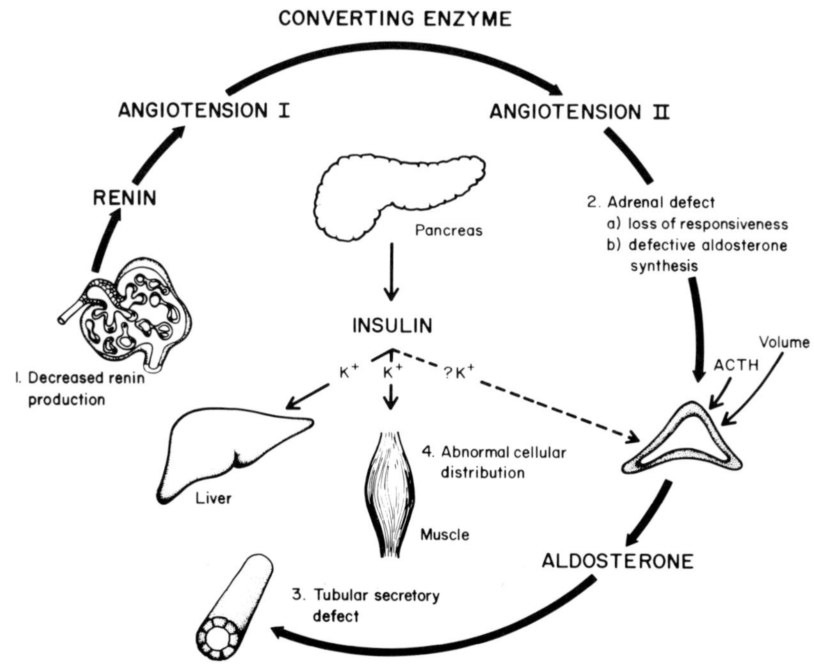

Fig. 5-6 Potential hormonal, renal, and extrarenal defects resulting in hyperkalemia in the diabetic. Hyperkalemia may result as a consequence of: (1) decreased renin production; (2) decreased aldosterone production despite normal renin secretion (adrenal defect); (3) a renal tubular secretory defect; (4) an abnormal distribution of potassium between intracellular and extracellular fluid compartments.

association with reduced levels of plasma renin activity in diabetic subjects.[53,219,220] These observations raise the possibility that in the diabetic hyporeninemia may result from impaired conversion of prorenin (or "big renin") to active renin. Decreased circulating catecholamine levels and/or autonomic neuropathy also have been suggested to explain the hyporeninemia in diabetic subjects with hypoaldosteronism. Sympathetic nerve terminals are known to innervate the juxtaglomerulosa apparatus, and epinephrine has been shown to stimulate renin secretion.[221] Because autonomic neuropathy is common in diabetics and longstanding diabetics may have decreased circulating levels of catecholamines,[222] decreased sympathetic activity has been implicated in the hyporeninemia in diabetic subjects. Support for this hypothesis was provided by Tuck et al,[212] who found a decreased plasma renin response to isoproterenol in five hyperkalemic diabetic patients with hyporeninemic hypoaldosteronism and evidence of autonomic and/or peripheral neuropathy. In contrast, previous studies described normal plasma and/or urinary catecholamines in six cases of selective hypoaldosteronism,[203] and deChatel et al.[54] found no relation between decreased plasma epinephrine levels and defects in the renin-aldosterone axis in 59 diabetic patients.

Decreased circulating prostaglandin levels have been suggested as a cause of the hyporeninemia in patients with selective hypoaldosteronism, but the evidence for this is not compelling.[203] Extracellular fluid volume expansion secondary to sodium retention has also been postulated to result in a state of physiological renin suppression.[20;3,216] However, in none of the studies in which volume contraction was induced with diuretics and/or a low sodium diet were changes in plasma potassium or total body potassium stores taken into account. Because hyperkalemia is known to suppress renin secretion, the simultaneous correction of this abnormality could, in part, have been responsible for the increase in plasma renin activity observed after volume contraction. Most importantly, even though many patients demonstrate a two- to three-fold increase in plasma aldosterone level after volume contraction, the absolute values are always well below those reported in healthy controls with a similar volume stimulus.

An interesting pathogenetic sequence that has not previously been discussed and which could lead to the development of hyporeninemia has to do with the concept of glomerular hyperfiltration and tubuloglomerular feedback.[205,223–225] In the diabetic with fasting hyperglycemia ($>$180 mg/dl) one would expect a translocation of fluid from the intracellular to the extracellular compartment. However, the intravascular volume expansion that results from this fluid shift is small, in the order of a few hundred milliliters, and one would not expect this to have a major effect on suppressing renin secretion. However, with fasting glucose levels in excess of 180 mg/dl, there would be a large increase in the filtered load of glucose, particularly postprandially; glucosuria would result, and sodium reabsorption by all segments of the nephron would be inhibited. According to the concept of tubuloglomerular feedback initially proposed by Schnermann et al.[226] and recently reviewed by Wright and Briggs,[227] increased tubular flow through the ascending limb, when it is associated with enhanced sodium/chloride reabsorption by the macula densa cells, provides a signal for increased renin production by the adjacent zona glomerulosa cells. This in turn enhances the local generation of angiotensin, which causes glomerular vasoconstriction and a decrease in the single nephron glomerular filtration rate (SNGFR). If sodium/chloride reabsorption by the macula densa cells is blocked with furosemide[227,228] or the osmotic agent mannitol,[227] the normal tubuloglomerular feedback mechanism is interfered with, the renin-angiotensin system is not activated, and SNGFR does not decline. One would expect that glucose, which has osmotic effects similar to those of mannitol, would also disrupt the normal tubuloglomerular feedback loop. In fact, studies by Blantz, Konnen, and co-workers[229–231] have shown just such an effect. If the macula densa is perfused with increasing rates of a glucose-free solution, there is a marked drop in SNGFR. If, however, glucose is added to the perfusion solution, the decrease in SNGFR is markedly blunted. These observations may help to explain the characteristically high rates of renal plasma flow and GFR observed early in the course of type I diabetes as well as the late development of hyporeninemia. We return to this construct later in the discussion.

In summary, it is likely that there are multiple factors which can affect both renin and aldosterone secretion in the diabetic. The complexity of the alterations in the renin-aldosterone axis in the diabetic is underscored by a recent report by deChatel et al.[54] They studied 59 normokalemic diabetics in an attempt to characterize the defect in the aldosterone axis at an early stage in the evolution of the syndrome (Table 5-5). In 31 of 59 patients (53 percent), both the renin and aldosterone responses to tilting were normal. In the other 28 patients, however, a variety of defects were observed. Five (8 percent) had diminished aldosterone responses with a normal renin response; 13 (22 percent) had impaired renin release with a normal aldosterone response; and 10 (17 percent) manifested impaired release of both renin and aldosterone. These results suggest that, at least in the diabetic patient, multiple defects are present in the renin-aldosterone axis and that the hyperkalemia is likely to be multifactorial in origin.

A variety of drugs have been shown to result in a state of functional hypoaldosteronism, and these should be avoided in the diabetic. Of these the beta-blockers are the most widely known. Propranolol and other beta-adrenergic antagonists inhibit plasma renin activity and, secondarily, plasma angiotensin II and aldosterone secretion. Despite their widespread use, however, it is surprising that so few cases of clinically

Table 5-5. Plasma Aldosterone and Renin Responses to Tilting in 59 Normokalemic Diabetic Patients

Parameter	No. of Patients
Aldosterone normal Renin normal	31 (53%)
Aldosterone decreased Renin normal	5 (8%)
Aldosterone normal Renin decreased	13 (22%)
Aldosterone decreased Renin decreased	10 (17%)

Data summarized from deChatel R, Weidmann P, Flammer J, et al: Sodium, renin, aldosterone, catecholamines and blood pressure in diabetes mellitus. Kidney Int 12:412, 1977.

significant hyperkalemia have been reported. Over the last 2–3 years, we have observed moderate hyperkalemia in several patients after the institution of propranolol therapy and disappearance of the hyperkalemia after discontinuation of the drug. All of these patients had underlying chronic renal disease, were on dialysis, or had diabetes mellitus. Propranolol also blocks cellular uptake of potassium by a $beta_2$-adrenergic mechanism. Therefore, if a beta-blocking agent is needed and hyperkalemia remains a problem, substitution of metoprolol, a specific $beta_1$ antagonist, may be tried.

Captopril, an antihypertensive agent that works by inhibiting the conversion of angiotensin I to angiotensin II, has also been shown to cause hyperkalemia.[203,216] In a prospective study Textor et al.[232] found that 23 of 33 hypertensive patients started on captopril experienced a rise in serum potassium concentration ($\Delta = 0.8 \pm 0.1$ mEq/L) in association with a decrease in aldosterone secretion. The rise in serum potassium was inversely related to the GFR, and severe hyperkalemia (>6.0 mEq/L) was observed only in patients with markedly impaired renal function.

The last group of drugs which have been shown to impair aldosterone biosynthesis are the prostaglandin inhibitors, particularly indomethacin. These agents act by decreasing renin release[233] but may also have a direct inhibitory effect on aldosterone synthesis.[234] Several well documented cases of indomethacin-induced hyperkalemia and hyporeninemic hypoaldosteronism[203,216,235] have been described. The syndrome is completely reversible when the medication is discontinued.

In conclusion, hyperkalemia in the diabetic may occur as the result of a variety of factors (Fig. 5-5), including impaired renin secretion, impaired aldosterone secretion, a renal tubular secretory defect, or abnormal cellular distribution of potassium.

Treatment of hyperkalemia is dependent on two factors: (1) the severity of the hyperkalemia; and (2) definition of the etiology. Whether aggressive therapy should be instituted is dictated by both the degree of hyperkalemia and the presence of cardiac or neuromuscular manifestations. Regardless of the electrocardiogram and clinical symptomatology, therapeutic intervention should be initiated when the serum postassium concentration has risen acutely to greater than 6.0 mEq/L. Acute therapy can be divided into three general categories[236]: measures designed to (1) oppose directly the effects of hyperkalemia at the level of the cell membrane (calcium and sodium); (2) enhance the transfer of potassium from the extracellular to the intracellular compartment (sodium bicarbonate and insulin/glucose); and (3) remove potassium from the body (cation-exchange resins, diuretics to increase renal excretion, and dialysis). Once the acute effects of hyperkalemia on cardiovascular and neuromuscular function have been reversed, the specific etiology of the hyperkalemia should be sought[203,216] and more specific therapy instituted. All diabetic patients with chronic hyperkalemia should be placed on a low potassium diet (less than 40–60 mEq/day). Any coexisting acidemia should be corrected with bicarbonate, which causes a shift of potassium into cells. Intravascular volume contraction should be avoided as decreased distal sodium and fluid delivery impair potassium secretion. Great care should be taken to avoid drugs (beta-adrenergic blockers, prostaglandin inhibitors, captopril, spironolactone, triamterene, amiloride) that inhibit the renin-angiotensin-aldosterone axis and renal tubular potassium secretion. Good diabetic control should be encouraged as hyperglycemia causes a shift of potassium out of cells. In the diabetic with documented aldosterone deficiency and hyperkalemia, treatment with fludrocortisone acetate, 0.1

mg/day, may be beneficial. In patients with a specific renal tubular potassium secretory defect, thiazide diuretics (but not the more potent loop diuretics) are often effective in promoting renal potassium excretion.[203,216]

Metabolic Acidosis

Metabolic acidosis is very common in IDDs (Table 5-6), and Halperin et al. reviewed this topic in depth.[237,238] From the clinical and pathophysiological standpoints, metabolic acidosis can be divided into two broad categories: anion gap and nonanion gap (hyperchloremic) acidosis. The anion gap is calculated by subtracting the sum of the serum concentrations of the two major anions (chloride and bicarbonate) from the major cation (sodium). The difference should not exceed 12 ± 2 mEq/L. If the value exceeds 14 mEq/L, an anion gap acidosis is present.

In the diabetic individual there are three causes of anion gap acidosis: ketoacidosis, lactic acidosis, and renal insufficiency (Table 5-6). Although chronic renal failure is associated with insulin resistance,[239–241] there does not seem to be any increase in the incidence of ketoacidosis in diabetic patients who develop renal disease. Lactic acidosis is more common in the diabetic population,[242] but the incidence in patients with renal failure is no greater than in those with normal renal function. In diabetic nephropathy, as in all other causes of chronic renal disease, when the GFR decreases to less than 20–25 ml/min the ability of the kidney to excrete titratable acid becomes impaired. The clinical manifestation of this is the development of an anion gap metabolic acidosis.[243]

The above causes of an anion gap acidosis in the diabetic are all well known to the clinician. What is less well recognized, however, is the frequent occurrence of a hyperchloremic (or nonanion gap) metabolic acidosis in patients with diabetes mellitus (Table 5-6). As discussed in the preceding section, the syndrome of hypoaldosteronism is frequently observed in diabetic patients, particularly those with renal impairment.[203,209–216] Numerous studies have shown that aldosterone is an important regulator of ammonia production and hydrogen ion secretion by the distal nephron.[244,245] Therefore it is not surprising that over half of the reported cases of hyporeninemic hypoaldosteronism have hyperchloremic metabolic acidosis[203,216] on initial presenta-

Table 5-6. Causes of Metabolic Acidosis in Insulin-Dependent Diabetic Patients.

Anion gap acidosis
Ketoacidosis
Lactic acidosis
Renal insufficiency
Hyperchloremic metabolic acidosis
Hypoaldosteronism (urine $pH<5.4$)
Distal RTA (urine $pH>5.4$)
Chronic interstitial nephritis (urine $pH<5.4$)
Increased plasma potassium concentration (inhibition of ammoniagenesis)
Loss of bicarbonate equivalents (ketones)—occurs in DKA when rate of ketone excretion exceeds the rate of NH_4^+ excretion
Expansion acidosis—occurs in treatment of DKA

tion. In humans[246] and animals[247,248] with pure aldosterone deficiency, the ability to acidify the urine (i.e., urine pH less than 5.4) is not impaired. The primary cause of the metabolic acidosis with aldosterone deficiency is impaired ammonium excretion.[246–248] By definition, therefore, the urine pH in patients with pure hypoaldosteronism and hyperchloremic metabolic acidosis should be acidic, i.e., less than 5.4. The constellation of hyporeninemia, hypoaldosteronism, hyperkalemia, and hyperchloremic metabolic acidosis has been termed "type IV renal tubular acidosis."[214,215,249,250] Although this terminology has gained widespread usage, it is somewhat misleading in that these individuals are able to elaborate a maximally acidic urine. In contrast, there are some diabetic subjects who also are hyperkalemic and have a hyperchloremic metabolic acidosis, yet are unable to acidify their urine (urine pH>5.4). By definition, therefore, they have a true distal renal tubular acidosis (RTA). They have received the label "hyperkalemic distal RTA."[215,250] Plasma aldosterone levels are normal in these individuals, and they fail to respond to exogenous mineralocorticoid administration. These patients have a primary renal tubular defect (independent of aldosterone) that involves both hydrogen and potassium secretion. In the diabetic patient this may be related to the prominent interstitial fibrosis and inflammatory response, to the marked tubular basement membrane thickening, or to an intracellular abnormality in any one of a number of steps involved in hydrogen and potassium ion secretion. It should be noted that some diabetic patients may have both hyperkalemic distal RTA and hypoaldosteronism.

Some diabetics may have a urinary acidification defect that closely resembles that observed in patients with chronic interstitial nephritis.[251,252] Such individuals have normal serum potassium levels, and aldosterone secretion is not impaired—yet they manifest hyperchloremic metabolic acidosis. Their urine pH is maximally acidic, indicating that the ability of the distal tubule and collecting duct to generate a steep pH gradient is intact. In these individuals the primary problem is one of ammonia production. Because the renal tubular cells are primarily responsible for ammoniagenesis, any disease process that destroys the integrity of these cells or interrupts the normal cycling of ammonia within the medullary interstitium[253] leads to a reduction in ammonia excretion. From a quantitative standpoint, ammonia is the most important urinary buffer. Therefore when ammonia excretion is diminished, the total amount of hydrogen ion that can be excreted is decreased. In the absence of ammonia, which is one of the major urinary buffers, the urine pH is maximally acidic. Hence this patient's acidification defect closely resembles that observed in the syndrome of hyporeninemic hypoaldosteronism. The diabetic with interstitial nephritis and the one with hypoaldosteronism can be differentiated from the patient with true renal tubular acidosis in that the first two can elaborate a maximally acidic urine. Determination of the urine pH is therefore an important diagnostic test in evaluating diabetic individuals with hyperchloremic metabolic acidosis.

Hyperkalemia is another important factor that needs to be considered when evaluating the etiology of hyperchloremic metabolic acidosis in the diabetic. Potassium per se is capable of inhibiting ammonia synthesis by the distal nephron.[253,254] If the plasma potassium concentration rises from any cause (i.e., hypoaldosteronism, a specific renal tubular secretory defect, or advanced renal insufficiency), ammoniagenesis is inhibited and the total amount of buffer in the urine, and therefore the total amount of hydrogen ion that can be secreted, is markedly reduced. Treatment of the hyperkalemia corrects the defect in hydrogen ion secretion and returns the blood pH to normal.

During treatment of diabetic ketoacidosis (DKA) the development of hyperchloremic metabolic acidosis is inevitable.[237,255] As ketoacidosis develops, the production of each ketone anion is quantitatively matched by the generation of one hydrogen ion. It is important to remember that each ketone anion represents a bicarbonate equivalent. When the ketoacidosis is corrected, the metabolism of the ketone anion is associated with the generation of one bicarbonate ion. If none of the ketone anions are lost from the body, reversal of the ketoacidosis leads to a quantitative correction of the metabolic acidosis. However, all diabetics in ketoacidosis, even those with advanced renal failure, have significant urinary losses of ketones. Consequently, when the ketoacidosis is reversed, there is a deficit of bicarbonate equivalents and hyperchloremic metabolic acidosis ensues. Because of the osmotic diuresis, most diabetic patients who develop ketoacidosis also are volume-depleted. Large amounts of saline are usually administered during the treatment of DKA, and this further lowers the plasma bicarbonate concentration by causing an expansion acidosis.

Proximal renal tubular acidosis may occur in diabetic patients but is quite unusual. It has been reported with severe phosphate depletion and in diabetics who are taking Diamox (a carbonic anhydrase inhibitor) for the treatment of glaucoma.

The treatment of metabolic acidosis in the diabetic with renal disease is no different from that in the nondiabetic with renal insufficiency. The mainstay of therapy is bicarbonate in amounts sufficient to return the plasma bicarbonate concentration to normal. When hyperkalemia is present, it should be corrected. This will have two beneficial effects: (1) it is associated with a shift of hydrogen ions into cells; and (2) it relieves the inhibition of ammonia production, thereby augmenting renal acid excretion. In patients with hypoaldosteronism, fludrocortisone acetate (0.1 mg/day) may prove helpful.

CLINICAL CORRELATIONS

It is commonly stated in most textbooks that it is unusual to observe diabetic nephropathy in the absence of retinopathy, neuropathy, and hypertension. Recent studies, however, have challenged the validity of such statements.

Diabetic Retinopathy

Diabetic retinopathy is present in the overwhelming majority of diabetics with end-stage renal failure who are admitted into dialysis/transplant programs.[5,6,;11,256–261] In such patients a careful ophthamological examination usually reveals the presence of hemorrhages, exudates, and proliferative retinopathy. However, at the time of the diagnosis of diabetic nephropathy (i.e., documentation of persistent proteinuria or initial elevation in the serum creatinine or urea nitrogen concentration), as many as 30–40 percent of patients do not have evidence of diabetic retinopathy by routine ophthamological examination.[14,25,177,262–264] As the renal disease progresses, however, there seems to be an acceleration of diabetic retinopathy.[177,263,264] In the study of Goldstein and Massry, evidence of retinopathy was present in only 61 of 150 diabetic patients when nephropathy was first diagnosed but developed in an additional 42 during the period of follow-up.[173] Part of the reason why investigators have failed to find a strong correlation between the presence of retinopathy and nephropathy may be related to observer differences in establishing the presence of retinal involvement. In a recent study[265] internists, diabetologists, ophthalmologists, and retinal specialists at a university hospital were asked to evaluate the eyes of IDDs, and their evaluation was contrasted to that obtained with stereofunduscopic photographs. "Serious errors" were made by 70 percent of internists, 50 percent of diabetologists, and 11 percent of ophthalmologists. It is not surprising, therefore, that many investigators have failed to find a correlation between diabetic retinopathy and diabetic nephropathy. It is likely that if fluorescein angiography were performed in all diabetic patients a stronger association between the presence of eye involvement and renal disease would be observed.

In diabetic patients placed on hemodialysis there seems to be a particularly rapid progression of diabetic retinopathy. Early reports indicated that 44 percent of the eyes of diabetics on chronic hemodialysis progressed to blindness within the first year.[266–268] However, later figures from the same group have indicated a considerable improvement, with only 9 percent of eyes developing blindness during the first 1.5 years after starting hemodialysis.[269] The reasons underlying the improved prognosis are not entirely clear.

The dissociation between retinopathy and nephropathy is even more impressive if one considers all diabetic patients with established retinopathy. After 15–20 years approximately 80 percent of diabetics have evidence of retinopathy.[270] However, only 40 percent have evidence of nephropathy. In several large series of patients with proliferative retinopathy[271,272] 30–50 percent of diabetic patients had no laboratory evidence of renal disease. A marked dissociation between retinopathy and nephropathy also has been documented in individuals who have had their diabetes for 40 years or more.[273,274] A discussion of the potential factors responsible for the dissociation between diabetic renal and retinal involvement has recently appeared.[275]

Diabetic Neuropathy

The association between diabetic nephropathy and neuropathy is much less impressive than between diabetic nephropathy and retinopathy. In addition, published data relating diabetic nephropathy and neuropathy are more difficult to interpret because uremia per se causes neuropathic changes that are similar to those observed in diabetes mellitus. Estimates of the overall incidence of diabetic neuropathy in diabetic patients have varied considerably. In individuals who have had their diabetes for 20 years or more, approximately 50 percent will have some clinical evidence of diabetic neuropathy.[145,273,275] As reviewed by McCrary et al.[139] and Goldstein and Massry,[173] the incidence of neuropathy in diabetics at the time of end-stage renal failure has ranged from 60 to 90 percent. However, the specificity of these neuropathological abnormalities must be questioned as dialysis often leads to their reversal. This suggests that much of the neuropathy may be uremic in origin. Among a group of diabetic patients who received kidney transplants at the University of Minnesota, the neuropathy was so severe that in 15 to 20 percent of these patients could walk only if assisted.[276,277] Within 2 years after renal transplantation over 70 percent had an improvement in muscle strength and ambulation. Such observations raise further questions concerning the specificity of the neuropathological changes observed in diabetic patients with neuropathy. As with retinopathy, it seems that uremia exacerbates the presence of diabetic neuropathy. In summary, it appears that at the time diabetic nephropathy is first diagnosed less than 50 percent of the patients have clinically evident diabetic neuropathy.

A special comment should be made about diabetic bladder involvement. This diagnosis is difficult to establish as the onset is insidious and often progresses without the patient being aware of its symptoms.[278] The initial clue to diagnosis is an increase in the interval between voidings, but this usually goes unrecognized. Eventually there develops hesitancy, straining while voiding, weakened urinary stream, and postvoid dribbling. At this time the bladder is distended, and significant postvoid residual is present. These symptoms are often misdiagnosed for prostatic obstruction. Because urinary tract obstruction and recurrent bladder infection with ascending pyelonephritis have the potential to accelerate the course of diabetic nephropathy, it is important to recognize these symptoms and institute appropriate therapy (see subsequent discussion on therapy). The diagnosis is established by cystometrogram, which demonstrates a long, low pressure tracing with increased bladder capacity and lack of feeling to void. Because of an increased incidence of acute renal failure in diabetic patients,[279–281] dye studies (intravenous pyelograms and retrograde pyelograms) should be avoided. The precise incidence of neurogenic bladder involvement in diabetic patients is unknown. Ellenberg and Weber estimated that approximately 80 percent of diabetic patients with clinically evident neuropathy have evidence of neurogenic bladder involvement as evidenced by an abnormal cystometrogram and grossly enlarged bladder.[282]

Hypertension

Contrary to what is stated in most textbooks, elevated blood pressure is distinctly uncommon at the time diabetic nephropathy is first diagnosed, being present in only 10–25 percent of such individuals.[11,20,144,174,177,283] In the report of Goldstein and Massry[173] hypertension was absent in 119 of 150 diabetics at the time evidence for renal disease was first detected. However, with the progression of renal disease, hypertension eventually developed in 103 of their patients. Many other studies have documented a progressive increase in the incidence of hypertension in diabetics with established nephropathy. At the time end-stage renal failure ensues, approximately 70–80 percent of diabetic individuals are hypertensive.[11,20,144,177,257,258,262,284] Patients with heavy proteinuria seem to be particularly prone to develop elevated blood pressures, and the incidence of hypertension seems to parallel the appearance and progression of proteinuria.[11,144,147,264,285,286] In most patients the hypertension seems to be volume-dependent and becomes relatively easy to control after patients are started on dialysis and dry weight is attained.[287,288] There is little evidence to suggest either high renin or autonomic hyperactivity as a cause of the elevated blood pressure.

Edema

The full-blown symptom complex in individuals with diabetic glomerulosclerosis includes edema, hypertension, proteinura, and azotemia. The latter three have already been discussed. In patients without renal disease or in those with early proteinuria (less than 0.5–1 g/day) and a normal GFR, edema is uncommon. However, as the GFR begins to decline and albuminuria exceeds 1–2 g/day, the incidence of edema increases precipitously. This is due to two factors: sodium retention and hypoalbuminemia. In many diabetic patients with advanced nephropathy significant atherosclerotic cardiovascular changes are also present, and diminished cardiac output may contribute to the salt and water retention. At the time end-stage renal failure is present, over 50–75 percent of individuals have some evidence of edema.[9,11,23,24,173]

TREATMENT OF DIABETIC NEPHROPATHY

At our present state of knowledge the treatment of diabetic nephropathy (Table 5-7) is largely preventive, i.e., avoiding those factors that are known to accelerate the natural progession of renal disease. When end-stage renal failure ensues, two options are available: dialysis or transplantation. In the present section we review those therapeutic options which have been shown to be of benefit in treating or preventing the development of renal insufficiency. Several hopeful but as yet unproved modalities of therapy are also discussed.

Hypertension

Once detected, aggressive treatment of hypertension is indicated. Parving et al.,[289,290] Mogensen,[144,291,292] and Christlieb et al.[293] demonstrated that normalization of the blood pressure may have a dramatic effect in slowing the progression of renal insufficiency in diabetic patients with established renal disease (Fig. 5-7). The importance of hemodynamic factors in determining the development of diabetic nephropathy is emphasized by a case report by Berkman and Rifkin.[294] In an IDD with renal artery stenosis, extensive diabetic glomerulosclerosis was found in the unprotected kidney. In contrast, only mild diabetic changes were present in the kidney with the stenotic renal artery. Similarly, in diabetic rats with Goldblatt hypertension, the kidney with the renal artery stenosis is largely protected from the development of diabetic glomerular changes; the contralateral kidney, which is exposed to hypertension, displays accelerated diabetic glomerulopathy.[295] In diabetic rats[296] and dogs[297] that have undergone unilateral nephrectomy, there also is marked acceleration of diabetic nephropathy in the remaining kidney even though systemic hypertension does not develop. This observation emphasizes the role of intrarenal hemodynamic factors in the initiation and progression of diabetic as well as other types of glomerulopathy.[223–225,298]

Because hypertension is known to accelerate the development of diabetic nephropathy and treatment of the hypertension is the only factor known to slow the rate of progression of renal disease, it is of paramount importance that all diabetic

Table 5-7. Treatment of Diametic Nephropathy

1. *Hypertension*—the single most important factor that has been shown to accelerate the progression of renal failure.
   a. Treatment = diuretic (very volume-sensitive) plus antihypertensive agent.
   b. Avoid captopril (hyperkalemia).
   c. Avoid propranolol (hyperkalemia, hypoglycemia, hyperglycemia).
2. *Urinary tract infection*—increased incidence, frequent cultures.
3. *Neurogenic bladder*—parasympathetic/adrenergic drugs, voiding maneuvers, bladder neck resection.
4. *Intravenous pyelography*—increased incidence of acute renal failure, particularly if heavy proteinuria and renal impairment are present.
5. *Blood glucose control*
   a. Uremia is associated with insulin resistance and increased insulin requirements.
   b. With advanced uremia, decreased insulin requirements may be observed. The kidney removes ~25% of the daily secreted insulin. When GFR decreases to less than 15–20 ml/min, the metabolic clearance rate of insulin (MCR_I) becomes impaired.
   c. Uremia also inhibits hepatic degradation of insulin, further contributing to the decreased MCR_I.
   d. After the institution of dialysis, the situation is quite complex. Insulin sensitivity improves (→hypoglycemia), but the MCR_I is enhanced (→hyperglycemia).
6. *Artificial pancreas*
   a. At present there is no evidence that tight metabolic control prevents or ameliorates the progression of established renal disease.
   b. Whether insulin pump theory instituted within the first 1–2 years after the diagnosis of diabetes mellitus prevents the development of renal disease remains to be established by prospective trials.
7. *Dialysis*
   a. *One in four patients beginning dialysis in the U.S. is diabetic.*
   b. *Diabetics do significantly worse on hemodialysis than do nondiabetics.*
   c. The increased mortality in diabetics treated with hemodialysis is largely due to cardiovascular deaths resulting from myocardial infarction. The incidence of stroke and infection is also significantly increased. Other complications include peripheral vascular disease, CHF, angina, psychiatric problems, and progressive retinopathy and neuropathy.
   d. Diabetic patients treated with peritoneal dialysis do not fare any better than those treated with hemodialysis.
   e. Chronic ambulatory peritoneal dialysis may offer some hope. With addition of insulin to the dialysate, several groups have reported survival rates as good as with hemodialysis.
   f. A major problem with CAPD remains the high incidence of infection.
8. *Transplantation*
   a. If a well-matched, living related donor can be found, renal transplantation is probably the preferable mode of therapy in type I (IDD) diabetics.
   b. Survival statistics with kidneys transplanted from a haplotype identical relative or unrelated donor are similar to those obtained with hemodialysis.
   c. With the advent of cyclosporin, however, it is likely that transplant statistics with unrelated kidneys will improve significantly.
9. *Protein restriction*
   a. There are good data in animals and preliminary data in man that a low-protein diet slows the progression of renal disease in nondiabetic individuals with advanced renal insufficiency. A similar beneficial effect has been reported in diabetics.
   b. It is unknown if protein restriction, instituted early in the course of renal disease, prevents or ameliorates the progression of either diabetic or nondiabetic nephropathy.

patients have their blood pressure *normalized.* Even mild hypertension (130/90 mm Hg) should not be tolerated in a diabetic patient. Because the hypertension is in large part volume-dependent, a low sodium diet and diuretics should be used to initiate therapy. Because most diabetic hypertensives also have some degree of renal insufficiency, a loop diuretic is usually necessary. Potassium-sparing diuretics should never be employed in diabetic patients. Beta-adrenergic antagonists, e.g., propranolol, are relatively contraindicated in diabetics for a number of reasons: they have a propensity

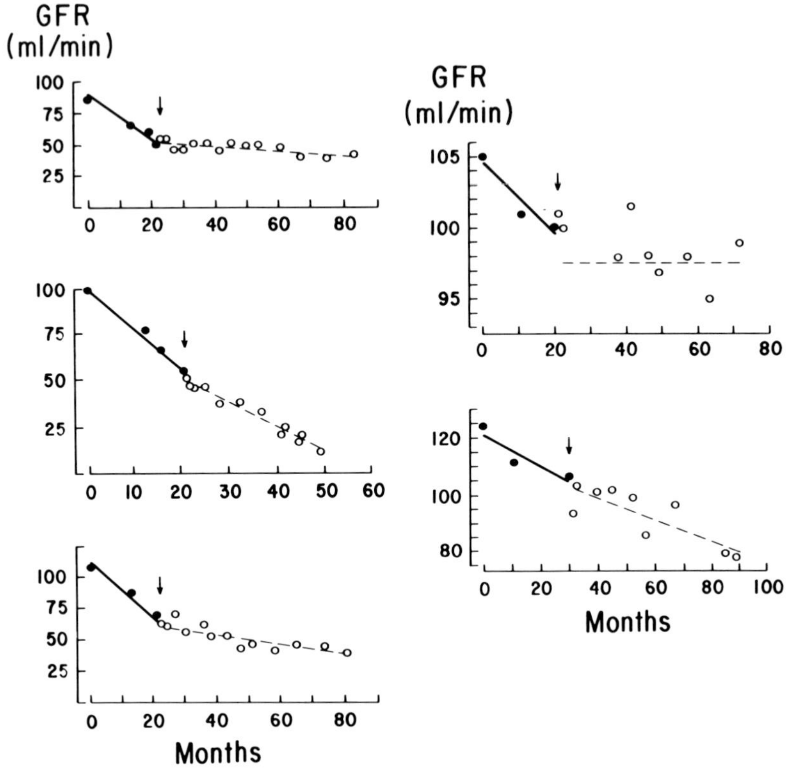

Fig. 5-7 Effect of antihypertensive therapy on the decrease in the GFR (ml/min) in five insulin-dependent diabetics before (closed circles) and after (open circles) the start (↓) of therapy. (Redrawn from Mogensen CE: Antihypertensive treatment inhibiting the progression of diabetic nephropathy. Acta Endocrinol (Copenh) [Suppl 238] 94:103, 1980.)

to cause hyperkalemia; they can cause hypoglycemia by inhibiting hepatic glucose production; they may mask the symptoms of hypoglycemia; in NIDDs they may cause hyperglycemia by inhibiting residual endogenous insulin secretion. If a beta-blocking drug is to be used, consideration should be given to a selective $beta_1$ agent. In the hypertensive diabetic with autonomic neuropathy, alpha-adrenergic antagonists should be used cautiously because of the propensity of these patients to develop severe orthostatic hypotension. In the absence of autonomic dysfunction, either an alpha-adrenergic antagonist or a vasodilating agent can be employed. For a more detailed discussion of the treatment of hypertension, the reader is referred to an excellent review by Black.[299]

Urinary Tract Infection

As discussed earlier, diabetics seem to have an increased incidence of urinary tract infection. Therefore it is imperative that a urinalysis be performed on each visit. If white blood cells or bacteriuria are noted, a urine culture should be obtained. Even in the absence of pyuria, periodic urine cultures are essential. Positive cultures should be treated with an appropriate bactericidal antibiotic based on the results of the culture sensitivity.

Neurogenic Bladder

The clinician must have a high index of suspicion to establish the diagnosis of neurogenic bladder. In addition to the history, recurrent urinary tract infections may provide a clue to the diagnosis. Once the presence of a neurogenic bladder has been confirmed by cystometrogram, the patient should receive instruction in the Crede manual voiding maneuver, which should be performed every 6–8 hr. This may be sufficient to prevent any significant postvoid residual. If necessary, parasympathetic agents, e.g., urecholine, may be tried. In some diabetics adrenergic drugs, e.g., phenoxybenzamine, have proved useful. The success of these various medical interventions should be evaluated by determining the postvoid residual volume. If medical therapy proves unsuccessful, intermittent straight catheterization should be performed at least two to three times daily. In some patients bladder neck resection has proved useful in promoting complete bladder emptying.[300] A more detailed review of this problem has been provided by Ellenberg.[301]

Intravenous Pyelography

Diabetic patients are at increased risk to develop acute renal failure after radiocontrast (arteriography, cholangiography, intravenous and retrograde pyelography, CAT scanning) procedures,[279–281] and this subject has been reviewed.[302] Patients with an elevated serum creatinine (greater than 2.0 mg/dl) and/or heavy proteinuria are at greatest risk. It should be noted that renal failure has also been reported despite adequate hydration before the study. In our opinion there is little indication for dye studies in diabetic patients. With the use of echography, radionucleotide studies and CAT scanning without contrast, most of the information necessary to ensure adequate diagnosis and treatment can be obtained. If contrast media must be administered, the least amount of dye necessary to perform the study should be given, and the patient should be adequately hydrated. An osmotic diuresis with mannitol should also be initiated in an attempt to prevent acute tubular necrosis. Renal function should be monitored closely after performing the contrast study with daily serum creatinine determinations for 2–3 days.

Blood Glucose Control

Changes in Insulin Degradation and Sensitivity. With the development of progressive renal insufficiency, moderate to severe insulin resistance can be found in all uremic individuals, be they diabetic or nondiabetic.[239–241] The site of this insulin resistance resides in peripheral tissues, primarily muscle.[303–315] In both insulin-dependent (type I) and noninsulin-dependent (type II) diabetics it is common to observe a marked deterioration in glucose control with the advent of renal insufficiency. Insulin requirements are increased in IDDs, and NIDDs may require the institution of insulin therapy to achieve adequate glucose control. However, as the GFR continues to decrease and reaches levels of less than 15–20 ml/min, the clearance of insulin becomes markedly reduced.[305–307] That insulin which is not degraded by the liver/kidney is returned to the circulation, and the glucose tolerance may improve. In fact, some IDDs may even cease to require insulin. After the institution of hemodialysis therapy, a very complex situation ensues. Dialysis enhances tissue sensitivity to insulin,[305] thereby decreasing insulin requirements. In contrast, dialysis also returns insulin degradation toward normal,[316] increasing the need for insulin. In any given uremic diabetic who is started on dialysis, it is difficult to predict what will happen to the insulin requirements. One must be cognizant of the fact that either an increase or a decrease in the daily insulin dose may be required.

Hypoglycemia in Chronic Renal Failure and Dialysis Patients. Spontaneous hypoglycemia is well documented in both diabetic[308–311] and nondiabetic patients[312–316] with chronic renal failure. Nonetheless, the pathogenetic mechanisms responsible for the low blood glucose concentration have been poorly characterized. With advancing renal failure (GFR $<$ 15–20 ml/min) the metabolic clearance rate of insulin becomes prolonged.[305–307] Therefore it has been suggested that the hypoglycemia is the result of hyperinsulinemia. However, plasma insulin levels have only rarely been reported at the time of hypoglycemia, and when reported they have been low to normal. Furthermore, several patients have been ketotic, suggesting insulin lack instead of excess. Such observations imply that defective hepatic glucose production may be the cause of the hypoglycemia.[311] Again, little information is available concerning abnormalities in hepatic glucose output (glycogenolysis or gluconeogenesis) in patients with chronic renal failure. A decrease in hepatic glucose production due to diminished alanine availability for gluconeogenesis has been documented in a single uremic diabetic patient with spontaneous hypoglycemia.[311] The frequency with which decreased alanine turnover contributes to spontaneous hypoglycemia is not clear, as most uremic patients have been reported to have increased alanine turnover and normal plasma alanine levels.[317] Hypoglycemia has been frequently reported in IDDs who develop renal insufficiency.[306] In this situation the hypoglycemia most likely results from diminished insulin degradation by the diseased kidney. The resultant hyperinsulinemia enhances peripheral glucose metabolism while simultaneously inhibiting hepatic glucose production.

It is our impression that symptomatic hypoglycemia occurs not infrequently in both diabetic and nondiabetic patients who are on chronic hemodialysis. However, few case reports have appeared in the literature. Grajower et al.[318] described severe symptomatic hypoglycemia in five nondiabetic patients on chronic maintenance hemodialysis. None of the individuals were malnourished and in none could hyperinsulinemia explain the low plasma glucose levels. All patients were on propranolol, and the authors implicated this agent in the pathogenesis of the hypoglycemia. Although propranolol is known to cause hypoglycemia by inhibiting hepatic glucose production, we have observed symptomatic hypoglycemia in both diabetic and nondiabetic patients on hemodialysis even though they were not taking beta-adrenergic blocking agents. Clearly, much more information is needed to define the incidence of, as well as the pathogenetic factors contributing to, the development of hypoglycemia in chronic hemodialysis patients, both diabetic and nondiabetic.

Peritoneal Dialysis, Glucose Absorption, and Insulin Requirements.

Standard hemodialysate solutions are devoid of glucose. In several studies, glucose-enriched dialysate has been employed in an attempt to prevent dialysis intolerance.[319,320] In nondiabetic patients a significant rise in plasma insulin concentration was observed during dialysis, and the increase in plasma glucose concentration was modest (50–75 mg/dl). Recently there has been considerable interest in continuous ambulatory peritoneal dialysis, especially in diabetic patients.[321–328] The major advantages of this technique are that it is adaptable to home care, minimizes the burden on the cardiovascular system, and provides excellent control of uremia and hypertension.[329] Because dialysis is performed 24 hr per day, every day of the week, glucose absorption is considerable and may provide an important source of calories to the uremic patient, who is often undernourished. Grodstein et al.[330] showed that the quantity of glucose absorbed each day is directly related to the amount of glucose instilled into the peritoneal cavity. In their patients the energy intake derived from the dailysate glucose absorption averaged approximately 8 kcal/kg body weight, which represented 20 percent of the total daily energy intake. Similar observations have been made by others.[331–333] Plasma glucose levels in excess of 160–180 mg/dl are uncommon in nondiabetic patients.

The use of continuous ambulatory peritoneal dialysis (CAPD) has been advocated in diabetic patients.[321–329] Using this technique survival rates similar to those with hemodialysis have been reported for insulin-requiring diabetics.[321,322,324,327,328] However, severe hyperglycemia presents a significant problem with this modality of therapy. To circumvent this problem, Crossley and Kjellstrand added insulin to the dialysis fluid,[325] a mode of insulin administration that has been employed effectively by several groups.[321–324,326–330,334] The most extensive experience with the use of CAPD in diabetics with end-stage renal disease was reported by Amair et al.[321] In 20 diabetic patients followed for a mean of 14.5 months, the insulin requirement ranged from 70 to 200 U/day. Glucose control was adequate, and the glycosylated hemoglobin concentration, although elevated by 80 percent compared to healthy controls, was no greater than in nondiabetic patients undergoing dialysis. In the diabetic group all insulin was administered peritoneally. Using this route, insulin requirements were two- to four-fold greater than the amount required before starting dialysis treatment. This is not surprising as dialysis is known to enhance insulin degradation,[305] and the liver extracts approximately 50 percent of the insulin delivered via the portal vein.[335] Additionally, a significant amount of insulin adheres to the peritoneum and mesentery, where it is locally degraded.[336] It is difficult to estimate the insulin requirements in any given diabetic patient started on CAPD.[321] Therefore we agree with Amair et al. that it is most efficacious to start such patients on CAPD in the hospital setting so that optimum glucose control can be achieved within the shortest time and without hypoglycemic complications.[321] The Toronto experience has been updated,[328] and they continue to report similar, encouraging results.

Artificial Pancreas

The use of chronic continuous subcutaneous insulin infusion (CSII) (insulin pump) regimens has been enthusiastically employed by numerous groups throughout the world. The cumulative experience from many diabetes centers has shown that this modality of insulin therapy can achieve excellent glycemic control with little or no increased morbidity. However, as previously discussed, there is at present no evidence that such tight metabolic control is capable of ameliorating or preventing the progression of established renal disease.[112–116] These results have been very discouraging considering the large volume of experimental data in animals (dogs, monkeys, rats, mice) indicating that good control can prevent the development of diabetic nephropathy and significantly reverse established renal disease.[67,69,71–73,91–98]

Although the results in man have been discouraging to date, there is still optimism that good control may have a major impact on altering the natural progression of diabetic nephropathy. All of the previous studies in man have examined the effect of insulin pump therapy in diabetic patients who have had their disease for more than 5–10 years and in whom clinical/laboratory evidence of renal involvement was already present. In this group significant renal hemodynamic (increased GFR, renal plasma flow, and filtration fraction) changes present for many years prior to the onset of renal functional impairment, and renal biopsy studies demonstrated evidence of moderately advanced histological changes. Therefore it is not surprising that the natural course of diabetic renal disease was not significantly altered. The true effect of tight metabolic control in preventing the development of diabetic nephropathy must await the results of prospective clinical trials in which newly diagnosed diabetics (within 1–2 years of diabetes onset or earlier) are closely regulated with insulin pump delivery systems or receive a pancreatic transplant that restores insulin secretory dynamics to normal.

Dialysis

For the diabetic with end-stage renal failure who choses dialysis, three options are currently available: hemodialysis, peritoneal dialysis, CAPD. The advantages of CAPD in the diabetic were discussed earlier and have been reviewed in detail by Nolph.[329] An excellent review of the complications and management of the diabetic patient on hemodialysis was published by Kjellstrand et al.[287]

The most important question that needs to be addressed is when to start dialysis in the diabetic patient with advanced renal insufficiency. We strongly agree with Kjellstrand et al.[287] that vascular access and dialysis should be instituted earlier in diabetic than in nondiabetic patients for a number of reasons: (1) once the serum creatinine concentration has risen to above 3.0–4.0 mg/dl, there is rapid deterioration in renal function and most diabetics will require dialysis within 6–12 months; (2) in general, IDDs tolerate uremia more poorly than nondiabetic uremic individuals; (3) there is accelerated deterioration of retinopathy during the later stages of renal failure in the diabetic; (4) uremia tends to exacerbate preexisting diabetic neuropathy; (5) diabetic control often becomes more difficult; (6) negative nitrogen balance and malnutrition become significant problems with advancing uremia; and (7) hypertension becomes more difficult to control. Shapiro and others have shown that all of these complications become easier to manage if dialysis is instituted earlier.[287,288,337–339] It seems reasonable to establish vascular access in diabetics when the serum creatinine reaches 4–5 mg/dl and to initiate dialysis at creatinine levels of 8–9 mg/dl.

There is no doubt that morbidity and mortality statistics are significantly worse in diabetics than in nondiabetic individuals. However, the survival statistics are not nearly as pessimistic as earlier reports suggested.[15,143,258,259,266,268,284,339–351] Results from the European Dialysis Registry (1966–1981) are representative and show that 40–50 percent of patients are alive at 2 years.[343,351] Furthermore, these statistics have not changed over the last 10 years. These results are similar to the overall experience reported by Kjellstrand et al.[287] in 303 diabetic patients who were dialyzed in Minnesota (Fig. 5-8). In contrast, nondiabetic patients on hemodialysis have 2-year survival rates of 70–80 percent.[15,343,351–358] This marked difference in survival between diabetic and nondiabetic patients on hemodialysis persists at 3–5 years. However, there is some evidence to suggest that the outlook for diabetic patients on dialysis may be improving. If one excludes elderly patients (over the age of 60 years) and examines those who have started dialysis during the period 1976–1981, the 2-year survival is 70–80 percent (Fig. 5-7). This compares favorably to mortality statistics in diabetic patients treated with transplantation from the same center (see subsequent discussion). This improvement in mortality reflects recent advances in dialysis technology as well as the selection of younger patients, who are likely to have fewer underlying cardiovascular complications. It is important to keep the age factor in mind when comparing results obtained with dialysis and transplantation. In general, surgeons tend to select younger, healthier patients for renal transplantation. Thus the mean age for all diabetic dialysis patients reported by Kjellestrand et al. is 50 years compared to only 35 years for patients accepted for transplantation at the same institution.[287] It will be of interest to see if updated reports from other centers which have

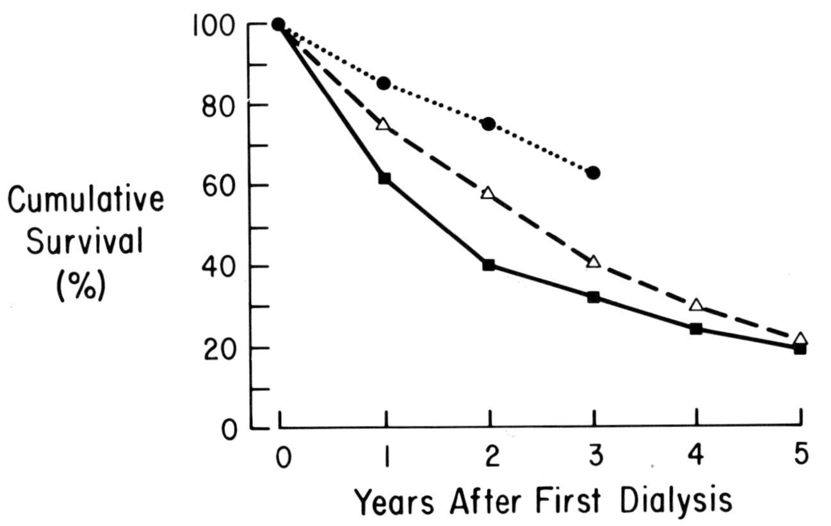

Fig. 5-8 Cumulative survival of diabetic patients from the European Dialysis Registry before 1980 (n = 2,851 patients) (squares), from the Hennepin County Medical Center from 1966 to 1981 (n = 303) (triangles), and from the Hennepin County Medical Center from 1976 to 1981 (n = 98) (circles). The later group includes only diabetic patients under the age of 60 years. (Redrawn from Kjellstrand CM, Whitley K, Comty CM, Shapiro FL: Dialysis in patients with diabetes mellitus. Diabetic Nephropathy 2:5, 1983.)

a large experience in treating diabetic patients with end-stage renal failure will document a similar improvement in survival statistics.

The causes of death in diabetic patients undergoing dialysis in the series of Shapiro et al.[259,266,287,337,350] are shown in Figure 5-9. During the first 18 months cardiac and cerebrovascular catastrophes account for 75 percent of all deaths. After 18 months, uremia and sepsis were responsible for most of the mortality.

There also seems to be an improvement in the quality of life for patients who have started dialysis more recently. Forty-three percent of all diabetic patients who began dialysis during the period 1966–1971 developed blindness.[268,287,337] During the period 1972–1975 the incidence of blindness decreased to 20 percent, and from 1976–1981 the incidence was less than 5 percent. The incidence of serious neuropathy and myopathy also seems to have improved in patients starting dialysis more recently.[287]

Nutritional management of the diabetic patient on dialysis continues to be a problem. Many of these patients are malnourished before starting dialysis, and it is difficult to put them into positive nitrogen balance and return them to their ideal body weight. Subjects should receive approximately 37.5–40 calories/kg of ideal body weight, with approximately 50 percent of the calories given as carbohydrate. Complex, rather than simple, sugars are preferable to assist in diabetic control. At least 1.5 g of high biological value protein per kilogram is needed to achieve positive nitrogen balance. The remaining calories are supplied as fat. In order to achieve adequate glucose control in diabetic patients on dialysis, a split, mixed insulin regimen is necessary. A morning and evening injection of long-acting insulin (i.e., NPH) is almost always required, and this should be administered with sufficient quantities of regular insulin to cover the postprandial glucose excursions. It is important to remember that once dialysis is started the total daily insulin requirement usually increases by 50–100 percent.[354] During the first several months after starting dialysis, it is advisable for the

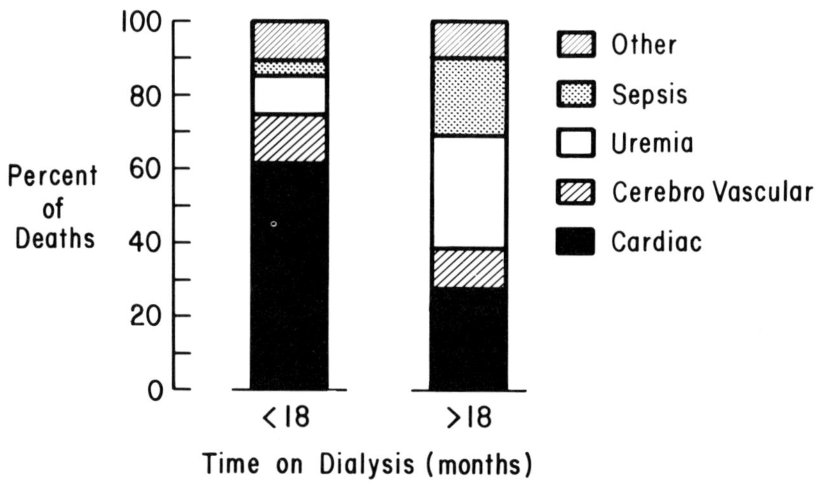

Fig. 5-9 Early (< 18 months) and late (> 18 months) causes of death in diabetic patients on dialysis. (Redrawn from Kjellstrand CM, Whitley K, Comty CM, Shapiro FL: Diagnosis in patients with diabetes mellitus. Diabetic Nephropathy 2:5, 1983.)

diabetic patient to perform home glucose monitoring. Glycosylated hemoglobin levels may be misleading in diabetic patients with advanced renal failure or who are on dialysis as they may be increased by uremia per se.[355] This is another reason for teaching the uremic diabetic to perform home glucose monitoring. Initial concerns about an increased risk of acute bleeding into the eye because of the administration of heparin during dialysis have not been borne out.[287]

Although hemodialysis is by far the most frequent form of dialysis employed in diabetic (as well as nondiabetic) patients with end-stage renal failure, it does not seem to be superior to any other dialytic technique. Morbidity and mortality statistics are similar with intermittent peritoneal[261,356–358] and chronic ambulatory peritoneal[311,322,324,326–328] dialysis. In fact, the most impressive results have been reported with CAPD.[311,328] Because of blindness, neuropathy, amputations, and the necessity for a family member, home dialysis is difficult to achieve in diabetic patients. Because CAPD considerably improves caloric intake and nitrogen balance,[287,329] it has been advocated in the diabetic patient. It also has been stated to be "gentler" and to provide less cardiovascular stress than hemodialysis in patients with underlying cardiovascular disease.[329] One important advantage is that vascular access, which represents a major problem in many diabetics, is not needed. The major problem with CAPD remains the high incidence of peritonitis.

Renal Transplantation

Because of the great diversity in survival statistics from different centers, it is difficult to compare the results. The cumulative survival statistics from the United States and European transplant registries[351,359] are reported in Figure 5-10. The results of the Minnesota experience are not included in the U.S. statistics; these dialysis survival statistics are also presented in Figure 5-10 for comparison.[351,360] There is no doubt that living related donor transplants are much superior to all others. Dialysis patients do slightly better than those with transplants at 1 year. After the first year transplant patients do significantly better in the European registries; there is little difference between dialysis and transplantation in the U.S. results.

The largest transplant experience in the United States has been reported by the Minnesota group.[267,361,362] Their results of renal transplants performed in HLA identical siblings, nonidentical HLA related relatives, and cadaveric transplants in diabetic and nondiabetic patients are shown in Figure 5-11. Several observations are evident: (1) For all groups, nondiabetic transplants do slightly better than diabetics. (2) In diabetics there is not much difference between related nonidentical HLA donors and cadaveric transplants, and with the advent of cyclosporin this difference is apt to become even less. (3) The overall dialysis and transplant experience (Fig. 5-11) from the Minnesota group has been compared by Kjellstrand et al.[269,287] Their results indicate that, as a whole, diabetic patients receiving a renal transplant (HLA identical patients excluded) do slightly better than dialysis patients after the first year (Fig. 5-12). (4) If only diabetic dialysis patients under the age of 60 and who have started on dialysis during the last 4 years are considered, there is little difference in short-term (3-year) survival between diabetic patients treated with dialysis and those who

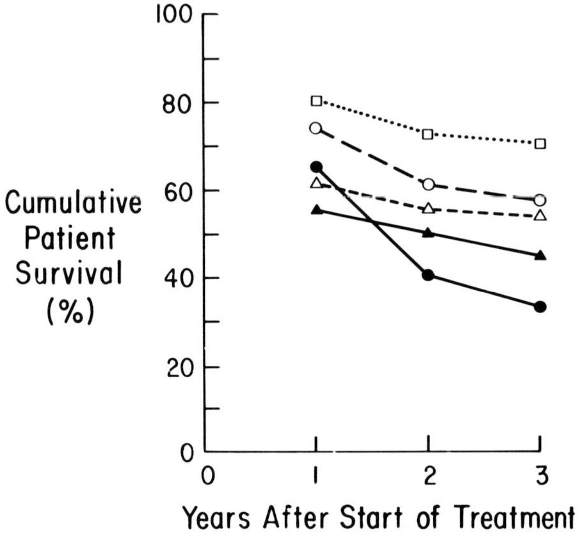

Fig. 5-10 Cumulative survival in diabetic patients from the United States and European transplant and dialysis registries. Open triangles = 13th U.S. transplant registry, cadaver donors (1976). Open circles = U.S. dialysis registry (1975). Open squares = 13th U.S. transplant registry, living related donors (1976). Closed circles = European dialysis registry (1981). Closed triangles = European transplant registry (1981)—cadaver and living related donor transplants are not listed separately. (Redrawn from Kjellstrand C, Comty C, Shapiro F: A comparison of dialysis and transplantation in insulin-dependent diabetic patients. In Friedman EA, L'Esperance FA (eds): Diabetic Renal-Retinal Syndrome. pp. 405–417. Grune & Stratton, New York, 1982.)

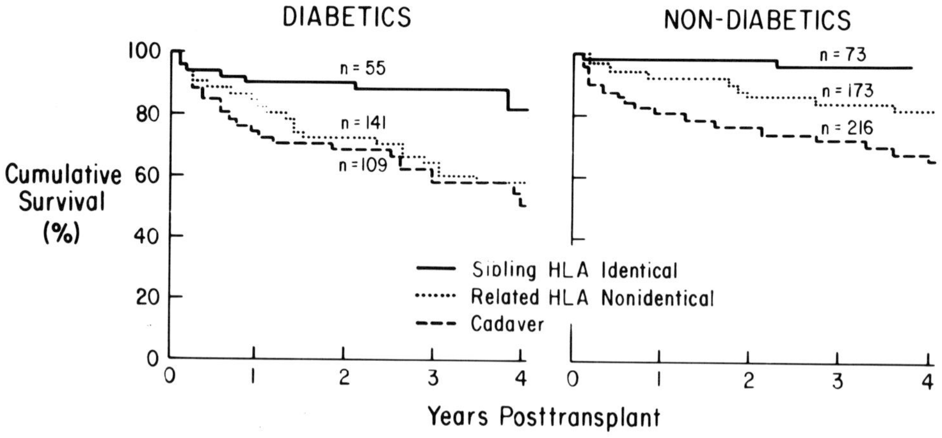

Fig. 5-11 Four-year patient survival in diabetic and nondiabetic patients treated by renal transplantation at the University of Minnesota. (Redrawn from Sutherland DER, Fryd DS, Morrow CE, et al: Kidney transplantation in diabetics at the University of Minnesota: an analysis of results by era. Transplant Proc 15:1110, 1983.)

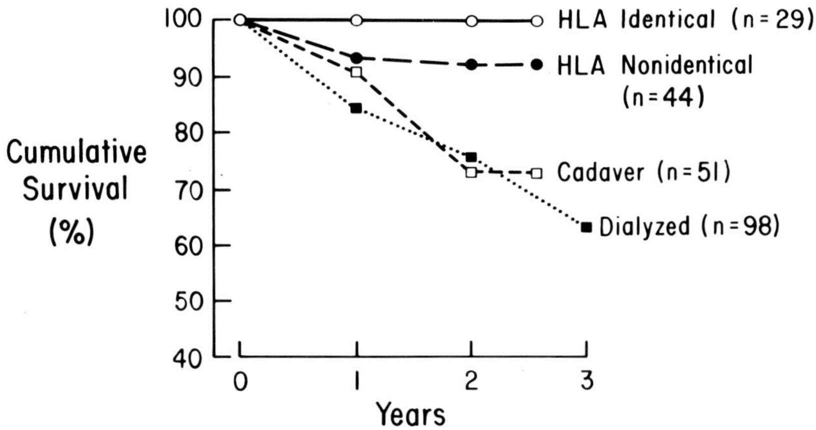

Fig. 5-12 Patient survival in diabetic patients treated by renal transplantation at the University of Minnesota and Hennepin County Medical Center during 1979–1981. Only diabetic patients who are less than 61 years of age are included in the dialyzed group. The mean age (35–37 years) for the HLA nonidentical transplants, cadaver transplants, and dialyzed patients is similar. HLA identical transplanted patients are significantly younger. Living related transplants clearly do better than cadaver transplants and dialysis patients. However, there is little difference between these last two groups. (Redrawn from Kjellstrand CM, Whitley K, Comty CM, Shapiro FL: Dialysis in patients with diabetes mellitus. Diabetic Nephropathy 2:5, 1983.)

receive a cadaveric renal transplant. Similar transplantation results in diabetics have been reported by other groups.[363–365]

In summary, there is no doubt that if an HLA identical donor can be found the chances of long-term patient and graft survival are much superior to the results with dialysis. HLA nonidentical recipients also seem to do better than diabetic patients treated with dialysis. However, there is little difference in long-term survival between dialysis and cadaveric renal transplantation. Therefore at present, in the absence of an HLA related donor, the choice of dialysis versus transplantation must be individualized for any given diabetic patient. However, with the advent of cyclosporin and other newer immunosuppressive regimens, it is not unreasonable to expect that patient survival after cadaveric renal transplantation will exceed that with dialysis. Furthermore, with the introduction of these newer immunosuppressive techniques, it is unlikely that either patient or graft survival will differ between cadaveric and nonidentical HLA related donors. This should lead to a significant decline in the number of non-HLA identical living related transplants.

Early rehabilitation after renal transplantation is much better than with dialysis. The results of long-term rehabilitation also are more encouraging than with dialysis.[267,269,366] A major problem after transplantation in diabetic patients is the frequency of amputations. Of 305 transplant recipients at the University of Minnesota, 45 (15 percent) have undergone 100 amputations.[267,269] Among patients treated with hemodialysis at the same institution, only 10 of 202 (5 percent) have undergone 13 amputations.[269] Development of blindness in patients on dialysis seems to be much greater than in those undergoing renal transplatation.[266–268] However, a significant decline in ophthalmological complications in diabetic patients on dialysis has been documented.[269] Improvements in diabetic gastroenteropathy[367,368] and neuropathy[367] represent other advantages associated with a well-functioning transplant. Two excellent and comprehensive reviews have appeared concerning the advantages and disadvantages of dialysis versus transplantation in diabetic individuals with end-stage renal failure[269,339] and are highly recommended for a more in-depth discussion of the problem

Protein Restriction

During the last 3 years there has been tremendous interest in the use of a low protein diet to prevent the progression of chronic renal failure.[225] The use of such protein-restricted diets is based on two assumptions: (1) the adaptive increases in glomerular pressures and blood flow that occur in response to a reduction in renal mass are responsible for the progressive injury to remaining nephrons; and (2) the adaptive increases in renal hemodynamics can be prevented by decreasing the dietary protein intake, which will have a protective effect on renal function. In this section we briefly review these assumptions.

In rats, if renal mass is reduced by any one of a number of experimental maneuvers,[223,224,369–374] there is an initial stabilization of renal function. However, this is followed by a progressive decline in GFR that eventually ends in end-stage renal failure and death. The data of Brenner and colleagues in the remnant kidney model is summarized in Table 5-8.[223–225] After a 75 percent reduction in total renal mass, there is a marked increase in GFR by each remaining nephron; that is, the SNGFR increases. This increase in SNGFR results from two factors: an increase in glomerular plasma flow rate and an increase in transhydraulic glomerular pressure difference (Table 5-8). These renal hemodynamic changes are associated with the development

Table 5-8. Effect of Protein Restriction in Preventing Progressive Renal Insufficiency in the Remnant Kidney Model in Rats

Model	SNGFR[a] (nl/min)	Glomerular Plasma Flow Rate (nl/min)	Glomerular Transcapillary Hydraulic Pressure Difference (mm Hg)	Proteinuria	Kidney Life Span	Renal Histology
Control rats	28	74	37	0	2 Years	Normal
Remnant kidney	63[b]	187[b]	44[b]	+ + + +	Weeks	Glomerulo-sclerosis
Remnant plus low protein	38	92	32	+	Months	Marked Improvement

Data are summarized from Hostetter TH, Rennke HG, Brenner BM: Compensatory renal hemodynamic injury: a final common pathway of residual nephron destruction. Am J Kidney Dis 1:310, 1982; Hostetter TH, Rennke HG, Brenner BM: The case for intrarenal hypertension in the initiation and progression of diabetic and other glomerulopathies. Am J Med 72:375, 1982; Brenner BM, Meyer TW, Hostetter TH: Dietary protein intake and the progressive nature of kidney disease. N Engl J Med 307:652, 1982.

[a] Single nephron glomerular filtration rate.

[b] Statistically significant compared to control rats.

of heavy proteinuria and prominent glomerular sclerosis. On the basis of these results Brenner and colleagues[223–225] postulated that chronic renal vasodilation and glomerular hyperfiltration are responsible for the progressive mesangial cell injury and glomerular sclerosis, eventuating in end-stage renal failure.

If rats with a remnant kidney are placed on a protein-restricted diet, the rise in SNGFR, glomerular plasma flow, and transcapillary hydraulic pressure are prevented; heavy proteinuria does not develop, glomerular histology is markedly improved, and kidney survival is significantly prolonged (Table 5-8).

Based on the above results obtained in animals, a number of studies have examined whether a low protein diet in man also will have a palliative effect on the progression of renal failure.[194,196,375–380] Most but not all of these studies have been retrospective in nature. Nonetheless, the results have been quite consistent and suggest that a low protein diet will slow the decline in GFR in patients with *advanced* renal failure of diverse etiology. The data of Barsotti et al.[196] are representative and are shown in Figure 5-13.

Although the above results are extremely interesting and exciting, several comments are indicated lest these results be interpreted out of context. First, most of the studies were retrospective and involved relatively small numbers of patients. Second, almost all patients had far-advanced renal failure with GFRs below 15–20 ml/min. Whether protein restriction will have the same beneficial effects in patients with less severely advanced renal insufficiency remains to be determined. Third, very few patients in the preceding studies were diabetic, and extrapolation of these results to di-

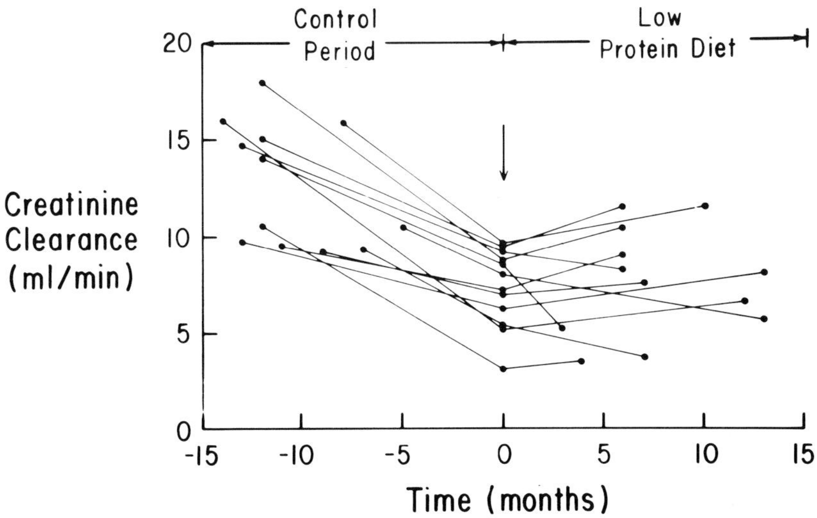

Fig. 5-13 Effect of a low-protein diet (essential amino acids plus keto analogues) on the progression of renal disease in patients with chronic glomerulonephritis and chronic interstitial nephritis of diverse etiology. (Redrawn from Barsotti G, Guiducei A, Ciardella F, Giovannetti S: Effects of renal function of a low nitrogen diet supplemented with essential amino acids and ketoanalogues and of hemodialysis and free protein in patients with chronic renal failure. Nephron 27:113, 1981.)

abetic patients with kidney failure may not be justified. Fourth, it is unknown if long-term protein restriction, particularly in the diabetic, is associated with any adverse side effects in the patient with advanced renal disease. For instance, one could imagine that in the diabetic, particularly if he is in poor metabolic control, a low protein diet could lead to negative nitrogen balance, accelerate the rate of muscle protein breakdown, and lead to the development of clinically manifest myopathy. Therefore at present it seems prudent to view low protein dietary therapy of chronic renal disease as an experimental maneuver that offers significant promise for the future.

HYPERFILTRATION HYPOTHESIS: IMPLICATIONS FOR THE DIABETIC

At the time of initial diagnosis, IDDs have a supernormal GFR and slightly elevated renal plasma flow.[20–22,144–153,172,174,297] These hemodynamic changes persist for many years, and the elevation in GFR is often present at the onset of proteinuria, some 15–20 years later.[20,21,144,174,175] In experimental animal models of diabetes mellitus, marked increases in SNGFR, renal plasma flow, and glomerular transcapillary hydraulic pressure have also been reported.[166–169] Renal hypertrophy and elevated kidney GFR are the most impressive features of experimentally induced diabetes mellitus in animals.[159] As can be seen in Table 5-9, changes in kidney weight and function after the induction of experimental diabetes in the rat are quite similar to those observed in the remnant (75 percent nephrectomy) model of renal insufficiency.[159,205,223,224] An increased transglomerular passage of albumin and neutral dextrans has also been demonstrated during the early phase of diabetes in man as well as in these experimentally induced diabetic animal models.[20,144,175,184,186–189,381] The increase in albumin excretion during this early phase is due entirely to an elevated transglomerular pressure; there is no change in pore diameter or the charge selective properties of the glomerular barrier. These changes in renal function and protein excretion occur at a time when there are no histological changes of diabetic nephropa-

Table 5-9. Summary of Changes in Kidney Weight and Function after Streptozotocin-Induced Diabetes Mellitus and 75% Nephrectomy in the Rat

	% Change	
Paramcter[a]	Nephrectomy	Diabetes
Kidney weight	48	31
GFR	50	34
SNGFR	84	43
SNGPF	79	71
Hydrostatic filtration pressure gradient	18	22

Data are from Seyer-Hensen K: Renal hypertrophy in experimental diabetes mellitus. Kidney Int 33:643, 1983.

[a]GFR = glomerular filtration rate. SNGFR = single nephron glomerular filtration rate. SNGPF = single nephron glomerular plasma flow.

thy and can readily be reversed with insulin therapy.[20,144,154,158–160,180–182] The primary cause(s) of renal hypertrophy and glomerular hyperfiltration in diabetes mellitus have been discussed,[159,224] but in our opinion none of the postulated mechanisms are adequate to explain the changes in renal function. As discussed earlier, we believe that loss of the normal tubuloglomerular feedback loop, due to the glucose-induced inhibition of chloride reabsorption at the macular densa segment, may be responsible for the elevation in renal plasma flow and GFR. According to the Brenner hypothesis,[223–225,382] the resultant increase in renal plasma flow and glomerular transcapillary hydraulic pressure, if sustained for a prolonged period of time, leads to direct cellular injury. The end result is an increase in mesangial matrix and glomerulosclerosis (Fig. 5-14). The increases in glomerular plasma flow and transcapillary hydraulic pressure also result in an increased transcapillary protein flux, which may further exacerbate the mesangial cell injury and proliferation of mesangial matrix material (Fig. 5-14). With progressive renal injury there are permselectivity changes in the glomerular barrier, further exacerbating the degree of proteinuria.

If the above theory is correct, one would predict that tight glucose control with insulin early in the course of diabetes would prevent all of the renal hemodynamic changes and stay the dvelopment of albuminuria. This has, in fact, been demonstrated in both man and animals.[20,144,154,158–160,180–182] Furthermore, in experimental animal models of diabetes, insulin treatment[71–73,91] or islet cell transplantation[67,92–97] is capable of preventing the typical histological changes of diabetic nephropathy.

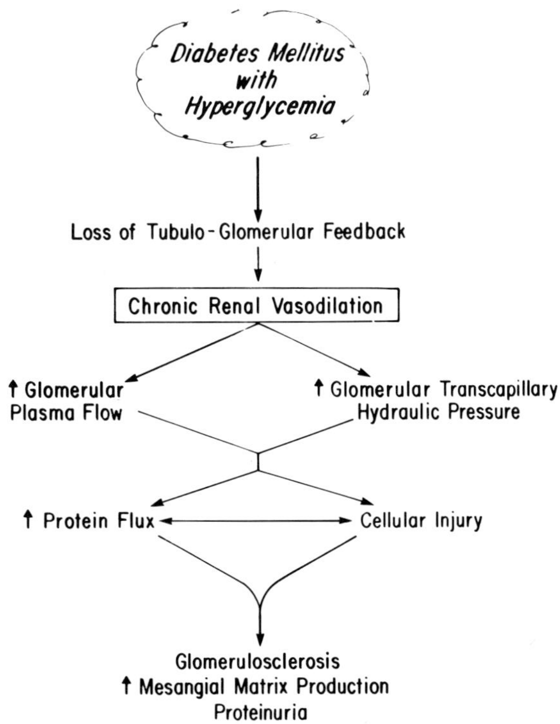

Fig. 5-14 Hypothetical sequence of events leading to end-stage diabetic nephropathy.

Whether tight metabolic regulation in man will similarly prevent the development of structural changes remains to be determined.

A second prediction of the above model is that late intervention with insulin therapy would be unlikely to have a major effect on progression of diabetic nephropathy. At this stage, fixed histological alterations would be present, and permselectivity changes and glomerular ultrastructural damage would be largely responsible for the proteinuria. Therefore after 5–10 years of established diabetes mellitus, one would not expect the institution of tight metabolic control to have a major impact on the natural progression of diabetic nephropathy. This hypothesis is consistent with the recent observation that insulin pump therapy fails to prevent the progression of renal disease in diabetic patients with proteinuria who have had their disease for 5–10 years or more.[112–114]

RENAL DISEASE IN NIDDM

Although our knowledge concerning functional and structural alterations in the insulin-dependent (type I) diabetic have proliferated rapidly during the last decade, there have been few good studies that have examined the course of renal involvement in the noninsulin-dependent (type II) diabetic. This is surprising since the great majority of diabetics are noninsulin-dependent. The most comprehensive study was published by Fabre et al.[7] They reported data on 510 patients whose diabetes was diagnosed after the age of 40. The majority were obese, and there was a very high incidence of angina pectoris, myocardial infarction, and cerebrovascular disease. Of the 510 patients, 114 were treated with diet alone, 231 with diet plus oral agents, and 165 with insulin. The indication for starting insulin in the latter group was not specified, and it is not possible to determine whether these diabetes were really insulin-dependent or insulin-independent. In Table 5-10 the laboratory findings in the 510 type II diabetics are compared with the typical findings reported in type I diabetics. At the time of initial diagnosis 48 percent of the NIDDs had urinary protein excretion rates in excess of 150 mg/day, but only 16 percent excreted more than 500 mg/day. In contrast, none of the controls excreted more than 150 mg of protein per day, and less

Table 5-10. Comparison of Renal Involvement in Insulin-Dependent (Type I) and Noninsulin-Dependent (Type II) Diabetes Mellitus

Parameter	Type I	Type II
Proteinuria at onset	<5%	48%
Proteinuria within first 10 years	~10–15%	64%
Progression of proteinuria after 10 years	Common	Uncommon
Degree of proteinuria	Large	Small
Nephrotic syndrome	~30–40%	<5%
End-stage renal failure	~40%	<5%
Hypertension (diastolic pressure >110 mm Hg)	46%	<5%
Renal histology[a]	Diffuse/nodular glomerular sclerosis with arteriolar hyalinosis	

[a]See text for a more detailed discussion of the histological findings and their significance.

han 5 percent of IDDs would be expected to have protein excretion rates in excess of 150 mg/day at the time of initial diagnosis. During the first 10 years after the diagnosis of diabetes mellitus, 64 percent of type II diabetics had proteinuria (>150 mg/day) compared to 10–15 percent of type I diabetics. After 10 years, however, there was a marked increase in the incidence of proteinuria in type I diabetics, the proteinuria was usually heavy, and the nephrotic syndrome was common. In contrast, in NIDDs progression of proteinuria after 10 years was uncommon, the proteinuria was usually not heavy, and the nephrotic syndrome was relatively infrequent. End-stage renal failure eventually occurred in approximately 40 percent of IDDs but in less than 5 percent of type II diabetics. A GFR less than 60 ml/min per 1.73 sq meters was observed in only 9 percent of the patients reported by Fabre et al.,[7] and most of these patients had moderate to severe hypertension. During a follow-up period of 8 years no patient had died of diabetic nephropathy whereas 24 percent had died of other causes, primarily coronary heart disease.[7] The incidence of hypertension was particularly high in the type II diabetic patients: 46 percent diastolic blood pressures in excess of 110 mm Hg and 79 percent greater than 95 mm Hg. In contrast, hypertension was distinctly uncommon in type I diabetics until renal insufficiency was well advanced. Renal tissue was available for histological analysis in 50 of the 510 patients reported by Fabre et al.,[7] and the authors stated that "all exhibited diffuse or nodular glomerulosclerosis and arteriolar hyalinosis." Unfortunately, these findings are not elaborated on, and it is not possible to ascertain the severity of these lesions or their relationship to any observed renal functional changes. Several other groups have reported on the histological changes, but in much smaller groups of NIDDs.[9,13,14,23,24] Although these authors also have described the typical changes of diabetic glomerulosclerosis, one has the distinct impression that the renal changes are not nearly as frequent as in IDDs and when present are much less severe. For instance, Takazakura et al.[14] reported the results of renal biopsies performed on 12 type II diabetics. Five had no evidence of diabetic glomerulosclerosis, four had mild diabetic glomerulosclerosis (grade 1 out of 4), and three had moderate diabetic glomerulosclerosis (grade 2 out of 4). Of these 12 only one had progressed to stage 3 changes after a mean follow-up of 53 months. In conclusion, our knowledge of renal involvement (with respect to frequency, severity, clinicopathologic correlations) in NIDDM remains incomplete and represents an area in need of further investigation.

ACKNOWLEDGMENTS

The author thanks Drs. Jerold Olefsky and Robert Sherwin for the opportunity to write this review on diabetic nephropathy. There has been a tremendous interest and proliferation of information in this area over the last 5 years, and it is hoped that the reader will derive as much enjoyment and knowledge in reviewing this manuscript as I did in writing it. I am indebted to Drs. C. Kjellstrand, J. Najarian, and G. Oreopoulos for supplying me with their most updated information concerning dialysis and transplantation in the treatment of end-stage diabetic renal disease.

REFERENCES

1. Harris M: The prevalence of diagnosed diabetes, undiagnosed diabetes, and impaired glucose tolerance in the United States. In Melish JS, Hana J, Baba F (eds): Genetic and Environmental Interactions in Diabetic Mellitus. Proceedings of the Third Symposium on Diabetes Mellitus in Asia and Oceana. International Congress Series 549. pp. 72–76. Excerpta Medica, Amsterdam, 1984
2. Marks HH: Longevity and mortality of diabetics. Am J Public Health 55:416, 1965
3. Balodimos MC: Diabetic nephropathy. In Marbel A, White P, Bradly RF (eds): Joslin's Diabetes Mellitus p. 526. Lea & Febiger, Philadelphia, 1971
4. Joslin EP: Diabetes in the future. Diabetes 10:148, 1961
5. Deckert T, Poulsen JE, Larsen M: Prognosis of diabetes with diabetes onset before the age of thirty one. I. Survival, causes of death, and complications. Diabetologia 14:363, 1978
6. Deckert T, Poulsen JE, Larsen M: Prognosis of diabetics with diabetes onset before the age of thirty one. II. Factors influencing the prognosis. Diabetologia 14:371, 1978
7. Fabre J, Balant LP, Dayer PG, et al: The kidney in maturity onset diabetes mellitus: a clinical study of 510 patients. Kidney Int 21:730, 1982
8. Kimmelstiel, P, Wilson C: Intercapillary lesions in glomeruli of kidney. Am J Pathol 12:83, 1936
9. Heptinstall RE: Pathology of the Kidney. pp. 1397–1953. 3rd Ed. Little, Brown, Boston, 1983
10. Churg J, Dolger H: Diabetic renal disease. In Early LE, Gottschalk CW (eds): Strauss and Welt's Diseases of the Kidney. 3rd Ed. Little, Brown, Boston, 1983
11. Ireland JT, Viberti GC, Watkins PJ: The kidney and renal tract. In Keen H, Jarrett J (eds): Complications of Diabetes. 2nd Ed. pp. 137–178. Edward Arnold, London, 1982
12. Osterby R, Gundersen HJG, Horlyck A, et al: Diabetic glomerulopathy: structural characteristics of the early and advanced stages. Diabetes, suppl. 2, 32:79, 1983
13. Brun C, Gormsen H, Hilden T, et al: Diabetic nephropathy: kidney biopsy and renal function tests. Am J Med 15:187, 1953
14. Takazakura E, Nakamoto Y, Hayakawa H, et al: Onset and progression of diabetic glomerulosclerosis: a prospective study based on serial renal biopsies. Diabetes 24:1, 1975
15. Arieff A: Kidney, water and electrolyte metabolism in diabetes mellitus. In Brenner BM, Rector FC (eds): The Kidney. 2nd Ed. pp. 1257–1296. Saunders, Philadelphia, 1981
16. Mauer, SM, Steffes MW, Brown DM: The kidney in diabetes. Am J Med 70:603, 1981
17. Osterby R: Early phases in the development of diabetic glomerulopathy. Acta Med Scand [suppl 574] 54:14, 1975
18. Westberg NG, Michael AF: Immunopathology of diabetic glomerulosclerosis. Diabetes 21:163, 1972
19. Tisher CC, McCoy RC: Diabetes mellitus and the kidney. In Suki WN, Eknoyan G (eds): The Kidney in Systemic Diseases. pp. 479–506, Wiley, New York, 1981
20. Mogensen CE, Christensen CK, Vittinghus E: The stages in diabetic renal disease. Diabetes, suppl. 2, 32:64, 1978
21. Gundersen HJG, Mogensen CE, Seyer-Hansen K, et al: Early and late changes in the diabetic kidney. In: Advances in Nephrology. pp. 1–27. Year Book, Chicago, 1978
22. Osterby R, Gundersen HJG: Glomerular size and structure in diabetes mellitus. I. Early abnormalities. Diabetologia 11:225, 1975
23. Gellman DD, Pirani CL, Soothill JF, et al: Diabetic nephropathy: a clinical and pathologic study based on renal biopsies. Medicine 38:321, 1959
24. Hatch FE, Watt MF, Kramer NC, et al: Diabetic glomerulosclerosis: a long-term follow-up study based on renal biopsies. Am J Med 31:216, 1961

25. Watkins PJ, Blainey JD, Brewer DB, et al: The natural history of diabetic renal disease: a follow-up study of a series of renal biopsies. Q J Med 41:437, 1972
26. Ireland JJ, Patnaik BK, Duncan LJP: Effect of pituitary ablation on the renal arteriolar and glomerular lesions in diabetics. Diabetes 16:636, 1967
27. Ireland JJ, Patnaik BK, Duncan LJP: Glomerular ultrastructure in secondary diabetes and normal subjects. Diabetes 16:623, 1967
28. Spiro RG: Studies on the renal glomerular basement membrane: preparation and chemical composition. J Biol Chem 242:1915, 1967
29. Spiro RG: Biochemistry of the renal glomerular basement membrane and its alteration in diabetes mellitus. N Engl J Med 288:1337, 1973
30. Kefalides NA: Structure and biosynthesis of basement membranes. Int Rev Connect Tissue Res 6:63, 1973
31. Farquhar MG, Wissig SL, Palade GE: Glomerular permeability. I. Ferritin transfer across the normal glomerular capillary wall. J Exp Med 113:47, 1961
32. Walker F: The origin, turnover, and removal of glomerular basement membrane. J Pathol 110:233, 1973
33. Price RG, Spiro RG: Studies on the metabolism of the renal glomerular basement membrane. J Biol Chem 252:8597, 1977
34. Westberg NG: Diabetic nephropathy: pathogenesis and prevention. Acta Endocrinol (Copenh) [Suppl 238] 94:85, 1980
35. Spiro RG, Spiro MJ: Effect of diabetes on the renal glomerular basement membrane: studies on the glucosyltransferase. Diabetes 20:641, 1971
36. Khalifa A, Cohen, MP: Glomerular protocollagen lysyl-hydroxylase activity in streptozotocin diabetes. Biochim Biophys Acta 386:332, 1975
37. Cohen MP, Vogt C: Evidence for enhanced basement membrane synthesis and lysine hydroxylation in renal glomerulus in experimental diabetes. Biochem Biophys Res Commun 49:1542, 1972
38. Grant ME, Harwood R, Williams IF: Increased synthesis of glomerular basement membrane collagen in streptozotocin diabetes. J Physiol (Lond) 257:56P, 1976
39. Caufield JP, Farquhar MG: Distribution of anionic sites in glomerular basement membranes: their possible role in filtration and attachment. Proc Natl Acad Sci USA 73:1646, 1976
40. Kanwar YS, Farquhar MG: Presence of heparin sulfate in the glomerular basement membrane. Proc Natl Acad Sci USA 76:1303, 1979
41. Michael AF, Blau EB, Vernier RL: Glomerular polyanion: alteration in aminonucleoside nephrosis. Lab Invest 23:649, 1970
42. Beisswenger PJ, Spiro RG: Human glomerular basement membrane: chemical alteration in diabetes mellitus. Science 168:596, 1970
43. Kefalides NA: Biochemical properties of human glomerular basement membrane in normal and diabetic kidneys. J Clin Invest 53:403, 1974
44. Westberg NG, Michael AF: Human glomerular basement membrane: chemical composition in diabetes mellitus. Acta Med Scand 194:39, 1973
45. Sato T Munakata H, Yoshinago K, Yosizawa Z: Comparison of the chemical composition of glomerular and tubular basement membranes obtained from human kidneys of diabetics and nondiabetics. Clin Chim Acta 61:145, 1975
46. Wahl P, Depperman D, Hasslacher C: Biochemistry of glomerular basement membrane of the normal and diabetic human. Kidney Int 21:744, 1982
47. Blownlee M, Cahill GF: Diabetic control and vascular complications: a review. Atheroscler Rev 4:29, 1979
48. Falk RJ, Scheinman JI, Mauer SM, Michael AF: Polyantigenic expansion of basement membrane constituents in diabetic nephropathy. Diabetes, suppl. 2, 32:34, 1983

49. DeBats A, Gordon AH, Rhodes EL: Variation in Glomerular sialic acid content in diabetes and as the result of aging. Clin Sci Mol Med 47:93, 1974
50. Uitto J, Perejda AJ, Grant GA, et al: Glycosylation of human glomerular basement membrane collagen: increased content of hexose in ketoamine linkage and unaltered hydroxylysine-O-glycosides in patients with diabetes. Connect Tissue Res 10:45, 1982
51. Cohen MP, Wu VY: Identification of specific amino acids in diabetic glomerular basement membrane collagen subject to nonenzymatic glucosylation in vivo. Biochem Biophys Res Commun 100:1549, 1981
52. Wahl P, Deppermann D, Deschner W, et al: The metabolism of the isolated renal glomerulus and its basement membranes. In Camerini-Davalos RA, Cole HS (eds): Vascular and Neurological Changes in Early Diabetes. p. 85. Academic Press, New York, 1973
53. DeLieta A, Christlieb R, Melby J, et al: Big renin and biosynthetic defect of aldosterone in diabetes mellitus. N Engl J Med 295:639, 1976
54. DeChatel R, Weidmann, P, Flammer J, et al: Sodium, renin, aldosterone, catecholamines and blood pressure in diabetes mellitus. Kidney Int 12:412, 1977
55. Shapiro AP, Perez-Stable E, Moutos SE: Coexistence of renal arterial hypertension and diabetes mellitus. JAMA 192:813, 1965
56. Miller K, Michael A: Immunopathology of renal extracellular membranes in diabetes mellitus. Diabetes 25:701, 1976
57. Thomsen AC: The significance of renal biopsy for the diagnosis of pyelo-nephritis in diabetic patients. In Wolstenholme GEW, Carmeton MP (eds): Ciba Foundation Symposium on Renal Biopsy. p. 281. Little, Brown, Boston, 1961
58. Vejlsgaard R: Studies on urinary tract infection in diabetics. Acta Med Scand 179:173, 1966
59. Batalla MA, Balodimos MC, Bradley RF: Bacteriuria in diabetes mellitus. Diabetologia 7:297, 1971
60. Eknoyan G, Qunibi WY, Grissom RJ, et al: Renal papillary necrosis: an update. Medicine 61:55, 1982
61. Mandel EE: Renal medullary necrosis. Am J Med 13:322, 1952
62. Lauler DP, Schreiner GE, and David A: Renal medullary necrosis. Am J Med 29:132, 1960
63. Kroustrup JP, Gundersen HJG, Osterby R: Glomerular size and structure in diabetes. III. Early enlargment of the capillary surface. Diabetologia 13:207, 1977
64. Becker D, Miller M: Presence of diabetic glomerulosclerosis in patients with hemochromatosis. N Engl J Med 263:367, 1960
65. Ennis G, Miller M, Unger FM: Intercapillary glomerulosclerosis in diabetes secondary to chronic relapsing pancreatitis. Diabetes 18:333, 1969 (abstract)
66. Mauer SM, Michael AF, Fish AJ, and Brown DM: Spontaneous immunoglobulin and complement deposition in glomeruli of diabetic rats. Lab Invest 27:488, 1972
67. Mauer SM, Sutherland DER, Steffes MW, et al: Pancreatic islet transplantation: effects on the glomerular lesions of experimental diabetes in the rat. Diabetes 23:748, 1974
68. Foglia VG, Mancini RE, Cardeza AF: Glomerular lesions in the diabetic rat. Arch Pathol Lab Med 50:75, 1950
69. Lee CS, Mauer SM, Brown DM et al: Renal transplantation in diabetes mellitus in rats. J Exp Med 139:793, 1974
70. Weil R III, Nozawa M, Koss M et al: The kidney in streptozotocin diabetic rats: morphologic, ultrastructure and function studies. Arch Pathol 100:37, 1976
71. Rasch R: Prevention of diabetic glomerulopathy in streptozotocin diabetic rats by insulin treatment: kidney size and glomerular volume. Diabetologia 16:125, 1979
72. Rasch R: Prevention of diabetic glomerulopathy in streptozotocin rats by insulin treatment: glomerular basement membrane thickness. Diabetologia 16:319, 1979

73. Hagg E: Influence of insulin treatment on glomerular changes in rats with longterm alloxan diabetes. Acta Pathol Microbiol Scad 82:228, 1974
74. Steffes MW, Brown DM, Mauer SM: Diabetic glomerulopathy following unilateral nephrectomy in the rat. Diabetes 27:35, 1978
75. Rosenmann E, Teitelbaum A, Cohen AM: Nephropathy in sucrose-fed rats: electron and light microscopic studies. Diabetes 20:803, 1971
76. Cohan AM, Teitelbaum A, Saliternik R: Genetics and diet as factors in development of diabetes mellitus. Metabolism 21:235, 1972
77. Orskov H, Steen Olsen T, Nielsen K, et al: Kidney lesions in rats with severe long-term alloxan diabetes. Diabetologia 1:172, 1965
78. Cameron DP, Amherdt M, Leuenberger P et al: Microvascular alterations in chronically streptozotocin-diabetic rats. In Camerini-Davalos RA, Cole HS (eds): Vascular and Neurological Changes in Early Diabetes. pp. 257–269. Academic Press, New York, 1973
79. Hagg E: Glomerular basement membrane thickening in rats with long-term alloxan diabetes: a quantitative electron microscopic study. Acta Pathol Microbiol Scand 82:211, 1974
80. Hagg E: Occurrence of immunoglobulin and complement in the glomeruli of rats with long-term alloxan diabetes. Acta Pathol Microbiol Scand 82:220, 1974
81. Kirose K, Osterby R, Nozawa M, Gundersen HG: Development of glomerular lesions in experimental long-term diabetes in the rat. Kidney Int 21:689, 1982
82. Wehner H, Hohn O, Faix-Schade U, et al: Glomerular changes in mice with spontaneous hereditary diabetes. Lab Invest 27:331, 1972
83. Like AA, Lavine RL, Poffenbarger PL, Chick WL: Studies in the diabetic mutant mouse. VI. Evolution of glomerular lesions and associated proteinuria. Am J Pathol 66:193, 1972
84. Coleman DL: Obese and diabetes: two mutant genes causing diabetes-obesity syndromes in mice. Diabetologia 14:141, 1978
85. Bower G, Brown DM, Steffes MW, et al: Studies of the glomerular mesangium and the juxtaglomerular apparatus in the genetically diabetic mouse. Lab Invest 43:333, 1980
86. Bloodworth JMB Jr, Engerman RL, Powers KL: Experimental diabetic microangiopathy. I. Basement membrane statistics in the dog. Diabetes 18:455, 1969
87. Luken FDW, Dohan FC: Experimental pituitary diabetes of five years duration with glomerulosclerosis. Arch Pathol 41:19, 1946
88. Bloodworth JMB Jr: Experimental diabetic glomerulosclerosis. II. The dog. Arch Pathol 79:113, 1965
89. Patz A, Berkow JW, Maumenee AE, Cox J: Studies on diabetic retinopathy. II. Retinopathy and nephropathy in spontaneous canine diabetes. Diabetes 14:700, 1965
90. Bloodworth JMB Jr, Engerman RL, Anderson PJ: Microangiopathy in the experimentally diabetic animal. In Camerini-Davalos RA, Cole HS (eds): Vascular and Neurological Changes in Early Diabetes. pp. 245–250. Academic Press, New York, 1973
91. Rasch R: Prevention of diabetic glomerulopathy in streptozotocin diabetic rats by insulin treatment: the mesangial regions. Diabetologia 17:243, 1979
92. Mauer SM, Steffes MW, Sutherland DER, et al: Studies of the rate of regression of the glomerular lesions in diabetic rats treated with pancreatic islet transplantation. Diabetes 24:280, 1975
93. Federlin K, Bretzel RG, Schmidtchen U: Islet transplantation in experimental diabetes of the rat. V. Regression of glomerular lesions in diabetic rats after intraportal transplantation of isogenic islets. Horm Metab Res 8:404, 1976
94. Weil R III, Nozawa M, Koss M, et al: Pancreatic transplantation in diabetic rats: renal function, morphology, ultrastructure and immunohistology. Surgery 78:142, 1975
95. Gray BN, Watkins E Jr: Prevention of vascular complications of diabetes by pancreatic islet transplantation. Arch Surg 111:254, 1976

96. Steffes MW, Brown DM, Basgen JM, et al: Glomerular basement membrane thickness following islet transplantation in the diabetic rat. Lab Invest 41:116, 1979
97. Steffes MW, Brown DM, Basgen JM, Mauer SM: Amelioration of mesangial volume and surface alterations following islet transplantation in diabetic rats. Diabetes 29:509, 1980
98. Mauer SM, Steffes MW, Brown DM: Animal models of diabetic nephropathy. In Hamburger J, Crosnier J, Grunfield JP, Maxwell MH (eds): *Advances In Nephrology*. Vol. 8. pp. 23–42. Yearbook, Chicago, 1979
99. Engerman R, Bloodworth JMB, Nelson S: Relationship of microvascular disease in diabetes to metabolic control. Diabetes 26:760, 1977
100. Mauer SM, Barbosa J, Vernier RL, et al: Development of diabetic vascular lesions in normal kidneys transplanted into patients with diabetes mellitus. N Engl J Med 295:916, 1976
101. Mauer SM, Miller K, Goetz FC, et al: Immunopathology of renal extracellular membranes in kidneys transplanted into patients with diabetes mellitus. Diabetes 25:709, 1976
102. Miller K, Michael AF: Immunopathology of renal extracellular membranes in diabetes mellitus: specificity of tubular basement membrane immunofluorescence. Diabetes 25:701, 1976
103. Abouna GM, Kremer GD, Daddah SK, et al: Reversal of diabetic nephropathy in human cadaveric kidneys after transplantation into non-diabetic recipients. Lancet 2:1274, 1983
104. Sutherland DER, Goetz FC, Elick BA, Najarian JS: Pancreas transplantation for diabetes: clinical experience and metabolic studies in 54 recent cases at the University of Minnesota. Transplant Proc 15:1322, 1983
105. Bondy PK, Felig P: Relation of diabetic control to development of vascular complications. Med Clin North Am 55:889, 1971
106. Colwell JA: Effect of diabetic control on retinopathy. Diabetes 15:497, 1966
107. Knowles HC Jr: The problem of the relation of the control of diabetes to the development of vascular disease. Trans Am Clin Climatol Assoc 76:142, 1964
108. Raskin P: Diabetic regulation and its relationship to microangiopathy. Metabolism 27:235, 1978
109. Stowers JM: Complications in relation to diabetic control: general review. In Keen H, Jarrett J (eds): *Complication of Diabetes*. pp. 1–5. Arnold, London, 1975
110. Tchobroutsky G: Metabolic control and diabetic complication. In Brownlee M (ed): Handbook of Diabetes Mellitus. Vol. 5. pp. 3–39. Garland STPM Press, New York, 1981
111. Kaplan MH, Feinstein AR: A critique of methods in reported studies of long-term vascular complications in patients with diabetes mellitus. Diabetes 22:160, 1973
112. Tamborlane WV, Puklin JE, Bergman M, et al: Long-term improvement of metabolic control with the insulin pump does not reverse diabetic microangiopathy. Diabetes Care, suppl. 1, 5:58, 1982
113. Viberti GC, Bilous RW, Mackintosh D, et al: Long term correction of hyperglycaemia and progression of renal failure in insulin dependent diabetics. Br Med J 286:598, 1983
114. Lawson P, White M, Rosenstock J, Kohner E: Failure of continuous subcutaneous insulin infusion as a therapeutic tool in severe forms of diabetic nephropathy. Diabetologia 21:510, 1981 (abstract)
115. Urizar RE, Schwartz A, Top F, Vernier RL: The nephrotic syndrome in children with diabetes mellitus of recent onset. N Engl J Med 281:173, 1969
116. Daysog A Jr, Dobson HL, Brennan JC: Renal glomerular and vascular lesions in prediabetes and in diabetes mellitus: a study based on renal biopsies. Ann Intern Med 54:672, 1961

117. Nash DA, Rogers PW, Langlinois PC, Bunn SM: Diabetic glomerulosclerosis without glucose intolerance. Am J Med 59:191, 1975
118. Linner E, Svanborg A, Zelander T: Retinal and renal lesions of diabetic type, without obvious disturbances in glucose metabolism, in a patient with family history of diabetes. Am J Med 39:298, 1971
119. Strauss, FG, Argy WP Jr, Schreiner GE: Diabetic glomerulosclerosis in the absence of glucose intolerance. Ann Intern Med 75:239, 1971
120. Harrignton AR, Hare HG, Chambers WN, Valtin H: Nodular glomerulosclerosis suspected during life in a patient without demonstrable diabetes mellitus. N Engl J Med 275:206, 1966
121. Collens WS, Silverstein JN, Dobkin GB: Case of a diabetic with a Kimmelstiel-Wilson syndrome and a normal glucose tolerance. Ann Intern Med 50:1282, 1959
122. Arnold JD, Tarlov AR, Spargo B, et al: Subclinical diabetes mellitus in patients presenting with clinical chronic "glomerulonephritis." Trans Assoc Am Physicians 71:186, 1958
123. Freedman LR: Inapparent diabetes mellitus as a cause of renal insufficiency due to Kimmelstiel-Wilson lesions. Johns Hopkins Med J 100:132, 1957
124. Siperstein MD, Unger RH, Madison LL: Studies of muscle capillary basement membranes in normal subjects, diabetic and prediabetic patients. J Clin Invest 47:1973, 1968
125. Siperstein MD Raskin P, Burns H: Electron microscopic quantification of diabetic microangiopathy. Diabetes 22:514, 1973
126. Siperstein MD, Feingold KR, Bennett PH: Hyperglycemia and diabetic microangiopathy. Diabetologia 15:365, 1978
127. Williamson JR, Vogler NJ, Kilo C: Microvascular disease in diabetes. Med Clin North Am 55:846, 1971
128. Williamson JR, Kilo C: Basement-membrane thickening and diabetic microangiopathy. Diabetes, suppl. 2, 25:925, 1976
129. Williamson JR, Rowold E, Hoffman P, Kilo C: Influence of fixation and morphometric technics on capillary basement-membrane thickening prevalence data in diabetes. Diabetes 25:604, 1976
130. Williamson JR, Kilo C: Current status of capillary basement-membrane disease in diabetes mellitus. Diabetes 26:65, 1977
131. Williamson JR, Kilo C: A common sense approach resolves the basement membrane controversy and the NIH Pima Indian study. Diabetologia 17:129, 1979
132. Jackson R, Guthrie R, Esterly J, et al: Muscle capillary basement membrane changes in normal and diabetic children. Diabetes, suppl. 2, 24:400, 1975 (abstract)
133. Sheikholislam BM, Irias JJ, Lin HT: Carbohydrate metabolism and capillary basement-membrane thickness in children. I. Cross sectional studies. Diabetes 25:650, 1976
134. Sheikholislam BM, Irias JJ, Lowry GH, et al: Carbohydrate metabolism and capillary basement-membrane thickness in children. 2. Longitudinal studies. Diabetes 25:661, 1976
135. Bundersen HJG, Osterby R, Lundbaek K: The basement membrane controversy. Diabetologia 15:361, 1978
136. Raskin P, Pietri AO, Unger R, Shannon WA: The effect of diabetic control on the width of skeletal-muscle capillary basement membrane in patients with type I diabetes mellitus. N Engl J Med 309:1546, 1983
137. Knowles HC Jr: Magnitude of the renal failure problem in diabetic patients. Kidney Int, suppl. 1, 6:S3, 1974
138. Knowles HC Jr: Long-term juvenile diabetes treated with unmeasured diet. Trans Assoc Am Physicians 84:95, 1971

139. McCrary RF, Pitts TO, Puschett JB: Diabetic nephropathy: natural course, survivorship and therapy. Am J Nephrol 1:206, 1981
140. Deckert T, Poulsen JE: Diabetic nephropathy: fault of destiny? Diabetologia 21:178, 1981
141. Paz-Guavara AT, White P: Juvenile diabetes mellitus after forty years. Diabetes 24:449, 1975
142. Paul JT, Presley SJ: Complications of long-term diabetes mellitus. Ann Intern Med 49:142, 1958
143. White P: Natural course and prognosis of juvenile diabetes. Diabetes 5:445, 1956
144. Mogensen CE: Abnormal physiological processes in the kidney. In Brownlee M (ed): Handbook of Diabetes Mellitus. Vol. 4. pp. 23–85. Garland STPM Press, New York, 1981
145. Mogensen CE: Kidney function and glomerular permeability in early juvenile diabetes. Scand J Clin Lab Invest 28:79, 1971
146. Mogensen CE: Glomerular filtration rate and renal plasma flow in short-term and long-term juvenile diabetes. Scand J Clin Lab Invest 28:91, 1971
147. Stalder G, Schmid R: Severe functional disorders of glomerular capillaries and renal haemodynamics in treated diabetes mellitus during childhood. Acta Paediatr Scand 193:129, 1959
148. Stalder G, Schmid R, von Wolff M: Funtionelle Mikroangiopathie der Nieren beim behandelten Diabetes mellitus in Kindsalter. Dtsch Med Wochenschr 85:346, 1960
149. Ditzel J, Schwartz M: Abnormally increased glomerular filtration rate in short-term insulin-treated diabetic subjects. Diabetes 16:264, 1967
150. Ditzel J, Junker K: Abnormal glomerular filtration rate, renal plasma flow and renal protein excretion in recent and short-term diabetics. Br Med J 2:13, 1972
151. Brochner-Mortensen J, Ditzel J, Mogensen CE, Rodbrer P: Microvascular permeability to albumin and glomerular filtration rate in diabetic and normal children. Diabetologia 16:307, 1979
152. Mogensen CE, Steffes MW, Deckert T, Christansen JS: Functional and morphological renal manifestations in diabetes mellitus. Diabetologia 21:89, 1981
153. Mogensen CE, Andersen MJF: Increased kidney size and glomerular filtration rate in early juvenile diabetics. Diabetes 22:706, 1973
154. Mogensen CE, Anderson MJF: Increased Kidney size and glomerular filtration rate in untreated juvenile diabetes: normalization by insulin treatment. Diabetologia 11:224, 1975
155. Kahn CB, Raman PG, Zic Z: Kidney size in diabetes mellitus. Diabetes 23:788, 1974
156. Mogensen CE, Osterby R, Gundersen HJG: Early functional and morphologic vascular renal consequences of the diabetic state. Diabetologia 17:71, 1979
157. Hirose K, Tsuchida H, Osterby R, Gundersen HJG: A strong correlation between glomerular filtration rate and filtration surface in diabetic kidney hyperfunction. Lab Invest 43:434, 1980
158. Parving HH, Noer I, Deckert T, et al: The effect of metabolic regulation on microvascular permeability to small and large molecules in short-term juvenile diabetics. Diabetologia 12:161, 1976
159. Seyer-Hansen K: Renal hypertrophy in experimental diabetes mellitus. Kidney Int 23:643, 1983
160. Seyer-Hansen K: Renal hypertrophy in streptozotocin diabetes rats. Clin Sci Mol Med 51:551, 1976
161. Seyer-Hansen K: Renal hypertrophy in experimental diabetes: relation to severity of diabetes. Diabetologia 13:141, 1977
162. Seyer-Hansen K: Renal hypertrophy in experimental diabetes: comparison to compensatory hypertrophy. Diabetologia 14:323, 1978

163. Seyer/Hansen K, Hansen J, Gundersen HJGG: Renal hypertrophy in experimental diabetes: a morphometric study. Diabetologia 18:501, 1980
164. Osterby R, Gundersen HJGG: Fast accumulation of basement membrane material and the rate of morphological changes in acute experimental diabetic glomerular hypertrophy. Diabetologia 18:493, 1980
165. Cohen MP, Klein CV: Glomerulopathy in rats with streptozotocin diabetes: assimulation of glomerular basement membrane analogous to human diabetic nephropathy. J Exp Med 149:623, 1979
166. Hostetter TH, Troy JL, Brenner BM: Glomerular hemodynamics in experimental diabetes mellitus. Kidney Int 19:410, 1981
167. Michels LD, Davidman M, Keane WF: Determinants of glomerular filtration and plasma flow in experimental diabetic rats. J Lab Clin Med 98:869, 1981
168. Jensen PK, Christiansen JS, Steven K, Parving H-H: Renal function in streptozotocin-diabetic rats. Diabetologia 21:409, 1981
169. Carney SL, Wong NLM, Dirks JHJ: Acute effects of streptozotocin diabetes on rat renal function. J Lab Clin Med 93:950, 1979
170. Cortes P, Levin NW, Dumler F, et al: Uridine triphosphate and RNA synthesis during diabetes-induced kidney growth. Am J Physiol 238:E349, 1980
171. Gotzsche O, Gundersen HJGG, Osterby R: Irreversibility of glomerular basement membrane accumulation despite reversibility of renal hypertrophy with islet transplantation in early experimental diabetes. Diabetes 30:481, 1981
172. Sandahl-Christiansen J, Gammelgaard J, Frandsen M, Parving HH: Increased kidney size, glomerular filtration rate and renal plasma flow in short-term insulin dependent diabetics. Diabetologia 20:451, 1981
173. Goldstein DA, Massry SG: Diabetic nephropathy: clinical course and effect of hemodialysis. Nephron 20:286, 1978
174. Mogensen CE: Diabetes mellitus and the kidney. Kidney Int 21:673, 1982
175. Mogensen CE: Kidney function and glomerular permeability to macromolecules in juvenile diabetes with special reference to early changes. Dan Med Bull, suppl. 3, 19:1, 1972
176. Mogensen CE: Renal function changes in diabetes. Diabetes, supp. 2, 25:872, 1976
177. Mogensen CE, Vittinghus E, Solling K: Increased urinary albumin, light chain and beta-2-microglobulin excretion after intravenous arginine adminstration in normal man. Lancet 2:581, 1975
178. Mogensen CE, Vittinghus E, Solling K: Abnormal albumin excretion after two provocative renal test in diabetes: physical exercise and lysine injection. Kidney Int 16:385, 1979
179. Viberti GC, Jarrett RJ, McCartney M, Keen H: Increased glomerular permeability to albumin induced by exercise in diabetic subjects. Diabetologia 14:293, 1978
180. Koivisto VA, Huttunen NP, Vienkko P: Continuous subcutaneous insulin infusion corrects exercise-induced albuminuria in juvenile diabetes. Br Med J 282:778, 1981
181. Viberti G, Pickup JC, Bilous RW, et al: Correction of exercise-induced microalbuminuria in insulin-dependent diabetics after three weeks of subcutaneous insulin infusion. Diabetes 30:818, 1981
182. Viberti GC, Pickup JC, Jarrett RJ, Keen H: Effect of control of blood glucose on urinary excretion of albumin and beta$_2$-microglobulin in insulin-dependent diabetics. N Engl J Med 300:638, 1979
183. Viberti GC, Jarrett RJ, Mahmud V, et al: Micro-albuminuria as a predictor of clinical nephropathy in insulin-dependent diabetes mellitus. Lancet 1:1430, 1983
184. Friedman S, Jones HW, Golbetz HV, et al: Mechanisms of proteinuria in diabetic

nephropathy. II. A study of the size selective glomerular filtration barriers. Diabetes, suppl. 2, 32:40, 1983
185. Winetz JA, Goldbetz HV, Spencer RJ, et al: Glomerular function in advanced human diabetic nephropathy. Kidney Int 21:750, 1982
186. Carrie BJ, Myers BD: Proteinuria and functional characteristics of the glomerular barrier in diabetic nephropathy. Kidney Int 17:669, 1980
187. Viberti GC, Mackintosh D, Keen H: Determinants of the penetration of proteins through the glomerular barrier in insulin-dependent diabetes mellitus. Diabetes, suppl. 2, 32:92, 1983
188. Parving HH, Rutili F, Granath K, et al: Effect of metabolic regulation on renal leakiness to dextran molecules in short-term insulin dependent diabetics. Diabetologia 17:157, 1979
189. Parving HH, Noer I, Deckert T, et al: The effect of metabolic regulation on microvascular permeability to small and large molecules in short-term juvenile diabetes. Diabetologia 12:161, 1976
190. Brenner BM, Hostetter TH, Humes HD: Molecular bases of proteinuria of glomerular origin. N Engl J Med 298:826, 833, 1978
191. Deen WM, Satvat B: Determinants of glomerular filtration of proteins. Am J Physiol 241:F162, 1981
192. Viberti GC, Bilous RW, Mackintosh D, Keen H: Monitoring glomerular function in diabetic nephropathy. Am J Med 74:256, 1983
193. Mitch WE, Lemann J, Buffington GA, Walser M: A simple method of estimating progression of chronic renal failure. Lancet 2:1326, 1976
194. Walser M, Mitch WE, Collier VU: The effect of nutritional therapy on the course of chronic renal failure. Clin Nephrol 11:66, 1979
195. Jones RH, Hayakawa M, Mackay JD, et al: Progression of diabetic nephropathy. Lancet 1:1105, 1979
196. Barsotti G, Guiducei A, Ciardella F, Giovannetti S: Effects on renal function of a low nitrogen diet supplemented with essential amino acids and ketoanalogues and of hemodialysis and free protein supply in patients with chronic renal failure. Nephron 27:113, 1981
200. Mogensen CE: Maximum tubular reabsorption capacity for glucose and renal hemodynamics during rapid hypertonic glucose infusion in normal and diabetic man. Scand J Clin Lab Invest 28:101, 1971
201. Robertson JA, Gray CH, Baynes AH: Renal function in diabetic nephropathy. Arch Intern Med 87:570, 1951
202. Lundbaek K: Long Term Diabetes. Munksgaard, Copenhagen, 1953
203. Smith D, Bia M, DeFronzo RA: Clinical disorders of potassium metabolism. In Arieff A, DeFronzo RA (eds): Fluid, Electrolyte, and Acid-Base Disorders. Churchill Livingstone, New York, 1984, pp 413–510
204. Bia MJ, DeFronzo RA: Extrarenal potassium homeostasis. Am J Physiol 240:F257, 1981
205. DeFronzo RA, Sherwin RS, Dillingham M, et al: Influence of basal insulin and glucagon secretion on potassium and sodium metabolism. J Clin Invest 61:472, 1978
206. Bia M, Tyler K, DeFronzo RA: Regulation of extrarenal potassium homeostasis by adrenal hormones in rats. Am J Physiol 242:F641, 1982
207. DeFronzo RA, Bia M, Birkhead G: The effect of epinephrine on potassium homeostasis. Kidney Int 20:83, 1981
208. DeFronzo RA, Lee R, Jones A, Bia M: Effect of insulinopenia and adrenal hormone deficiency on acute potassium tolerance. Kidney Int 7:586, 1980
209. DeFronzo RA: Hyperkalemia and hyporeninemic hypoaldosteronism. Kidney Int 17:118, 1980

210. DeFronzo RA, Sherwin RS, Felig P, Bia M: Nonuremic diabetic hyperkalemia: possible role of insulin deficiency. Arch Intern Med 137:842, 1979
211. Schambelan M, Sebastian A, Biglieri E: Prevalence, pathogenesis, and functional significance of aldosterone deficiency in hyperkalemic patients with chronic renal insufficiency. Kidney Int 17:89, 1980
212. Tuck ML, Sambhi MP, Levin L: Hyporeninemic hypoaldosteronism in diabetes mellitus. Diabetes 28:237, 1979
213. Tuck ML, Mayes DM: Mineralocorticoid biosynthesis in patients with hyporeninemic hypoaldosteronism. J Clin Endocrinol Metab 50:351, 1980
214. Arruda JAL, Battle DC, Sehey JT, et al: Hyperkalemia and renal insufficiency: role of selective aldosterone deficiency and tubular unresponsiveness to aldosterone. Am J Nephrol 1:260, 1981
215. Battle DC: Hyperkalemic hyperchloremic metabolic acidosis associated with selective aldosterone deficiency and distal renal tubular acidosis. Semin Nephrol 1:260, 1981
216. DeFronzo RA, Bia M, Smith D: Clinical disorders or hyperkalemia. Annu Rev Med 33:521, 1982
217. Fredlund P, Saltman S, Dando J, et al: Aldosterone production by isolated glomerulosa cells: modulation of sensitivity to angiotensin II and ACTH by extracellular potassium concentration. Endocrinology 100:481, 1977
218. Tait JF, Tait SAS: The effect of changes in potassium concentration on the maximal steroidogenic response of purified zona glomerulosa cells to angiotensin II. J Steroid Biochem 7:687, 1976
219. Day RP, Leutscher JA, Gonzales CM: Occurance of big renin in human plasma, amniotic fluid, and kidney extracts. J Clin Endocrinol Metab 40:1078, 1975
220. Sealey JE, Atlas SA, Laragh JH: Prorenin and other large molecular weight forms of renin. Endocr Rev 1:365, 1980
221. Gordon R, Kuchel O, Liddle G, Island D: Role of the sympathetic nervous system in regulating renin and aldosterone production in man. J Clin Invest 46:599, 1967
222. Christensen NJ: Plasma catecholamines in long-term diabetes with and without neuropathy and in hypophysectomized subjects. J Clin Invest 51:779, 1972
223. Hostetter TH, Rennke HG, Brenner BM: Compensatory renal hemodynamic injury: a final common pathway of residual nephron destruction. Am J Kidney Dis 1:310, 1982
224. Hostetter H, Rennke HG, Brenner BM: The case for intrarenal hypertension in the initiation and progression of diabetic and other glomerulopathies. Am J Med 72:375, 1982
225. Brenner BM, Meyer TW, Hostetter TH: Dietary protein intake and the progressive nature of kidney disease. N Engl J Med 307:652, 1982
226. Schnermann J, Persson AEG, Agerup B: Tubuloglomerular feed-back: nonlinear relation between glomerular hydrostatic pressure and loop of Henle perfusion rate. J Clin Invest 52:862, 1973
227. Wright FS, Briggs JP: Feedback control of glomerular blood flow, pressure, and filtration rate. Physiol Rev 59:958, 1979
228. Wright R, Schnermann J: Interference with feedback control of glomerular filtration rate by furosemide, triflocin, and cyanide. J Clin Invest 53:1695, 1974
229. Blantz RC, Konnen KS: The relation of distal tubular delivery and reabsorptive rate to nephron filtration. Am J Physiol 223:F315, 1977
230. Tucker BJ, Peterson OW, Gushwa LC, Blanz RC: Mechanism of diuresis with modest hyperglycemia. Clin Res 29:478A, 1981
231. Blantz RC, Peterson OW, Gushwa L, Tucker BJ: Effect of modest hyperglycemia on tubuloglomerular feedback activity. Kidney Int 22:S206, 1982
232. Textor SC, Bravo EL, Fouad FM, Tarazi RC: Hyperkalemia in azotemic patients during

angiotensin-converting enzyme inhibition and aldosterone reduction with captopril. Am J Med 73:719, 1982
233. Franco-Saenz R, Suzuki S, Tan ST: Prostaglandins and renin production: a review. Prostaglandins 20:1131, 1980
234. Saruta T, Kaplan NM: Adrenocortical steroidgenesis: the effects of prostaglandins. J Clin Invest 51:2246, 1972
235. Tan SY, Shapiro R, Franco R, et al: Indomethacin-induced prostaglandin inhibition with hyperkalemia. Ann Intern Med 90:783, 1979
236. DeFronzo RA, Thier SO: Fluid and electrolyte disturbances: hypo- and hyperkalemia. In Martinez-Maldonado M (ed): Handbook of Renal Therapeutics. pp. 25–55. Plenum, New York, 1983
237. Halperin ML, Bear RA, Hannaford MC, Goldstein MB: Selected aspects of the pathophysiology of metabolic acidosis in diabetes mellitus. Diabetes 30:781, 1981
238. Halperin ML, Goldstein MB, Josse RG: In Arieff A, DeFronzo RA (eds): Fluid, Electrolyte, and Acid-Base Disorders. Churchill Livingstone, New York, 1984, pp 933–967
239. DeFronzo RA, Andres R, Edgar P, Walker WG: Carbohydrate metabolism in uremia: a review. Medicine 52:469, 1973
240. DeFronzo RA: Pathogenesis of glucose intolerance in uremia. Metabolism, suppl. 2, 27:1866, 1978
241. DeFronzo RA, Alvestrand A: Glucose intolerance in uremia: site and mechanism. Am J Clin Nutr 33:1438, 1980
242. Kreisberg RA: Lactate homeostasis and lactic acidosis. Ann Intern Med 92:227, 1980
243. Emmett M, Narrins RG: Clinical use of the anion gap. Medicine 56:38, 1977
244. Tannen RL: Ammonia metabolism. Am J Physiol 235:F265, 1978
245. Tannen RL: Relationship of renal ammonium production and potassium homeostasis. Kidney Int 11:453, 1977
246. Sebastian A, Sutton JM, Hulter HN, et al: Effect of mineralocorticoid replacement on renal acid-base homeostasis in adrenalectomized patients. Kidney Int 18:762, 1980
247. DiTella PJ, Sodhi B, McCreary J, et al: Mechanism of metabolic acidosis of selective mineralocorticoid deficiency. Kidney Int 14:466, 1978
248. Hulter HN, Ilnicki LP, Harbottle JA, Sebastian A: Impaired renal hydrogen secretion and ammonia production in mineralocorticoid-deficient glucocorticoid replete dogs. Am J Physiol 232:F136, 1977
249. Vaamonde CA, Perez GO, Oster JR: Syndromes of aldosterone deficiency. Mineral Electrolyte Metab 5:121, 1981
250. Arruda JAL, Kurtzman NA: Mechanisms and classification of deranged distal urinary acidification. Am J Physiol 8:F515, 1980
251. Lathem W: Hyperchloremic acidosis in chronic pyelonephritis. N Engl J Med 258:1031, 1958
252. Harrington JJ, Cohen JJ: Metabolic acidosis. In Cohen JJ, Kassiner JP (eds): Acid/Base. pp. 121–225. Little, Brown, Boston, 1982
253. Sonnenberg H, Cheema-Dhadli S, Goldstein MB, et al: Quantitation of ammonia addition to the medullary collecting duct of the rat. Kidney Int 19:281, 1981
254. Szylman P, Better OS, Chaimowitz C, Roseler R: Role of hyperkalemia in the metabolic acidosis of isolated hypoaldosteronism. N Engl J Med 294:361, 1976
255. Oh MS, Banerji MA, Carroll HJ: The mechanism of hyperchloremic acidosis during the recovery phase of diabetic ketoacidosis. Diabetes 30:310, 1981
256. Renal transplantation in insulin-dependent diabetics: a joint Scandinavian report. Lancet 2:915, 1978
257. Andersen AR, Andersen JK, Christiansen JS, Deckert T: Prognosis for juvenile diabetics with nephropathy and failing renal function. Acta Med Scand 302:131, 1978

258. Ma KW, Masler DS, Brown DC: Hemodialysis in diabetic patients with chronic renal failure. Ann Intern Med 83:215, 1975
259. Comty CM, Kjellstrand D, Shapiro FL: Results of treating diabetic patients by chronic hemodialysis. Dialysis Transplant 5:20, 1976
260. Huang C, Greco FD, Ivanovich P, Krumbovsky FA, et al: Maintenance dialysis for diabetic nephropathy with uremia. J Chronic Dis 28:365, 1975
261. Mitchell JC, Frohnert PP, Kurtz SB, Anderson CF: Chronic peritoneal dialysis in juvenile-onset diabetes mellitus: a comparison with hemodialysis. Mayo Clin Proc 53:775, 1978
262. Pirart J: Diabetes mellitus and its degenerative complications: a prospective study of 4,400 patients observed between 1947 and 1973 [in three parts]. Diabete Metab 3:97, 173, 245, 1977 [English translation: Diabetes Care 1:168, 1978]
263. Deckert T, Paulsen JE: Prognosis for juvenile diabetics with late diabetic manifestations. Acta Med Scand 183:351, 1968
264. Malins JM: Clinical Diabetes Mellitus. Eyre & Spottiswoode, London, 1968
265. Sussman EJ, Tsiaras WG, Soper KA: Diagnosis of diabetic eye disease. JAMA 247:3231, 1982
266. Leonard A, Comty C, Raij I, et al: The natural history of regularly dialyzed diabetics. Trans Am Soc Artif Intern Organs 19:282, 1973
267. Najarian JS, Sutherland DE, Simmons RL, et al: Ten year experience with renal transplantation in juvenile onset diabetics. Ann Surg 190:487, 1979
268. Shapiro FL, Leonard A, Comty CM: Mortality, morbidity and rehabilitation results in regularly dialyzed patients with diabetes mellitus. Kidney Int [Suppl. 1] 6:S8, 1974
269. Kjellstrand C, Comty C, Shapiro F: A comparison of dialysis and transplantation in insulin-dependent diabetic patients. In Friedman EA, L'Esperance FA (eds): Diabetic Renal-Retinal Syndrome. pp. 405–417. Grune & Stratton, New York, 1982
270. Kahn HA, Bradley FR: Prevalence of diabetic retinopathy: age, sex, and duration of diabetes. Br J Ophthalmol 59:345, 1975
271. Feldman JN, Kirsch SR, Beyer MM, et al: Prevalence of diabetic nephropathy at the time of treatment for diabetic retinopathy. In Friedman EA, L'Esperance FA (eds): Diabetic Renal-Retinal Syndrome. pp. 9–22. Grune & Stratton, New York, 1982
272. Root HF, Mirsky S, Ditzal J: Proliferative retinopathy in diabetes mellitus. JAMA 169:903, 1959
273. Oakley WG, Dyke DA, Tattersall RB, Watkins PJ: Long-term diabetes: a clinical study of 92 patients after 40 years. Q J Med 43:145, 1974
274. Chahal PS, Kohner EM: The relationship between diabetic retinopathy and diabetic nephropathy. Diabetic Nephropathy 2:4, 1983
275. Thomas PK, Ward JD, Watkins PJ: Diabetic neuropathy. In Keen H, Jarrett J (eds): Complications of Diabetes. 2nd Ed. pp. 108–136. Arnold, London, 1982
276. Najarian JS, Sutherland DER, Simmons RL, et al: Kidney transplantation for the uremic diabetic patient. Surg Gynecol Obstet 144:682, 1977
277. Barbosa J, Burke B, Buselmeier TJ, et al: Neuropathy, retinopathy and biopsy findings in the transplanted kidney in diabetic patients. Kidney Int [Suppl 1] 6:S32, 1974
278. Ellenberg M: Diabetic neurogenic vesical dysfunction. Arch Intern Med 117:348, 1966
279. Kamdar A, Weidmann P, Makoff DL, Massry SG: Acute renal failure following intravenous use of radiographic contrast dyes in patients with diabetes mellitus. Diabetes 26:643, 1977
280. Bryd L, Sherman RL: Radio-contrast-induced renal failire: a clinical and pathophysiologic review. Medicine 58:270, 1979
281. Krumlovsky FA, Simon N, Santhanam S, et al: Acute renal failure—association with administration of radiographic material. JAMA 239:125, 1978

282. Ellenberg M, Weber H: The incipient asymptomatic diabetic bladder. Diabetes 16:331, 1967
283. Hatch FE, Parish AE: Apparent remission of a severe diabetic on developing the kimmelstiel Wilson syndrome. Ann Intern Med 54:544, 1961
284. Blagg CR: Visual and vascular problems in dialyzed diabetic patients. Kidney Int [Suppl 4] 6:S27, 1974
285. Honey GE, Pryse-Davies J, Roberts DM: Nephropathy in young diabetics. Q J Med 31:473, 1962
286. Freedman P, Moulton R, Spencer AG: Hypertension and diabetes mellitus. Q J Med 27:293, 1958
287. Kjellstrand CM, Whitley K, Comty CM, Shapiro FL: Dialysis in patients with diabetes mellitus. Diabetic Nephropathy 2:5, 1983
288. Massry SG, Feinstein EI, Goldstein DA: Early dialysis in diabetic patients with chronic renal failure. Nephron 23:2, 1979
289. Parving H-H, Smidt UM, Friisberg B, et al: A prospective study of glomerular filtration rate and arterial blood pressure in insulin-dependent diabetics with diabetic nephropathy. Diabetologia 20:457, 1981
290. Parving H-H, Andersen AR, Smidt UM, et al: Reduced albuminuria during early and aggressive antihypertensive treatment of insulin-dependent diabetic patients with diabetic nephropathy. Diabetes Care 4:459, 1981
291. Mogensen CE: Progression of nephropathy in long-term diabetics with proteinuria and effects of initial anti-hypertensive treatment. Scan J Clin Lab Invest 36:383, 1976
292. Mogensen CE: Antihypertensive treatment inhibiting the progression of diabetic nephropathy. Acta Endocrinol (Copenh) [Suppl 238] 94:103, 1980
293. Christlieb AR, Warram JH, Krolewski AS, et al: Hypertension: the major risk factor in juvenile-onset insulin-dependent diabetes. Diabetes, suppl. 2, 30:90, 1981
294. Berkman J, Rifkin H: Unilateral nodular diabetic glomerulosclerosis (Kimmelsteil-Wilson): report of a case. Metabolism 22:175, 1973
295. Mauer SM, Steffes MW, Azar S, et al: The effect of Goldblatt hypertension on the development of glomerular lesions of diabetes mellitus in the rat. Diabetes 27:738, 1978
296. Steffes MW, Brown DM, Mauer SM: Diabetic glomerulopathy following unilateral nephrectomy in the rat. Diabetes 27:35, 1978
297. Steffes MW, Buchwald H, Wigness BD, et al: Diabetic nephropathy in the uninephrectomized dog: microscopic lesions after one year. Kidney Int 21:721, 1982
298. Paving H-H, Viberti GC, Keen H, et al: Hemodynamic factors in the genesis of diabetic microangiopathy. Metabolism 32:943, 1983
299. Black HR: Evaluation and treatment of the hypertensive patient. Primary Care 10:3, 1983
300. Ellenberg M: Neuropathy in long-standing insulin-dependent diabetic patients. Kidney Int, suppl. 1, 6:S77, 1974
301. Ellenberg M: Diabetic Neuropathy. In Ellenberg M, Rifkin H (eds): Diabetes Mellitus: Theory and Practice. pp. 777–801. Medical Examination Pub., New Hyde Park, NY, 1983
302. Shieh SD, Hirsch SR, Boshell BR, et al: Low risk of contrast media-induced acute renal failure in nonazotemic type 2 diabetes mellitus. Kidney Int 21:739, 1982
303. DeFronzo RA, Alvestrand A, Smith D, et al: Insulin resistance in uremia. J Clin Invest 67:563, 1981
304. Smith D, DeFronzo RA: Insulin resistance in uremia is mediated by postbinding defects. Kidney Int 22:54, 1982
305. DeFronzo RA, Tobin JD, Rowe JW, Andres R: Glucose intolerance in uremia: quanti-

fication of pancreatic beta cell sensitivity to glucose and tissue sensitivity to insulin. J Clin Invest 62:425, 1978

306. Rubenstein AH, Mako ME, Horowitz DL: Insulin and the kidney. Nephron 15:306, 1975
307. Rabkin R, Simon NM, Steiner S, Colwell JA: Effect of renal disease on renal uptake and excretion of insulin in man. N Engl J Med 282:182, 1970
308. Runyan JW, Hurwitz D, Robbins SL: Effect of Kimmelstiel-Wilson syndrome on insulin requirements in diabetes. N Engl J Med 252:385, 1955
309. Rabu M, Dor J, Adar R, et al: Spontaneous hypoglycemia in a diabetic patient with renal failure. Isr J Med Sci 9:1036, 1973
310. Block MB, Rubenstein AH: Spontaneous hypoglycemia in diabetic patients with renal insufficiency. JAMA 213:1863, 1970
311. Garber AJ, Bier D, Cryer PE, Pagliara AS: Hypoglycemia in compensated chronic renal insufficiency: substrate limitation of gluconeogenesis. Diabetes 23:982, 1974
312. White MG, Kutzman NA: Hypoglycemia in non-diabetics with renal failure. JAMA 215:117, 1971
313. Frizzell M, Larsen PR, Field JB: Spontaneous hypoglycemia associated with chronic renal failure. Diabetes 23:493, 1973
314. Pietsman SJ, Agarnal BN: Spontaneous hypoglycemia in end-stage renal failure. Nephron 19:131, 1977
315. Rutsky EA, McDaniel HG, Thorpe DL, et al: Spontaneous hypoglycemia in chronic renal failure. Arch Intern Med 138:1364, 1978
316. Mutaverde A, El-Rani R, Cohen M: Spontaneous hypoglycemia in chronic renal failure. Clin Res 22:475A, 1974
317. Rubenfeld S, Garber AJ: Abnormal carbohydrate metabolism in chronic renal failure: the potential role of accelerated glucose production, increased gluconeogenesis, and impaired glucose disposal. J Clin Invest 62:20, 1978
318. Grajower M, Walter L, Albin J: Hypoglycemia in chronic hemodialysis patients: association with propranolol use. Nephron 26:126, 1980
319. Leski M, Niethammer T, Wyss T: Glucose-enriched dialysate and tolerance to maintenance hemodialysis. Nephron 24:271, 1979
320. Rodrigo F, Shideman J, McHugh R, et al: Natural history, clinical correlations and influence of dialysate glucose and intravenous mannitol. Ann Intern Med 86:554, 1977
321. Amair P, Knanna R, Leibel B, et al: Continuous ambulatory peritoneal dialysis in diabetics with end stage renal disease. N Engl J Med 306:625, 1982
322. Moncrief JW, Popovich RP, Nolph KD, et al: Clinical experience with continuous ambulatory peritoneal dialysis. Am Soc Artif Intern Organs 2:114, 1979
323. Flynn CT, Anason JA: Intraperitoneal insulin with CAPD—artificial pancreas. Trans Am Soc Artif Intern Organs 25:114, 1979
324. Katirtzoglou A, Elzatt S, Oreopoulos D, et al: Chronic peritoneal dialysis in diabetics with endstage renal failure. In L'Esperance FA, Friedman EA (eds): *The Diabetic Renal-Retinal Syndrome*. pp. 317–331. Grune & Stratton, New York, 1980
325. Crossley K, Kjellstrand GM: Intraperitoneal insulin for control of blood sugar in diabetic patients during peritoneal dialysis. Br Med J 1:269, 1971
326. Madden MA, Zimmerman SW, Simpson DP: Continuous ambulatory peritoneal dialysis in diabetes mellitus. Am J Nephrol 2:133, 1982
327. Rottenbourg J, el Shahat Y, Agrefiotis A, et al: Continuous ambulatory peritoneal dialysis in insulin dependent diabetic patients: a 40 month experience. Kidney Int 23:40, 1983
328. Khanna R, Wu G, Chisholm L, Opeopoulos DG: Further experience with CAPD in diabetics with end stage renal disease. Diabetic Nephropathy 2:8, 1983

329. Nolph KD: Chronic peritoneal dialysis in a patient with diabetes mellitus and heart disease. Kidney Int 15:698, 1979
330. Grodstein GP, Blumenkrantz MJ, Kopple JD, et al: Glucose absorption during continuous ambulatory peritoneal dialysis. Kidney Int 19:564, 1981
331. Desanto NG, Capodicasa G, Senatore R, et al: Glucose utilization from dialysate in patients on continuous ambulatory peritoneal dialysis (CAPD). Int J Artif Organs 2:119, 1978
332. Nolph KD, Rosenfield PS, Powell JT, Danforth E: Peritoneal glucose transport and hyperglycemia during peritoneal dialysis. Am J Med Sci 259:272, 1970
333. Andersson G, Bergquist-Poppen M, Bergstrom J, et al: Glucose absorption from the dialysis fluid during peritoneal dialysis. Scand J Urol Nephrol 5:77, 1971
334. Wideroe TE, Smeby LC, Berg KJ, et al: Intraperitoneal insulin absorption during intermittent and continuous peritoneal dialysis. Kidney Int 23:22, 1983
335. Blackard WG, Nelson NC: Portal and peripheral vein immunoreactive insulin concentrations before and after glucose infusion. Diabetes 19:302, 1970
336. Shapiro DJ, Blumenkrantz MJ, Levin SR, Coburn JW: Absorption and action of insulin added to peritoneal dialysate in dogs. Nephron 23:174, 1979
337. Shapiro FL, Comty CM: Hemodialysis in diabetics—1981 update. In Friedman EA, L'Esperance FA (eds): Diabetic Renal-Retinal Syndrome. pp. 309–320. Grune & Stratton, New York, 1982
338. Robin JE, Friedman EA: Dialysis and transplantation of diabetics in the United States. Nephron 18:309, 1977
339. Friedman EA: Strategy in diabetic nephropathy. In Brownlee M (ed): Handbook of Diabetes Mellitus. Vol. 5. pp. 213–241. Garland STPM Press, New York, 1981
340. Ghavamian M, Gutch CF, Kopp KF, Kolff JW: The sad truth about hemodialysis for end-stage diabetic nephropathy. JAMA 222:1386, 1972
341. Blagg CR, Esback JW, Sawyer TK, Casaretto AA: Dialysis for end-stage diabetic retinopathy. Proc Clin Dialysis Transplant Forum 1:133, 1973
342. Chazan BI, Rees SB, Balodimos MC, et al: Dialysis in diabetics: a review of 44 patients. JAMA 209:2026, 1969
343. Drukker W, Haaggma-Schouten WAG, Alberts CHR: Report of regular dialysis treatment in Europe. Proc Eur Dialysis Transplant Assoc 7:3, 1970
344. Goetz FC, Kjellstrand CM: The treatment of diabetic disease. Diabetologia 17:267, 1979
345. White N, Snowden SA, Parsons V, et al: The management of terminal renal failure in diabetic patients by regular dialysis therapy. Nephron 11:261, 1973
346. Schupak E, Neff MS, Slifkin R, et al: Hemodialysis and diabetic nephropathy. JAMA 223:1157, 1973
347. Comty CM, Leonard A, Shapiro FL: Psychosocial problems in dialyzed diabetic patients. Kidney Int [Suppl 1] 6:S144, 1974
348. Kassissieh SD, Yes MC, Lazarus JM, et al: Hemodialysis-related problems in patients with diabetes mellitus. Kidney Int [Suppl 1] 6:S100, 1974
349. Shideman JR, Buselmeier TJ, Kjellstrand CM: Hemodialysis in diabetics: complications in insulin-dependent patients accepted for renal transplantation. Arch Intern Med 136:1126, 1976
350. Comty CM, Kjellstrand D, Shapiro FL: A reassessment of the prognosis of diabetic patients treated by chronic hemodialysis (CHD). Trans Am Soc Artif Intern Organs 22:404, 1976
351. Jacobs C, Broyer M, Brunner FP, et al: Combined report on regular dialysis and transplantation in Europe XI, 1980. Proc Eur Dialysis Transplant Assoc 18:2, 1981

352. Wineman RJ: Edn-stage renal disease: 1978. Dialysis Transplant 7:1034, 1978
353. Wing AJ, Brunner FP, Burck HC, et al: Dialysis and transplantation in Europe. Clin Nephrol 3:123, 1975
354. Comty CM, Leonard A, Shapiro FL: Nutritional and metabolic problems in dialyzed patients with diabetes mellitus. Kidney Int [Suppl 1] 6:S51, 1974
355. Kovarik J, Stummvoll HK, Graf H, Muller MM: Glucose intolerance and hemoglobin A_1, in chronic renal insufficiency. Nephron 28:209, 1981
356. Blumenkrantz MJ, Shapiro DJ, Mimura N, et al: Maintenance peritoneal dialysis as an alternative in the patient with diabetes mellitus and end-stage uremia. Kidney Int [Suppl 1] 6:S108, 1974
357. Rubin J, Orepoulos DG, Blair RDG, et al: Chronic peritoneal dialysis in the management of diabetics with terminal renal failure. Nephron 19:265, 1977
358. Quellhorst E, Schuenemann B, Mietzsch G, Jacob I: Haemo- and peritoneal dialysis treatment of patients with diabetic nephropathy—a comparative study. Proc Eur Dialysis Transplant Assoc 15:205, 1978
359. Advisory Committee to the Renal Transplant Registry 13th Report of the Human Transplant Registry. Transplant Proc 9:926, 1977
360. Bryan FA: National Dialysis Registry 7th Annual Progress Report AK-CUP, NIAMD Report No. AK-7-7-1387. Research Triangle Park, NC 27709
361. Najarian JS, Sutherland DER, Morrow CE, et al: Kidney transplants for high-risk patients. Kidney Int [Suppl 14] 23:S10, 1983
362. Sutherland DER, Fryd DS, Morrow CE, et al: Kidney transplantation in diabetics at the University of Minnesota: an analysis of results by era. Transplant Proc 15:1110, 1983
363. Belzer FO, Miller DT, Sollinger HW, Glass NR: Renal transplantation—a review of the 1980's. Semin Nephrol 2:99, 1982
364. Larsson O, Brynger H: Transplantation in patients with diabetic nephropathy. Acta Endocrinol (Copenh) 238:113, 1980
365. Zincke H, Woods JE, Sterioff S, et al: Renal transplantation in patients with diabetes mellitus—revisited. Transplant Proc 11:55, 1979
366. Simmons RG, Kamstra-Hennen L, Thompson CR: Psychosocial adjustment five to nine years posttransplant. Transplant Proc 13:40, 1981
367. Bakshanden K, Picacheh R, Bastounis E, et al: Renal transplantation complications in patients with juvenile diabetes. Urology 5:21, 1975
368. Mitchell JC: End-stage renal failure in juvenile diabetes mellitus: a five year follow up of treatment. Mayo Clin Proc 52:281, 1977
369. Chanutin A, Ferris E: Experimental renal insufficiency produced by partial nephrectomy. Arch Intern Med 49:767, 1932
370. Purkerson ML, Hoffsten PE, Klahr S: Pathogenesis of the glomerulopathy associated with renal infarction in rats. Kidney Int 9:407, 1976
371. Shimamura T, Morrison AB: A progressive glomerulosclerosis occurring in partial five-sixths nephrectomy. Am J Pathol 79:95, 1975
372. Ibels LS, Alfrey AC, Haut L, Hoffer WE: Preservation of function in experimental renal disease by dietary phosphate restriction. N Engl J Med 298:122, 1978
373. Karlinsky ML, Haut L, Buddington B, et al: Preservation of renal function in experimental glomerulonephritis. Kidney Int 17:293, 1980
374. Tomford RC, Karlinsky ML, Buddington B, Alfrey A: Effect of thyroparathyroidectomy and parathyroidectomy on renal function and nephrotic syndrome in rat nephrotoxic serum nephritis. J Clin Invest 68:655, 1981
375. Alvestrand A, Ahlberg M, Bergstrom J, Furst P: The effect of nutritional regimens on

branched chain amino acid (BCAA) antagonism in uremia. In Walser M, Williamson JR (eds): Metablism and Clinical Implications of Branched Chain Amino and Ketoacids. p. 60. Elsevier/North-Holland, New York, 1981

376. Furst P, Alvestrand A, Bergstrom J: Effects of nutrition catabolic stress on intracellular amino acid pools in uremia. Clin Nutr 33:1387, 1980
377. Mitch WE, Bras E, Walser M: Long-term effects of a new ketoacid-amino acid supplement in patients with chronic renal failure. Kidney Int 22:371, 1982
378. Maschio G, Oldrizzi L, Tessitore N, et al: Effects of dietary protein and phosphorus restriction on the progression of early renal failure. Kidney Int 22:371, 1982
379. Walser M: Nutritional management of chronic renal failure. Am J Kidney Dis 5:261, 1982
380. Giordano C: Protein restriction in chronic renal failure. Kidney Int 22:401, 1982
381. Pennell JP, Hwang KH, Millard MM, Bourgoignie JJ: Glomerular selective permeability to macromolecular neutral dextrans in experimental diabetes. Diabetologia 20:223, 1981
382. Brenner BM: Hemodynamically mediated glomerular injury and the progressive nature of kidney disease. Kidney Int 23:647, 1983

6 Diabetic Neuropathy

Douglas A. Greene
Michael A. Pfeifer

Although first recognized as a clinical entity almost 200 years ago,[1] diabetic peripheral neuropathy remains an unsolved medical problem of enormous proportions.[2] The very prominent neurological concomitants of diabetes led many nineteenth century observers, including Claude Bernard, to conclude that diabetes was itself a neurological disorder.[3] The general concept of diabetic neuropathy as a complication rather than a cause of diabetes evolved only recently[4] but is now accepted in both diabetes care and research. Although definitive prevention and treatment are still not generally available, research toward these goals has been greatly accelerated. New and specific therapeutic agents for diabetic neuropathy are finally undergoing clinical trials, and for the first time significant pathogenetic insight into the disorder has been gained.

Diabetic neuropathy encompasses several somatic and autonomic peripheral nerve syndromes, each having a characteristic clinical presentation and course. Clinical neuropathy, defined as "symptoms plus either signs or objective measurement of peripheral neural impairment," must accompany currently accepted diagnostic criteria for diabetes, and other causes of peripheral neuropathy must be excluded (Table 6-1). Confirmatory clinical signs or objective measurements of peripheral nerve dysfunction must accompany any subjective neuropathic symptoms, which are often nonspecific and vague.

Diabetic neuropathy is subclassified into diffuse and focal somatic neuropathies and autonomic neuropathy; these are further subdivided neuroanatomically using descriptive terms which sometimes carry pathophysiological connotations that are inappropriate for diabetic neuropathy. Sensitive diagnostic procedures have now also defined a subclinical stage of diabetic neuropathy (e.g., slowed nerve conduction[4–8]) not discernible by careful history and physical examination alone.

Table 6-1. Common Important Differential Diagnoses of Diabetic Neuropathy

Distal symmetrical polyneuropathy
Metabolic disorders
Diabetes mellitus
Uremia
Folic acid/cyanocobalamin deficiency
Hypothyroidism
Acute intermittent porphyria
Toxins
Alcohol
Heavy metals (lead, mercury, arsenic)
Industrial hydrocarbons
Drugs
Infiltrative/inflammatory disorders (nerve biopsy often helpful)
Amyloidosis
Leprosy
Sarcoidosis
Periarteritis nodosa
Refsum's disease
Other diseases
Connective tissue diseases, e.g., SLE
Dys- and paraproteinemias
Leukemias/Lymphomas
Paraneoplastic syndrome
Pains and paresthesias without neurological deficit
Depression
Hysteria
Early small fiber sensory neuropathy
Autonomic neuropathy without somatic component
Shy-Drager syndrome (progressive autonomic failure)
Diabetic neuropathy with mild somatic involvement
Riley-Day syndrome
Idiopathic orthostatic hypotension
Diffuse motor neuropathy without sensory deficit
Guillain-Barré syndrome
Primary myopathies
Myasthenia gravis
Heavy metal toxicity
Femoral neuropathy
Degenerative spinal disc disease
Paget's disease of the spine
Intrinsic spinal cord mass lesion
Equina cauda lesions
Coagulopathies
Cranial neuropathy
Carotid aneurysm
Intracranial mass
Elevated intracranial pressure
Mononeuropathy multiplex
Vasculitides
Amylyoidosis
Hypothyroidism
Acromegaly
Coagulopathies

EPIDEMIOLOGY

The true prevalence and incidence of clinical diabetic neuropathy are obscured by inconsistencies in terminology, diagnostic criteria, and study populations.[9,10] Surveys of neurology clinic populations introduce substantial selection and referral biases. Hence prevalence estimates for diabetic neuropathy range between 0 and 93 percent, with the highest figures including those diabetic patients with subclinical neuropathy alone.[11]

Pirart's unique 25-year prospective study of 4,400 unselected patients in a diabetic clinic provides a more balanced clinical view of diabetic neuropathy.[12] Clinical neuropathy was present in 12 percent of patients at the time diabetes was diagnosed with prevalence increasing linearly with duration of diabetes to nearly 50 percent after 25 years.[12,13] Because of its high prevalence, diabetic neuropathy probably has a significant impact on the nation's health care costs, especially when indirect costs (loss of work time, early retirement, disability) are included.[14]

Relationship to Type of Diabetes

The prevalence and incidence of neuropathy, corrected for duration of diabetes, did not differ substantially as a function of the age at which the diagnosis of diabetes was made in Pirart's study.[13] Neuropathy is well described in childhood diabetes of over 5 years' duration[15] and occurs in secondary forms of diabetes (pancreatectomy, nonalcoholic pancreatitis, and hemochromatosis).[10] Therefore diabetic neuropathy represents a concomitant or consequence of the diabetic state per se.

Relationship to Duration of Diabetes

Clinically detectable neuropathy is rarely reported within the first 5 years of diabetes[15] except in type II diabetes where preexisting asymptomatic hyperglycemia is difficult to exclude.[12,13] Thus the prevalence of diabetic neuropathy is initially low but increases progressively with duration of diabetes.[2,12,16,17]

Relationship to Diabetic "Control"

The relationship between blood glucose control and the development of diabetic neuropathy is shrouded in controversy and misinterpretation. Ellenberg dismissed what he referred to as "the widely accepted" notion "that neuropathy in diabetes uniformly follows a prolonged period of poor diabetic control" and pointed out that "neuropathy may be unrelated to the duration and severity of diabetes."[2] Because the development of clinically overt neuropathy represents a late stage in a chronic underlying process ("subclinical neuropathy"), temporal dissociation between the quality of glucose control and the development of neuropathic signs and symptoms is not unexpected. The occasionally paradoxical precipitation of painful neuropathic symptoms after institution of good control probably reflects repair and regeneration of damaged nerve fibers rather than disease progression.[11,16] Hence the frequency of clinical neuropathy seems to be related to the duration and severity of diabetes.[11,12,16,17]

On the other hand, the onset of clinically overt diabetic neuropathy in a given patient is unpredictable, neither reflecting concurrent metabolic control[9] nor following inexorably from even prolonged and severe hyperglycemia,[12] suggesting the presence of other independent pathogenetic variables, e.g., genetic, nutritional, toxic (e.g., alcohol),[18] and mechanical (entrapment and compression)[10,11] factors.

The isolated but unconfirmed reports of improvement in neuropathy with rigorous glucose control[11,19] support a prominent role for the altered metabolism in the pathogenesis of diabetic neuropathy; however, the efficacy of metabolic control in the prevention or treatment of human clinical diabetic neuropathy has not yet been firmly established by well-designed and controlled studies.

Relationship to Other Diabetic Complications

Because the prevalence of diabetic retinopathy and nephropathy also increase with duration of diabetes, patients with neuropathy are more likely to have a second complication,[12,13] leading to the speculation that all three cardinal complications of diabetes represent separate manifestations of a global ''microvascular'' process. On the other hand, it is quite clear that individual patients may be discordant for diabetic renal or retinal disease and neuropathy. Furthermore, independent variables implicated in the pathogenesis or progression of renal and/or retinal disease (e.g., hypertension[20]) are not related to the course of diabetic neuropathy, whereas the reverse is true for other variables (e.g., alcoholism[18]). To further complicate this issue, renal insufficiency accelerates not only diabetic retinopathy but diabetic neuropathy as well.[20] Therefore the three cardinal complications of diabetes are all related to longstanding underlying hyperglycemia and/or insulin deficiency but are differentially affected by independent variables and are accompanied by distinctly different histopathological hallmarks; however, they may mutually interact in their later course and progression.

SYNDROMES OF DIABETIC NEUROPATHY

Diabetic neuropathy is usually subdivided into a set of distinct syndromes, each having a characteristic clinical presentation and course (Table 6-2); however, these syndromes overlap clinically and frequently occur simultaneously, precluding rigid classification of individual cases.[21] Hence classification should be regarded primarily as descriptive, with each subtype representing an idealized rather than a discrete clinical syndrome, and with most cases representing amalgamations of these various subtypes.

Focal and Multifocal Neuropathies

Focal and multifocal diabetic neuropathies are characterized by neurological deficits confined to the distribution of single or multiple peripheral nerves (''mononeuropathy'' or ''mononeuropathy multiplex'') or to focal lesions at the level of the bra-

Table 6-2. Classification of Diabetic Neuropathies

Focal and multifocal neuropathies
Cranial neuropathy
Mononeuropathy or mononeuropathy multiplex
Entrapment neuropathy
Other mononeuropathies
Radiculopathy (intercostal neuropathy)
Plexopathy (asymmetrical motor neuropathy)
Distal symmetrical polyneuropathy
Mixed sensory-motor neuropathy
Predominantly sensory neuropathy
Mixed large and small fiber involvement
Predominantly large fiber involvement
Predominantly small fiber involvement
Predominantly motor neuropathy
Autonomic neuropathy

chial or lumbosacral plexes (''plexopathy'') or nerve roots (''radiculopathy''). Onset is typically acute, and complete or partial recovery is the rule. Although these characteristics suggest a vascular or traumatic etiology, supporting pathoanatomical evidence is fragmentary at best (see below).[11]

Cranial Neuropathies. Isolated cranial neuropathies occur most frequently in elderly diabetic patients[21] and rarely in diabetic children.[22] Though generally unaccompanied by signs and symptoms of generalized diabetic neuropathy,[21] the cranial palsies may be recurrent or bilateral.[10]

The third cranial nerve is most commonly involved, characteristically with pupillary sparing (with carotid aneurysms, pupillary dilatation is usually an early feature).[21] The classic presentation is unilateral ophthalmoplegia (sparing lateral eye movement) and headache.[22] The pain is typically intense and referred above or behind the eye, but may be mild or absent.[21] The responsible nociceptors are thought to be either perineurial or in the adjacent first and second divisions of the trigeminal nerve, as the third nerve is essentially purely motor.[21] Progressive diminution of pain and return of oculomotor function is the rule, even in elderly patients.

The presumed vascular basis of focal diabetic neuropathy is most convincingly demonstrated for isolated third nerve palsy. Dreyfus et al.[23] and Asbury et al.[24] each demonstrated focal fusiform central destructive lesions involving the cavernous sinus portion of the third nerve in individual autopsied cases of isolated diabetic third nerve palsy. Central nerve fibers were most heavily damaged, with distal Wallerian degeneration, whereas superficial fibers (thought to innervate the pupil[21]) were relatively spared. Both fusiform lesions were associated with significant disease of the vasa nervorum, although frank vascular occlusion was not documented. Asbury et al. demonstrated that the intracavernous portion of the third nerve represents a vascular ''watershed'' region between the intra- and extracranial circulation, where the vascular supply is most tenuous.[24]

Other cranial nerves which are less commonly involved in diabetic neuropathy include the sixth, the fourth (usually in combination with other cranial nerves rather than alone), and the seventh cranial nerves,[21] presumably also on a vascular basis.[16]

Mononeuropathy or Mononeuropathy Multiplex. Isolated peripheral nerve palsies occur more commonly in diabetics but a causal versus coincidental relationship is difficult to distinguish.[10] However, 40 percent of unselected patients with clinically overt diffuse diabetic neuropathy have either electrophysiological or clincial evidence of superimposed focal nerve damage at common entrapment or compression sites, suggesting that diffuse diabetic neuropathy predisposes to focal nerve damage.[11] Compression and entrapment palsies in diabetic patients respond to standard conservative or surgical management, i.e., protection against additional mechanical trauma, or surgical release procedures.[16] Nerves not commonly exposed to compression or entrapment damage occasionally develop focal impairment in patients with diabetes, but this may simply reflect coincidental occurrence.

Radiculopathy (Intercostal Neuropathy). Diabetic radiculopathy presents with dermatomal pain and loss of cutaneous sensation. Hypesthesia or paraesthesia may be inapparent initially but usually develops during the course of the disorder.[25,26] Symptoms are often attributed to a compressive lesion, e.g., a herniated nucleus pulposus, but radiographic studies and myelography are negative.[25] When pain is prominent and hypesthesia subtle, truncal radiculopathy is frequently misdiagnosed as an acute medical emergency, e.g., myocardial infarction, cholecystitis, peptic ulcer, or appendicitis, entailing fruitless diagnostic and/or exploratory surgical procedures before the correct diagnosis is recognized.[11,25,26] Electromyography of the paraspinus muscles is usually diagnostic.[26] Although generally ascribed to acute nerve root infarction, confirmatory histopathological evidence in humans is totally lacking. Subtle signs of diffuse distal symmetrical polyneuropathy are often present.[26] Spontaneous resolution of both symptoms and signs is the rule.

Plexopathy (Asymmetrical Proximal Motor Neuropathy, Femoral Neuropathy). Femoral neuropathy arises in nondiabetics from unilateral injury to the femoral nerve or its origins within the lumbar plexus, usually in association with pelvic or abdominal surgery, parturition, or various bleeding disorders.[27] Pain and sensory impairment in the distribution of the femoral nerve (anterior thigh and medial calf) accompany disabling weakness of thigh flexion and knee extension.[27] The diabetic syndrome occurs spontaneously, and sensory loss is usually less marked.[21,28] Pain, which classically extends from the hip to the anterior and lateral surface of the thigh, may radiate into the foot, or it may originate in the sacroiliac region and extend down the leg dorsally.[21,28] The pain may develop gradually or episodically, and it may be worse at night.[28] Muscle weakness most often affects the iliopsoas, quadriceps, and adductor muscles but usually spares the hip extensors and hamstrings. The anterolateral muscles in the calf may also be involved, mimicking an "anterior compartment syndrome."[21] The plantar response may be extensor.[21] Nearly complete recovery is the rule[28] though not universal,[21] and the syndrome may persist or recur.[28] Diabetic plexopathy is a diagnosis of exclusion; space-occupying lesions, trauma, nondiabetic vasculopathies, and skeletal abnormalities must be carefully eliminated. Treatment is supportive pending spontaneous recovery, and the benefit of improved "diabetic control"[21,28] remains unsupported.

A focal pathogenesis has been inferred from rarely associated femoral nerve tenderness,[28] but the meager sensory deficit[28] and more generalized muscle involvement of diabetic femoral neuropathy imply a more diffuse pathogenetic process.[21] The cerebrospinal fluid protein level is usually elevated,[21,28] suggesting very proximal involvement, but femoral nerve conduction velocity is also prolonged, implying some peripheral damage as well.[21] Detailed histopathological study[29] of a single autopsy case of diabetic femoral neuropathy revealed multiple necrotic-appearing lesions in the lumbosacral plexus and the femoral, obturator, lateral femoral cutaneous, sciatic, common peroneal, and posterior tibial nerves accompanied by both distal Wallerian degeneration and segmental demyelination.[29] Atherosclerosis was moderate and generalized, but serial sections of the vasa nervorum revealed only a single small occluded vessel which could not "account for the majority of infarcts."[29] Hence unequivocal histopathological proof of the putative vascular basis of diabetic femoral neuropathy remains elusive, but the disorder is still generally considered to have a vascular basis,[11] probably involving the femoral nerve and/or sacral plexus.

Distal Symmetrical Polyneuropathy

In the most widely recognized form of diabetic peripheral neuropathy,[21] distal symmetrical polyneuropathy, neurological impairment involves all somatic nerves ("polyneuropathy") but demonstrates a distinct predilection for the most distal innervated sites, producing a "stocking–glove" pattern ("distal symmetrical"). The distal symmetrical pattern, shared by other "metabolic" neuropathies, including uremia and various nutritional deficiencies,[30] can be explained by two entirely separate theoretical constructs. Diffuse intraneuronal disturbances might selectively damage the most vulnerable part of the axon, i.e., that furthest away from the cell body. Hence distal parts of long axons would be damaged first, followed by more proximal sites of long axons and distal sites of shorter axons, producing a "dying-back neuropathy."[30] Alternatively, focal lesions distributed randomly along nerve fibers might selectively impair longer fibers, which amass more lesions by virtue of their greater length.[31] In either case, neurological impairment begins distally, usually in the feet or toes, and marches proximally up both the upper and lower extremities. Finally a coexisting vertical anterior chest band of sensory deficit develops as the tips of the shorter truncal nerves become involved[11] (Fig. 6-1).

The diffuseness of peripheral nervous damage is evident by both electrophysiological and histological studies.[21] The generalized conduction slowing and the axonal degeneration and demyelination characteristic of chronic diabetes are exaggerated in patients with distal symmetrical polyneuropathy.[32,33] Conduction slowing and histological fiber loss correlate both in their earlier and more pronounced distal distribution[34–37] and in individual patients.

Clinically detectable neurological deficits evolve only when diffuse peripheral nerve damage outstrips compensatory collateral reinnervation, usually as a late stage in a chronic underlying process.[38] The signs, symptoms, and neurological and electrophysiological deficits of distal symmetrical polyneuropathy vary depending on the spectrum of nerve fiber involvement.[11] Symptoms and signs always appear distally and spread proximally in a fiber-length-dependent fashion, however. Because the signs and symptoms of diabetic distal symmetrical polyneuropathy are shared by other distal symmetrical neuropathies (Table 6-1), the clinical diagnosis is one of exclusion.

Pathology. Histopathology in distal symmetrical diabetic polyneuropathy is similar to but more pronounced than that in longstanding nonneuropathic diabetes.[33]

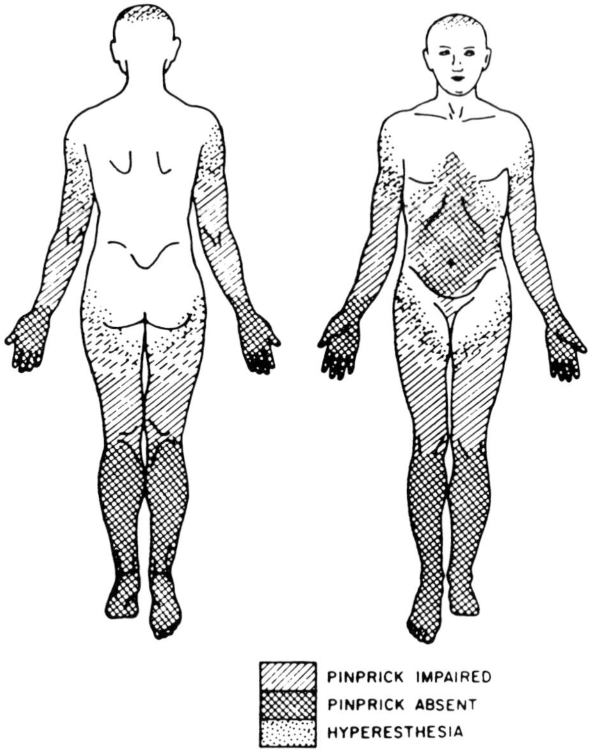

Fig. 6-1 Sensory deficits in distal symmetrical polyneuropathy. (Reprinted with permission from Sabin TD, Geshchwind N, Waxman SG: Patterns of clinical deficits in peripheral nerve disease. Pp. 431–438. In Waxman SG (ed): Physiology and Pathobiology of Axons. Raven Press, New York, 1978.)

Within weeks after the onset of type I diabetes, subtle neurogenic atrophy is detectable in muscle biopsy specimens[35]; but contemporaneous nerve biopsies have never been obtained. Histological damage in longstanding type I or II diabetes is nonspecific and involves all major peripheral nerve components.[11] Myelinated and unmyelinated nerve fibers are reduced in number with a relative preservation of smaller fibers, suggesting either coexisting regeneration or thinning of nerve fiber diameter.[11] Demyelination and remyelination are usually mild[11,33,34,37] except in rare cases.[21] The axonopathy alone accounts for the bulk of clinical and electrophysiological impairment in diabetic polyneuropathy, whereas the Schwann cell changes are usually considered incidental[11,34] and possibly secondary to the axonal alterations.[21] Accompanying endoneurial fibrosis, connective tissue proliferation,[34,37] and thickening and reduplication of endoneurial capillary[11,21,34] and subperineurial[39] basement membranes are seen in various other peripheral neuropathies as well.[11] Hence nerve biopsy is rarely diagnostically helpful in distal symmetrical diabetic neuropathy except when other treatable forms of neuropathy with characteristic histologic appearances are suspected (Table 6-1).

Electrophysiology. Maximum nerve conduction velocity (MNCV), which primarily reflects the integrity of the largest and most rapidly conducting nerve fibers, is only minimally decreased with selective fiber loss but is dramatically reduced by diffuse demyelination which interrupts saltatory conduction. MNCV is also reversibly slowed by metabolic perturbation of peripheral nerves in the absence of histologically demonstrable structural change.[11]

MNCV is slightly reduced at the time of diagnosis of type I diabetes but normalizes with institution of insulin therapy, suggesting a direct metabolic influence.[40,41] Thereafter, MNCV becomes progressively but modestly reduced in type I and II diabetes as a function of duration.[42,43] In chronic stable type II diabetes, MNCV is inversely correlated with glycohemoglobin[44] but improves slightly and proportionately with glycohemoglobin level in response to successful metabolic therapy,[45] suggesting a direct metabolic component to conduction slowing in established diabetes. Furthermore, morphometric-electrophysiological correlations in sural nerves from patients with advanced diabetic distal symmetrical polyneuropathy suggest that nerve conduction slowing exceeds that which can be accounted for by nerve fiber loss, presumably reflecting a direct metabolic component to conduction slowing in overt diabetic neuropathy.[34] A small subgroup of diabetics with seriously slowed nerve conduction[46] either have a large demyelinating component to their diabetic neuropathy or an independent explanation for their electrophysiological impairment. Thus nerve conduction velocity impairment in diabetes reflects a combination of processes in diabetic nerve which cannot be easily differentiated by standard electrophysiological techniques. Although conduction slowing is usually more pronounced in diabetic patients with clinically overt neuropathy, the predictive value of conduction impairment for either the subsequent development or clinical course of diabetic neuropathy has not been established.[47] Furthermore, if diffuse diabetic neuropathy primarily involves smaller-diameter nerve fibers, maximal conduction velocity may not be slowed significantly, in which case electrodiagnostic studies may be somewhat deceiving (see below).

Clinical Signs, Symptoms, and Syndromes. The signs and symptoms of distal symmetrical polyneuropathy vary depending on the spectrum of nerve fiber involvement.

Mixed Sensorimotor Neuropathy. Fiber damage is most commonly diffuse, with a predominance of sensory (versus motor) involvement.[11] Usually both large and small sensory fibers are involved, with the former diminishing position and light touch and the latter diminishing pain and temperature sensation. Motor weakness is usually not marked, involving only the most distal intrinsic muscles of the hands and feet as a rather late feature. However, diminished deep tendon reflexes, especially of the Achilles tendon, is often an early feature.[11]

Large Fiber Sensory Neuropathy. Patients with more selective fiber damage present with variations of this general theme. Patients with predominantly large fiber sensory loss develop impaired balance, diminished proprioceptive and position sense, and absent or reduced vibration sensation. Subjective sensory symptoms are usually absent, and the neuropathy may surface with late neuropathic complications, e.g., a Charcot joint or a neuropathic ulceration (see below). In the most severe form, a sensory ataxia may develop, referred to as "pseudotabetic" diabetic neuropathy. Nerve conduction slowing is usually clearly evident owing to the involvement of the large, rapidly conducting fiber population.[11]

Small Fiber Sensory Neuropathy. Small sensory fiber neuropathy may present with undetected trauma of the extremities (unnoticed burns of the fingers from cigarettes or of the feet from hot bath water, acute ulcerations of the feet from small undetected objects retained inside the shoe, etc.). Alternatively, subjective symptoms of pain or numbness or feelings of "cold feet" or "dead feet" may develop. Most commonly, the patients experience typical neuropathic distal paresthesias (spontaneously occurring uncomfortable sensations) or dysesthesias (contact paresthesias).[11] Some patients complain of exquisite cutaneous contact hypersensitivity to light touch. At times the pain is described as superficial and burning, shooting or stabbing, or bone-deep and aching or tearing. Often the pains are noticed more at night, producing associated insomnia. Pain can become an overriding and disabling feature of diabetic neuropathy. Muscle cramps, which begin distally and slowly ascend, are similar to those reported in other muscle denervation disorders.[11] Because disease may be primarily confined to the small myelinated nerve fibers,[48] conduction velocity may not be dramatically impaired, vibration sensation may be intact, and motor weakness may be absent; moreover, if subjective symptoms bring the neuropathy to the physician's attention early in its course, objective sensory loss may not be striking. The presence of painful symptoms in the absence of striking neurological deficit seems somewhat paradoxical; however, pain may reflect increased fiber regeneration,[11] which may commence before degeneration is sufficiently severe to present marked sensory deficit. Most patients with diabetic neuropathy experience minimal subjective symptoms and present primarily with neurological deficits detected on physical examination or with complications resulting from asymptomatic sensory deficits.[12]

Distal Motor Neuropathy. Distal motor neuropathy is very rare in diabetes and should suggest an alternate etiology, e.g., Guillain-Barré syndrome.[11] A primary motor neuropathy has been associated with insulin-induced hypoglycemia in psychiatric patients and in those with insulinoma; animal experiments support the concept of a hypoglycemic peripheral neuropathy.[11] Hence recurrent iatrogenic hypoglycemia should be considered in any diabetic presenting with a primarily motor distal neuropathy.[11,49]

Complications of Distal Symmetrical Polyneuropathy. With the exception of the generally mild subjective sensory symptoms and rare motor weakness, diabetic distal symmetrical polyneuropathy would constitute only an incidental finding on clinical examination were it not for secondary complications. These mechanical and traumatic complications of sensory and/or motor denervation are almost entirely preventable but constitute a major risk to the neuropathic patient. Their prophylaxis is a major goal of diabetes patient education, foot care, and hygiene.

Neuropathic Foot Ulceration. Repeated traumatic skin and soft tissue damage to the foot results from most sensory neuropathies including diabetic polyneuropathy.[2] Insensitivity to pain is a central element in diabetic foot ulceration, although diminished proprioception, muscle strength, and vascularity may play contributing roles. In the classic plantar ulcer, neurogenic atrophy of the intrinsic foot muscles, which normally oppose the more proximal foot flexors and extensors, results in chronic flexion of the metatarsal-phalangeal joints, drawing the toes into a cocked-up position

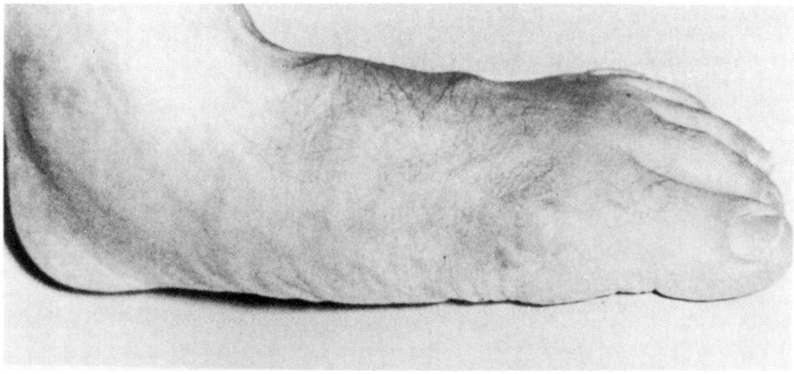

Fig. 6-2 'Claw toe'' (intrinsic-minus) deformity in a neuropathic diabetic foot. (Reprinted with permission from Lippmann HI, Perotto A, Farrar R: The neuropathic foot of the diabetic. Bull NY Acad Sci 52:1159, 1976.)

(claw toe deformity)[2] (Fig. 6-2). Weight-bearing is then shifted to the now uncovered metatarsal heads, leading to thinning and atrophy of the normal fat pad. Thick protruding calluses form over the exposed metatarsal bony prominences, further shifting weight-bearing to the metatarsal heads. The calluses thicken, split, and develop central ulcerations which may remain unnoticed in the absence of pain sensation even when secondary infection develops. Such plantar ulcers are predictably located at callused sites of maximal walking pressure[2] (Fig. 6-3).

Neuropathic foot ulcers develop at other noncallused locations through other mechanisms. The deformed neuropathic foot conforms poorly to the shape of the standardly constructed shoe, leading to pressure lesions and/or abrasions at non-weight-bearing locations.[10] The generally thin dorsal dermis of the foot may be abraded within hours or minutes in the absence of pain sensation, so that repeated self-examinations are mandatory with new footwear or prolonged weight-bearing.

Ischemic factors have been invoked in diabetic foot ulceration, but their role is controversial. Ischemic gangrene may be hastened in neuropathic feet as ischemic rest pain may go unnoticed. Proximal atherosclerotic vascular insufficiency undoubtedly delays healing of neuropathic foot ulcers. However, the neuropathic ulcerated foot is characteristically warm, with easily palpable dorsalis pedis pulses, militating against an important ischemic component.[2] Recent doppler flow studies confirm that blood flow to the neuropathic foot is increased but suggest that increased flow results from abnormal local arteriovenous shunting, which may paradoxically decrease oxygen delivery to the tissues of the foot.[10] Whether arteriovenous shunting is a consequence of the neuropathy itself remains to be determined.[10]

The major element in the treatment of diabetic foot ulcers is removal of traumatic elements which contribute to the ulcer formation. Readjustment of weight-bearing with appropriate orthopedic devices is essential, and in some cases partial or complete elimination of weight-bearing is required (decreased ambulation, support with a cane or crutches, use of a wheelchair, or enforced bed rest). When callous protrusions interfere with weight-bearing, appropriate débridement, trimming, and abrasion

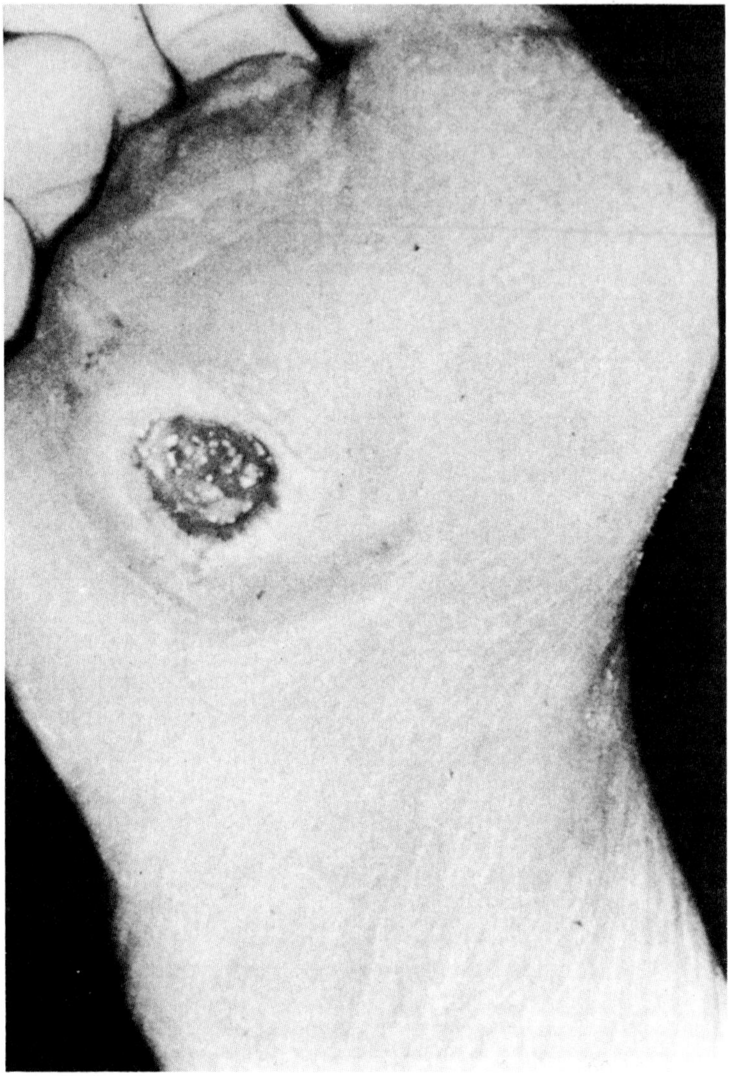

Fig. 6-3 Neuropathic foot ulcer. (Reprinted with permission from Ellenberg M: Diabetic neuropathy: clinical aspects. Metabolism 25:1627, 1976.)

is indicated. Complicating infection should be treated with antibiotics. In refractory cases, removal of the offending metatarsal head and amputation of the toe may be necessary.[2]

Neuroarthropathy (Charcot's Joint). Neuroarthropathy can occur in any nervous system disease which leaves motor function relatively intact but impairs sensation.[50] The primacy of nociceptive impairment in the pathogenesis of neuroarthropathy is supported by its reported occurrence in the congenital indifference to pain syndrome and by the almost complete absence of pain in diabetic neuroarthropathy.[50]

Whereas tabetic neuroarthropathy classically involves large weight-bearing joints, diabetic neuroarthropathy primarily involves small joints of the foot (tarsal-metatarsals or metatarsal-phalangeals) or the ankle.[50] In recent-onset diabetic neuroarthropathy, the foot is usually painless, swollen, and red; fever and leukocytosis are absent; and a distal symmetrical sensory deficit with absence of pain sensation is clearly demonstrable. The differential diagnosis is usually cellulitis or osteomyelitis, depending on coexistent radiographic bony destruction. Unhealed painless fractures are often radiographically present, and a recent history of painless trauma is sometimes elicited.[50] In later stages the disorder presents as gross architectural distortion of the foot, with shortening and widening of the joint. In its most advanced stage, there are multiple painless fractures accompanied by extensive bone demineralization and reabsorption, so that the foot appears to the examiner as "a bag of bones"[2] (Fig. 6-4). As with other forms of neuroarthropathy, the pathogenetic mechanism is presumed to be multiple recurrent traumatic insults to the joint and surrounding bony structures which are not noticed by the patient because of insensitivity to pain. The therapy is directed at removal of continued trauma by decreasing weight-bearing, by either decreasing ambulation or providing other means of ambulation, e.g., a cane, crutches, or wheelchair.

Treatment of Distal Symmetrical Diabetic Neuropathy. Current therapy for diabetic polyneuropathy is symptomatic, palliative, and supportive. Sensory deficits are usually only mildly symptomatic unless complications develop; hence their management is primarily prophylactic (see above). Paresthesias and dysesthesias are usually well tolerated once they are understood as indicative of reparative processes. Troubling painful symptoms are generally thought to improve spontaneously within a matter of months,[2,11] though disagreement exists with this conclusion.[19]

Various pharmacotherapeutic measures have been recommended for painful diabetic neuropathy, including standard analgesics, phenytoin (Dilantin) or carbamazepine (Tegretol) in anticonvulsive doses, and amitriptyline (Elavil) in subantidepressive doses (50–150 mg p.o. at bedtime) either alone or in combination with fluphenazine (Prolixin) 1 mg three times a day.[11] The lack of supporting well-controlled clinical trials[51,52] is especially troubling in view of the dramatic analgesic placebo response which occurs with intensely perceived pain.[53] Depression with associated anorexia is a major factor in painful diabetic neuropathy and seems to exceed that which can be attributed entirely to the painful symptoms alone, suggesting that simultaneous antidepressant therapy might be efficacious.[2,54] An exaggeration of this interaction probably accounts for the syndrome of diabetic neuropathic cachexia described by Ellenberg in 1974.[55] This syndrome in elderly male diabetics combines severe weight loss with mild diabetes and painful neuropathy; weight loss is sufficient (up to 60 percent of total body weight) to suggest an underlying malignancy.[55] Improved diabetic control, counseling, and amitriptyline plus fluphenazine are all recommended therapies.

Improved glycemic control as treatment for clinically overt diabetic distal symmetrical polyneuropathy has been recommended by many but proved efficacious by none.[11,19,43–45,47] Hence the diabetologist has no rational clinical basis on which to select among various alternatives of metabolic control for patients with distal symmetrical polyneuropathy. Prospective clinical trials, e.g., the Diabetes Control and Complications Trial, will hopefully resolve the role of intensive insulin regimens in

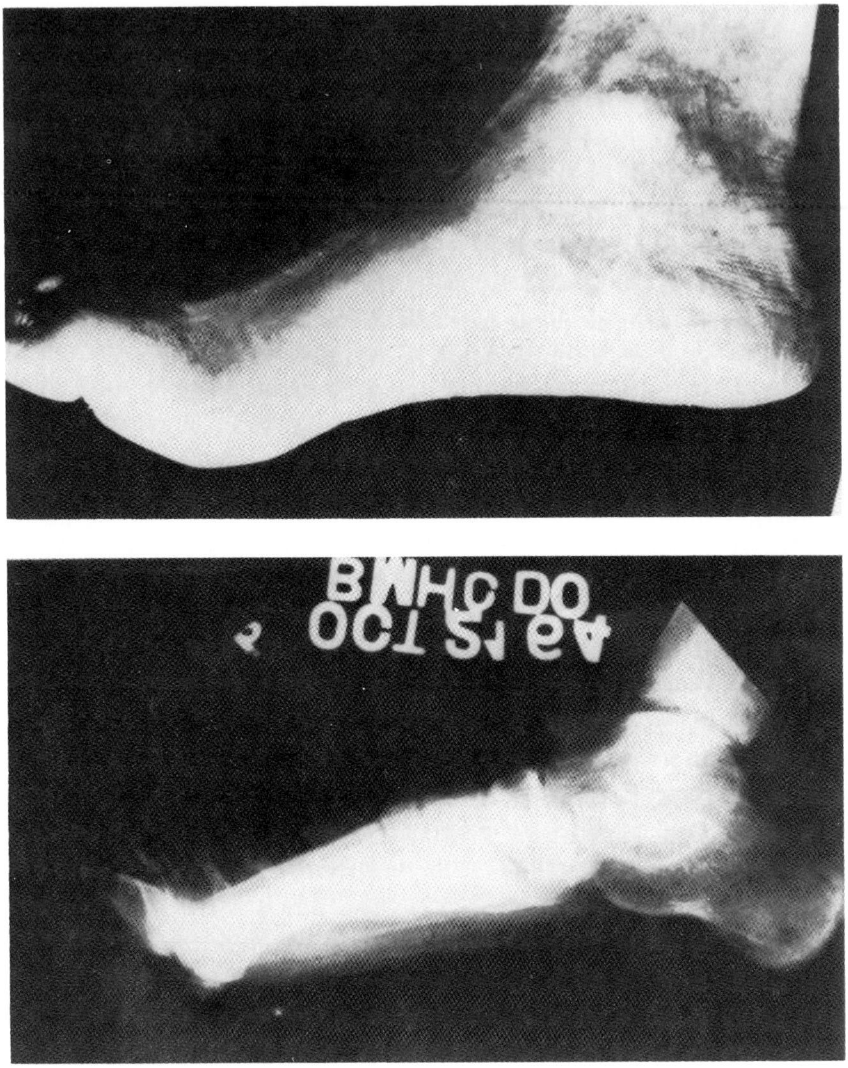

Fig. 6-4 Advanced diabetic neuroarthropathy. (Reprinted with permission from Ellenberg M: Diabetic neuropathy: clinical aspects. Metabolism 25:1627, 1976.)

the treatment or prevention of distal symmetrical polyneuropathy.[56] Furthermore, various specific pharmacological interventions, based on specific metabolic pathogenetic hypotheses for diabetic neuropathy, have been attempted, with conflicting and/or marginal success, in part due to the limitations in assessing clinical response in distal symmetrical polyneuropathy.[47] However, some of these agents are now undergoing or will shortly undergo carefully constructed large-scale clinical trials to establish their potential efficacy in the treatment and/or prevention of diabetic neuropathy; these issues are discussed more fully in a later section.

Autonomic Neuropathy

Diabetic autonomic neuropathy, with its insidious onset and protean multiple-organ involvement, may go completely unrecognized by patient and physician alike, or it may receive intense diagnostic and therapeutic attention. Like other forms of diabetic neuropathy, it is a diagnosis of exclusion. Subclinical abnormalities may be widespread, whereas clinical symptoms and signs may be focused within a single organ.

The autonomic nervous system (ANS) consists of individual composite reflex arcs each comprised of a sensor, afferent nerve, ganglionic and/or central nervous system association component, efferent nerve, nerve ending, and effector organ. ANS function tests, which generally stimulate entire reflex arcs and record end-organ responses, cannot localize defects within the composite reflex pathway. ANS function is usually divided between opposing sympathetic and parasympathetic innervation, so that an ANS response might reflect either decreased parasympathetic or increased sympathetic nervous system stimulation. ANS fibers are widely dispersed in web-like arrays not easily accessible for nerve conduction studies. Thus dual innervation, composite reflex arcs, and anatomical dispersion greatly complicate ANS testing.

Despite these limitations, the ANS has been extensively studied in diabetes during the last 10 years. Although subtle ANS dysfunction may be widespread, clinical involvement in diabetic autonomic neuropathy is primarily restricted to a few discrete organ systems, which have been analyzed in greater detail. However, correlation of discrete clinical organ involvement with generalized ANS function has not been well studied.

Sudomotor. The primary manifestation of diabetic autonomic sudomotor dysfunction is distal anhidrosis, usually confined to the lower extremity and producing diminished thermoregulatory reserve.[21] The strikingly distal symmetrical distribution suggests a relationship with distal symmetrical somatic polyneuropathy.[21] Symptoms include excessive compensatory truncal and facial sweating, and heat intolerance; distal anhidrosis is usually unnoticed unless elicited by a careful history. Management is aimed at the prevention of heat stroke and hyperthermia and consists primarily of heat stress avoidance.

A curious manifestation of diabetic sudomotor dysfunction is gustatory sweating,[21] which has been attributed to abnormal nerve regeneration. Gustatory sweating, which can be quite incapacitating, is often traced to specific foods, e.g., cheese, whose simple avoidance usually provides adequate symptomatic relief. Anticholinergic drugs, e.g., propantheline and poldine methylsulfate are occasionally efficacious but are often poorly tolerated.

Bladder Dysfunction. The bladder is triply innervated by sympathetic, parasympathetic, and somatic nerve fibers. Contraction of the bladder fundus during micturition is stimulated via direct parasympathetic innervation. Sympathetic innervation of the trigone area and the internal urethral sphincter mediate involuntary relaxation during micturition. Somatic pudendal innervation of the external urethral sphincter provides voluntary control. In the basal state, parasympathetic activity is low, and sympathetic and pudendal activities are increased. Fullness is sensed by stretch receptors in the bladder wall and transmitted to the central nervous system via both sympathetic and parasympathetic pathways,[57] initiating a mixed autonomic and somatic response, which lowers sympathetic and pudendal nervous activity and stimulates bladder parasympathetic activity, thereby initiating micturition.

In early diabetic autonomic neuropathy, afferent autonomic activity from the bladder is selectively diminished, blunting sensation without impairing motor function.[58] Urological symptoms are relatively rare, although many patients report diminished urinary frequency and nocturia. Bladder function tests reveal impaired bladder sensation, however.[58] Subsequent autonomic efferent involvement leads to complaints of infrequent urination, incomplete or difficult bladder emptying, dribbling, and overflow incontinence. Urodynamic studies reveal bladder residual volumes exceeding 150 ml, predisposing to recurrent urinary tract infections.

Management strategies[58] include regularly scheduled urination (every 2–3 hr while awake), cholinergic stimulation (bethanecol 10–20 mg orally three to four times per day), chronic catheterization, and bladder neck resection of the internal sphincter. (Continence is retained because the external sphincter is left intact; however, premature ejaculation in men and cystourethrocele in women are possible surgical complications.) Complicating prostatic hypertrophy should be excluded in elderly men by appropriate laboratory tests.

Sexual Dysfunction. The prevalence of sexual dysfunction approaches 50 percent in diabetic males and 25–35 percent in diabetic females, a difference which may primarily reflect limitations in the assessment of female sexual dysfunction (a single study reported no excess sexual dysfunction in diabetic women over age-matched controls).[59] Neuropathic sexual dysfunction in diabetic males includes retrograde ejaculation and impotence. Ejaculation requires simultaneous closure of the internal vesicle sphincter and relaxation of the external vesicle sphincter, both mediated by efferent sympathetic innervation. Erection, orgasm, and libido are normal with retrograde ejaculation, but ejaculate volume and fertility are reduced. Ejaculate azospermia plus recovery of live, mobile sperm in the postcoital urine is diagnostic. Mechanical, especially postoperative, causes of retrograde ejaculation should be excluded. Brompheniramine (8 mg p.o. b.i.d.) may ameliorate retrograde ejaculation,[58] but controlled studies are not available. Artificial insemination of sperm recovered from fresh urine samples may circumvent infertility in retrograde ejaculation.[58]

Neurogenic erectile impotence, the most common form of organic sexual dysfunction in male diabetics, is a diagnosis of exclusion. Organic and psychogenic impotence are distinguished by a detailed sexual history and/or appropriate laboratory tests. Psychogenic impotence is characteristically rapid in onset and partner-specific, whereas organic impotence is marked by the absence of morning erections. Documentation of rapid-eye-movement sleep (REMS)-associated nocturnal penile tumescence and erection in an appropriately equipped sleep laboratory excludes organic impotence.[60] Penile tumescence may be assessed less reliably by the patient at home with a variety of portable penile tumescence devices which, however, cannot document the simultaneous presence of REM sleep. Because some psychiatric disorders impair REM sleep, organic impotence may be mimicked by psychiatric disorders during ambulatory testing. Psychogenic impotence demands psychological treatment,[61] and organic impotence requires a more definitive diagnosis. Drug-related organic impotence is common (Table 6-3) and is treated by modification of drug regimens. Pel-

Table 6-3. Drugs Causing Erectile Impotence

Antihypertensives
Guanethidine
Reserpine
Propranolol
Alpha-methyldopa
Anticholinergics
Antipsychotics
Phenothiazines
Butyrophenones
Antidepressants
Tricyclics
MAO inhibitors
Narcotics
Heroin
Methadone
Morphine
Cocaine
Other CNS drugs
Barbiturates
Alcohol
Amphetamines

vic and lumbosacral mechanical disorders (e.g., injuries, prostatectomy, certain congenital malformations) may cause erectile dysfunction. Endocrine impotence is usually marked by decreased libido and is unlikely if the serum testosterone is normal; an abnormal serum testosterone level requires further investigation including gonadotropin levels. Because testosterone levels and pituitary gonadotropin dynamics are normal in most diabetic patients with erectile dysfunction,[62] testosterone treatment is reserved for clearly documented hypogonadism. Elevated prolactin may cause erectile dysfunction despite normal gonadotropins in some patients. Vascular insufficiency can cause penile erectile dysfunction in diabetic patients,[63] but usually only in the presence of atherosclerosis that is sufficiently generalized to reduce femoral pulses (although selective penile artery insufficiency has been reported). Penile blood pressure may be measured directly by means of a doppler and penile blood pressure cuff.[63] Penile artery insufficiency is often surgically correctable.[64] Only when organic impotence occurs in the absence of disease processes independently associated with impotence and is accompanied by other concomitants of diabetic neuropathy should impotence be regarded as neurogenic.

Therapy for neurogenic impotence should be guided by a detailed assessment of sexual attitudes and family interrelationships. Should erectile dysfunction be judged to significantly impinge on the quality of life of the patient and/or his family, a penile prosthesis should be considered. Protheses are either semirigid and permanently erect or inflatable. The former may be embarrassing and physically uncomfortable for some patients but are relatively inexpensive and easy to operate; the latter are approximately three to four times as expensive and subject to mechanical failure. Surgical complications, e.g., skin breakthrough, have become much more infrequent with increased surgical experience. Several papers attest to the improved quality of life and patient satisfaction with penile prostheses.[65,66]

Impaired Glucose Counterregulation. Glucose counterregulation, defined as those mechanisms which maintain blood glucose in the physiological range during substrate deprivation or increased insulin action, is partly mediated by the ANS. This regulatory function is extremely important in diabetic patients in whom endogenous counterregulation must compensate for the impreciseness of exogenous insulin administration to prevent serious hypoglyemia.

Short-term glucose counterregulation is primarily mediated by the action of two hormones, glucagon and epinephrine (growth hormone and cortisol may be important for chronic glucose regulation).[67] In the nondiabetic, hypoglycemia is a potent stimulus for glucagon secretion; this hypoglycemic response is blunted in type I diabetes as a function of duration of disease, becoming almost totally undetectable after 14–31 years of diabetes.[67] The blunted response has been attributed to diabetic autonomic neuropathy,[68] iatrogenic hyperinsulinism,[69] and an intrinsic alpha-cell defect.[70] Regardless of its etiology, the blunted glucagon secretory response to hypoglycemia increases reliance on remaining adrenergic counterregulation, which is also progressively impaired in diabetics, though usually somewhat less rapidly.[71]

Blunted epinephrine response to hypoglycemia in chronic diabetes is generally ascribed to autonomic neuropathy of the adrenal medulla, though it occasionally occurs as an isolated finding. Combined glucagon and adrenal medullary counterregulatory impairment presents clinically as hypoglycemic unawareness, a syndrome marked by absence of the usual adrenergic warning signs of impending neuroglucopenia. This syndrome may be complicated by coexistent generalized sympathetic autonomic neuropathy, which further blunts the palpitations and diaphoresis which normally signal hypoglycemia. Hypoglycemic unawareness may significantly increase the risk of intensive insulin therapy and can be diagnosed by reduced glucagon and epinephrine responses to a controlled insulin-induced hypoglycemia.[71]

Gastrointestinal Problems. The ubiquitous ANS gastrointestinal innervation is comprised of both extrinsic (sympathetic and parasympathetic) and intrinsic [myenteric (Auerbach's) and submucosal (Meissner's) plexus] components. The extrinsic sympathetic and parasympathetic components are, respectively, stimulatory and inhibitory, whereas the intrinsic component plays a coordinating role. The striated muscles of the upper esophagus are innervated by both the voluntary glossopharyngeal and the vagus nerves, and smooth muscle innervation in the lower esophagus is primarily vagal; hence esophageal peristalsis is predominantly controlled by the vagus but coordinated by the myenteric plexus. (Sympathetic adrenergic and dopaminergic esophageal innervation is present but poorly understood.) The gastric muscularis receives vagal parasympathetics and both adrenergic and dopaminergic sympathetics from the celiac plexus. Liquid-phase gastric emptying is mediated primarily by gravity and gastroduodenal pressure gradients, whereas peristalsis is primarily adjunctive. Solid-phase emptying requires coordinated integration of all gastric autonomic components and is impaired by sympathetic adrenergic or dopaminergic hyperactivity or by decreased parasympathetic tone. In contrast, acid production is primarily parasympathetic. Intestinal parasympathetics from the vagus and hypogastric plexus stimulate intestinal motility, whereas adrenergic sympathetics from the celiac, superior mesenteric, and hypogastric plexuses inhibit motility; dopaminergic intestinal innervation is not well understood.

Gastrointestinal symptoms are extremely common in diabetic patients and often reflect diabetic gastrointestinal autonomic neuropathy[72]; however, their pathophysiology varies along the length of the gastrointestinal (GI) tract and is often poorly documented.

Esophagus. Asymptomatic esophageal motility disorders are common in long-standing diabetes and represent a subclinical component of autonomic neuropathy.[21,58] Although minor ultrastructural abnormalities exist in the esophageal myenteric plexus, convincing denervation supersensitivity has never been demonstrated, and their pathophysiological implications are controversial.[58,73] Delayed esophageal emptying, disordered peristalsis, primary aperistalsis, and decreased lower esophageal sphincter tone are detected by conventional manometry in roughly 50 percent of diabetic patients, but newer, more sensitive, less invasive radionucleotide techniques may be even more revealing. Referable symptoms, including dysphagia, retrosternal discomfort, and heartburn, occur to a much lesser degree than might be predicted by esophageal motility studies.[73] Symptoms usually ascribed to delayed gastric emptying (e.g., dysphagia and early satiety) may reflect esophageal dysfunction in diabetics and may respond to metoclopramide[74] when lower esophageal sphincter tone and/or disordered motility is present.

Stomach. Diabetic autonomic neuropathy may cause both acid-secretion and motility disorders. Impaired gastric acid secretion has been invoked to explain the reduced frequency of duodenal ulceration in diabetics.[73] Parietal cell response to direct stimulation is normal,[73] and decreased acid secretion is attributed to vagal impairment. Gastric motility abnormalities produce anorexia, nausea, vomiting, postprandial fullness, early satiety, and a gastric ''splash'' on physical examination and may complicate diabetic control owing to delayed postprandial caloric absorption.

Gastric emptying is assessed by either a standard barium meal or the more sophisticated radionucleotide studies which can distinguish solid- from liquid-phase emptying disorders. Because these may occur independently, a normal upper GI series does not exclude solid-phase gastric motility disorders. Management includes small, frequent meals comprised primarily of calorie-rich liquids and appropriate adjustment of antihyperglycemic therapy. Pharmacotherapy includes dopaminergic antagonists (metoclopramide)[74] or the less-well-tolerated parasympathetic agonists (bethanecol), which may produce increased salivation. Metoclopramide therapy may be initiated parenterally until oral administration is feasible. High-fiber diets may delay gastric emptying and should be avoided in patients with gastric motility disorders.

Gallbladder. Gallbladder atony ascribed to diabetic autonomic neuropathy produces both enlargement and poor contractility, but predisposition to neither infection nor cholelithiasis has been established; however, resulting bile salt malabsorption may contribute to diabetic diarrhea (see below).[73]

Intestine. Constipation, the most frequent gastrointestinal symptom in diabetes, occurs in 60 percent of patients.[72] Conservative treatment includes stool softeners, laxatives, or cathartics, and metoclopramide may be efficacious.[75]

Diarrhea in the diabetic, which can be multifactorial, may reflect intestinal hypermotility from decreased sympathetic inhibition, hypomotility with bacterial overgrowth, pancreatic insufficiency, diabetic ''sprue'' (steatorrhea with mucosal histology resembling gluten sensitivity), and bile salt malabsorption. The classic neuropathic syndrome is characterized by nocturnal diarrhea and fecal incontinence, 20–30 bowel movements per day,[2,73] and greater than 300 g of stool per 24 hr,[58,72] but presentation may vary depending on various etiological factors. Loss of sphincter control reflects impaired rectal sensation.[73] Therapy is empirical and may include broad-spectrum antibiotics, bile salt sequestrants, and diphenoxylate hydrochloride (Lomotil) 5–20 mg/day.

Cardiovascular Problems. The cardiovascular ANS includes baroreceptor afferents, central nervous system processing, and efferent sympathetic and parasympathetic innervation of the heart and blood vessels. Cardiac sympathetics are both chronotropic and ionotropic, and parasympathetics slow the heart rate. The basal heart rate mirrors parasympathetic activity, whereas basal vascular tone reflects sympathetic activity. (The role of parasympathetic peripheral vascular innervation is not known.) Adrenergic sympathetic innervation of peripheral vessels modulates vasoconstriction and is primarily responsible for circulating concentrations of norepinephrine.

Exercise Intolerance. Graded cardiovascular exercise initially decreases cardiac parasympathetic and increases peripheral sympathetic tone, thereby augmenting both heart rate and peripheral resistance, and diverting blood flow from viscera to skeletal muscle. As maximal performance is approached, cardiac sympathetic tone increases ionotropically and chronotropically, augmenting cardiac output and raising peripheral blood pressure. With near-exhaustion, copious adrenal epinephrine release further enhances vascular tone and cardiac stimulation. Exercise intolerance in diabetic autonomic neuropathy is mediated by a reduced capacity to augment cardiac output due to diminished cardiac sympathetic activity and an inability to redirect peripheral blood flow to skeletal muscle due to reduced parasympathetic activity.[76]

Postural Hypotension. Postural hypotension (a decrease in diastolic blood pressure of >20 mm Hg with standing) is the most widely recognized sign of diabetic autonomic cardiovascular neuropathy. The normal postural reflex, mediated by a baroreceptor-initiated increase in cardiac and peripheral vascular sympathetic efferent activity, maintains blood pressure and cardiac output in the face of dependent venous pooling and is normally accompanied by a rise in circulating norepinephrine. Hence autonomic neuropathy with orthostatic hypotension is marked by a blunted or absent rise in circulating norepinephrine upon standing (orthostatic hypotension accompanied by supranormal norepinephrine responses in a subclass of diabetic patients is presently ascribed to subclinical vascular hypovolemia[77]). Orthostatic hypotension in diabetic autonomic neuropathy is generally thought to reflect ANS dysfunction; however, some observers have invoked primary baroreceptor dysfunction or inappropriate cardiac chronotropic or ionotropic catecholamine response to explain euvolemic orthostatic hypotension that is accompanied by either blunted norepinephrine levels or a subnormal response to normal norepinephrine levels.[78,79] Various medications (e.g., nitroglycerin and insulin) may potentiate orthostatic hypotension in neuropathic diabetics,[58,73] and symptoms of hypotension and hypoglycemia are often difficult to distinguish. Management of orthostatic hypotension in diabetic patients includes volume repletion and control of glycosuria, elastic stockings, high salt intake, mineralocorticoids, military antigravity suits, and atrial pacing. The response to mineralocorticoid therapy—α-fluorohydrocortisone (Florinef) 0.1–0.3 mg/day—may be primarily mediated by increased sensitivity to norepinephrine rather than increased intravascular volume.[80] Long-duration vasoconstrictors usually produce supine hypertension, but nasal Neo-Synephrine (10 percent ophthalmic solution, 1–3 drops every 4 hr while upright) avoids this effect and may be efficacious; however, definitive clinical trials are not available.

Cardiac Denervation Syndrome. An invariant pulse rate of 80–90 beats/min unresponsive to stress, exercise, or sleep indicates near-complete cardiac denervation.[58,73] Sudden cardiac death, painless myocardial infarction, and coronary artery spasm have all been attributed to this syndrome in diabetics.[58,73] Sudden death occurred in 8 percent of a diabetic autonomic neuropathy cohort followed for 3 years, but the cause remains unclear. Because diabetic autonomic neuropathy is characterized by cardiac adrenergic supersensitivity,[81] excess cardiovascular arrythmias and/or coronary artery spasm remains a plausible explanation. Furthermore, painless myocardial infarction may place the diabetic with autonomic neuropathy at greater cardiovascular risk as well. Management of cardiac denervation is expectant, requiring a high index of suspicion for cardiac ischemic symptoms and avoidance and/or prophylaxis of stress situations (e.g., hypoglycemia, sudden exercise, imprudent cardiac stress testing, general anesthesia). Recognition of cardiac denervation is facilitated by bedside physiological testing.[73]

Pupillary Abnormalities. Pupillary constriction is predominantly parasympathetic, and pupillary dilatation is primarily sympathetic. Small pupillary size (decreased sympathetic tone) is a component of autonomic neuropathy which reflects duration of diabetes, metabolic factors, and the presence of other diabetic complications.[58,73] This finding has little direct clinical significance, however.

Relationship to Other Neuropathic Syndromes. Although symptomatic autonomic neuropathy is classically regarded as a late diabetic complication, new autonomic function tests have revealed early autonomic defects in the cardiovascular system, iris, esophagus, and bladder which antedate clinical disease. Furthermore, subclinical involvement is widespread in diabetic autonomic neuropathy when clinical manifestations are limited to a single organ.[82] Therefore both autonomic and somatic neuropathy represent related, generalized, and progressive peripheral nervous system disorders which emerge clinically only at a late stage in a chronic underlying process.

PATHOGENESIS

Result or Cause of Diabetes?

The notion that neuropathy was the consequence rather than the cause of diabetes, proposed as early as 1864,[83] remained an issue of controversy[3] until type I diabetes was recognized as a primary disorder of the islets of Langerhans.[4] The role of the nervous system in type II diabetes is still actively debated. Claude Bernard produced hyperglycemia in animals by manipulation of the ventromedial hypothalamus (VMH),[84] and others have since demonstrated that VMH stimulation or ventrolateral hypothalamic nuclei (VLH) ablation reduces circulating insulin levels, presumably via sympathetic (VMH) or parasympathetic (VLH) pathways.[85] Because blunted glucose-mediated insulin secretion without manifest islet pathology characterizes type II diabetes,[86] altered autonomic control of insulin secretion is a potential etiologic factor (present evidence strongly suggests a multifactorial pathogenesis for type II diabetes). Pancreatic polypeptide secretion to hypoglycemia, a vagally influenced islet cell phenomenon,[85] is blunted in patients with diabetic autonomic neuropathy.[68] Two major insulin secretory defects in type II diabetes—absence of first-phase glucose-induced insulin secretion and impaired glucose potentiation of nonglucose secretagogues—could result from increased sympathetic stimulation to the pancreatic islets.[86] Hence the 100-year long debate of diabetic neuropathy as a cause or consequence of diabetes continues today, although in modified form which takes into account the complex and multifactorial pathogenesis of diabetes and our rapidly expanding knowledge of neuroendocrinology.

Vascular Hypothesis

The role of vascular disease in the pathogenesis of diabetic neuropathy has also been a chronically confusing and controversial question for many years. Numerous pathoanatomical studies demonstrated the concurrence of neuropathic and macrovascular disease in longstanding diabetics.[87] More modern studies demonstrating that severe large blood vessel occlusive disease alone does not produce peripheral neuropathy led to the rejection of a macrovascular ischemic pathogenesis for diffuse diabetic neuropathy.[32,33] Occlusive disease of medium-sized intraneural blood vessels has been invoked in the pathogenesis of focal neuropathy in diabetes[29] and various forms of necrotizing arteritis,[21] however. Structural abnormalities of the endoneurial microvasculature (capillary endothelial cells, basement membranes, and supporting connective tissue) have been invoked to explain diffuse diabetic polyneuropathy; these changes are not specific for diabetic neuropathy, however, and occur in various other neuropathic syndromes as well but with somewhat less frequency.[87] Three-dimensional computer reconstructions of proximal peripheral nerve trunks from diabetic autopsy specimens reveal a distinct spatial heterogeneity of nerve fiber loss consistent with a generalized ischemic phenomenon in the absence of frank vascular occlusion (heterogeneity is lost in the more distal regions of the peripheral nervous system due to nerve fiber dispersion).[31] This last observation suggests that regions of peripheral nerve fascicles most susceptible to ischemic damage may be selectively involved in diabetic neuropathy, either reflecting deranged microvascular function or altered metabolic requirements of diabetic nerve fibers. Thus neural vascular and metabolic factors may interact in the pathogenesis of diabetic neuropathy (see below).

Metabolic Hypothesis

Neuropathy and other long-term complications of diabetes are thought to result from the interaction of multiple metabolic, genetic, and environmental factors. An important role for chronic hyperglycemia and/or insulin deficiency in the causation of most forms of diabetic neuropathy is strongly suggested by histopathological, epidemiological, physiological, and clinical observations. The peripheral neuropathology characteristic of chronic diabetes resembles that seen in various other "metabolic" neuropathies.[11,21] The prevalence of diabetic neuropathy in both type I and type II diabetes is related to the duration and severity of hyperglycemia and/or insulin deficiency.[12] Subclinical nerve dysfunction in diabetic patients not only correlates with the severity and/or duration of hyperglycemia and/or insulin deficiency,[44,87] it improves with metabolic therapy.[40,41,45,87] Finally, intensive metabolic therapy may improve neuropathic symptoms in diabetic polyneuropathy,[19] although this has not been confirmed in appropriately controlled studies. Thus deficient insulin action and its metabolic concomitants (including hyperglycemia) seem to be major (but not the sole) factors in the development of diabetic neuropathy. The inability to reliably predict the development of clinical diabetic neuropathy in individual patients from their degree and duration of hyperglycemia or insulin deficiency favors additional independent metabolic, genetic, and/or environmental factors in the pathogenesis of diabetic neuropathy (see below).

The pathogenetically relevant metabolic alterations in diabetic peripheral nerve resulting from insulin deficiency and/or hyperglycemia have been difficult to study because: (1) structurally intact human peripheral nerve in early diabetes has not been readily accessible for biochemical study; and (2) the regulation of peripheral nerve metabolism has been poorly understood. Recent studies employing animal models of human diabetes, *in vitro* tissue preparations derived from animal peripheral nerve, and human peripheral nerve samples have significantly advanced the study of nerve metabolism in diabetes. These studies have led to the generation of a cogent hypothesis which relates biochemical alterations induced in peripheral nerve by hyperglycemia to the biophysical events which alter nerve function. The relevance of these experimental observations to human diabetic neuropathy derives from the assumption that the metabolic mediators of acute nerve dysfunction are pathogenetically relevant to chronic diabetic peripheral neuropathy.

Impaired Nerve Conduction in Experimental Diabetes. Acute slowing of nerve conduction in the streptozocin or spontaneously diabetic rat is a consequence of insulin deficiency and occurs in the absence of structural nerve changes.[87] Subtle axonal changes in the more chronically diabetic rat, however, resemble those of early human diabetic neuropathy.[88] Although a variety of biochemical peripheral nerve defects have been uncovered in experimental diabetes, thus far only one sequence—that involving altered neural sorbitol and *myo*-inositol metabolism, and sodium-potassium (Na-K)-ATPase—is directly implicated in acute nerve conduction slowing in experimental diabetes.[89–92] This association is based on the observed parallel responses of nerve *myo*-inositol content, Na-K-ATPase activity, and motor nerve conduction velocity to specific metabolic intervention in the streptozocin and spontaneously diabetic rat. This parallelism persists with both insulin deficiency and insulin replacement,[87,91] *myo*-inositol supplementation,[87,93] and aldose reductase inhibition.[92–95] These observations thus support the contention that acute nerve conduction slowing in diabetic animals is mediated by biochemical events linking nerve *myo*-inositol content to the function of Na-K-ATPase, which in the axon develops the sodium gradient necessary for nerve depolarization.

Relationship of Na-K-ATPase and *Myo*-inositol. Although insulin does not directly limit peripheral nerve glucose metabolism, oxidative metabolism in nerve is reduced 25–30 percent by experimental diabetes despite augmented endogenous tissue substrate stores.[96] This reduced energy utilization has been traced to a 40 percent reduction in activity of nerve Na-K-ATPase,[91] an enzyme which is normally responsible for a major fraction of resting peripheral nerve energy utilization. The Na-K-ATPase defect in diabetic peripheral nerve is not influenced acutely by insulin *in vitro*.[96] However, the defect is entirely prevented or reversed by *in vivo myo*-inositol supplementation or aldose reductase inhibition, both of which prevent the characteristic fall in *myo*-inositol level and motor conduction velocity in diabetic rat sciatic nerve.[89,92–95] Thus the impairment of diabetic rat Na-K-ATPase activity can be explained on the basis of altered diabetic nerve *myo*-inositol metabolism, which seems to alter the structure and/or function of the Na-K-ATPase-membrane complex (the effect persists in broken cell preparations[89]). Because *myo*-inositol is a substrate for the synthesis of membrane phosphatidylinositol (and the higher polyphosphoinositides), it is tempting to speculate that the effect of *myo*-inositol on nerve Na-K-ATPase is membrane-phosphatidylinositol-mediated. (Support for this contention comes from the observation of Simmons et al.[97] that free *myo*-inositol levels may limit phosphatidylinositol turnover in peripheral nerve.)

Peripheral nerve normally maintains a tissue-to-plasma *myo*-inositol concentration gradient of 90- to 100-fold, which is reduced in both human[98] and animal diabetes, probably by the action of glucose as a competitive inhibitor of *myo*-inositol transport into peripheral nerve.[99] The characteristics of this sodium-dependent *myo*-inositol transport system suggest that factors which influence passive efflux of *myo*-inositol might also greatly influence the *myo*-inositol concentration gradient in nerve (see below).

This peripheral nerve *myo*-inositol transport system is driven by the sodium gradient generated by the Na-K-ATPase[99] so that reduced Na-K-ATPase activity in diabetic peripheral nerve might further impair sodium-dependent *myo*-inositol uptake. Recent experiments confirm this suggestion.[91] These relationships thus set the stage for a self-reinforcing cyclic metabolic derangement involving *myo*-inositol and the Na-K-ATPase in diabetic peripheral nerve (Fig. 6-5). Furthermore, other sodium-gradient-dependent processes are also likely to be impaired in diabetic nerve, possibly leading to a range of biochemical and physiological abnormalities which might well contribute to structural alterations in peripheral nerve culminating in clinical diabetic neuropathy.

Other Effects of Hyperglycemia on Nerve Metabolism. Although the major pathways of nerve glucose metabolism are unaffected by high ambient glucose concentrations *in vitro*,[96] several potentially important peripheral nerve intracellular biochemical alterations are directly attributable to elevated extracellular glucose levels. These include increased polyol pathway activity and nonenzymatic protein glycosylation.

Increased Polyol (Sorbitol) Pathway Activity. The reduction of glucose to sorbitol by the enzyme aldose reductase and the oxidation of sorbitol to fructose by the enzyme sorbitol dehydrogenase are primarily regulated by the intracellular glucose and sorbitol concentrations, respectively. Hence these two linked reactions are accelerated when tissue glucose concentrations are elevated by hyperglycemia, and they comprise the ''sorbitol'' or ''polyol'' pathway in peripheral nerve. Peripheral nerve

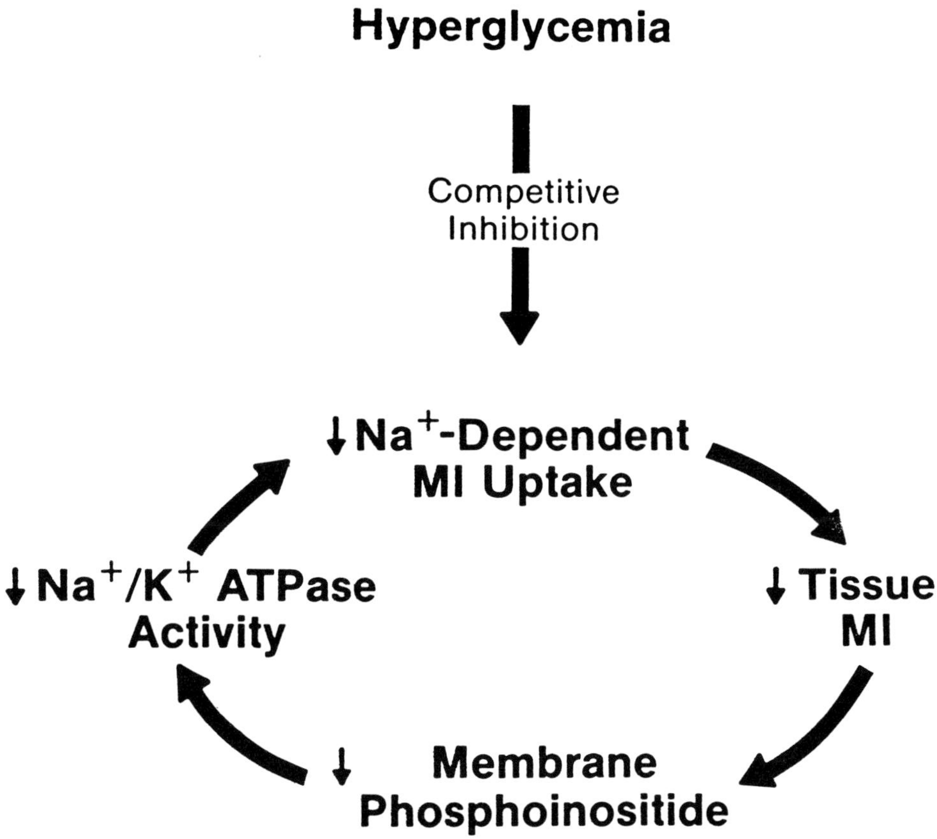

Fig. 6-5 A self-reinforcing cycle of metabolic abnormality in diabetic peripheral nerve. (Reprinted with permission from Greene DA, Lattimer SA: Action of sorbinil in diabetic peripheral nerve: relationship of polyol (sorbitol) pathway inhibition to a myo-inositol-medicated defect in sodium-potassium ATPase activity. Diabetes 33:712, 1984.)

glucose, sorbitol, and fructose levels are raised in both human and experimental diabetes—but only in the micromolar range, which is too low to be osmotically significant (unless sorbitol were highly localized to a minute tissue fraction). Although polyol osmotic effects are unlikely to contribute prominently to diabetic peripheral nerve dysfunction, other manifestations of increased polyol pathway activity may be pathogenetically relevant. Specific aldose reductase inhibitors improve nerve function in diabetes,[100,101] although the effects in humans are small. Furthermore, aldose reductase inhibitors prevent the fall in diabetic peripheral nerve *myo*-inositol content[93–95] and Na-K-ATPase activity.[92] Thus increased peripheral nerve polyol pathway activity may contribute to the derangement in diabetic nerve *myo*-inositol metabolism; or, alternatively, aldose reductase inhibitors may have effects on peripheral nerve metabolism other than that mediated by inhibition of aldose reductase. In either case, aldose reductase inhibitors seem to influence diabetic nerve function at least in part by a *myo*-inositol-related Na-K-ATPase-mediated mechanism.

Nonenzymatic Protein Glycosylation. Nonenzymatic protein glycosylation occurs in a variety of tissue proteins as a result of increased ambient glucose concentration, and in some instances protein function is secondarily altered. Peripheral nerve protein glycosylation is increased by acute experimental diabetes.[102] Of significant interest is the recent discovery that brain tubulin may be nonenzymatically glycosylated *in vitro* and *in vivo,* with dramatic alteration in its self-assembly and solubility characteristics.[103] Glycosylation of peripheral nerve tubulin might well have important consequences on both fast and slow axonal transport, which are altered in experimental diabetes,[104] and on the physical characteristics of the axon cylinder.

Unifying Metabolic Hypothesis. Hyperglycemia alters nerve metabolism in several ways. Competitive inhibition of sodium-dependent *myo*-inositol uptake and/or increased polyol (sorbitol) pathway activity reduces nerve *myo*-inositol content, alters nerve phosphoinositide metabolism, and impairs Na-K-ATPase activity, further reducing sodium-gradient-dependent *myo*-inositol uptake and thereby intiating a self-reinforcing cycle (Fig. 6-5). Elevated tissue glucose levels also result in nonenzymatic glycosylation of nerve proteins, potentially impairing their function. Although the latter pathophysiological mechanism has not yet been critically examined, the possibility that tubulin glycosylation might impair axonal microtubular function (and perhaps axonal transport or intracellular *myo*-inositol binding) is intriguing. Impairment of the electrogenic Na-K-ATPase secondarily and acutely reduces nerve conduction velocity[105] while probably also inhibiting other sodium-gradient-dependent processes, e.g., amino acid uptake and intracellular water hemostasis. Other membrane defects may also occur as a consequence of altered inositol phospholipid metabolism, independent of the Na-K-ATPase, possibly involving other membrane-bound proteins, e.g., the voltage-dependent sodium channel, or other membrane cationic ATPases. These abnormalities may become self-reinforcing cyclic defects with potentially widespread pathophysiological implications, leading to impaired nerve conduction, axonal transport, intermediary metabolism, water balance, and possibly later structural effects in diabetic peripheral nerve as well.

However, the clinical variability of diabetic neuropathy independent of degree and duration of hyperglycemia suggests the involvement of additional environmental and/or inherited pathogenetic factors. Some of these factors (nerve compression and entrapment, alcohol[18]) are readily identifiable, whereas others are probably completely unknown.

Definitive Metabolic Prevention and Treatment

The potential efficacy of general antidiabetic therapy in the prevention and treatment of diabetic neuropathy is dependent on the pathogenetic role of insulin deficiency and/or hyperglycemia. The efficacy of enhanced "diabetic control" in the treatment of clinically overt diabetic neuropathy, a rather late stage in a chronic underlying process, is in addition dependent on the reversibility of the metabolically derived pathogenetic components but is potentially enhanced by the generally great regenerative capacity of the peripheral nervous system. As the pathogenetic sequence(s) linking the diabetic milieu to impaired nerve function and overt neuropathy are unraveled, prophylaxis and treatment may become much more focused and specific than general antidiabetic regimens, and perhaps more potent.

Metabolic Treatment of Subclinical Neuropathy. Elements of subclinical neuropathy, particularly impaired nerve conduction in both newly diagnosed type I diabetes[40,41] and chronic stable type II diabetes,[45] respond to general antidiabetic treatment. Whether these therapeutic effects merely reflect the improved diabetic milieu directly or represent reversal of intraneural metabolic or structural abnormalities is not entirely clear. However, similar improvement in nerve conduction with specific metabolic therapy, e.g., administration of aldose reductase inhibitors in the absence of improved antidiabetic treatment, strongly implicates intraneural metabolic or structural factors.[100] Whether chronically maintained improvement in subclinical neuropathy insures against the subsequent development of clinically overt diabetic neuropathy is not presently known. Long-term, prospective clinical trials of the effect of various levels of diabetic control on the development and progression of subclinical and clinically overt diabetic neuropathy, such as that incorporated in the Diabetes Control and Complications Trial (DCCT) sponsored by the National Institutes of Health, will be required to answer this important question.[56]

Metabolic Treatment of Clinically Overt Neuropathy. Although emphasized by some[19] and dismissed by others,[2] the role of metabolic control in the treatment of established diabetic neuropathy remains an important but unanswered question.[10] The reversibility of neuropathic damage with metabolic control in overt neuropathy seems to vary widely and unpredictably, with published reports of both impressive therapeutic success[19] and failure. With increasing evidence linking nerve metabolism and nerve function in experimental diabetes, and the absence of convincing evidence to the contrary, metabolic regulation of hyperglycemia remains a viable therapeutic alternative in the treatment of diabetic neuropathy.

Specific Metabolic Therapy. Several specific avenues of metabolic treatment are implicit in the biochemical pathogenetic sequence currently favored for diabetic neuropathy. Although reduced nerve *myo*-inositol content, now documented in both human[98] and animal diabetes, is central to this scheme, *myo*-inositol supplementation remains unproved as either treatment or prophylaxis for diabetic neuropathy. Existing clinical trials of *myo*-inositol treatment have either involved small numbers of carefully selected patients and yielded suggestively positive but inconclusive results or have involved large and heterogeneous populations of diabetic patients with decidedly negative results.[87] A well-controlled, well-designed large prospective clinical trial of *myo*-inositol supplementation in diabetic neuropathy remains to be done.

An industry-supported placebo-controlled crossover multicenter clinical trial of the aldose reductase inhibitor sorbinil has demonstrated a small but significant acute effect on nerve conduction slowing in human diabetics,[100] consistent with the view that a small fraction of conduction slowing resides directly in intraneural metabolic disturbances in diabetic nerve.[34] The actions of aldose reductase inhibitors on nerve function in experimental diabetes are entirely attributable to their effects on nerve *myo*-inositol content,[92–95] although the mechanism(s) linking aldose reductase and nerve *myo*-inositol metabolism remain in doubt. These observations support the notion that alterations in nerve *myo*-inositol metabolism may influence nerve conduction in human diabetes. Furthermore, sorbinil and other aldose reductase inhibitors are now undergoing large-scale industry-sponsored clinical trials which test their efficacy in the prevention and/or treatment of diabetic neuropathy. Preliminary but unconfirmed data[101,106] suggest that these new agents may prove beneficial in the therapy of diabetic neuropathy.

REFERENCES

1. Rollo J: Cases of Diabetes Mellitus. C. Dilly, London, 1978
2. Ellenberg M: Diabetic neuropathy: clinical aspects. Metabolism 25:1627, 1976
3. Bernard C: Lecons sur le Diabete et al Glycogenese Animale. Baillière, Paris, 1877
4. Rundles RW: Diabetic neuropathy: general review with a report of 125 cases. Medicine (Baltimore) 24:111, 1945
5. Sundkvist G: Autonomic nervous system function in asymptomatic diabetic patients with signs of peripheral neuropathy. Diabetes Care 4:529, 1981
6. Pfeifer MA, Cook D, Brodsky J, et al: Quantitative evaluation of cardiac parasympathetic activity in normal and diabetic man. Diabetes 31:339, 1982
7. Pfeifer MA, Cook D, Brodsky J, et al: Quantitative evaluation of sympathetic and parasympathetic control of iris function. Diabetes Care 5:518, 1982
8. Pfeifer MA, Weinberg CR, Cook DL, et al: Autonomic neural dysfunction in recently diagnosed diabetic subjects. Diabetes Care (in press)
9. Winegrad AI, Morrison AD, Greene DA: Late complication of diabetes. In DeGroot LJ, Cahill GF, Martini L (eds): Endocrinology. Vol. 2. Grune & Stratton, New York, 1979
10. Thomas PK, Ward JD, Watkins PJ: Diabetic neuropathy. In Keen H, Jarrett J (eds): Complications of Diabetes. Edward Arnold, London, 1982
11. Brown MJ, Greene DA: Diabetic neuropathy: pathophysiology and management. In: Neurology, Peripheral Nerve Disorders: A Practical Approach. (in press)
12. Pirart J: Diabetes mellitus and its degenerative complications: a prospective study of 4,400 patients observed between 1947 and 1973. Diabetes Care 1:168, 252, 1978
13. Pirart J: Diabetic neuropathy: a metabolic or a vascular disease? Diabetes 14:1, 1965
14. Johsson B: Diabetes—the cost of illness and the cost of control. Acta Med Scand [Suppl] 671:19, 1983
15. Eng GD, Hung W, August GP, Smokvina MD: Nerve conduction velocity determinations in juvenile diabetes: continuing study of 190 patients. Arch Phys Med Rehabil 57:1, 1976
16. Brown MJ, Asbury AK: Diabetic neuropathy. Ann Neurol (in press)
17. Ward JD: Abnormal processes in the nerve. In Brownless M (ed): Diabetes Mellitus. Vol. 4. Garland STPM Press, New York, 1981
18. McCulloch DK, Campbell IW, Prescott RJ, Clarke BP: Effect of alcohol intake on symptomatic peripheral neuropathy in diabetic men. Diabetes Care 3:245, 1980
19. Boulton AJM, Drury J, Clarke B, Ward JD: Continuous subcutaneous insulin infusion in the management of painful diabetic neuropathy. Diabetes Care 5:386, 1982

20. De Venecia G: The eye in accelerated hypertension. 3. Accelerated hypertension in patients with diabetic retinopathy. In Friedman EA, L'Esperance AL (eds): Diabetic Renal-Retinal Syndrome. Grune & Stratton, New York, 1980
21. Thomas PK, Eliasson S: Diabetic neuropathy. In Dyck PJ, Thomas PK, Lambert EH (eds): Peripheral Neuropathy. Saunders, Philadelphia, 1975
22. Jackson, WPU: Ocular nerve palsy with severe headaches in diabetics. Br Med J 2:408, 1955
23. Dreyfus PM, Hakim S. Adams RD: Diabetic ophthalmoplegia. Arch Neurol Psychiatry 77:337, 1957
24. Asbury AK, Aldredge H, Hershberg R, Fisher CM: Oculomotor palsy in diabetes mellitus: a clinico-pathological study. Brain 93:555, 1970
25. Locke S: The nervous system and diabetes. Marble A, White P, Bradley RF (eds): In Joslin's Diabetes Mellitus, 11th ed. Lea & Febiger, Philadelphia, 1971
26. Longstreth GG, Newcomer AD: Abdominal pain caused by diabetic radiculopathy. Ann Intern Med 86:166, 1977
27. Calverley JR, Mulder DW: Femoral neuropathy. Neurology 10:963, 1960
28. Goodman JI: Femoral neuropathy in relation to diabetes mellitus: report of 17 cases. Diabetes 3:266, 1954
29. Raff MC, Sangalang V, Asbury AK: Ischemic mononeuropathy multiplex associated with diabetes mellitus. Arch Neurol 18:487, 1968
30. Spencer PS, Schaumburg, HH: Central-peripheral distal axonopathy: the pathology of dying-back polyneuropathies. Prog Neuropathol 3:253, 1976
31. Sugimura K, Dyck PJ: Multifocal fiber loss in proximal sciatic nerve in symmetrical distal diabetic neuropathy. J Neurol Sci 53:501, 1982
32. Chopra JS, Hurwitz, LJ: A comparative study of peripheral nerve conduction in diabetes and non-diabetic chronic occulsive peripheral vascular disease. Brain 92:83, 1969
33. Chopra JS, Hurwitz LJ, Montgomery DAD: The pathogenesis of sural nerve changes in diabetes mellitus. Brain 92:391, 1969
34. Behse F, Buchthal F, Carlsen F: Nerve biopsy and conduction studies in diabetic neuropathy. J Neurol Neurosurg Psychiatry 40:1072, 1977
35. Reske-Nielsen E, Aage H, Vorre P: Ultrastructure of muscle biopsies in recent, short-term and long-term juvenile diabetes. Acta Neurol Scand 55:345, 1977
36. Kimura J, Yamada T, Stevland NP: Distal slowing of motor nerve conduction velocity in diabetic polyneuropathy. J Neurol Sci 42:291, 1979
37. Chopra JS, Fannin T: Pathology of diabetic neuropathy. J Pathol 104:175, 1971
38. Hansen S, Ballantyne JP: Axonal dysfunction in the neuropathy of diabetes mellitus: a quantitative electrophysiological study. J Neurol Neurosurg Psychiatry 40:555, 1977
39. Johnson PC, Brendel K, Meezan E: Human diabetic perineurial cell basementmembrane thickening. Lab Invest 44:265, 1981
40. Gregersen G: Variations in motor conduction velocity produced by acute changes of the metabolic state in diabetic patients. Diabetologia 4:273, 1968
41. Ward JD, Fisher DJ, Barnes CG, Jessop JD: Improvement in nerve conduction following treatment in newly diagnosed diabetics. Lancet 1:428, 1971
42. Eng GD, Nellington H, August GP: Nerve conduction velocity determination in juvenile diabetes. Mod Probl Paediatr 12:213, 1975
43. Gregersen, G: Diabetic neuropathy: influence of age, sex, metabolic control and duration of diabetes on motor conduction velocity. Neurology 17:972, 1967
44. Graf RJ, Halter JB, Halar E, Porte D Jr: Nerve conduction abnormalities in untreated maturity-onset diabetes: relation to levels of fasting plasma glucose and glycosylated hemoglobin. Ann Intern Med 90:298, 1979

45. Graf RJ, Halter JB, Pfeifer MD, et al: Glycemic control and nerve conduction abnormalities in non-insulin-dependent diabetic subjects. Ann Intern Med 94:307, 1981
46. Gilliat RW, Willison, RG: Peripheral nerve conduction in diabetic neuropathy. J Neurol Neurosurg Psychiatry 25:11, 1962
47. Greene DA, Brown MJ, Braunstein SN, et al: Comparison of clinical course and sequential electrophysiological tests in diabetics with symptomatic polyneuropathy and its implications for clinical trials. Diabetes 30:139, 1981
48. Brown MJ, Martin JR, Asbury AK: Painful diabetic neuropathy: a morphometric study. Arch Neurol 33:164, 1976
49. Jaspan JB, Wollman RL, Bernstein L, Rubenstein AH: Hypoglycemic peripheral neuropathy in association with insulinoma: implication of glucopenia rather than hyperinsulinism. Medicine 61:33, 1982
50. Sinha S, Munichoodappa CS, Kozak GP: Neuro-arthropathy (''Charcot joints'') in diabetes mellitus: clinical study of 101 cases. Medicine (Baltimore) 51:191, 1972
51. Davis JL, Lewis SB, Gerich JE, et al: Peripheral diabetic neuropathy treated with amitriptyline and fluphenazine. JAMA 238:2291, 1977
52. Saudek CD, Werns S, Reidenberg MM: Phenytoin in the treatment of diabetic symmetrical polyneuropathy. Clin Parmacol Ther 22:196, 1977
53. Levin JD, Gordon NC, Bornstein JC, Fields HL: Role of pain in placebo analgesia. Proc Natl Acad Sci USA 76:3528, 1979
54. Turkington RW: Depression masquerading as diabetic neuropathy. JAMA 243:1147, 1980
55. Ellenberg M: Diabetic neuropathic cachexia. Diabetes, 23:5, 1974
56. Protocol for the Diabetes Control and Complications Trial. Diabetes Branch, NIADDK, National Institutes of Health, Bethesda, MD
57. DeGroat WC, Booth AM: Physiology of the urinary bladder and urethra. Ann Intern Med 92:312, 1980
58. Hosking DJ, Bennett T, Hamptom JR: Diabetic autonomic neuropathy. Diabetes 27:1043, 1978
59. Ellenberg M: Sexual function in diabetic patients. Ann Intern Med 92:331, 1980
60. Karacan I, Salis PJ, Williams RL: The role of the sleep laboratory in the diagnosis and treatment of impotence. Williams RL, Laracan I (eds): In Sleep Disorders: Diagnosis and Treatment. Wiley, New York, 1978
61. Schiavi RC: Psychological treatment of erectile disorders in diabetic patients. Ann Intern Med 92:337, 1980
62. Wright AD, London DR, Holder G, et al: Luteinizing release hormone tests in impotent diabetic males. Diabetes 25:975, 1976
63. Jevtich MJ, Edson M, Jarmn WD, Herrera HH: Vascular factor in erectile failure among diabetics. Urology 19:163, 1982
64. Michal V, Kramer R, Pospichal J, Hejhal L: Direct arterial anastomosis to the cavernous body in the treatment of erectile impotence. Rozhl Chir 52:587, 1973
65. Beaser RS, Vanderhock C, Jacobson AM, et al: Experience with penile prostheses in the treatment of impotence in diabetic men. JAMA, 248:943, 1982
66. Pfeifer MA, Reenan A, Berger R, Best J: Penile prosthesis and quality of life. Diabetes, suppl 1, 32:307, 1983
67. Cryer PE, Gerich JE: Relevance of glucose counter-regulatory systems to patients with diabetes: critical roles of glucagon and epinephrine. Diabetes Care 6:95, 1983
68. Hilsted J, Madsbad S, Krarup T, et al: No response of pancreatic hormones to hypoglycemia in diabetic autonomic neuropathy. J Clin Endocrinol Metab 54:815, 1982
69. Samols E: Glucagon and insulin secretion. In Lafebvre P (ed): Handbook of Experimental Pharmacology. Springer-Verlag, Berlin, 1982

70. Gerich JE, Langlois M, Noacco C, et al: Lack of glucagon response to hypoglycemia in diabetes: evidence for an intrinsic pancreatic alpha cell defect. Science 182:171, 1973
71. Boden G, Reichard GA Jr. Hoeldtke RD, et al: Severe insulin-induced hypoglycemia associated with deficiencies in the release of counter-regulatory hormones. N Engl J Med 305:1200, 1981
72. Feldman M, Schiller LR: Disorders of gastrointestinal motility associated with diabetes mellitus. Ann Intern Med 98:378, 1983
73. Clarke BF, Ewing DJ, Campbell IW: Diabetic autonomic neuropathy. Diabetologia, 17:195, 1979
74. Pinder RM, Brogden RN, Sawyer PR, et al: Metoclopramide: a review of its pharmacological properties and clinical use. Drugs 12:81, 1976
75. Snape WJ, Battle WM, Schwartz SS, et al: Metoclopramide to treat gastroparesis in diabetes mellitus. Ann Intern Med 96:444, 1982
76. Hilsted J: Pathophysiology in diabetic autonomic neuropathy: cardiovascular, hormonal, and metabolic studies. Diabetes 31:730, 1982
77. Tohmeh JF, Shah SD, Cryer PE: The pathogenesis of hyperadrenergic postural hypotension in diabetic patients. Am J Med 67:772, 1979
78. Olshan AR, O'Connor DT, Cohen IM, et al: Baroreflex dysfunction in patients with adult-onset diabetes nd hyptension. Am J Med 74:233, 1983
79. Sundkvist G, Lilja B, Almer L-O: Abnormal diastolic blood pressure and heart rate reactions to tilting in diabetes mellitus. Diabetologia 19:433, 1980
80. Chobanian AV, Volicer L, Tifft CP, et al: Mineralocorticoid-induced hypertension in patients with orthostatic hypotension. N Engl J Med, 301:68, 1979
81. Christensen NJ: Catecholamine and diabetes mellitus. Diabetologia 16:211, 1979
82. Pfeifer MA, Weinberg CR, Cook DL, et al: Proportional changes of autonomic and somatosensory neural function in untreated noninsulin dependent diabetics. (submitted)
83. Calvi M de: Recherches sur les Accidents Diabetique. P Asselin, Paris, 1864
84. Bernard C: Clines rendus diabetique. Soc Biol 1:60, 1849
85. Miller RE: Pancreatic neuroendocrinology: peripheral neural mechanisms in the regulation of the islets of Langerhans. Endocr Rev 2:471, 1981
86. Ward WK, Beard JC, Halter JB, et al: Pathophysiology of insulin secretion in noninsulin dependent diabetes mellitus. Diabetes Care (in press)
87. Clements RS: Diabetic neuropathy—new concepts of its etiology. Diabetes 28:604, 1979
88. Sima AAF: Peripheral neuropathy in the spontaneously diabetic BB-Wistar rat. Acta Neuropathol (Berl) 51:223, 1980
89. Greene DA, Lattimer SA: Impaired rat sciatic nerve sodium-potassium ATPase in acute streptozocin diabetes and its correction by dietary myo-inositol supplementation. J Clin Invest 72:1058, 1983
90. Greene DA: Metabolic abnormalities in diabetic peripheral nerve: relation to impaired function. Metabolism, suppl. 1, 32:118, 1983
91. Greene DA, Lattimer SA: Impaired energy utilization and sodium-potassium ATPase in diabetic peripheral nerve. Am J Physiol 246:E311, 1984
92. Greene DA, Lattimer SA: Action of sorbinil in diabetic peripheral nerve: relationship of polyol (sorbitol) pathway inhibition to a myo-inositol-mediated defect in sodium-potassium ATPase activity. Diabetes 33:712, 1984
93. Mayer JH, Tomlinson DR: The influence of aldose reductase inhibition and nerve myo-inositol on axonal transport and nerve conduction velocity in rats with experimental diabetes. J Physiol (Lond) 340:25, 1983
94. Gillon KRW, Hawthorne JN: Sorbitol, inositol and nerve conduction in diabetes. Life Sci, 32:1943, 1983

95. Finegold D, Lattimer SA, Nolle S, et al: Polyol pathway activity and myo-inositol metabolism: a suggested relationship in the pathogenesis of diabetic neuropathy. Diabetes 32:988, 1983
96. Greene DA, Winegrad AI: Effects of acute experimental diabetes on composite energy metabolism in peripheral nerve axons and Schwann cells. Diabetes 30:967, 1981
97. Simmons DA, Winegrad AI, Martin DB: Significance of tissue myo-inositol concentrations in metabolic regulation in nerve. Science 217:848, 1982
98. Mayhew JA, Gillon KRW, Hawthorne JN: Free and lipid inositol, sorbitol and sugars in sciatic nerve obtained post-mortem from diabetic and control subjects. Diabetologia 24:10, 1983
99. Greene DA, Lattimer SA: Sodium- and energy-dependent uptake of myo-inositol by rabbit peripheral nerve. J Clin Invest 70:1009, 1982
100. Judzewitsch RG, Jaspan JB, Polonsky KS, et al: Aldose reductase inhibition improves nerve conduction velocity in diabetic patients. N Engl J Med 308:119, 1983
101. Fagius J, Jameson S: Effects of aldose reductase inhibitor treatment in diabetic polyneuropathy—a clinical and neurophysiological study. J Neurol Neurosurg Psychiatry 44:991, 1981
102. Vlassara H, Brownlee M, Cerami A: Nonenzymatic glycosylation of peripheral nerve protein in diabetes mellitus. Proc Natl Acad Sci USA 78:5190, 1981
103. Williams SK, Howarth NL, Devenny JJ, Bitensky MW: Structural and functional consequences of increased tubulin glycosylation in diabetes mellitus. Proc Natl Acad Sci USA 79:6546, 1982
104. Sidenius P: The axonopathy of diabetic neuropathy. Diabetes 31:356, 1982
105. Brismar T, Sima AAF: Changes in nodal function in nerve fibres of the spontaneously diabetic BB-Wistar rat: potential clamp analysis. Acta Physiol Scand 113:499, 1981
106. Jaspan J, Maselli R, Hevold K, Bartkus C: Treatment of severely diabetic neuropathy with an aldose reductase inhibitor: relief of pain and improved somatic and autonomic nerve function. Lancet 8353:758, 1983

7 The Diabetic Foot

Andrew J. M. Boulton
John H. Bowker

An association between diabetes mellitus and foot problems has been recognized for many years. In 1887 Pryce, an English surgeon, described a diabetic patient who developed peripheral neuropathy and, later, ulcers on the plantar surfaces of his feet.[1] He concluded that "diabetes may of itself be a cause of perforating ulcers." Although many early studies attributed the frequent findings of foot lesions in diabetic patients to large-vessel disease and sepsis, Martin reemphasized the importance of neuropathy as a major cause of foot problems and pointed out that with proper therapy prevention of amputation is possible.[2] Despite an increased awareness of the long-term diabetic complications, 20 percent of diabetic admissions during the 1980s are for foot problems secondary to neuropathy or peripheral vascular disease,[3] and diabetic patients have recently been shown to have a 15 times higher overall risk of amputation than their nondiabetic counterparts.[4] It has been estimated that a 50–75 percent reduction in the amputation rate among diabetic patients could be achieved with the widespread application of patient education and preventive foot care.[5] The expense to the patient and the community of hospital treatment for diabetic foot problems is well recognized,[6] and the annual cost of diabetes-related peripheral vascular disease (PVD) alone in 1978 exceeded $100 million in the United States.[7] Recognition of etiological and pathogenetic factors in diabetic foot disease is therefore of paramount importance, so that with increased patient education and preventive care we might begin to see a reduction in the prevalence of these dreaded complications.

The etiological factors which lead to characteristic foot lesions seen in the diabetic patient are considered in this chapter. Useful investigations for the detection of the foot at risk of ulceration are described and methods of patient education in preventive foot care discussed. Finally, medical and surgical management of the patient with active foot ulceration is considered.

DIABETIC NEUROPATHIES

Although the diabetic neuropathies are fully discussed in the previous chapter, their importance in the etiology and pathogenesis of diabetic foot lesions is such that a review of the relevant facts is presented here. It is only during the last 30 years that the major role of neuropathy in the causation of diabetic foot ulceration has been accepted, for prior to this foot lesions had generally been attributed to vascular disease.[8–10] Kelly and Coventry[9] studied patients with neuropathic ulcers of diverse etiologies presenting to the Mayo Clinic, and demonstrated that half of these were in diabetic patients. The lack of any clinical evidence of occulsive vascular disease in many of these patients was recognized by Ellenberg.[10]

Peripheral symmetrical sensory neuropathy is the most common of the neuropathies and is characterized by painful and unpleasant sensations (burning pains, paresthesias, numbness, and altered temperature sensation, most symptoms having nocturnal exacerbations) occurring mainly in the lower limbs. Despite these symptoms, many subjects have a marked reduction in pain sensation in the feet, the "painful-painless" leg.[11] The natural history of symptomatic neuropathy is controversial; however, it seems that painful symptoms of short duration have a good prognosis for recovery,[12] whereas the more chronic, longstanding symptoms carry a guarded prognosis.[13] A significant number of patients lose their unpleasant symptoms but develop insensitive feet and must be regarded as being at high risk of painless trauma. There seem to be a small number of diabetic patients who develop progressive loss of sensation in a stocking distribution in the absence of other sensory symptoms: thus the lack of a history of painful or paresthetic symptoms does not exclude the presence of significant neuropathy.

Although the symptoms of peripheral neuropathy are predominantly sensory (Table 7-1), there is invariably evidence of motor dysfunction on examination. Wasting and weakness of the intrinsic muscles of the foot are frequently found, which may lead to an imbalance of the toe flexors and extensors. The result of this imbalance is frequently the "intrinsic minus" foot, characterized by claw toes and prominent metatarsal heads.[14,15] More proximal muscles may be affected in more advanced cases, e.g., the dorsiflexors of the foot, which leads to footdrop.

The contribution of autonomic neuropathy to the pathogenesis of diabetic foot ulcer has only recently been emphasized,[16,17] though the importance of diabetic autonomic neuropathy was originally described by Rundles.[18] Sympathetic denervation

Table 7-1. Common Findings in the Neuropathic Foot at Risk of Ulceration

Well perfused, warm, apparently healthy foot on inspection
Palpable foot pulses, prominent dorsal foot veins
Decreased pain sensation, vibration perception, and joint position sensation.
Absent ankle reflex
Diabetic dermopathy on lower leg
Dry, thickened skin
Calluses under high-pressure area
"Intrinsic minus" foot

in the lower limb leads to a reduction or complete absence of normal sweating and has been shown to be a major contributory factor to increased blood flow in the foot.[11,19] A reduction in sweating causes dryness in the keratin layer of the skin, which in turn is responsible for brittle skin, which loses the ability to stretch.[20] Such skin on the sole of the foot, which is subjected to frequent stress during standing and walking, is liable to crack, causing fissures that can form a portal of entry for infection. A collection of dry skin under pressure areas leads to the formation of callus. Two studies have demonstrated a significant assocation between a lack of sweating and foot ulceration.[17,21] In one study, sweating was absent in all feet with neuropathic ulceration.[21] There has also been much interest in the increased blood flow which is commonly seen in neuropathic feet,[11,19] and it seems likely that increased arteriovenous shunting is occurring in many such feet, probably secondary to sympathetic neuropathy.[11,19,22] A useful physical sign in the neuropathic foot at risk of ulceration is the presence of distended, turgid veins on the dorsum of the feet of supine patients.[22,23] Furthermore, these veins remain distended on elevation of the leg, suggesting the presence of shunting.[22] Further direct and indirect evidence for increased blood flow and shunting has been presented. Doppler sonograms have demonstrated increased diastolic flow,[24] and elevated venous oxygenation in the doral foot veins has been shown.[23] Partsch confirmed the presence of an increase shunt volume by using intraarterially injected labeled albumin microspheres.[25]

It is not possible to state whether shunting is occurring through preexisting shunts normally found in the periphery or through a distended abnormal capillary bed. However, this abnormal blood flow does explain the frequent finding of a warm foot in the neuropathic subject, and it may also explain the rare syndrome of neuropathic edema and the Charcot changes occasionally seen in neuropathic feet.[19]

PERIPHERAL VASCULAR DISEASE

Peripheral vascular disease (PVD) is more common among diabetic patients than in the nondiabetic population,[26] with a prevalence rate of 15.9 percent for this complication reported by Janka et al.[27] Other controllable risk factors, e.g., smoking and hypercholesterolemia, are important in the pathogenesis of PVD, though age and duration of diabetes are also significant factors.[3] As in the nondiabetic, the earliest symptoms of PVD are those of pain in the muscles of the leg induced by exercise and relieved by rest. The absence of foot pulses supports the diagnosis of intermittent claudication, but occasionally such symptoms are present with bounding foot pulses and warm extremities. It has been suggested that in these rare cases the claudication may be an unusual manifestation of neuropathy.[11] However, nocturnal rest pain in the foot is usually easily distinguishable from neuropathic pain. It is generally relieved by hanging the foot over the edge of the bed, i.e., in a cooler environment than under the covers, but is aggravated by walking. Conversely, nocturnal exacerbation of neuropathic pain is associated with hyperesthesias and bedclothes irritation, and may be relieved by walking. Pain sensation is commonly preserved in uncomplicated vascular disease, with foot ulceration in the ischemic foot (Table 7-2) usually secondary to inflammation (e.g., infection or sunburn), which leads to increased de-

Table 7-2. Common Findings in the Ischemic Foot

Cold feet
Dry, atrophic skin
Rubor of toes
Dystrophic nails
Reduced capillary filling

mands for blood supply that cannot be met. The combination of neuropathy and vascular disease is particularly dangerous, as large painless ulcers can form which are resistant to treatment.

All subjects presenting with symptoms and signs of vascular disease should be investigated using the noninvasive vascular laboratory. Simple tests, e.g., the ankle pressure or ischemic index[28] (ratio of ankle to brachial systolic pressure), can be performed at the bedside using the doppler ultrasound stethoscope. The results of these investigations must be compared with the clinical findings, as the frequent occurrence of vascular calcification in the diabetic leg can cause false elevation of the doppler systolic pressures.[29] Indeed, because of the peculiar nature and distribution of arterial disease in the diabetic patient, clinical judgment remains a good predictor of the success of amputation.[30]

Management of the patient with exercise-induced pain in the leg and foot remains controversial.[15] There is no place for vasodilator drugs, though simple measures such as stopping smoking, losing weight, and adequate exercise may be beneficial.[15,31] Those patients with more severe lower limb ischemia, including rest pain or ischemic necrosis, should be investigated with angiography by the vascular surgeon. The diagnosis of diabetes should not deter an aggressive surgical approach,[32] especially as a recent study found no difference in the morbidity among diabetic and nondiabetic patients after major peripheral vascular surgery.[33] Finally, it should be recognized that because of the frequency of autonomic dysfunction in the diabetic leg[17] and the peripheral distribution of atherosclerotic lesions there is virtually no indication for sympathectomy in the surgical management of the diabetic patient.

SKIN DISORDERS

Infections are the most common skin disorders seen in the diabetic foot, and if treated incorrectly they may lead to serious ulceration in neuropathic or ischemic feet. Intertriginous tinea pedis (athlete's foot, ringworm) is seen most frequently in the spaces between the third, fourth, and fifth toes. Accurate diagnosis is essential, as a trial of steroid cream could cause rapid spread of the infection. Topical antifungal therapy is preferred in this site, though this is not effective if the nails are involved in the infective process. Bacterial infections in the foot usually follow skin breaks, which may be caused by painless trauma in the neuropathic patient. All skin infections, with the exception of fungal nail infections, can be prevented by adequate hygiene and daily inspection. Necrobiosis lipoidica diabeticorum occasionally occurs on the dorsum of the foot and may ulcerate. There is, at present, no proved intervention which alters the course of this condition.[34]

PATHOGENESIS OF DIABETIC FOOT ULCER

It is unusual for any of the above conditions in isolation to cause foot ulceration; but when they occur in combination or with trauma, ulceration frequently follows (Fig. 7-1). It is therefore important to consider the pressures and loads under the normal foot during standing and walking, and how alterations caused by neuropathy may lead to excessive loads and ultimately ulceration. When standing, the body weight is transmitted through the tibia to the talus, and it is then distributed to the calcaneum and the forefoot. During each footstep, one leg carries the total body weight for a short time. The calcaneum actually takes more than body weight on initial foot-strike, followed by the cuboid, the fifth metatarsal head, and the rest of the metatarsal heads. The heel leaves the ground, and the metatarsal heads and toes absorb the weight during lift-off.[14,35,36] There have now been several studies of the pressures and loads under the neuropathic foot during standing and walking, and all confirm the findings of increased pressure at the sites of neuropathic foot ulcers.[21,37–39] The combined effects of motor and sensory changes in these feet lead to this redistribution of pressure. Motor changes, with the formation of the "intrinsic minus" foot cause a reduction in toe-loading, leading to increased pressure under the metatarsal heads during the weight-bearing and lift-off phases of the footstep.[21,39] The fat pads also move distally from beneath the metatarsal heads as the toes subluxate dorsally. The imbalance of the toe flexors and extensors[14,15] and the lack of proprioception and joint-

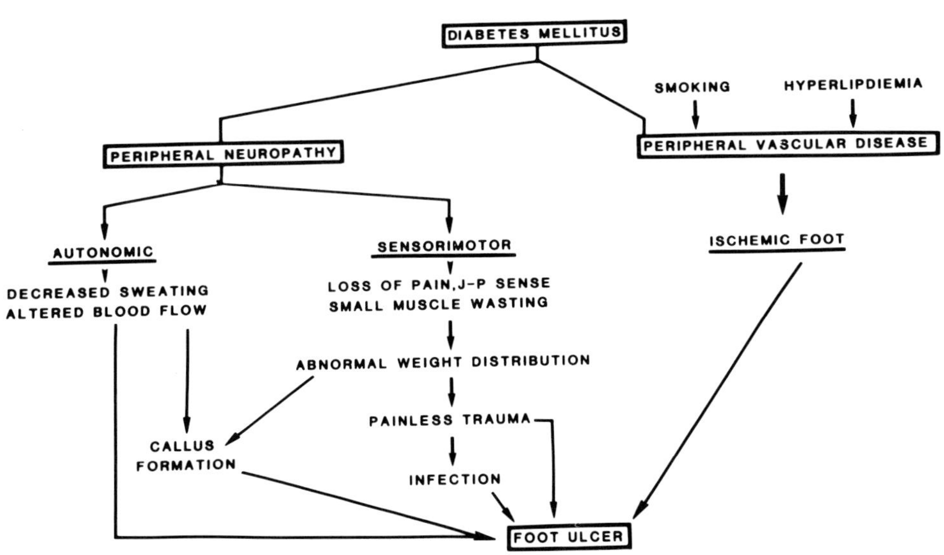

Fig. 7-1 Pathogenesis of the diabetic foot ulcer. Peripheral vascular disease and neuropathy may coexist.

position sensation cause further redistribution of pressures. Using an optical system with a microprocessor, Boulton et al. demonstrated that pressures as high as 30 kg/sq cm (normal less than 10 kg/sq cm) occurred under the metatarsal heads of patients with neuropathy[21,39] (Figs. 7-2 and 7-3). It is the combination of repeated high pressure in this area of the foot with the dry, inelastic skin that leads to callus formation. High-pressure areas can therefore be detected clinically in many subjects, though more quantitive assessment can be made by pressure-sensitive devices, thermography,[36–40] or semiquantitative methods, e.g., the Harris footprint map.[20]

Increased pressure can lead to neuropathic ulceration by several mechanisms. Pressure equals force divided by area; thus a very high pressure is produced by standing on objects such as nails or thumb tacks which have a small surface area (Fig. 7-4). In the normal foot such pressure is extremely painful, but in insensitive feet the pain is not felt and the subject continues to walk (Fig. 7-4). At the other extreme, ulceration may be caused by constant exposure to low static pressures. This situation exists when a patient with insensitive feet wears shoes that are too tight; after many hours, ulceration may occur, e.g., on the lateral border of the fifth metatarsal head. A similar situation exists when a plaster cast is applied too tightly and ulceration occurs over the malleoli. The most common cause of neuropathic ulceration, however,

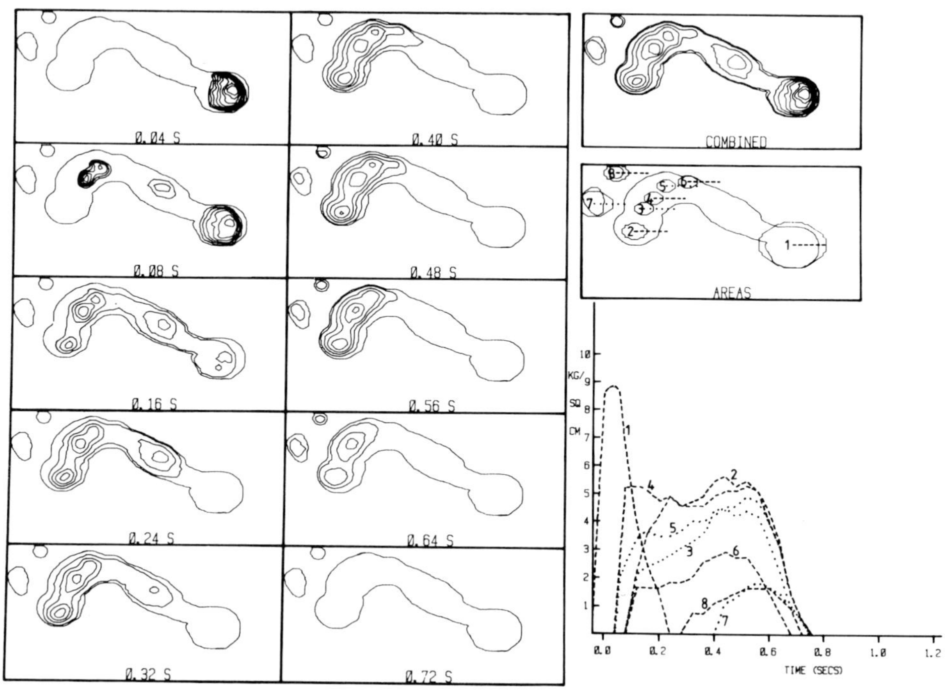

Fig. 7-2 The pressure/time record from a dynamic foot pressure study of a normal, nondiabetic subject. Note that at no time do the pressures under the metatarsal heads exceed 10 kg/sq cm. (Courtesy of Medical Illustration Department, Royal Hallamshire Hospital, Sheffield, UK.)

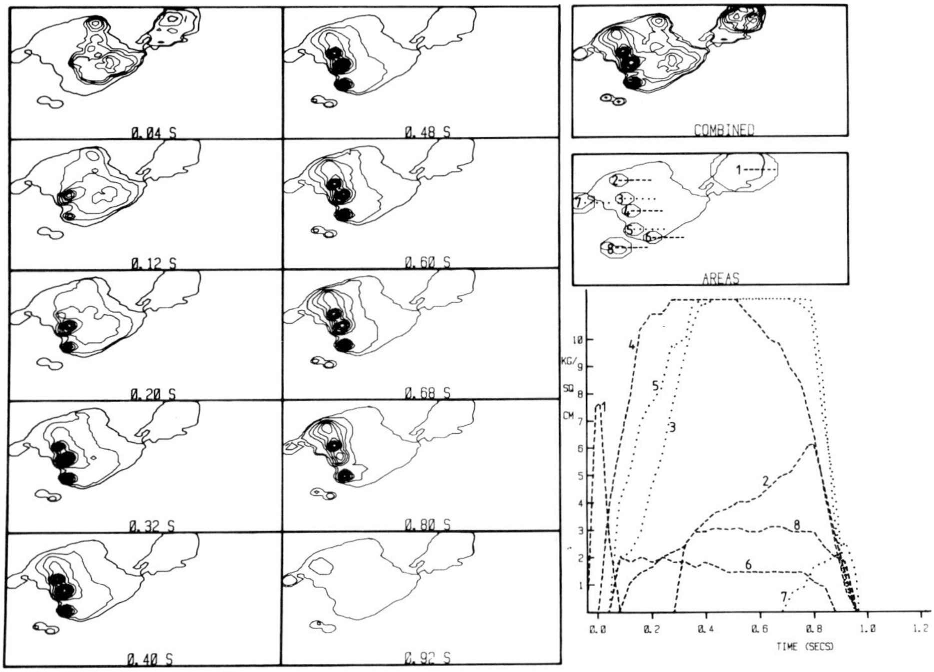

Fig. 7-3 The pressure/time record from a dynamic foot pressure study of a subject with a history of neuropathic foot ulceration. Note the abnormal distribution of pressure with high results under the 2nd, 3rd, and 4th metatarsal heads. (Courtesy of Medical Illustration Department, Royal Hallamshire Hospital, Sheffield, UK.)

is repeated moderate pressure, as might occur under the metatarsal heads. In the presence of normal sensation, this pressure induces pain so the subject alters his gait; the subject with insensitive feet, on the other hand, continues to apply the same pressure, unaware of the evolving damage to his foot. In the presence of infection, this repeated pressure can lead to ''pumping'' and spread of the infection into other tissue compartments.[41]

The ultimate catastrophic event in the diabetic neuropathic foot is the development of painless destruction of bones and joints, the Charcot foot. The striking feature in these cases is the degree of clinical deformity that is present in the absence of painful symptoms. The patient has usually had diabetes for many years, together with peripheral and autonomic neuropathy. They may not present to the physician until ulceration is present because of the lack of symptoms. Ulcers may be found in unusual sites because of the loss of normal architecture in such feet. It is now thought that painless trauma, rather than chronic infection, is the most important etiological factor. Sinha et al.[42] reported that 60 percent of this neuroarthropathy occurs in the tarsal and tarsometatarsal joints, 30 percent in the metatarsophalangeal joints, and 10 percent in the ankle joint (Fig. 7-5). The diagnosis is made on clinical grounds together with radiologic features of joint destruction.

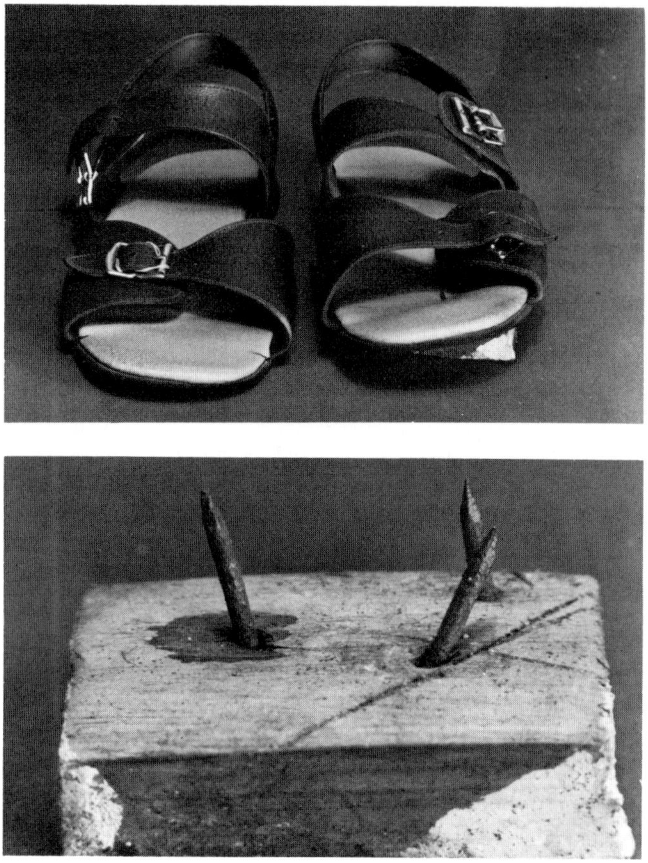

Fig. 7-4 A block of wood with three rusty nails protruding (bottom), and the same block with the nails embedded in the patient's left shoe. The patient, who had insensitive feet, walked for several hours without realizing that (1) his left foot was 2 inches higher than the right one and (2) a nail was piercing the sole of his foot. Note that these shoes are completely inappropriate for a patient with insensitive feet. (Courtesy of Medical Illustration Department, Royal Hallamshire Hospital, Sheffield, UK.)

IDENTIFICATION OF THE PATIENT "AT RISK" OF FOOT ULCERATION

It is thus apparent that the subject with insensitive feet as a result of diabetic peripheral neuropathy is a major candidate for foot ulceration. The development of the ulcer may be accelerated by coexisting vascular disease and skin infection. Males are more commonly affected than females, and the patients tend to be heavier than matched controls.[10,21] In addition to a full clinical evaluation, certain noninvasive investigations may help in the identification of patients prone to foot ulceration.

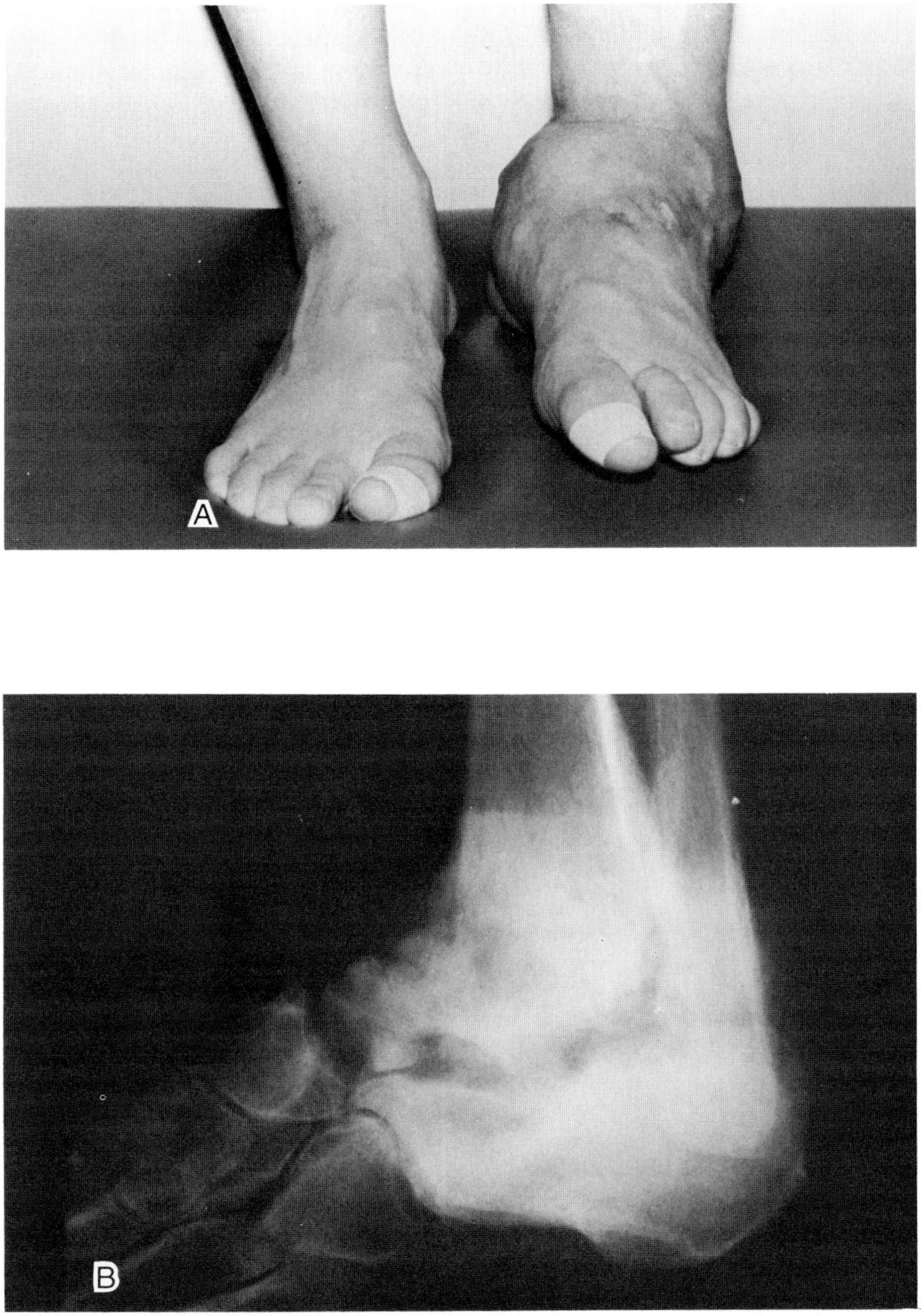

Fig. 7-5 **(A)** Charcot ankle following a routinely treated fracture in a 32-year-old type I diabetic with severe neuropathy. (B) Radiograph of the same patient showing talar fragments but total absence of talar structure in the typical Charcot joint.

Vibration Perception Threshold

A recent study of predictive factors for neuropathic foot ulcers reported that measurement of the vibration perception threshold (VPT) in the great toe using a Biothesiometer (Biomedical Instruments Co., Newbury, Ohio) was the most discriminative test for identification of the foot ulcer patient: a VPT of over 35 correlated with the presence of foot ulceration.[21] This simple, inexpensive test can be carried out at an office visit; a VPT over 35 is equivalent to a marked reduction in vibration sensation using a standard 128-cps tuning fork.

Electrophysiological Assessment

Sural nerve action potentials are not usually recordable in foot ulcer patients, and marked reduction in motor conduction velocities are observed in the upper and lower limbs.[43]

Assessment of Sweating

The degree of sweating on the feet can be assessed using a skin resistance meter[17,21] or simply application of quinizarin powder.[6]

Tests of Central Autonomic Function

The valsalva response and beat-to-beat variation,[44] measures of autonomic function, are invariably abnormal in diabetic subjects with insensitive feet.[17,21]

Radiologic Studies

Radiographs of the foot contribute greatly to the diagnosis and management of foot lesions.[45] Edmonds et al. demonstrated that medial arterial calcification was significantly associated with peripheral neuropathy: All the neuropathic subjects had either Charcot's arthropathy or foot ulceration.[46] Unsuspected foreign bodies in the foot, asymptomatic fractures, and neuroarthropathy are all readily diagnosed by radiographic studies.

These simple techniques may help in the identification of those at risk of ulceration. Such patients may then be further studied using the previously described methods to locate specific high-pressure areas under the foot. Education of the patient in preventive medicine ideally occurs at this stage.

PREVENTION OF FOOT ULCERATION

The majority of diabetic foot ulcers occur in insensitive feet and are precipitated by trauma, infection, or both. Thus most foot ulcers follow a series of preventable events. The major obstacle to prevention lies in the lack of education of the patient and the primary health care team. The patient with an insensitive foot is prone to deny its existence and rejects this part of the anatomy: This represents a form of denial that any problem exists. Walsh et al.[47] described an extreme example of this denial—a group of 47 patients who tolerated severe trophic foot ulcers for a considerable period of time before they eventually presented to a clinic. Education of the health care team in the principles of foot care is mandatory if any preventive foot care program is to succeed. Brand[20] reported the necessity of persuading physicians to remove their patients' shoes as a first recommendation in a campaign to reduce amputation. This has received further support from Cohen,[48] who showed that physicians are three times more likely to examine their patients' feet if the nurse or aide had the patient remove his or her shoes before being seen. Several institutions are now establishing special insensitive-foot clinics where special education in foot care can be given by nurse-clinicians. Emphasis on group therapy may also help patients to accept that they are at major risk of foot ulceration. Furthermore, other centers have set up diabetic foot clinics which bring together physician and surgeon as well as a team of allied health specialists. The foot has often been neglected in the past, as it falls "between" specialties.

At Jackson Memorial Hospital, diabetic foot care is a multiphasic, multidisciplinary program under the aegis of the Rehabilitation Center. It is multiphasic in that it provides preventive, acute, and rehabilitative care in a true continuum with all phases interdigitating closely. The program is multidisciplinary with strong representation from diabetology, orthopedics, rehabilitation nursing, nursing education, psychology, social work, dietetics, therapeutic recreation, physical therapy, and pedorthics (custom shoe-fitting).

Patients at risk for development of foot ulcers because of significant neuropathy are referred by our diabetologists to the patient/family education clinic run by the nurse-educators who provide a number of services including foot self-care instruction and nail and callus trimming. They have been instructed in the latter procedures by the orthopedist. If ulcers or infection are present upon referral or ensue while the disorder is being followed by the patient/family education group, the patient goes to the insensitive-foot clinic that is staffed by the full team or is seen by the orthopedist alone if the clinic is not in session. Upon resolution of the problem, the patient is more closely followed in the patient/family education clinic. Extra-depth shoes with necessary modifications are provided in the clinic setting. Patients with deep ulcers or abscesses are admitted directly to the hospital and upon resolution of the problem are referred back to the clinic for continuing preventive care. A "hot line" number open 24 hr a day is given to each patient to encourage compliance with the team requesting that they be contacted at the earliest sign of a foot lesion.

However, despite intense education, the patient with the insensitive foot frequently ignores advice, i.e., until the occurrence of the first ulcer. As Brand pointed out, the person with insensitive feet who develops his first ulcer now learns that he is truly at risk of ulceration.[36] This is certainly an appropriate time to concentrate on education of the patient, who is often receptive to classes in preventive medicine. The principles of preventive foot care are summarized in Table 7-3, and are outlined below.

1. *Inspect feet daily.* This is carried out at home by the patient or a relative if the patient has poor vision. A mirror is very useful for careful inspection of the plan-

Table 7-3. Patient Instructions

Dos	Don'ts
1. Inspect feet daily using mirror (especially between toes, pressure areas)	1. Walk barefoot
2. Wash feet daily in tepid water	2. Smoke
3. Apply lotion/oil to feet after washing	3. Use keratolytics
4. Wear roomy leather shoes	4. Step into bathtub *before* checking temperature
5. Change shoes often	5. Use hot water bottles or heating pads
6. Have physician check feet at each visit	6. Buy plastic shoes
7. Inspect shoes daily for defects	7. Perform bathroom surgery

tar surfaces. Those subjects with dry skin should soak their feet in warm (*not* hot) water for 15–20 min after the careful inspection. After drying, petroleum jelly or olive oil is applied to the feet to preserve the moistness of the skin and prevent drying and consequent cracking of keratin. If the skin breaks or infections are detected, the patient is instructed to attend his clinic as a matter of urgency.

2. *Avoid extremes of temperatures.* Scalding and burns are frequent causes of ulceration in insensitive feet. Patients are advised to use bed socks if their feet are cold, not hot water bottles. Heating pads likewise should not be used.

3. *Avoid keratolytics.* These proprietary products are chemicals, e.g., salicylic acid, which can burn normal skin after removing callus and corns. The neuropathic patient is unable to feel the burning and continues to apply them after the callus has been removed.

4. *Do not walk barefoot.* Barefoot diabetics with insensitive feet are at great risk in any environment. Splinters from wood floors, needles hidden in pile carpets, and hot grids from floor furnaces are a few of the common home hazards. Hot pavement or beach sand demands that sandals be worn to the water's edge by diabetic swimmers.

5. *Beware of new shoes.* Shoes can present many dangers as well as basic protection to the insensitive foot. They can cause ulcers because they are too tight (constant exposure to low static pressure) or too loose (friction). Nails used in shoe construction can impinge on the foot and cause painless ulcers. Thus new shoes should be made of soft leather, joined with stitching or adhesive but not nails. No new shoes should be worn for more than a few hours at a time, and, in principal, all neuropathic subjects are advised to change their shoes at midday. If insoles are needed to provide softness, this is suggestive that extra-depth shoes are required. The danger of placing an insole in a regular shoe is that the foot will have less room within the shoe, with increased pressure applied to the dorsal surface of the foot and toes, which may ulcerate following ischemic necrosis of the shin.

6. *Attend clinic regularly.* This is essential for patients with neuropathic feet, to enable regular examination of the feet to be performed. Nail care can be attended to at a podiatrist's office or foot care clinic. Patients should be instructed to cut the nails straight across, not at angles.

The following true case history is illustrative of the problems seen in patient education:

A 56-year-old lawyer had a 15-year history of type II diabetes complicated during the last 5 years by peripheral neuropathy. He was found to have insensitive feet on examination. He attended an inpatient unit program for education and optimized control of his diabetes. Two months later he took a vacation and spent the days walking (barefoot) along a stony beach. He awoke on the third morning of his vacation and noted blood stains on the sheets at the foot of his bed; to his surprise, he found a deep laceration on the plantar surface of his right fourth toe. After returning from his vacation a day later he took some broad-spectrum antibiotics which he happened to have at home to try to avoid infection in his foot. He called the clinic but ignored advice to come to see the doctor until several days later. At this time he had extensive cellulitis and radiologic signs of osteomyelitis in his toe. He required 3 weeks of hospital treatment, and his right fourth toe was amputated.

The above case demonstrates that even informed patients who have just attended a program in patient education are prone to deny that the problem of insensitive foot exists. The man in this case ignored many "dos and don'ts" for diabetic feet of which he was supposedly aware.

MANAGEMENT OF THE PATIENT PRESENTING WITH A FOOT LESION

Successful management of any diabetic foot lesion depends on determination of its full extent, evaluation of its potential for healing, selection of the surgical or nonsurgical procedure likely to preserve maximum function of the foot with the least likelihood of failure, and good diabetic control.

Determining the extent of a given lesion requires close observation of several signs. The depth and lateral extent of an ulcer may be measured by a sterile probe, e.g., a cotton applictor stick. Before probing, it is helpful to remove most of the callused edge of the ulcer with a callus trimmer. The diameter of the ulcer is also measured and recorded. Any ulcer extending to a joint or to bone is immediately cultured. If pus is discovered, the limb is gently milked from above the ankle toward the toes to see if the infection tracks along the tendon sheaths. Radiographs are very helpful at this point to identify bone and joint destruction as well as soft tissue swelling. Calcification of the arterial tree, well into the digits, is commonly seen in diabetics[46] but alone is not an indication that tissue perfusion is inadequate for healing.

Once the physical extent of the lesion has been ascertained, its potential for healing must be gauged. This potential is multifactorial and includes, in addition to the usual elements of bacterial virulence and resistance to antibiotics, the multifloral nature of diabetic infections, with two to six organisms (aerobic and anaerobic, gram-positive and gram-negative) being the rule rather than the exception.[49,50] Host resistance in diabetics is further compromised by a decrease in diffusible oxygen at the tissue level. This may be related to precapillary shunting as shown by increasd venous oxygen[23] in the foot, local microvascular disease, or both.

Neuropathy plays a role in several ways: Infection spreads rapidly by intermit-

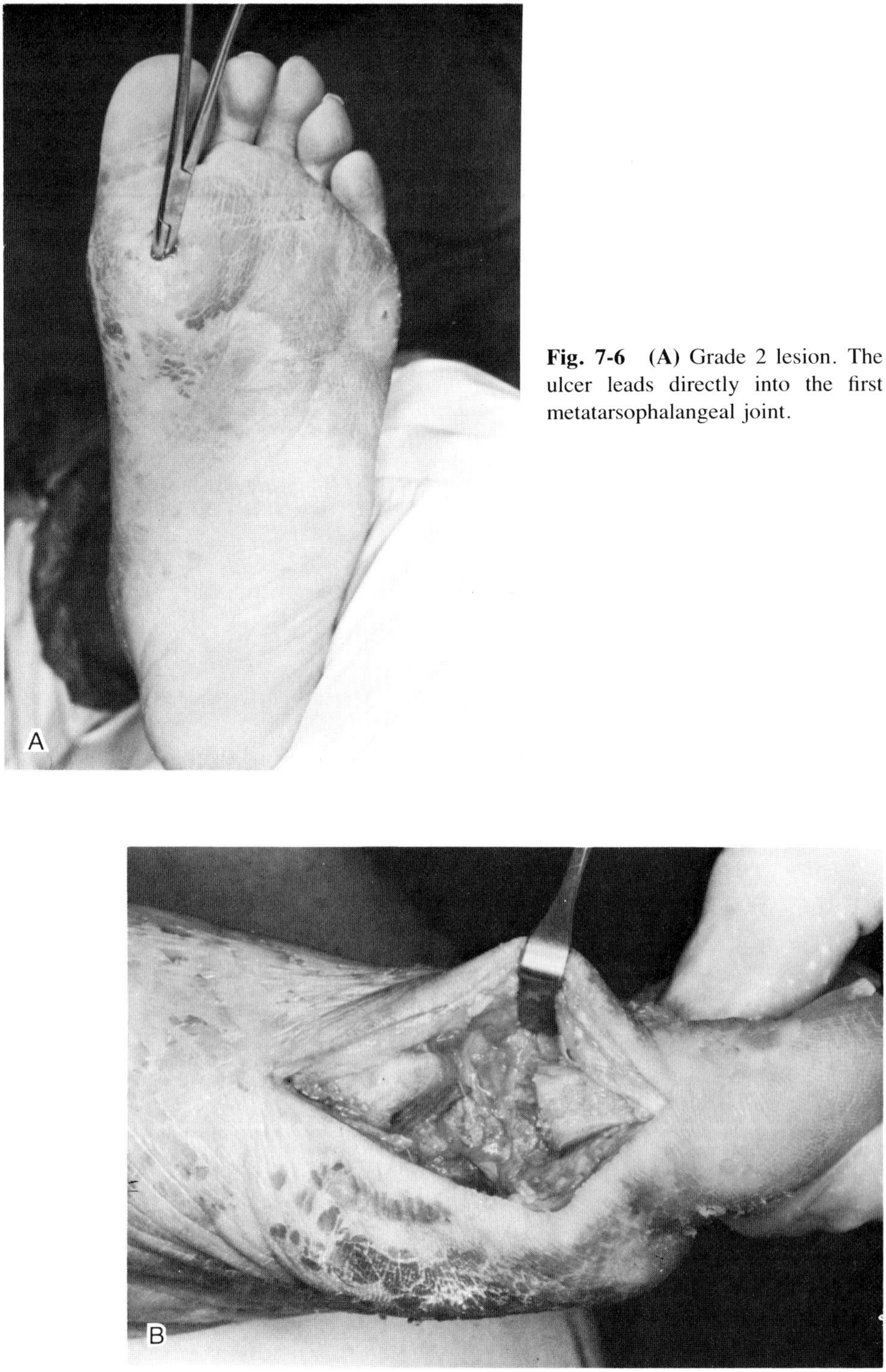

Fig. 7-6 (A) Grade 2 lesion. The ulcer leads directly into the first metatarsophalangeal joint.

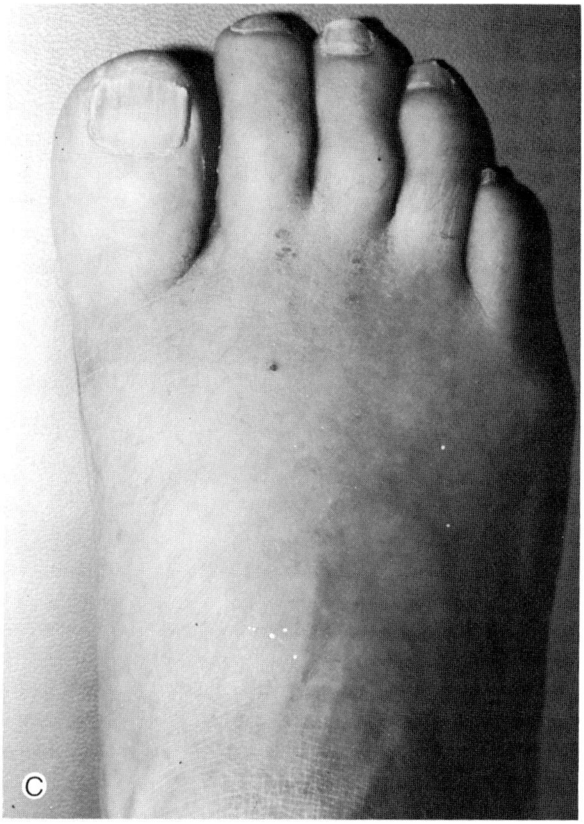

Figs. 7-6 (cont.) **(B)** Joint excision and soft tissue débridement completed. Joint space is exaggerated by traction on the toe. The wound was closed loosely over the Kritter irrigation system. **(C)** Dorsal view of the foot several months later. The great toe is slightly shorter but possesses enough active dorsiflexion to allow normal gait.

tent compression along natural routes, e.g., fascial planes and tendon sheaths, as a diabetic continues to walk on the infected but insensitive foot. Significant atherosclerosis is additive by further denying blood flow to tissue with an increased oxygen demand due to infection.

Few of these factors can be directly measured at this time. Bacteriological studies are of value, however, as are quantitative blood pressure determinations in the lower limb.[28] These are easily done as far distal as the toe web spaces. Systolic pressures obtained at locations in the lower limb are compared with the brachial systolic pressure to provide an ischemic index. According to Wagner's studies, an index of 0.45 indicates good healing potential, provided the infection can be controlled.[51] If a substantial pressure drop is found between the groin and popliteal fossa, vascular surgery consultation should be sought.

Direct measurement of skin blood flow may have more relevance to healing in diabetics. This is being actively investigated by measurements of transcutaneous oxygen flow and use of the laser doppler at a number of centers.

Wagner has developed a simple classification of diabetic foot lesions based on their extent.[51] Combining this with the ischemic index at the level of the lesion, a reasonable plan of treatment can be formulated. Grade 0 feet have no open lesions but may have calluses and/or bony prominences. These calluses should always be shaved to be sure that an ulcer has not formed beneath an apparently intact callus. Treatment consists of proper relief of pressure points by padding in roomy shoes with soft leather uppers. Usually a commercially available extra-depth shoe can be adequately modified. Otherwise, a custom-molded shoe is indicated.

A grade 1 lesion is a skin ulcer which has not penetrated the deep fascia of the foot. With an ischemic index of 0.45 or above, conservative débridement and avoidance of pressure on the ulcer by use of crutches or a snug weight-bearing cast should produce healing.[20] If the ulcer recurs despite proper shoes, prophylactic excision of the bony prominence may be indicated once healing occurs again.

Grade 2 lesions are ulcers which penetrate to joint capsule, joint, or bone (Fig. 7-6). Tissue necrosis without abscess formation is characteristic, and bacterial colonization is common. Treatment consists of excision of all necrotic tissue, including affected joints with loose closure of larger wounds over an irrigation system de-

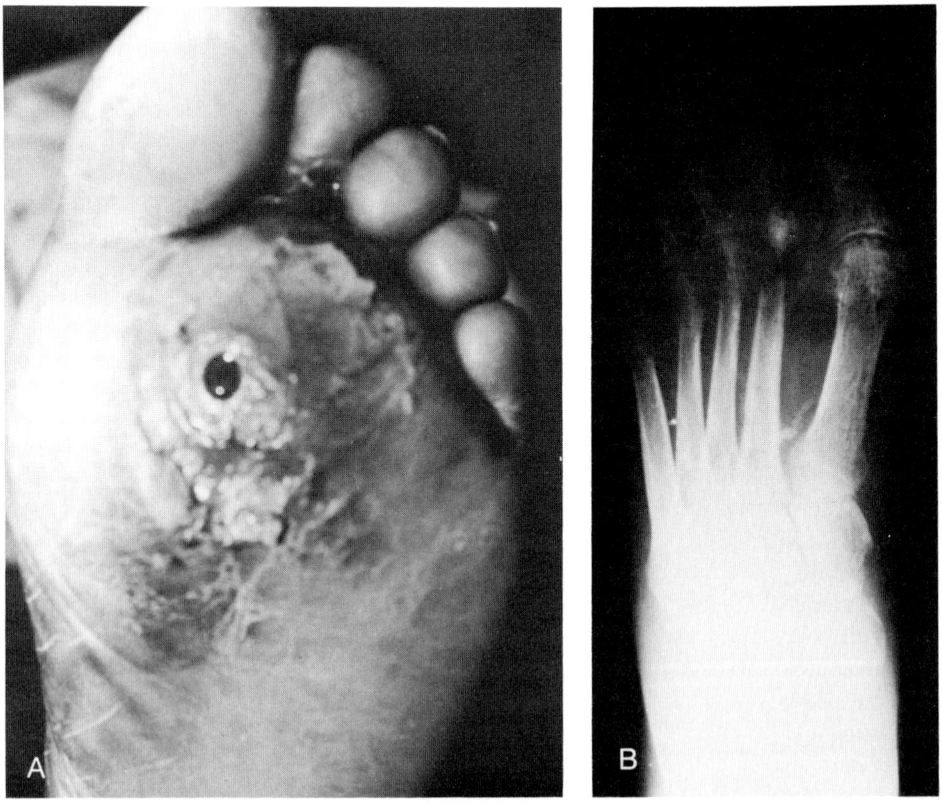

Fig. 7-7 **(A)** Grade 3 lesion. Note the ulceration through the heavy callus beneath the second metatarsal head. The ischemic index is adequate. **(B)** Radiograph showing marked destruction of the second metatarsophalangeal joint and second ray osteomyelitis. Note the widespread calcification of the distal arterial tree.

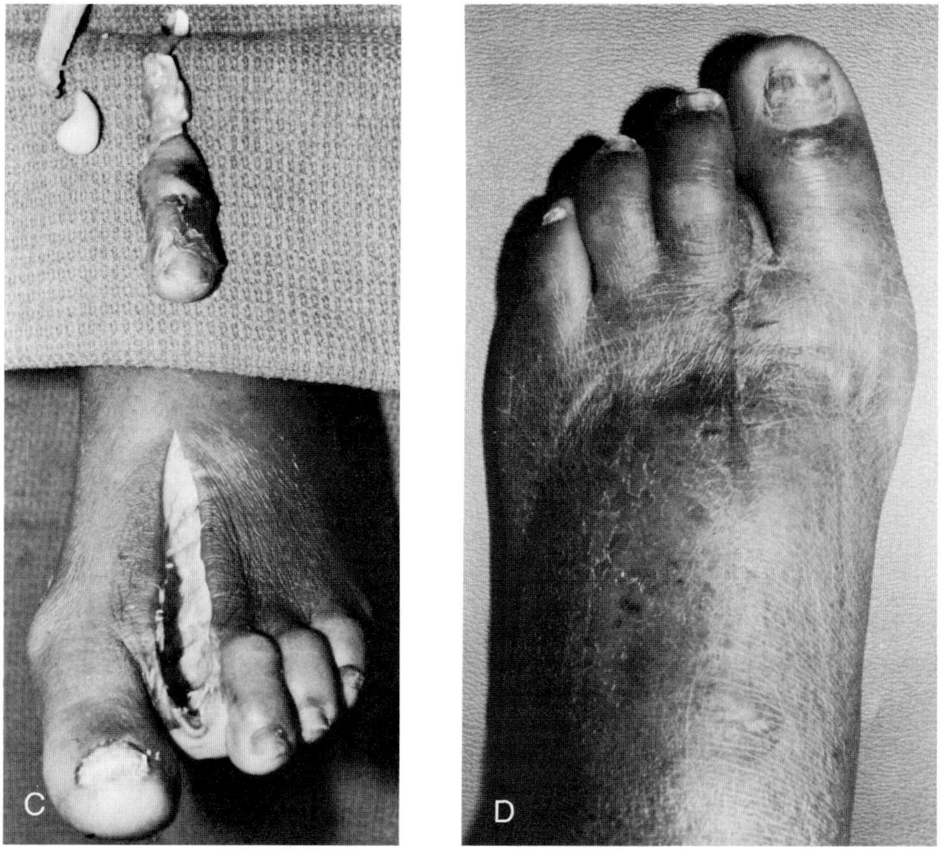

Figs. 7-7 (cont.) **(C)** Operative view at conclusion of abscess débridement, including second ray resection. Note the separation of the metatarsal head as found. **(D)** Dorsal view of foot 5 months later. Note the approximation of the first and third rays with good cosmesis.

scribed more fully below. A snug weight-bearing cast can be used for smaller wounds. These procedures should be undertaken only in the presence of an adequate ischemic index. Antibiotic coverage is necessary, and a combination of parenteral cloxacillin or metronidazole is recommended until results of organism sensitivity are available, at which point appropriate changes may be made if indicated.

Grade 3 lesions are penetrating ulcers associated with deep abscess formation, osteomyelitis, and if a joint is involved septic arthritis (Fig. 7-7). Multiple organisms are usually cultured, and extensive débridement of all necrotic tissue is mandatory. All extensions of the abscess must be widely opened through multiple incisions if necessary.

In selected cases in which a partial or complete toe amputation or single ray resection has removed all visible evidence of disease and good bleeding is evident, the wound may be loosely closed over a subclavian catheter, using the method described by Kritter.[52] The normal saline irrigant fluid exits between the widely spaced

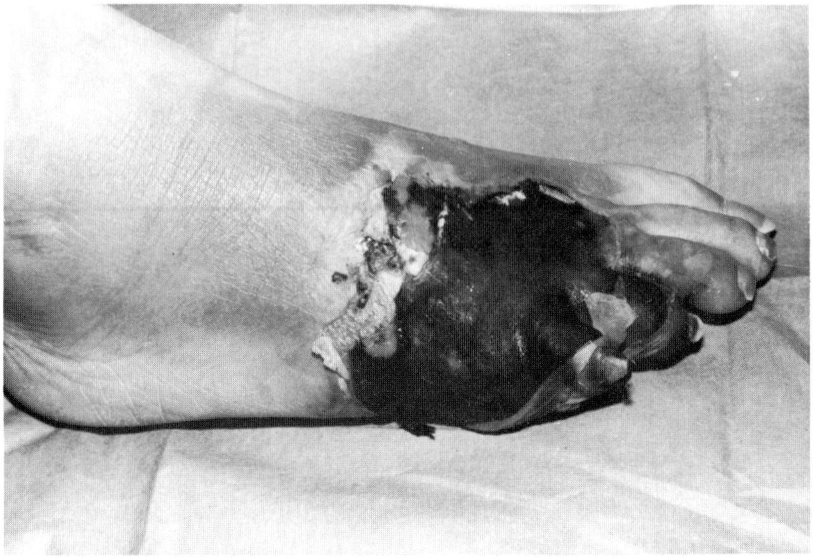

Fig. 7-8 Grade 4 lesion. This 46-year-old man completely denied both his diabetes and the presence of gangrene in his foot. The ischemic index was marginal. Syme amputation failed, resulting in revision to below-knee level.

sutures carrying hematoma and other detritus into the voluminous absorbent bandage. Intravenous antibiotics are an essential part of the regimen. Weight-bearing is not allowed until the wound is securely healed, a process requiring 4–8 weeks or longer. Wound packing technique is taught to the patient and/or family early postoperatively to allow for discharge as soon as the wound has passed from the exudative to the proliferative phase. The surgery is best done without a tourniquet in order to determine the exact extent of the necrosis. Weekly wound cultures are done to ensure continuing appropriateness of antibiotic coverage.

The level of amputation in grade 4 (gangrenous) lesions is dependent on the ischemic index, as gross infection may not be a factor (Fig. 7-8). Every attempt is made to salvage at least a Syme amputation, which is an ankle disarticulation with preservation of the heel pad for the proprioceptive benefits of end-weight-bearing. Occasionally a below-knee amputation is unavoidable.

Prosthetic management following limited amputation may require nothing more than shoe fillers, with or without sole stiffeners or rocker soles. These modifications are generally made in extra-depth shoes. Increased energy costs of ambulation do not become significant until the below-knee level is reached.

There are two overriding criteria of success in the rehabilitation of diabetic patients with foot lesions. The first is preservation of an intact foot or doing the least disabling amputation possible. The second criterion—prevention of recurrent lesions—is much more difficult to achieve. The keys to success are education and adjustment. Because so many diabetic patients with sensory impairment deny that a painless lesion is a threat, intensive counseling may be required to (1) break the pattern of denial and (2) deal with the resulting depression that comes with acceptance of the problem and the need for responsible self-care.

REFERENCES

1. Pryce TD: A case of perforating ulcers of both feet associated with diabetic and ataxic symptoms. Lancet 2:11, 1887
2. Martin MM: Neuropathic lesions of the feet in diabetes mellitus. Proc R Soc Med 47:139, 1953
3. Levin ME; Diabetic peripheral vascular desease. In Rifkin H, Raskin P (eds): Diabetes Mellitus, Vol. V. Robert J. Brady, Bowie, MD, 1981
4. Most RS, Sinnock P: The epidemiology of lower extremity amputation in diabetic individuals. Diabetes Care 6:87, 1983
5. U.S. Department of Health and Human Services: The Treatment and Control of Diabetes: A National Plan to Reduce Mortality and Morbidity. p. 25. NIH Publication 81-2284. Government Printing Office, Washington, DC, 1980
6. Levin ME, O'Neal LW: The Diabetic Foot. 3rd ed. Mosby, St. Louis, 1983
7. West KM: Specific morbid effects (complications). In: Epidemiology of Diabetes and Its Vacular Lesions. Elsevier, New York, 1978
8. Oakley W, Catterall RCF, Martin MM: Aetiology and management of lesions of the feet in diabetes. Br Med J 2:953, 1956
9. Kelly PJ, Coventry MB: Neurotrophic ulcers of the feet: a review of 47 cases. JAMA 168:388, 1958
10. Ellenberg M: Diabetic neuropathic ulcer. J Mt Sinai Hosp 35:585, 1968
11. Ward JD: The diabetic leg. Diabetologia 22:141, 1982
12. Archer AJ, Watkins PJ, Thomas PK, et al: The natural history of acute painful neuropathy in diabetes mellitus. J Neurol Neurosurg Psychiatry 46:491, 1983
13. Boulton AJM, Armstrong WD, Scarpello JHB, Ward JD: The natural history of painful diabetic neuropathy: a four year study. Postgrad Med J 59:556, 1983
14. Lippmann HI, Perotto A, Farrar R: The neuropathic foot of the diabetic. Bull NY Acad Med 52:1159, 1976
15. Lippmann HI: Must loss of limb be a consequence of diabetes millitus? Diabetes Care 2:432, 1979
16. Ozeran RS, Wagner GR, Reimer TR, Hill RA: Neuropathy of the sympathetic nervous system associated with diabetes mellitus. Surgery 68:953, 1970
17. Deanfield JE, Daggett PR, Harrison MJG: The role of antonomic neuropathy in diabetic foot ulceration. J Neurol Sci 47:203, 1980
18. Rundles RW: Diabetic neuropathy: general review with a report of 125 cases. Medicine (Baltimore) 24:111, 1945
19. Watkins PJ, Edmonds ME: Sympathetic nerve failure in diabetes. Diabetologia 25:73, 1983
20. Brand PW: The diabetic foot. In Ellenberg M, Rifkin H (eds): Diabetes Mellitus, Theory and Practice. 3rd ed. Medical Examinations Publications, New York, 1983
21. Boulton AJM, Hardisty CA, Betts RP, et al: Dynamic foot pressure and other studies as diagnostic and management aids in diabetic neuropathy. Diatetes Care 6:26, 1983
22. Ward JD, Boulton AJM, Simms JM, et al: Venous distension in the diabetic neuropathic foot. J Roy Soc Med 76:1011, 1983
23. Boulton AJM, Scarpello JHB, Ward JD: Venous oxygenation in the diabetic neuropathic foot. Diabetologia 22:9, 1982

24. Edmonds ME, Roberts VC, Watkins PJ: Blood flow in the diabetic neuropathic foot. Diabetologia 22:9, 1982
25. Partsch H: Neuropathien vom ulzero-mutilierenden. Vasa, suppl., 6:1, 1977
26. Jarrett RJ: Diabetes, hyperglycemia and arterial disease. Acta Diabetol Lat, suppl. 1, 8:7, 1971
27. Janka HU, Standl E, Mehnert H: Peripheral vascular disease in diabetes mellitus and its relation to cardiovascular risk factors: screening with doppler ultrasound technique. Diabetes Care 3:207, 1980
28. Yao JST, Hobbs JT, Irvine WT: Ankle systolic pressure measurements in arterial disease affecting the lower extremities: Br J Surg 56:676, 1969
29. Emanuele MA, Buchanan BJ, Abraira C: Elevated leg systolic pressure and arterial calcification in diabetic occulsive vascular disease. Diabetes Care 4:288, 1981
30. Gibbons, GW, Wheelock FC, Hoar CS, et al: Predicting success of forefoot amputations in diabetics by noninvasive testing. Arch Surg 114:1034, 1979
31. Editorial: Management of intermittent claudication. Lancet 1:404, 1980
32. Reichle FA, Rankin KP, Tyson RR, et al: Longterm results of femoroinfrapopliteal bypass in diabetic patients with severe ischemia of the lower extremity. Am J Surg 137:653, 1979
33. Hjortrup A, Rasmussen BF, Kehlet H: Morbidity in diabetic and nondiabetic patients after major surgery. Br Med J, 287:1107, 1983
34. Alexander S: Skin disorders associated with diabetes. In Keen H, Jarrett RJ (eds): Complications of Diabetes. 2nd ed. Edward Arnold, London, 1982
35. Lippmann HI, Farrar R: Prevention of amputation in diabetics. Angiology 30:649, 1979
36. Brand PW: Insensitive Feet: A Practical Handbook on Foot Problems in Leprosy. Leprosy Mission, London, 1977
37. Stokes IAF, Farris IB, Hutton WC: The neuropathic ulcer and loads on the foot in diabetic patients. Acta Orthop Scand 46:839, 1975
38. Ctercteko GC, Dhanedran M, Hutton WC, Le Quesne LP: Vertical forces acting on the feet of diabetic patients with neuropathic ulceration. Br J Surg 68:608, 1981
39. Boulton AJM, Franks CI, Betts RP, et al: Reduction of abnormal foot pressures in diabetic neuropathy using a new polymer insole material. Diabetes Care 7:42, 1984
40. Berfthold HT, Brand PW: Thermography: an aid in the management of insensitive feet and stumps. Arch Phys Med Rehabil 56:205, 1975
41. Thompson DE: Pathomechanics of soft tissue damage. In Levin ME, O'Neal LW (eds): The Diabetic Foot. 3rd ed. Mosby, St. Louis, 1983
42. Sinha SK, Frykberg RG, Kozak GP: Neuroarthropathy in the diabetic foot. In Kozak GP (ed): Clinical Diabetes Mellitus. Saunders, Philadelphia, 1982
43. Harrison MJG, Faris IB: The neuropathic factor in the aetiology of diabetic foot ulcers. J Neurol Sci 28:217, 1976
44. Ewing DJ, Clarke BF: Diagnosis and management of diabetic autnomic neuropathy. Br Med J 285:916, 1982
45. Staple TW: Radiography of the diabetic foot. In Levin ME, O'Neal LW (eds): The Diabetic Foot. 3rd ed. Mosby, St. Louis, 1983
46. Edmonds ME, Morrison N, Laws JW, Watkins PJ: Medial arterial calcification and diabetic neuropathy. Br Med J 284:928, 1982
47. Walsh CH, Soler MG, Fitzgerald MG, Malins JM: Association of foot lesions with retinopathy in patients with newly diagnosed diabetes. Lancet 1:878, 1975
48. Cohen SJ: Potential barriers to diabetes care. Diabetes Care 6:499, 1983
49. Pabhakar P, Rao AB, Hira J: Bacteriological study of diabetic foot ulcers. Trop Geogr Med 33:249, 1981

50. Sapico FL, Carawati H, Witte JL, et al: Quantitative aerobic and anaerobic bacteriology of infected diabetic feet. J Clin Microbiol 12:413, 1980
51. Wagner FW: Transcutaneous doppler ultrasound in the prediction of healing and the detection of surgical level of dysvascular lesions of the toes and forefoot. Clin Orthopaed 142:110, 1979
52. Kritter AE: A technique for salvage of the infected diabetic gangrenous foot. Orthop Clin North Am 4:21, 1973

8 Cutaneous Signs of Diabetes

Irwin M. Braverman

At least 30 percent of diabetics have some type of cutaneous involvement during the course of their chronic illness.[1,2] Some eruptions are caused by infectious agents; some result from vascular, metabolic, or nutritional disturbances; some arise as side effects of medications; and some are idiopathic. In addition, the skin of juvenile diabetics has an appearance that is different from that of adults with mature-onset disease. The skin of the former is frequently pale with a translucent quality, whereas the skin texture of the latter is usually identical to that of nondiabetics of the same ages. Recently a number of authors have described a new association: the diabetic hand syndrome in juvenile diabetes, which consists of insulin dependence, nonfamilial short stature, joint stiffness and thickened, and waxy skin of the palms and digits. Affected individuals are unable to flatten their hands completely on a table top because of mild flexion contractures of the fingers. Dupuytren's contractures have not been present. The cause of the disorder is unknown, although some of the patients have had diabetic neuropathy of the upper extremities. In a clinical study of 229 adolescents with diabetes, 65 displayed this syndrome.[3]

INFECTIONS

Diabetic patients probably do not have a predisposition to cutaneous bacterial or mycotic infections, but when these infections occur they are usually more severe and more difficult to bring under control than if they developed in a healthy person.[4] The necessity for preventing and vigorously treating bacterial infections stems from the fact that they frequently cause diabetes mellitus to go out of control. It is not unusual for diabetic acidosis to be precipitated by cellulitis and furuncles. Mycotic infections, whether caused by *Candida albicans* or a dermatophyte, are dangerous because they produce breaks in the skin that serve as portals for pathogenic bacteria.

Diabetics in ketoacidosis are especially prone to develop mucormycosis, a saprophyte fungal infection involving the paranasal sinuses and central nervous system. In the early phase of the infection, the nasal turbinates are inflamed and the mucosae necrotic. The eye is painfully inflamed. As the infection progresses, proptosis and ophthalmoplegia develop. Involvement of the cavernous sinus produces headache, lethargy, and cerebral infarction. The fungus spreads through the vascular channels, producing thromboses. Although this infection was originally thought to be caused only by the genus *Mucor,* other phycomycete species, e.g., *Rhizopus,* can also be pathogenic. Phycomycosis is a more accurate term to describe this dreaded complication of diabetic ketoacidosis. Although almost all cases have occurred in association with ketoacidosis, Sandler et al. described an instance of this infection in a patient with well-controlled diabetes.[5] These organisms can also produce hemorrhagic cutaneous infarction secondary to hematogenous dissemination.[6]

VASCULAR DISEASE

Premature peripheral vascular insufficiency secondary to arteriosclerosis is a frequent complication of diabetes mellitus. The earliest signs are loss of hair, shininess, atrophy, and coolness of the skin over the toes. As the condition progresses, gangrene and ulceration secondary to trauma may develop. Bacterial cellulitis and lymphangitis secondary to mycotic infections only aggravate these complications. When peripheral neuropathy is also present, ulcerations may develop because of loss of sensation. The sole is a frequent site for neurotropic ulcers, which are sometimes called malum perforans.

PRURITUS

Generalized pruritus is not a feature of diabetes mellitus, but it is common for patients to have pruritus vulvae and ani. Usually the perineal pruritus is associated with candidiasis (Fig. 8-1), but glycosuria must also be an important factor because when it is reduced the itching promptly disappears. Pruritus from any cause, especially in association with dry skin (xerosis), should be vigorously and quickly treated to prevent excoriations that can lead to secondary bacterial infections.

CAROTENEMIA

One textbook of endocrinology states that yellow discoloration of the skin secondary to carotenemia is present in 10 percent of diabetics,[7] but experience at the Yale–New Haven Medical Center does not support this statement. The statistic must have been obtained many years ago when diabetics were treated with diets low in carbohydrates and high in vegetables and protein. In 1945 Mosenthal and Loughlin

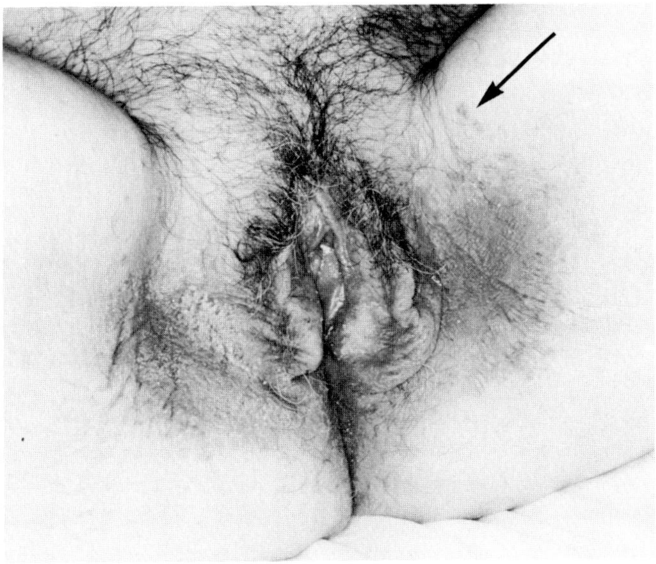

Fig. 8-1 Candidiasis. Note the satellite vesicopustular lesions characteristic of candidiasis (arrow). (Reprinted with permission from Braverman IM: Skin Signs of Systemic Disease. Saunders, Philadelphia, 1971.)

reported that only 24 percent of diabetics in their studies had elevated serum levels of carotene; this is in contrast to investigations carried out in 1930 when 85 percent of diabetics were so affected.[8] Carotenemia in diabetes mellitus is probably related more often to an increased dietary intake of carotene than to liver dysfunction or uncontrolled hyperlipemia. The hyperlipemia of diabetes usually represents hypertriglyceridemia and not hypercholesterolemia. Carotene is transported in the blood by β-liporotein, the carrier of cholesterol.

REACTIONS TO THERAPY

The therapy of diabetes mellitus can result in cutaneous complications. The sulfonylurea drugs produce a variety of drug reactions: urticaria, erythema multiforme, and photosensitivity eruptions. Lipoatrophy or lipohypertrophy may result from repeated injections of insulin into the same area. These abnormalities of the subcutaneous fat may disappear when the sites of infection are rotated. Lipoatrophy produces large hollow depressions in the skin that are thought to result from a local immunological reaction caused by contaminants in the less pure bovine insulin and/or local pH and tissue reactivity. Lipohypertrophy produces overgrowth of fat that clinically and histologically simulates lipomas (Fig. 8-2).

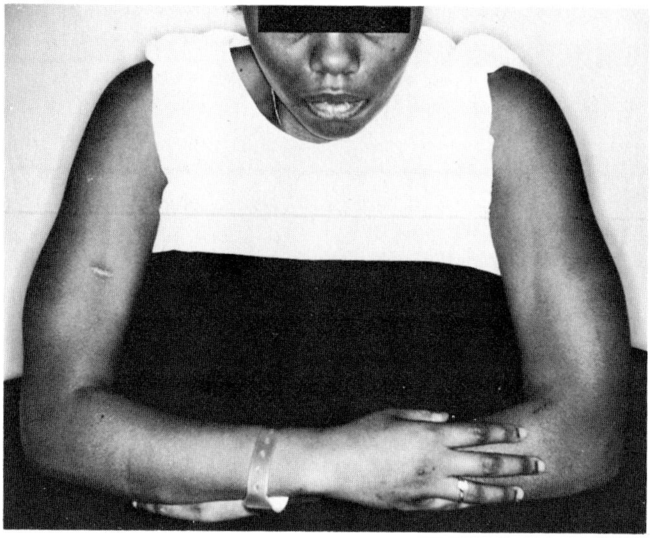

Fig. 8-2 Lipohypertrophy in biceps areas from repeated injections of insulin into the same sites. (Reprinted with permission from Braverman IM: Skin Signs of Systemic Disease. Saunders, Philadelphia, 1971.)

MICROANGIOPATHIC CUTANEOUS DISORDERS

The defect in carbohydrate metabolism is not the only abnormality in diabetes. Angiopathy of small vessels is another important feature. Currently two types are recognized.[9–13] The capillaries in the eye, kidney, and skeletal muscles frequently have thickened walls secondary to increased deposition of basement membrane material. These morphological changes may be the basis for the retinal disease and be partly responsible for the renal disease. The arterioles in the nerves and skin may be affected by obliterative endarteritis. Endothelial swelling and intimal proliferation lead to luminal narrowing of the affected arterioles. In addition, the vascular walls are thickened because of the deposition of mucopolysaccharides within the basement membrane material. This type of angiopathy may contribute to the peripheral neuropathy of diabetes and its most characteristic cutaneous lesions, necrobiosis lipoidica diabeticorum (NLD) and shin spots.[14,15]

Necrobiosis Lipoidica Diabeticorum

NLD occurs three times more often in women than in men. In 90 percent of patients it is localized to one or both shins; in the remaining individuals it may be on the trunk, arms, face, or scalp. The glans penis was affected in one of our patients. NLD usually develops during the third or fourth decade, but it may be seen in younger or older individuals; it was observed at birth in one patient. NLD appears in 0.1 to 0.3 percent of diabetics.[16]

NLD is a sharply demarcated plaque that has a shiny atrophic surface. It begins as a red or red-brown flat lesion that expands slowly. It can be as small as 0.5 cm or as large as 25 cm. The lesions tend to be oval, and several may coalesce to form a large plaque (Figs. 8-3 through 8-5). The active border remains erythematous, but the red-brown center becomes yellow as lipid is deposited. However, the yellow color is almost certainly produced by the accompanying carotene. A vascular pattern develops within the plaque. Dermal vessels become telangiectatic, and the subcutaneous vessels also become visible. NLD precedes the onset of diabetes in about 15 percent of patients by about 2 years (range 0.5–14 years). In 25 percent of the patients, NLD and diabetes mellitus appear concomitantly; in the rest, NLD appears after diabetes has been diagnosed. In two-thirds of the latter group of patients, the interval is less than 6 years. Spontaneous resolution occurs in 13–19 percent of cases after an average of 6–12 years. Resolution or progression of NLD does not seem to be related to the activity of the diabetes. Minor trauma may produce ulcerations in lesions of NLD, with healing taking as long as a year.

Muller and Winkelmann studied 171 patients with NLD.[16] Sixty-five percent of the patients had diabetes mellitus when they were examined initially. Nineteen of the remaining 60 persons were restudied several years later: Three had developed diabetes; five had abnormal glucose tolerance tests after pretreatment with prednisone; and six reported that diabetes had developed in a close relative. One of their patients had NLD for 17 years before diabetes mellitus developed. Only 5 of the 19 were untainted by the stigmata of diabetes mellitus. These data suggest that 90 percent of persons with NLD are either diabetic, will develop diabetes, or have a family history

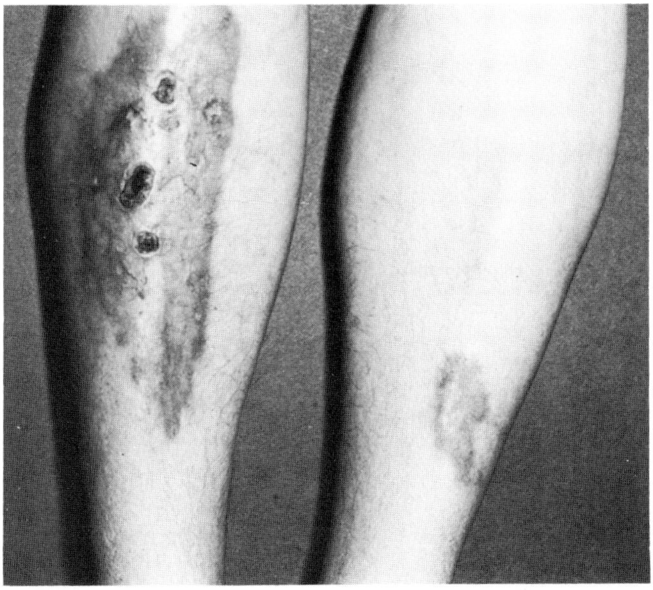

Fig. 8-3 NLD. Fully developed lesion with prominent dilated vessels and chronic ulcers. (Reprinted with permission from Braverman IM: Med Clin North Am 1971.)

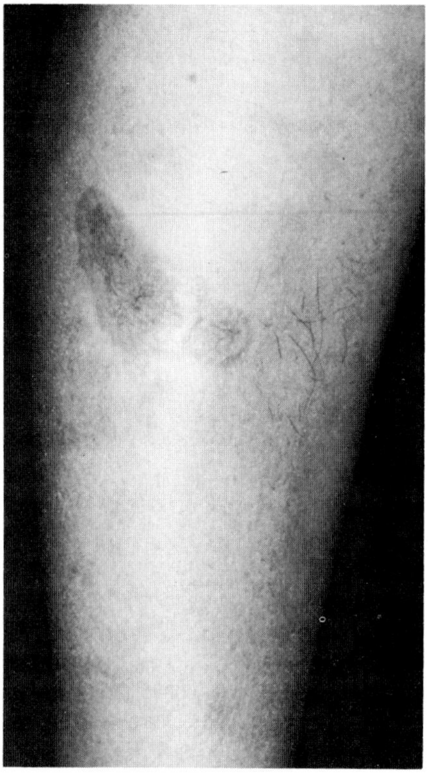

Fig. 8-4 NLD. Two plaques with dilated vessels. (Reprinted with permission from Braverman IM: Med Clin North Am 1971.)

of the disease. Muller and Winkelmann observed that diabetes occurred at an earlier age in those persons with NLD.[16]

The histopathology of NLD is that of obliterative endarteritis, characteristic of diabetic microangiopathy, with secondary necrobiotic changes in the bundles of collagen. However, on examination by electron microscopy the morphology of the collagen is normal. Instead the elastic fibers are missing, presumably having been destroyed by the inflammatory cells present in these necrobiotic foci.[17] A granulomatous reaction with giant cells may also occur.[18,19] The pathogenesis of the endarteritic lesion in NLD has not been established, although two hypotheses have been offered. Some investigators have suggested that an immune complex vasculitis is responsible for the angiopathy because immunoglobulins and complement have been detected in the vascular walls in some cases.[20] However, none of the other histologic features of vasculitis was present: neutrophils, nuclear dust, and fibrin deposition. A more attractive hypothesis implicates platelet abnormalities.[21] Platelets from diabetics show an increased sensitivity to aggregate both spontaneously and when stimulated by ADP, epinephrine, and collagen. In experimental animals, platelet interaction with the endothelial lining of large vessels results in the release of a mitogen from platelets that stimulates smooth muscle cell proliferation. This phenomenon is believed to cause intimal proliferation. Clinical observations have suggested that the sensitivity of platelets to aggregation in response to ADP and epinephrine may be correlated with progres-

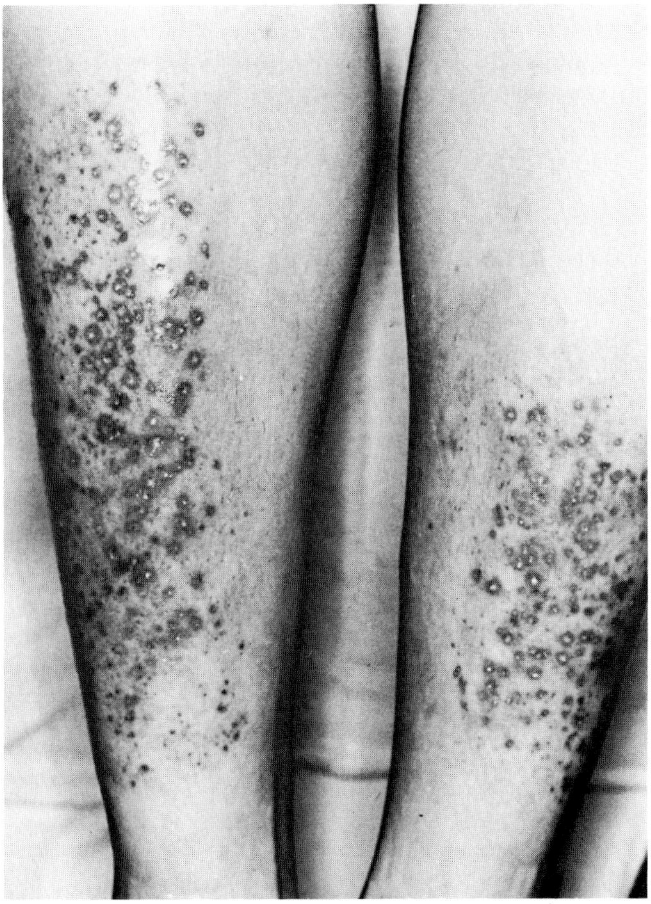

Fig. 8-5 NLD. Multiple small lesions are present on both shins. (Reprinted with permission from Braverman IM: Skin Signs of Systemic Disease. 2nd ed. Saunders, Philadelphia, 1981.)

sive retinopathy and neuropathy. Biopsies of sural nerves in diabetic patients have shown thromboses in the small vessels.

Therapy of NLD is generally unsatisfactory except in some early lesions or in those with advancing active borders which may respond to topical application or local injection with corticosteroids. Significant improvement or clearing may result. It is likely that the inflammatory cells with their proteolytic enzymes are affected by the corticosteroids. Eldor et al. produced resolution in a lesion of NLD by using antiplatelet aggregating agents, e.g., aspririn and dipyridamole.[22] The lesion had been present for 4 years and was ulcerated. The ulcer healed in 3 weeks, and the entire plaque of NLD disappeared within 6 weeks, leaving behind a scar. No new lesions appeared during the succeeding 8 months while the patient was on therapy. This interesting observation needs to be confirmed.

Diabetic Dermopathy

A second cutaneous sign of diabetes has been described under the following terms: shin spot, pigmented pretibial patch, and diabetic dermopathy. This marker begins as red or red-brown papules that evolve into sharply circumscribed atrophic patches which are often hyperpigmented and scaly (Fig. 8-6). Sometimes only depressed areas with normal skin color are present. Although these lesions are found almost exclusively on the shins, they have also been observed on the forearms. A quick glance at them suggests that trauma is responsible for their development, but this is not the correct explanation. According to Melin,[23] Binkley,[24] and Graham et al.,[15] the histologic findings in these lesions were identical to the microangiopathy of diabetes mellitus. Melin and Binkley also believed that these spots were correlated with diabetic retinopathy, nephropathy, and neuropathy. However, Danowski and co-workers were unable to confirm these associations except in men in whom the shin spots seemed to be related to neuropathy.[25] Danowski et al. observed identical cutaneous lesions in 1.5 percent of normal medical students and in 20 percent of patients with a variety of endocrinopathies but in whom the glucose tolerance test was normal. About 50 percent of their juvenile and adult diabetics had shin spots. Melin and Binkley observed that these spots occurred in 10–30 percent of female diabetics and in 60–65

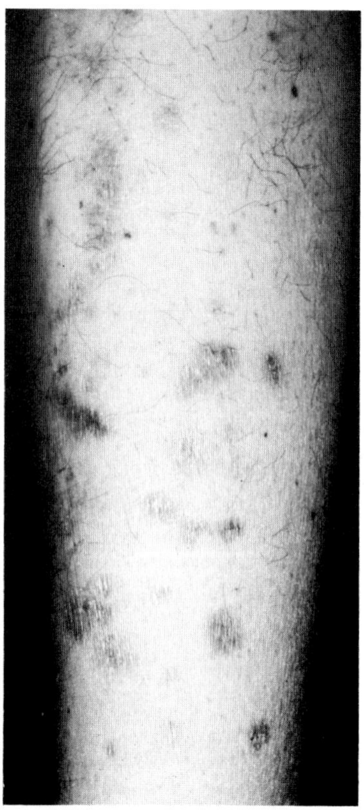

Fig. 8-6 Diabetic dermopathy. Hyperpigmented depressed spots on the shin. (Reprinted with permission from Braverman IM: Skin Signs of Systemic Disease. Saunders, Philadelphia, 1971.)

percent of male diabetics past the age of 30. The age and sex distribution of diabetic dermatopathy is different from that of NLD.

Fisher and Danowski studied the shin spots by light and electron microscopy and histochemical techniques.[26] Although they did not find obliterative endarteritis as others have, they did observe thickening of the arteriolar walls secondary to mucopolysaccharide deposition. All workers agree that the necrobiotic changes of collagen found in NLD are lacking in the shin spots.

GRANULOMA ANNULARE

Granuloma annulare has always been considered a dermatologic curiosity. Its morphology is that of rings with clear centers and an elevated border composed of contiguous papules. The etiology is unknown, and the disorder occurs at all ages. Spontaneous resolution is not uncommon and may follow biopsy of a lesion. The histopathology resembles NLD and the rheumatoid nodule in terms of both the angiopathy and the necrobiotic changes of the collagen. Deep subcutaneous lesions of granuloma annulare have been mistaken for rheumatoid nodules.[27] Granuloma annulare may occur as a generalized papular eruption in addition to the classic ringed form (Figs. 8-7 and 8-8).

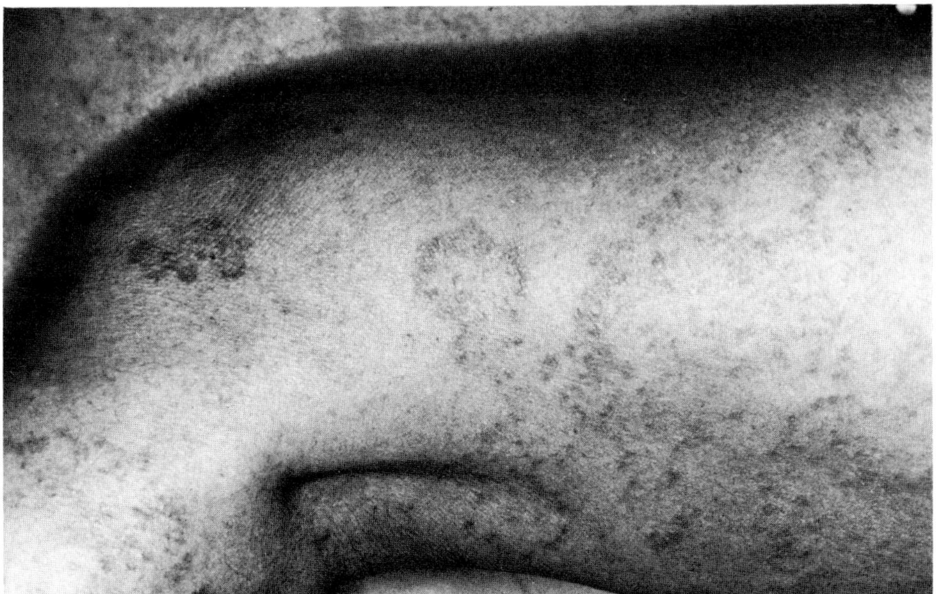

Fig. 8-7 Disseminated granuloma annulare. The disseminaed papules tend to form rings, but the centers are not completely free of the papules. (Reprinted with permission from Braverman IM: Skin Signs of Systemic Disease. 2nd ed. Saunders, Philadelphia, 1981.)

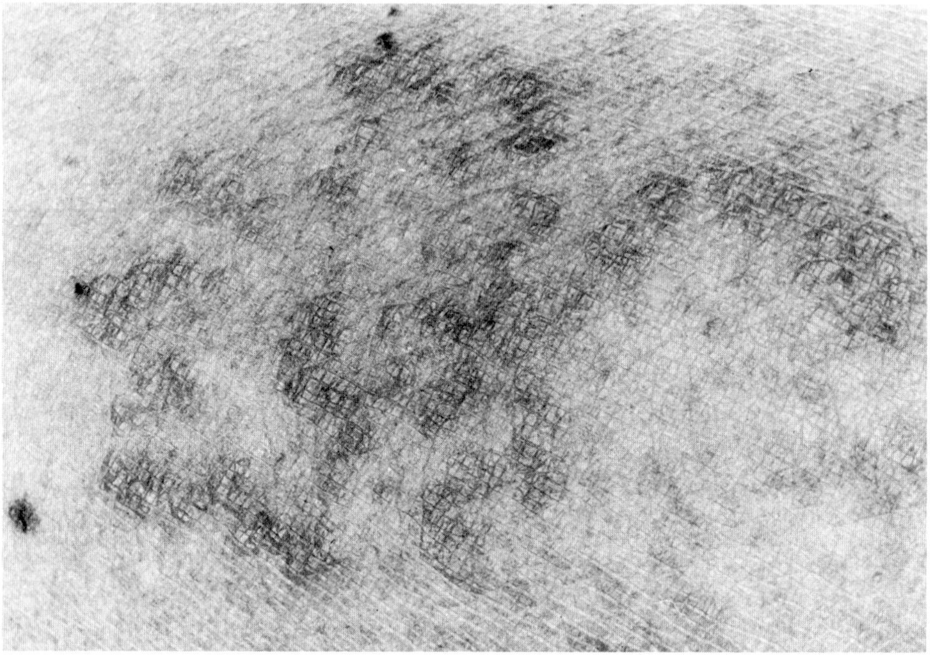

Fig. 8-8 Disseminated granuloma annulare. Close-up view of the granuloma annulare papules in Fig. 8-7. (Reprinted with permission from Braverman IM: Skin Signs of Systemic Disease. 2nd ed. Saunders, Philadelphia, 1981.)

Reports have suggested that disseminated granuloma annulare may be a sign of diabetes mellitus in adults. However, these observations have not been universally confirmed, and the issue needs further study.[28–30] Controversy also exists whether the angiopathy seen in granuloma annulare represents a vasculitis. Although some workers have demonstrated immunoglobulins and complement by direct immunofluorescence in some vessels, the other important histological features of leukocytoclasic vasculitis have been missing.[31] Other workers have suggested that granuloma annulare may represent a granulomatous disorder produced through the mechanism of delayed hypersensitivity.[32] Because the vascular changes in granuloma annulare resemble those found in NLD and diabetes mellitus, it would be worthwhile to determine if a disturbance in platelet aggregation could be related to the obliterative endarteritis found in both localized and disseminated granuloma annulare.

VITILIGO

The studies of Dawber suggest that there may be an increased prevalance of vitiligo in diabetes mellitus.[33] He found that 4.8 percent of 520 patients with diabetes had vitiligo, compared to 0.7 percent of 443 control subjects. The prevalance of vitiligo in the general population in the United States of America and in Europe is thought to range from 0.14 to 1.0 percent.[34] Vitiligo was twice as frequent in female as in male diabetics. Also, the vitiligo appeared after age 40 in 76 percent of the diabetics and frequently preceded the onset of the diabetes mellitus. Vitiligo usually developed before age 40 in 89 percent of individuals with this pigmentary disorder. Macaron et al. reported that the prevalance of vitiligo seemed to be increased in type I diabetics as well,[35] perhaps because of the association of type I diabetes and other autoimmune abnormalities.

DIABETIC BULLAE

Several investigators have described an unusual blistering dermatosis in approximately 30 patients.[35–40] These blisters appear suddenly without accompanying erythema on the fingers, toes, feet, and forearms (Fig. 8-9). They can range in size from several millimeters to several centimeters and may be recurrent. Typically the blister is tense and enlarges to its eventual maximum size within a few days. In my experience, the blister fluid has been viscous and clear. The chemical nature of the fluid has not been determined. The blisters heal without scarring over a 6-week period. The etiology is unknown, but trauma is not believed to play a role. Although many

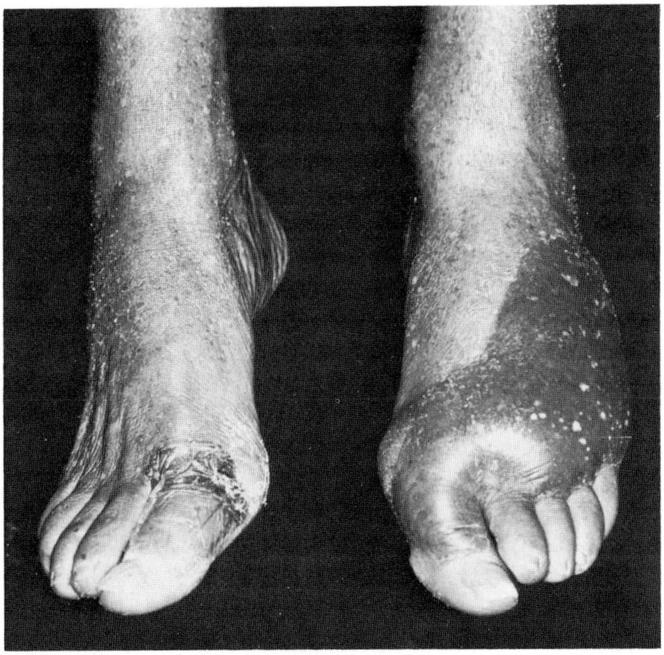

Fig. 8-9 Bullous lesions of diabetes mellitus. Extensive blister involving entire dorsum left foot. The blister at the base of the right great toe has broken and collapsed. (Reprinted with permission from Braverman IM: Skin Signs of Systemic Disease. 2nd ed. Saunders, Philadelphia, 1981.)

patients have had an accompanying peripheral neuropathy, this complication has not been considered to be important in the genesis of this bullous dermatosis.

The blisters have been shown by routine histological methods to be intraepidermal, subcorneal, and subepidermal. In a few cases with subepidermal blisters, the overlying epidermis was markedly edematous and exhibited foci of epidermal cell degeneration with vesicle formation. An electron microscopic study of one case showed that the blister formation began in the lamina lucida, the zone between the plasma cell membrane of the basal cells and the basal lamina itself.[40] Photosensitivity has been suggested as the initiating factor. In one case the lesions were provoked by exposure to the sun,[40] and in all cases the lesions have occurred in sun-exposed areas. Bernstein et al. suggested that an imbalance of Mg^{2+} and Ca^{2+} created by the underlying diabetes might contribute to a weakening of the dermal–epidermal interface so that sunlight and other stimuli might be able to induce separation with blister formation.[40] Porphyrin abnormalities and bullous pemphigoid have been excluded in this entity.

XANTHOMAS

Eruptive xanthomas arise during the hypertriglyceridemic phase of uncontrolled diabetes mellitus and spontaneously disappear over several weeks after the serum lipid levels have returned to normal (Figs. 8-10 and 8-11). Virtually all instances of eruptive xanthomas can be related to the hypertriglyceridemic phase of uncontrolled diabetes mellitus. If this underlying cause is not recognized and treated appropriately,

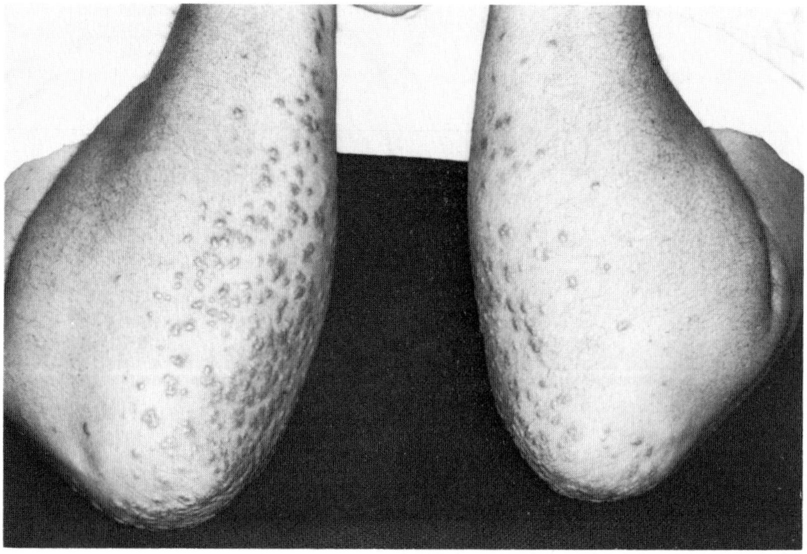

Fig. 8-10 Eruptive xanthomas in patient with uncontrolled diabetes mellitus. (Reprinted with permission from Braverman IM: Med Clin North Am 1971.)

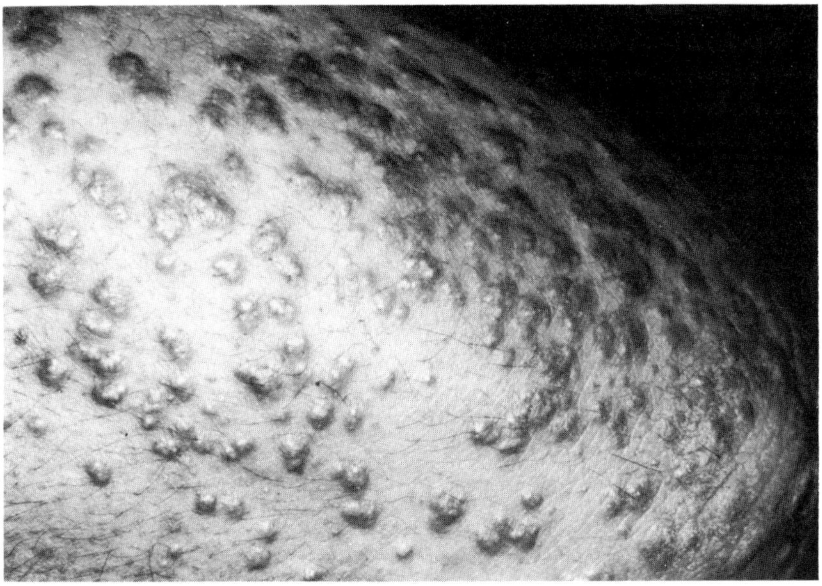

Fig. 8-11 Eruptive xanthomas. Close-up view of xanthomas shown in Fig. 10. (Reprinted with permission from Braverman IM: Med Clin North Am 1971.)

the eruptive xanthomas coalesce into large tuberous xanthomas which tend to persist. The xanthomas arise as erythematous papules which develop a yellow color in their evolution.

LIPODYSTROPHIES

The lipodystrophies comprise a group of uncommon disorders in which there is partial or total absence of subcutaneous fat. (The term lipoatrophy is used interchangeably with lipodystrophy in the literature.) A significant number of affected individuals develop insulin-resistant diabetes. Acanthosis nigricans is the striking cutaneous marker in some forms of lipodystrophy as well as in some individuals with only insulin-resistant diabetes.

Congenital total lipodystrophy (generalized lipodystrophy) is either present at birth or develops within the first 2 years of life. In the latter case, the subcutaneous fat disappears over the course of several months. Acquired generalized lipodystrophy has appeared during the first to third decades in a few individuals.[41–43] The two forms are considered to be variants of the same entity, even though the acquired form lacks some of the clinical features of the congenital variety. They are often referred to as the Lawrence-Seip syndrome. The syndrome is thought to be recessively inherited because of its presence in siblings and its association with parental consanguinity in several cases.

The disorder is characterized by acanthosis nigricans; accelerated somatic growth and bone maturation; increased muscle mass; enlarged penis, clitoris, or labia minora; and generalized hirsutism and hyperpigmentation. In addition, the individuals usually develop hypertriglyceridemia and hepatomegaly secondary to fatty infiltration that can lead to cirrhoisis and fatal hepatic failure. In some, dilatation of cerebral ventricles, cerebral atrophy, seizures, and mental retardation have been present. Insulin-resistant diabetes develops several years after the onset of the syndrome. In addition to complete atrophy of subcutaneous fat, the mesenteric, retroperitoneal, and epicardial fat has also disappeared in some individuals. Only the mammary fat remains. Idiopathic enlargement of the heart and kidney, nephrotic syndrome, and proteinuria with hypertension have been observed in a few patients. The acquired form of the disease lacks the features of hirsustism, hyperpigmentation, genital enlargement, and central nervous system involvement.[41]

Although the etiology and pathogenesis are not known, it has been suggested that lipodystrophy may be secondary to hypothalamic dysfunction. It is well recognized that the hypothalamus exerts important regulatory effects on glucose homeostasis and lipid metabolism.[44] Upton and colleagues implicated the hypothalamus in generalized lipodystrophy more directly by detecting increased concentrations of hypothalamic releasing factors for corticotropin and luteinizing hormone in the blood of these patients.[45,46] They proposed that the defect in this disorder may be a hypophyseal disturbance secondary to an abnormality in dopamine-β-hydroxylase activity, which is the rate-limiting step for the conversion of dopamine to norepinephrine. Dopamine and norepinephrine are believed to modulate the secretion of hypothalmic releasing factors. However, the manner in which the hypersecretion of these releasing factors would produce lipoatrophy or the metabolic disturbances is not understood. These investigators treated one patient with pimozide, a cerebral dopaminergic blocking agent. Within 2 years after treatment, the blood levels of releasing factors for corticotropin and luteinizing hormone had returned to normal and the sucutaneous fat had begun to reappear in the reverse order in which it had disappeared.[45]

Partial lipodystrophy is much more common and not genetically determined, appearing at any time from childhood to early adult life. It may appear idiopathically, after a febrile childhood illness, e.g., measles or scarlet fever, or after a nonspecific febrile illness.[41,47–49] As in the other forms of lipodystrophy, women are affected more often than men. The face is almost always affected. The neck, arms, chest, and trunk are involved in varying degrees. The fat from the hips or upper thighs to the feet remains. In some individuals there seems to be an increased deposition of fat around the hips. Variants of partial lipodystrophy exist but are uncommon. Subcutaneous atrophy may involve only the buttocks, arms, and legs, with sparing of the face and trunk.[50] Hemilipoatrophy affecting half the face or trunk has been described.[48] Figure 8-12 illustrates a patient in whom only the buttocks and upper thighs were affected. The lipoatrophy is usually permanent, although in one case following scarlet fever in which the face and arms were affected there was spontaneous reappearance of the fat 8 years later.[47] Generalized hirsutism, hyperpigmentation, and hepatomegaly have been observed in a few patients with partial lipodystrophy, but acanthosis nigricans has not been mentioned.[47] It is not clear whether acanthosis nigricans is truly absent or it has simply not been specifically looked for in this variety of lipoatrophy.

Membranoproliferative glomerulonephritis secondary to circulating immune

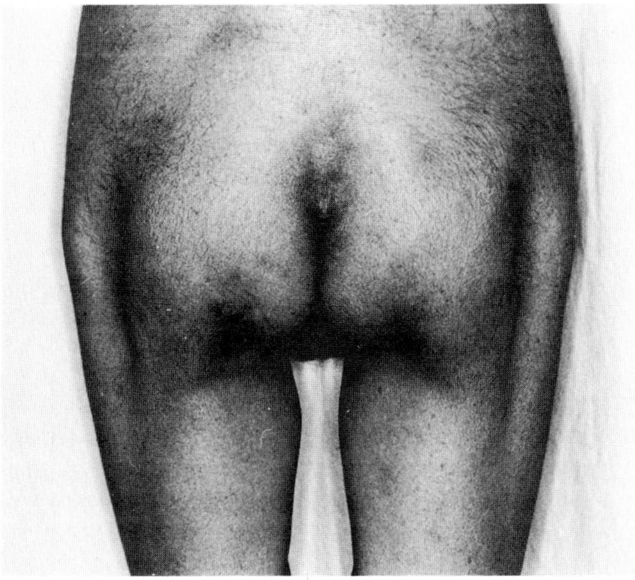

Fig. 8-12 Partial lipodystrophy. This woman had lipodytrophy only of the buttocks and upper thighs in association with insulin-resistant diabetes mellitus. (Reprinted with permission from Braverman IM: Skin Signs of Systemic Disease. 2nd ed. Saunders, Philadelphia, 1981.)

complexes can be detected in 40–50 percent of cases.[47,50] Usually there is an associated decrease in serum C3 levels with normal levels of C4 and C2, indicating activation of the alternative complement pathway. However, renal disease has developed in the absence of complement abnormalities.[51] In addition, the complement abnormalities are often present without renal disease, suggesting that they precede its development. Because a few patients have had an increased frequency of infections, it has been postulated that the renal disease may be related to immune complexes generated by repeated viral infections.[50] The relationship between lipodystrophy and the complement abnormalities is obscure.

Insulin-resistant diabetes associated with the lipodystrophy syndromes is produced by a reduced concentration or reduced affinity of the insulin receptor sites in some patients[52] and by as-yet-unidentified mechanisms in others.[53] Antibodies to insulin receptors have not been detected in any of these patients by the currently available assay.[53]

Insulin-resistant diabetes has also been reported in association with acanthosis nigricans. Kahn et al. described two groups of women with this syndrome which he termed types A and B.[53,54] Type A were adolescent girls, some of whom had increased body hair, enlargement of the clitoris, and accelerated somatic growth in addition to acanthosis nigricans. They had features found in congenital lipodystrophy, except for the absence of lipoatrophy. The insulin resistance was associated with a decreased number of receptors to insulin. Type B were women aged 10–60 who had circulating antibodies against insulin receptors in association with features suggesting an underlying autoimmune disease. Pulini et al. described an instance of the Type B variant in a 64-year-old black man.[55] Field et al. reported the case of a nonobese black woman with insulin-resistant diabetes and acanthosis nigricans developing at age 15.[56] Over the course of the succeeding 18 months, both diabetes mellitus and acanthosis nigricans spontaneously disappeared, and her response to insulin also returned to normal.

SCLEREDEMA ADULTORUM

A syndrome of cutaneous induration known as scleredma adultorum (Buschke) is frequently associated with diabetes mellitus. The syndrome often follows an infection and may persist for months to years. A firm, nonpitting edema develops on the face, neck, and trunk. The hands and feet are spared. The edema, which is caused by increased amounts of acid mucopolysaccharides in the dermis, may impart a peau d'orange appearance to the skin. Virtually all the cases diagnosed during the past decade at our medical center have been in diabetic men who were being trained to cope with their blindness secondary to diabetic retinopathy. There is no satisfactory therapy for scleredema.

REFERENCES

1. Braverman IM: SKin Signs of Systemic Disease. 2nd ed. p. 654. Saunders, Philadelphia, 1981
2. Allen GE: Diabetes mellitus and the skin. Practitioner 203:189, 1969
3. Grgic A, Rosenbloom AL, Weber FT, et al: Joint contracture: common manifestations of childhood diabetes mellitus. J Pediatr, 88:584, 1976
4. Thornton GF: Infections and diabetes. Med Clin North Am, 55:931, 1971
5. Sandler R, Tallman CB, Kearny DG, Irving WR: Successfully treated rhinocerebral phycomycosis in well controlled diabetes. N Engl J Med, 285:1180, 1971
6. Kramer BS, Hernandez AD, Reddick RL, Levine AS: Cutaneous infarction: manifestation of disseminated mucormycosis. Arch Dermatol 113:1075, 1977
7. Williams RH: The pancreas. In Williams RH (ed): Textbook of Endocrinology. 4th ed. p. 781. Saunders, Philadelphia, 1968
8. Mosenthal HO, Loughlin WC: Plasma vitamin A and carotene in diabetes mellitus. J Mt Sinai Hosp NY 12:523, 1945
9. Bloodworth JMB: Diabetic microangiopathy. Diabetes 12:99, 1963
10. Dolman CL: The morbid anatomy of diabetic neuropathy. Neurology 13:135, 1963
11. LeCompte PM: Vascular lesions in diabetes mellitus. J Chronic Dis 2:178, 1955
12. Bloodworth JMB Jr, Molitor DL: Ultrastructural aspects of human and canine diabetic retinopathy. Invest Ophthalmol 4:1037, 1965
13. Siperstein MD, Raskin P, Burns H: Electron microscopic quantification of diabetic microangiopathy. Diabetes 22:514, 1973
14. Bauer MF, Hirsch P, Bullock WK, Abul-Haj SK: Necrobiosis lipoidica diabeticorum. Arch Dermatol 90:558, 1964
15. Graham JH, Marques AS, Johnson WC, Gray HR: Stasis dermatitis. In Graham JH, John-

son WC, Helwig EB (eds): Dermal Pathology. p. 352. Harper & Row, Hagerstown, MD, 1972

16. Muller SA, Winkelmann, RK: Necrobiosis lipoidica diabeticorum: a clinical and pathologic investigation of 171 cases. Arch Dermatol 93:272, 1966
17. Braverman IM: Unpublished data.
18. Rollins TG, Winkelmann RK: Necrobiosis lipoidica granulomatosis: necrobiosis lipoidca in the non-diabetic. Arch Dermatol 82:537, 1960
19. Gray HR, Graham JH, Johnson WC: Necrobiosis lipoidica, necrobiosis lipoidica diabeticorum, and granuloma annulare. In Graham JH, Johnson WC, Helwig EB (eds): Dermal Pathology. p. 417. Harper & Row, Hagerstown, MD, 1972
20. Ullman S, Dahl MV: Necrobiosis lipoidica: an immunofluorescence study. Arch Dermatol 113:61, 1977
21. Mustard JF, Packham MA: Platelets and diabetes mellitus. N Engl J Med 297:1345, 1977
22. Eldor A, Diaz EG, Naparstek E: Treatment of diabetic necrobiosis with aspirin and dipyridamole. N Engl J Med 298:1033, 1978
23. Melin H: An atrophic circumscribed skin lesion in the lower extremities of diabetics. Acta Med Scand [Suppl 423] 176:1, 1964
24. Binkley GW: Dermopathy in the diabetic syndrome. Arch Dermatol 92:625, 1965
25. Danowski TS, Sabeh G, Sarver ME, et al: Shin spots and diabetes mellitus. Am J Med Sci 251:570, 1966
26. Fisher ER, Danowski TS: Histologic, histochemical and electron microscopic features of the shin spots of diabetes mellitus. Am J Clin Pathol 50:547, 1968
27. Taranta A: Occurrence of rheumatic-like subcutaneous nodules without evidence of joint or heart disease. N Engl J Med 266:13, 1962
28. Romaine R, Rudner EJ, Altman J: Papular granuloma annulare and diabetes mellitus. Arch Dermatol 98:152, 1968
29. Dicken CH, Carrington SG, Winkelmann RK: Generalized granuloma annulare. Arch Dermatol 99:556, 1969
30. Haim S, Friedman-Birnbaum R, Shafrir A: Generalized granuloma annulare: relationship to diabetes mellitus as revealed in 8 cases. Br J Dermatol 83:302, 1970
31. Dahl MV, Ullman S, Goltz RW: Vasculitis in granuloma annulare: histopathology and direct immunofluorescence. Arch Dermatol 113:463, 1977
33. Dawber RPR: Vitiligo in mature-onset diabetes mellitus. Br J Dermatol 80:275, 1968
34. Lerner AB: Vitiligo. J Invest Dermatol 32:285, 1959
35. Macaron C, Winter RJ, Traisman HS, et al: Vitiligo and juvenile diabetes mellitus. Arch Dermatol 113:1515, 1977
36. Rocca RP, Pereyra E: Phlyctenar lesions in the feet of diabetic patients. Diabetes 12:220, 1963
37. Cantwell AR, Martz W: Idiopathic bullae in diabetics: bullosis diabeticorum. Arch Dermatol 96:42, 1967
38. Allen GE, Hadden DR: Bullous lesions of the skin in diabetes. Br J Dermatol 82:216, 1970
39. Kurwa A, Roberts P, Whitehead R: Concurrence of bullous and atrophic skin lesions in diabetes mellitus. Arch Dermatol 103:670, 1971
40. Bernstein JE, Mendenica M, Soltani K, Griem SF: Bullous eruption of diabetes mellitus. Arch Dermatol 115:324, 1979
41. Senior B, Gellis SS: The syndromes of total lipodystrophy and of partial lipodystrophy. Pediatrics 33:593, 1964
42. Gordon H, Pimstone BL, Keary PM, Gordon W: Congenital generalized lipodystrophy with abnormal growth hormone homeostasis. Arch Dermatol 104:551, 1971

43. Reed WB, Ragsdale W Jr, Curtis AC, Richards HJ: Acanthosis nigricans in association with various genodermatoses. Acta Derm Venereol (Stockh) 48:465, 1968
44. Frohman LA: The hypothalamus and metabolic control. Pathobiol Annu 1:353, 1971
45. Corbin A, Uton GV, Mabry CL, Hollingsworth DR: Diencephalic involvement in generalized lipodystrophy: rationale and treatment with the neuroleptic agent pimozide. Acta Endocrinol (Copenh) 77:209, 1974
46. Upton GV, Corbin A: Hypothesis: hypothalamic dysfunction and lipoatrophic diabetes. Yale J Biol Med 46:314, 1973
47. Eisinger AJ, Shortland JR, Moorehead PJ: Renal disease in partial lipodystrophy. Q J Med 41:343, 1972
48. Poley JR, Stickler GB: Progressive lipodystrophy: a clinical study of 50 patients. Am J Dis Child 106:356, 1963
49. West RJ, Fosbrooke AS, Lloyd JK: Metabolic studies and autonomic function in children with partial lipodystrophy. Arch Dis Child 49:627, 1974
50. Sissons JGP, West RJ, Fallows J, et al: The complement abnormalities of lipodystrophy. N Engl J Med 294:461, 1976
51. Mery J Ph, Kowrilsky O, Morel-Maroger L, Adam C: Partial lipodystrophy and glomerulonephritis without complement activation. N Engl J Med 298:1034, 1978
52. Oseid S, Beck-Nielsen H, Pedersen O, Søvik O: Decreased binding of insulin to its receptor in patients with congenital generalized lipodystrophy. N Engl J Med 296:245, 1977
53. Flier JS, Kahn R, Roth J: Receptors, antireceptor antibodies and mechanisms of insulin resistance. N Engl J Med 300:413, 1979
54. Kahn CR, Flier JS, Bar RS, et al: The syndromes of insulin resistance and acanthosis nigricans. N Engl J Med 294:739, 1974
55. Pulini M, Raff SB, Chase R, Gordon EE: Insulin resistance and acanthosis nigricans: report of a case with antibodies to insulin receptors. Ann Intern Med 85:749, 1976
56. Field JB, Johnson P, Herring B: Insulin resistant diabetes with increased endogenous plasma insulin followed by complete remission. J Clin Invest 40:1672, 1961

9 Treatment of Hypertension in the Diabetic Patient

Robert V. Farese

Physicians are frequently confronted with patients who have coexisting hypertension and diabetes mellitus. In some cases the hypertension seems to be a specific consequence of diabetes mellitus, whereas in others it may antedate and provide a setting conducive to the development of diabetes mellitus; in still other cases these disorders may simply coexist (Table 9-1). In any case, the hypertensive-diabetic patient is at greater risk for developing arteriosclerotic and diabetic microvascular sequelae, and the physician providing care to these patients must be concerned with a number of diagnostic and therapeutic problems which are peculiar to this clinical subset of patients.

PREVALENCE OF COEXISTING HYPERTENSION AND DIABETES MELLITUS

Many studies have shown an increased prevalence of hypertension in diabetic patients, but the true prevalence is not certain. In several relatively large population studies, e.g., the Framingham,[1,2] Tecumseh,[3] and Joslin[4] studies, mean systolic blood pressures were 10–12 mm Hg higher, and the prevalence of hypertension in diabetic patients was observed to be approximately 1.5- to 2-fold above that of the general population. In selected groups, the prevalence of hypertension may be even greater. For example, in longstanding (>30 years) insulin-dependent diabetes mellitus, hypertension occurs secondary to diabetic glomerulopathy, and the prevalence ap-

Table 9-1. Potential Reasons for the High Prevalence of Coexisting Hypertension and Diabetes Mellitus

High prevalence of essential hypertension and noninsulin-dependent diabetes mellitus in the older population
Hypertensinogenic factors in diabetes mellitus
Altherosclerosis causing systolic hypertension
Hyperglycemia (without osmotic diuresis) causing hypervolemia
Recurrent Pyelonephritis
Diabetic glomerulopathy causing fluid retention
Diabetogenic factors in hypertensive states
Diabetogenic effects (impaired insulin secretin and/or resistance) of thiazides and β-blockers
Resistance to insulin secondary to ''adrenergic excess'' or hypertension per se
Other undefined (? genetic) factors
Primary clinical conditions causing (or associated with) secondary hypertension and diabetes mellitus (see Table 8-2)

proaches 50 percent[5]; moreover, in patients over 60 years of age, where the prevalence of hypertension is approximately 30 percent in the nondiabetic population, the prevalence in diabetic patients may be as high as 60 percent.[4]

The conclusion that is generally derived from the above studies (and from considerations discussed below) is that patients with diabetes mellitus have an increased risk for developing hypertension. The converse question may also be asked: Is the hypertensive patient at greater risk for developing diabetes mellitus? This question was addressed in the Tecumseh study,[3] and it was found that hypertensive patients have significantly more hyperglycemia than normotensive patients. In newly diagnosed hypertensive patients, Berglund and associates[6] observed an increased incidence of glucose intolerance with associated mild hyperinsulinemia but not overt diabetes mellitus; interestingly, effective treatment of blood pressure diminished this glucose intolerance, and the authors postulated that hypertension with attendant ''increased sympathetic discharge'' may have diminished the sensitivity of peripheral tissues to insulin. Although overt diabetes mellitus may not be more common at the outset in newly diagnosed hypertensive patients, with the passage of time its prevalence may increase; for example, in a recent Veterans Administration (VA) Cooperative Study, the incidence of frank fasting hyperglycemia was 3 percent in newly diagnosed hypertensives but had risen to 6 percent after 1 year of treatment with thiazides. Obviously, this increase in diabetes mellitus may have been the result of indiscriminate use of thiazides. Although the above studies suggest at least two nongenetic mechanisms whereby hypertensive patients may be at greater risk than nonhypertensive patients for development of diabetes mellitus (i.e., a decrease in insulin sensitivity and diabetogenic effects of commonly used antihypertensive agents), there presently is little or no information to suggest a genetic linkage of factors which are conducive to the development of both disorders.

PATHOGENESIS OF HYPERTENSION IN PATIENTS WITH DIABETES MELLITUS

There are several ways in which diabetes mellitus may lead to the development of hypertension: (1) hyperglycemia itself may expand plasma volume; (2) diabetes-related atherosclerosis may increase blood pressure, particularly systolic pressure, through a decrease in vascular wall resilience; (3) recurrent, sometimes silent pyelonephritis, which is common in diabetes mellitus, may lead to the development of hypertension through poorly understood mechanisms; and (4) longstanding diabetic glomerulopathy may diminish the ability to excrete salt and result in plasma volume expansion. Each of these is discussed separately.

The effect of hyperglycemia per se on blood pressure is unknown. Although hypertension is generally not thought of as a specific consequence of hyperglycemia, there are no published data to be certain that this is the case. Indeed, it would be expected that moderate hyperglycemia (in the absence of osmotic diuresis) would lead to expansion of plasma volume, and the latter has been documented in diabetic patients[4,7]; occasionally it is severe enough to precipitate pulmonary edema in patients with congestive heart failure.[8] This phenomenon might explain cases in which blood pressure seems to be improved after correction of hyperglycemia.

Age-related increases in blood pressure are thought to be at least partly due to diminished blood vessel wall resilience secondary to artherosclerosis. Diabetes mellitus clearly increases the risk for developing atherosclerosis[1–3] and may therefore be an important contributor to the development of hypertension in the older diabetic patient. This increase in blood pressure, which is provoked by a decrease in vascular distensibility, is primarily systolic in nature but nevertheless is an important risk factor for the development of cerebrovascular disease, coronary artery disease, and peripheral vascular disease.

The mechanism whereby pyelonephritis leads to hypertension is obscure. Decreased production of depressor substances, increased production of pressor substances, and/or neural reflex mechanisms whereby the kidney increases the adrenergic discharge from the central nervous system have been suggested as possible underlying mechanisms, but there is little direct or convincing evidence to support these postulations.

In longstanding and severe diabetes mellitus, particularly insulin-dependent diabetes mellitus for over 25 years, microvascular damage and thickening of the mesangium leads to sclerosis of the renal glomeruli. As a result, glomerular capillary perfusion is diminished, and the ability to excrete solutes and water is impaired, resulting in plasma volume expansion and hypertension. This hypertension generally also involves increases in both cardiac output and, eventually, peripheral vascular resistance. As a result of plasma volume expansion, renal renin production and secretion are frequently diminished.[9] In addition, renin secretion may be compromised further by diabetic neuropathy affecting the β-adrenergic nerves in the kidney or by direct pathological changes in the juxtaglomerular cells (which produce and secrete renin). This low-renin form of hypertension which is associated with diabetic glomerulopathy has been aptly referred to as "diabetic hypertension."[10] Understanding the pathogenesis of this form of hypertension is important because, as will become apparent, therapy should be directed primarily at improvement of the plasma volume overload, and the hyporeninemic state may predispose to the development of hypoaldosteronism and hyperkalemia.

DIAGNOSTIC CONSIDERATIONS

There are a number of primary clinical entities which provoke or are associated with secondary increases in blood pressure and either impaired glucose tolerance or frank diabetes mellitus (Table 9-2). These include: azotemic renal insufficiency of any etiology, obesity, oral contraceptive therapy, acromegaly, pheochromocytoma, aldosterone or other mineralocorticoid excess, and Cushing's syndrome or glucocorticoid excess. When evaluating patients with coexisting hypertension and diabetes, the physician must at least consider these disorders and employ appropriate diagnostic tests if necessary. With respect to renal disease, obesity, and oral contraceptive therapy, a simple history, physical examination, and routine laboratory tests bring these problems into focus. In most cases of the above-mentioned endocrine disorders (i.e., acromegaly, pheochromocytoma, mineralocorticoid excess, and Cushing's syndrome), the diagnosis is usually suggested by a careful history and physical examination, but in some cases the clinical findings may be much more subtle. For example, patients with early acromegaly may have only mild acromegaloid changes; patients with pheochromocytoma may not have paroxysmal hypertension; patients with mineralocorticoid excess may have only very mild muscle weakness and no symptoms related to hypokalemic alkalosis (e.g., carpopedal spasm, paresthesias, trismus); and patients with glucocorticoid excess, caused by corticosteroid therapy, hypersecretion of pituitary ACTH (Cushing's disease), autonomous adrenal tumors, or the ectopic ACTH syndrome, may have only mild cushingoid features on physical examination. Fortunately, simple laboratory screening tests usually provide ready answers to de-

Table 9-2. Primarily Clinical Conditions Causing (or Associated With) Secondary Hypertension and Diabetes Mellitus or Glucose Intolerance

Condition	Screening Test or Procedure
Azotemic renal insufficiency	BUN, creatinine
Obesity	Physical examination
Oral contraceptive therapy	History
Acromegaly	Physical examination; rarely, requires serum growth hormone level 2 hr after glucose administration or serum somatomedin C determination
Pheochromocytoma	History; occasionally requires urinary metanephrine determination
Aldosteronism or mineralocorticoid excess	Serum K^+ determination ($\pm$ salt loading)
Cushing's disease or syndrome	Physical examination; overnight dexamethasone suppression test

termine if the patient has these endocrinopathies. The major problem for the physician is knowing when to apply these screening tests. In the interest of cost-effectiveness, the tests should not be done on all patients who simply have hypertension and diabetes; they should be done only when there are one or more additional clinical findings to suggest the diagnosis, e.g., an increase in hand, foot, or head size for acromegaly; recurrent headaches, palpitations, or sweating for pheochromocytoma; and obesity, hirsutism, easy bruisability, osteoporosis, or menstrual abnormalities for Cushing's syndrome. Appropriate screening tests for each disorder are discussed below.

With respect to aldosterone or mineralocorticoid excess syndromes, most physicians routinely screen for this disorder by measuring serum K^+ prior to instituting antihypertensive therapy. This practice is relatively simple and inexpensive, and should be continued not only to diagnose aldosteronism or mineralocorticoid excess but also to detect decreases in serum K^+ (subsequent to diuretic therapy), which may profoundly influence insulin secretion and aggravate or provoke glucose intolerance or frank diabetes. Unprovoked hypokalemia (i.e., without diuretics, laxatives, or other causative factors) in a hypertensive patient is highly suggestive of aldosterone or mineralocorticoid excess. In patients who have been salt-restricted (voluntarily or therapeutically), however, serum K^+ may not be definitively abnormal. If the patient has been salt-restricted or if borderline values are obtained, supplemental salt ($>$ 10 g/day) should be given for 3–5 days before determining the serum K^+. With documentation of hypokalemia, further diagnostic testing is required, e.g., determining plasma aldosterone (i.e., its suppressibility) after administration of 2 L of normal saline intravenously over a 4-h period.

Two simple screening tests for acromegaly are the measurement of serum growth hormone 2 hrs after administration of an oral glucose load (normal $<$ 2 or 5 ng/ml in males and females, respectively) and measurement of serum somatomedin C. Normal values would in most cases rule out the possibility of acromegaly, but elevated values may be more difficult to interpret as they may occur in diabetic patients who are not optimally controlled.

The urinary metanephrine determination is recommended for screening patients in whom pheochromocytoma is suspected; this test is less affected by drugs and diet than the urinary vanillylmandelic acid (VMA) assay and can be used to check "spot urines" during paroxysms by expressing the metanephrine value as a function of the urinary creatinine.

The best screening test for Cushing's disease or syndrome is the overnight dexamethasone suppression test, i.e., measurement of plasma cortisol (normal $<$5 μg percent) between 8 and 9 AM after the administration of 1 mg dexamethasone between 11 PM and midnight on the preceding evening. In a general clinic setting, this screening procedure has very few false-positives ($<$10%) or false-negatives ($<$5%) and is simple to perform, inexpensive, and clinically reliable. However, it should be kept in mind that poor suppressibility (false-positives) may be encountered in patients with poorly controlled diabetes mellitus and those who are obese. In poorly controlled diabetes mellitus, secondary heightened activity of the hypothalamic-pituitary-adrenal axis may be difficult to distinguish from primary Cushing's disease by many of the commonly used clinical tests; fortunately, metyrapone testing (heightened response in Cushing's disease versus poor response in poorly controlled diabetes) or improved diabetic control will settle the issue. In obesity, the poor suppressibility of plasma cortisol can be distinguished from that observed in Cushing's disease by measuring (1) the 24-hr urinary free cortisol level; or (2) the 24-hr urinary 17-hydroxysteroids (normal <3 mg as Porter-Silber chromogens) after a 2-day, low-dose (0.5 mg every 6 hr) dexamethasone suppression test (both tests are normal in simple obesity).

PATHOLOGICAL INTERACTIONS OF HYPERTENSION AND DIABETES MELLITUS

Hypertension and diabetes are both well-known risk factors for the development of atherosclerotic macrovascular disease.[1–3] Other cardiovascular risk factors that are frequently present in hypertensive or diabetic patients include obesity, increases in serum cholesterol, and decreases in high density lipoproteins (HDLs). Of these factors, only treatment of hypertension has been shown to diminish the risk for developing cardiovascular complications. In view of the greater risk, antihypertensive therapy should be more aggressive in diabetic patients.

In addition to macrovascular disease, the coexistence of diabetes and hypertension leads to potentiation of microvascular disease. There are probably multiple mechanisms for this potentiation. Increased basement membrane thickening and "leakiness" (as evidenced by an increase in transcapillary escape rate of labeled albumin) of capillaries occurs in both diabetes mellitus and hypertension.[11] Albuminuria, an excellent clinical marker for leakiness of capillaries in the glomerular tuft, is a well-known consequence of both diabetic glomerulopathy[12] and hypertension.[13] Of great importance is the fact that improvement of either hyperglycemia or hypertension may be attended by considerable improvement in experimentally measured vascular leakiness and clinical albuminuria. Compromise of the glomerular filtration rate (GFR) is a relatively late and ominous consequence of kidney involvement due to either diabetes or hypertension; interestingly, the steady decrease in the GFR which occurs in end-stage diabetic glomerulopathy has been shown to be improved by antihypertensive therapy.[12] Diabetic retinopathy has also been found to be correlated with systolic blood pressure,[14] and hypertension is known to increase retinal leakiness of fluorescein.[11]

TREATMENT

In patients who have glucose intolerance or relatively mild noninsulin-dependent diabetes mellitus, there may be considerable pancreatic insulin reserve, and the defect in insulin secretion may be partly or wholly reversible; clearly, a major objective of antihypertensive therapy is to avoid further embarrassment of the insulin secretory mechanism in these patients. In patients who have more severe impairment of insulin secretion, e.g., in late stages of noninsulin-dependent diabetes mellitus or in most patients who have insulin-dependent diabetes mellitus, there is little or no pancreatic insulin reserve, the patient is already committed to life-long insulin therapy (which can be increased as needed), and it is unlikely that antihypertensive therapy will aggravate the diabetic state substantially through further compromise in insulin secretion.

Before discussing antihypertensive therapy further in diabetic patients, it is worthwhile to review a few important points which relate to insulin secretion. The secretion of insulin is provoked by a variety of agents which increase intracellular Ca^{2+} with or without increases in cyclic AMP. Glucose, the primary insulin secretagogue, provokes both changes, presumably as a result of its metabolism within the beta cell.[15] The plasma membrane plays a crucial role in the release and transport of Ca,$^{2+}$ and the polarization and functional integrity of the plasma membrane are profoundly dependent on K^+. Even slight decreases in serum K^+ may provoke rapid decreases in the ability to secrete insulin.[16,17] Insulin secretion is further modulated by the adrenergic nervous system[18]; α_2-adrenergic substances inhibit and β_2-adrenergic agents increase the insulin secretory response in basal and postprandial conditions.

Diuretic Therapy

For most physicians, thiazides continue to be the first step in antihypertensive therapy (Table 9-3). Unfortunately, thiazide usage presents important problems for the diabetic patient. First, thiazides can diminish glucose tolerance and provoke or aggravate overt diabetes mellitus by two mechanisms, i.e., inhibition of insulin secretion or peripheral action. Thiazide-induced inhibition of insulin secretion is probably largely due to a decrease in serum K^+, even of mild degree,[16,17] but it may also be due to a direct inhibitory effect on islet function. The mechanism whereby thiazides decrease tissue responsiveness to insulin is uncertain but may also be done to hypokalemia. As a result of inhibition of insulin secretion or action, serum insulin levels may be diminished[16,18] or increased.[19,20]

The reported severity of diabetogenic effects of thiazide diuretics has varied considerably. In some reports[19–21] glucose tolerance was found to decrease significantly in groups of nondiabetic patients who were placed on antihypertensive therapy for long periods. (It should be noted that these mean glucose values of groups obscure the fact that some individuals manifest much more dramatic blood sugar elevations, whereas most individuals show little or no appreciable change.) In other reports,[22] particularly if thiazides are used in low dosage and with careful avoidance of hypokalemia (e.g., by K^+ supplementation), there has been little or no decrease in glucose tolerance, even after 6 years of therapy. In overt diabetes mellitus[17] thiazides were found to provoke blood sugar increases in one-third of the patients challenged, but in this study relatively high dosages of thiazides were employed, and there was no attempt to avoid decreases in serum K^+.

A second major problem that has been observed with thiazides is mild (10–20 percent) increases in serum cholesterol and triglycerides, and associated increases in very low density lipoproteins (VLDL) and the total serum cholesterol/HDL cholesterol ratio.[20,23] These changes in serum lipids, although seemingly mild, may be of great importance, particularly in diabetic patients, over long periods of time. From

Table 9-3. Potential Problems for Diabetic Patients During Treatment with More Commonly Used Antihypertensive Agents

Diuretics
- Thizaides
  - Decreased insulin secretion (hyperglycemia)
  - Decreased insulin effectiveness in peripheral tissues (hyperglycemia)
  - Increased serum cholesterol (increased total cholesterol/HDL cholesterol ratio)
  - Increased serum triglycerides (VLDL)
  - Cardiac rhythm disturbances with hypokalemia or hypomagnesemia
- K^+-sparing diuretics
  - Hyperkalemia and cardiac disturbances

β-Blockers
- Decreased insulin secretion (hyperglycemia)
- Increased insulin effectiveness in peripheral tissues (hypoglycemia)
- Decreased responses to catecholamines (loss of warning symptoms during treatment and prolongation of hypoglycemia)
- Increased serum triglycerides
- Decreased HDL cholesterol
- Decreased renin release (hyporeninemia and hypoaldosteronism)
- Vasoconstriction (aggravation of peripheral vascular disease, paradoxical pressor responses)
- Decreased cardiac output (fluid retention, decreased GFR, congestive heart failure)

α-Blockers
- Postural hypotension

Centrally acting agents
- Clonidine: decreased insulin secretion (acutely), impotence
- Aldomet: impotence
- Guanethidine: postural hypotension, impotence

Peripheral vasodilators (hydralazine, minoxidil)
- Postural Hypotension, reflex tachycardia

Converting enzyme inhibitors (captopril)
- Hypoaldosteronism and hyperkalemia
- False-positive ketone reactions

analysis of large populations studies, in fact, it has been questioned[24] why mortality due to coronary heart disease has not significantly decreased in certain groups given antihypertensive therapy despite improved blood pressure and decreased death rates due to other causes, cerebrovascular disease in particular. The failure to observe improvement in coronary artery disease mortality may conceivably be due to the increases in serum lipids which were provoked by these agents. Further work is needed to evaluate this problem. In the meantime, physicians should be aware of the problem and monitor serum lipids carefully in patients who are placed on thiazides; if lipid elevations occur, there should be intensification of dietary measures to reverse these increases or consideration given to changing therapy.

With the above thoughts in mind, it may be questioned whether thiazides should be employed as first-line agents in patients with diabetes mellitus. As stated above, in patients who have insulin-dependent diabetes mellitus, where there is little or no appreciable pancreatic insulin reserve, thiazides will probably not further compromise the diabetic state and indeed may be effective in the treatment of hypertension associated with glomerulopathy-induced plasma volume expansion. In diabetic or glucose-intolerant patients who still have insulin secretory reserve, thiazides may still be used as the first line of antihypertensive therapy, but they should be used more cautiously. Because the therapeutic benefit/risk ratio decreases with increasing doses of thiazides, these agents should be used at the lowest possible dosage (e.g., hopefully 25–50 mg hydrochlorthiazide per day). Similarly, decreases in K^+ should be avoided; to this end, consideration should be given to using thiazide–triamterene or thiazide–spironolactone (K^+-sparing) combinations or prophylactic K^+ supplements. In most patients with milder forms of diabetes mellitus (where remaining insulin secretory reserve should be preserved as much as possible), the K^+-sparing diuretics or K^+ supplementation are well tolerated. However, in some patients, particularly those with even early renal impairment, there may be overt or incipient hyporeninemic (or occasionally hyperreninemic) hypoaldosteronism, and K^+-sparing diuretics or K^+ supplements may be harmful, provoking clinically dangerous hyperkalemia. Obviously, the decision to employ these agents must be arrived at after careful consideration of all factors; and, if used, serum K^+ and renal function must be monitored closely.

The question is frequently asked whether furosemide is less diabetogenic than thiazide diuretics. This may be the case, as furosemide does not directly diminish insulin secretion; on the other hand, diabetogenic effects have certainly been observed[19] and are presumably due to hypokalemia. Along these lines, it may also be noted that although furosemide is theoretically less diabetogenic than thiazides the more prolonged action of the latter agents make them more ideal for treating hypertension.

Beta-Blockers

During recent years β-blockers have been used extensively as first- or second-line agents for the treatment of hypertension; as such, these agents have proved very useful because of their clinical effectiveness and low incidence of troublesome side effects. The mechanisms whereby β-blockers diminish blood pressure include decreases in cardiac output, sympathetic discharge from the central nervous system (a "central effect"), and renal renin secretion. Unfortunately, peripheral resistance does not diminish with most β-blockers, although a new agent, pindolol, reportedly diminishes peripheral resistance, perhaps by virtue of its mild β-adrenergic agonistic properties. Along these lines, it should be noted that endogenous and exogenous β-adrenergic agonists promote vasodilatation in many vascular beds, not vasoconstriction; on the other hand, α-adrenergic agonists cause vasoconstriction. The latter explains why: (1) peripheral resistance generally increases during β-blockade; (2) hypertensive crises can occur in situations (e.g., during stress, hypoglycemia, and release of catecholamines) where α-adrenergic activity is increased and unopposed (as during drug-induced β-blockade); and (3) vasospastic disease may be aggravated by β-blockers.

In patients who have diabetes mellitus, there a number of potential problems which may be provoked or aggravated by the β-blockers. First, with respect to blood sugar regulation, as stated above, the blockade of β_2-adrenergic receptors diminishes insulin secretion, both basally and in response to a glucose challenge, in normal and diabetic individuals. In diabetic patients who have a partially compromised insulin secretory mechanism, this may lead to an increase in blood glucose; for example, in some studies[25] blood glucose increases of 15–25 mg percent on the average have been observed in diabetic patients who are treated with β-blockers (in a few patients the increases were much more striking). In other studies,[26] however, there were little or no changes in blood glucose levels in diabetic patients treated with metoprolol, and this may reflect the use of a selective β_1-blocker, a greater insulin secretory reserve in these patients, or a counterbalancing increase in peripheral glucose utilization.[27] The latter increase in peripheral glucose utilization, which may occur during β_2-adrenergic blockade, on the other hand, may contribute to the development and prolongation of hypoglycemia observed in response to insulin therapy.[27] Along these lines, β-blockers may intensify insulin-induced hypoglycemia in diabetic patients[28] by other mechanisms as well, e.g., decreased action of catecholamines, which mobilize hepatic carbohydrate stores.

In addition to glucose metabolism, a second problem associated with β-blocker therapy, and particularly worrisome in the diabetic patient, is a significant increase in serum triglycerides and a decrease in HDLs[23,29] (which are thought to have a protective influence for development of coronary artery disease). Further work is required to determine if these changes in serum lipids are of long-term importance.

Other problems frequently encountered in diabetic patients and which can be aggravated by use of β-blockers include: (1) peripheral vascular disease; (2) congestive heart failure; (3) hyporeninemia and consequent hypoaldosteronism and hyperkalemia; and (4) paradoxical pressor responses during hypoglycemic episodes.

Although there may be problems associated with the use of β-blockers in diabetic patients, these agents are nonetheless very useful for treating hypertension in the general population and occasionally must be used in diabetic patients. Because cardioselective (β_1) blockers are less likely to diminish insulin secretion or impair vasodilatation, these agents may be of greater value than nonselective (β_1 + β_2) agents in treating diabetic hypertensive patients. However, it should be realized that there is never an exclusively complete separation of β_1 and β_2 receptors in various target tissues; moreover, β_1-blocking agents may affect β_2 receptors, particularly at higher dosages.

If β-blocker therapy is employed in diabetic patients who have insulin reserve, attention should be given to the possibility that glycemic control may be impaired as a result of decreases in insulin secretion. If β-blockers are employed in patients who are being treated with insulin, the patient should be told that hypoglycemia may be a particular problem in terms of its severity and the failure to have certain warning symptoms (palpitations, tremors). The patient should be admonished not to miss meals or supplemental feedings and should be instructed that although palpitations may no longer serve as a warning signal for hypoglycemia the sweating response should remain intact. The physician should also closely monitor serum lipids, and if changes occur appropriate dietary measures should be intensified or the therapeutic regimen changed.

α-Blockers

During recent years prazosin, a selective α_1-blocker, has become available for treatment of hypertension. This agent is much more useful than nonselective α_1 + α_2-blockers, which had been available previously, e.g., regitine and dibenzyline. The latter agents, by inhibiting α_2 receptors, concomitantly block the normal feedback loop whereby norepinephrine inhibits its own secretion from nerve endings, and this leads to inordinate increases in norepinephrine secretion and consequent increases in blood pressure and heart rate. With the selective α_1-blockers, the inhibitory feedback loop remains intact, and there is a better blood-pressure-lowering effect and a decrease in bothersome symptoms, e.g., reflex tachycardia. The α_1-blockers have been shown to have no detrimental effects on insulin secretion, glucose metabolism, or serum lipids.[30] Thus α_1-blockers seem to be particularly well suited for use in diabetic patients.

Although prazosin has primarily been used as a "second line" antihypertensive agent and is more effective in the presence of a diuretic, it has been used effectively as a first-line antihypertensive agent and alone is capable of decreasing blood pressure by approximately 15–20 mm Hg.[30] Hence, this agent may be particularly useful in patients whose diabetic state is aggravated by more diabetogenic agents, e.g., thiazides or β-blockers.

The only major side effect of prazosin has been the development of postural hypotension, particularly with the first dose. Consequently, the patient should be told to take the first dose at bedtime and should avoid interruptions in therapy, as the "first dose" phenomenon may recur with resumption of treatment. In patients who have diabetic neuropathy and postural hypotension, prazosin should be avoided.

α_2-Adrenergic Agonists

As stated above, α_2-adrenergic agents may diminish insulin secretion. Clonidine, an α_2-agonist, lowers blood pressure through its "central effect," causing a decrease in total sympathetic discharge. In short-term studies this agent has been found to impair insulin secretion, apparently via direct effects on β-cells of the pancreatic islets.[31] In long-term studies, however, diabetogenic effects of clonidine have not been reported,[32] and this may reflect the fact that direct inhibitory effects of clonidine on islets may be counterbalanced by decreases (via a central effect) in endogenously liberated α-adrenergic catecholamines. In any event, it would be prudent to closely monitor blood sugar in diabetic patients who are treated with clonidine.

Other Antihypertensive Agents

Methyldopa, another centrally acting agent, is not known to influence insulin secretion or glucose metabolism. The only special considerations that relate to diabetes mellitus are that methyldopa may cause sexual impotence and decrease serum HDLs.[23,29]

Hydralazine, a peripheral vasodilator, is also without significant effect on insulin secretion, glucose metabolism, or lipid metabolism. This agent is used cautiously in patients who have postural hypotension or coronary artery disease.

Converting enzyme inhibitors, e.g., captopril, may aggravate any tendencies to develop hypoaldosteronism, and these agents have been reported to produce a false-positive reaction for urinary ketones.

There is conflicting information concerning the effects of Ca^{2+} channelblockers on insulin secretion and glucose homeostasis; in some studies insulin secretion, as might be expected, was impaired, but in other studies no untoward effects were observed.

Generalizations and Special Considerations

Patients With Glucose Intolerance or Mild to Moderate Noninsulin-Dependent Diabetes Mellitus. Although thiazides and β-blockers may have diabetogenic properties, as stated above, careful use of these agents in hypertensive patients may actually improve glucose tolerance (see above). Small doses of thiazides coupled with K^+ supplements or K^+-sparing diuretics (providing there is no renal impairment, and serum K^+ is monitored closely to avoid hyperkalemia) or small doses of cardioselective β_1-blockers or prazosin may be employed as first-line agents or used in combination as needed to control blood pressure. Of these, prazosin is the only agent that can be used without risk for impairment of glucose tolerance. Methyldopa and hydralazine can also be added as second- or third-line agents as needed, with no apparent risk for impairment of glucose tolerance.

Insulin-Dependent Diabetes Mellitus or Severe Noninsulin-Dependent Diabetes Mellitus With Little Pancreatic Insulin Reserve. When there is little or no pancreatic insulin reserve and it is clear that the patient is going to be on lifelong insulin treatment, there is less concern that antihypertensive agents will compromise insulin secretion. Thiazides (without K^+-sparing combinations or K^+ supplements—unless required for hypokalemia—as these patients are not infrequently susceptible to develop hyperkalemia) (see above) and β_1-blockers can then be used with less concern for their diabetogenic properties. However, the other effects of these agents on diabetes mellitus should not be disregarded. For example, careful attention should be given to changes in serum lipids. Moreover, β_1-blockers may be used but only with extreme caution in patients who are on insulin (see above); obviously if hypoglycemia is a recurrent problem, it is best to avoid the β-blockers entirely. Other antihypertensive agents can be employed in these diabetic patients as in the general nondiabetic population.

Diabetic Nephropathy. Because hypertension associated with diabetic nephropathy is largely due to sodium retention and plasma volume expansion, the major thrust of therapy is to alleviate this problem. A low-salt diet and diuretic therapy are of greatest importance. In early stages, thiazides (without K^+-sparing combinations or K^+ supplements because these patients commonly develop hyporeninemic hypoaldosteronism and hyperkalemia) may be employed, but stronger loop diuretics may be required with the progression of renal disease (e.g., large doses of furosemide may be required, up to 160 mg p.o. twice daily). Other agents may be added, including prazosin, β_1-blockers (if hypoglycemia is not a problem), combinations of prazosin and β_1-blockers, hydralazine, methyldopa, clonidine, and minoxidil. If β-blockers or angiotensin-converting enzyme blocking agents are employed, serum K^+ should be monitored, as these antihypertensive agents may aggravate or unmask latent hyporeninemic hypoaldosteronism. In late stages (particularly with azotemia) where diuretic therapy cannot effect significant natriuresis, dialysis may be helpful in removing excess fluids and improving blood pressure.

Diabetic Patients With Autonomic Neuropathy and Postural Hypoten-

sion. The problem of coexisting hypertension and orthostatic hypotension occurs occasionally in hypertensive diabetic patients who develop peripheral autonomic neuropathy. Unfortunately, it is very difficult to treat these problems effectively. Virtually every antihypertensive agent can aggravate postural hypotension, but centrally acting agents (clonidine and to a lesser extent methyldopa) are less likely to be serious offenders. Of the β-blockers, which are also generally not associated with severe postural hypotension, pindolol (perhaps because of its intrinsic sympathomimetic agonist properties) is even less likely to cause postural hypotension. Those agents which provoke maximum peripheral vasodilatation (prazosin, hydralazine, minoxidil) are most likely to provoke or aggravate postural hypotension; guanethidine is another serious offender. Severe volume depletion by diuretic therapy may also compound the problem. Measures which may be helpful in treating postural hypotension include: elevation of the head of the bed during sleep; use of elastic stockings and abdominal binders; and avoidance of rapid changes in position. Occasionally it is necessary to employ Fluorinef to expand plasma volume and couple this with centrally active antihypertensive agents. Very rarely, short-acting nasal Neo-Synephrine preparations may be taken in small amounts in anticipation of arising from the supine to the standing position.

Sexual Dysfunction. Virtually every antihypertensive agent has been incriminated as impairing the ability to have erections or ejaculate. Guanethidine, for example, commonly causes the latter problem. To date, adverse effects of prazosin on sexual function have not been noted. Other agents which are less likely to be offenders are thiazide or loop diuretics, β-blockers, and hydralazine. Along with guanethidine, methyldopa and clonidine are most likely to be associated with changes in potency and sexual function.

SUMMARY

It seems clear that diabetic patients who have hypertension are particularly vulnerable to the development of macrovascular and microvascular disease; aggressive and effective antihypertensive treatment is therefore of utmost importance in these patients. In addition, the physician is confronted initially with problems in diagnosing those primary disorders which may cause secondary hypertension and diabetes mellitus and is challenged thereafter in devising a therapeutic regiment which effectively controls blood pressure without aggravating the diabetic state or its complications. There are a number of therapeutic options which are available to accomplish the latter goal, but unfortunately none is without fault. For the latter reason, it is imperative that the physician pay even more attention to factors which are often neglected, viz., attainment and maintenance of ideal body weight and diminution of dietary sodium chloride intake, at least to reasonable levels (e.g., 4g/day). These factors cannot be emphasized too strongly, as they not only may of themselves decrease blood pressure mildly (5–10 mm Hg) but, moreover, diminish the tendency to develop hypokalemia with diuretic therapy and decrease the dosage of hypertensive medication (of any sort) required to effect normal blood pressure. Exercise is another important adjunct that should be stressed, as this may also have salutory effects on both blood pressure (perhaps through volume depletion secondary to sweating-induced salt loss) and hyperglycemia. Another factor which should not be overlooked is the control of hyperglycemia, which, as stated above, may be associated with expansion of plasma volume. Fortunately, when these general measures are combined with careful and judicious use of antihypertensive agents, diabetic patients can usually be rendered normotensive with minimal side effects.

REFERENCES

1. Garcia MJ, McNamara PM, Gordon T, Kannell WB: Morbidity and mortality in diabetes in the Framingham population. Diabetes 23:105, 1974
2. Kannel WB, McGee DL: Diabetes and glucose tolerance as risk factors for cardiovascular disease: the Framingham study. Diabetes Care 2:120, 1979
3. Ostrander LD, Francis T Jr, Hayner NS, et al: The relationship of cardiovascular disease to hyperglycemia. Ann Intern Med 62:118, 1965
4. Christlieb AR, Warram JH, Krolewski AS, et al: Hypertension: the major risk factor in juvenile-onset insulin-dependent diabetics. Diabetes 30:90, 1981
5. White P: Natural course and prognosis of juvenile diabetes. Diabetes 5:445, 1956
6. Berglund G, Larsson B, Andersson O, et al: Body composition and glucose metabolismm in hypertensive middle-aged males. Acta Med Scand 200:163, 1976
7. Mackay JD, Hayakawa H, Watkins PJ: Cardiovascular effects of insulin: plasma volume changes in diabetics. Diabetologia 15:453, 1978
8. Axelrod L: Response of congestive heart failure to correction of hyperglycemia in the presence of diabetic nephropathy. N Engl J Med 293:1243, 1975
9. Christlieb AR, Kaldany A, D'Elia JA: Plasma renin activity and hypertension in diabetes mellitus. Diabetes 25:969, 1976
10. Christlieb AR: The hypertensions of diabetes. Diabetes Care 5:50, 1982
11. Parving H-H: Microvascular permeability to plasma proteins in hypertension and diabetes mellitus in man—on the pathogenesis of hypertensive and diabetic microangiopathy. Dan Med Bull 22:217, 1975
12. Mogensen CE: Renal function changes in diabetes. Diabetes 25:872, 1976
13. Parving H-H, Andersen AR, Smidt UM, et al: Reduced albuminuria during early and aggressive antihypertensive treatment of insulin-dependent diabetic patients with diabetic nephropathy. Diabetes Care 4:459, 1981
14. Knowler WC, Bennett PH, Ballintine EJ: Increased incidence of retinopathy in diabetics with elevated blood pressure. N Engl J Med 302:645, 1980
15. Wollheim CB, Sharp GWG: Regulation of insulin release by calcium. Physiol Rev 61:919, 1981
16. Gorden P: Glucose intolerance with hypokalemia: failure of short-term potassium depletion in normal subjects to reproduce the glucose and insulin abnormalities of clinical hypokalemia. Diabetes 22:544, 1973
17. Goldner MG, Zarowitz H, Akgun S: Hyperglycemia and glycosuria due to thiazide derivatives administered in diabetes mellitus. N Engl J Med 262:403, 1960
18. Robertson RP, Porte D Jr: Adrenergic modulation of basal insulin secretion in man. Diabetes 22:1, 1973
19. Breckenridge A, Wellborn TA, Dollery CT, Fraser R: Glucose tolerance in hypertensive patients on long-term diuretic therapy. Lancet 1:61, 1967

20. Ames RP: Negative effects of diuretic drugs on metabolic risk factors for coronary heart disease: possible alternative drug therapies. Am J Cardiol 51:632, 1983
21. Lewis PJ, Petrie A, Kohner EM, Dollery CT: Deterioration of glucose tolerance in hypertensive patients on prolonged diuretic treatment. Lancet 1:564, 1976
22. Berglund G, Andersson O: Beta-blockers or diuretics in hypertension? A six year follow-up of blood pressure and metabolic side effects. Lancet 1:744, 1981
23. Ames RP, Hill P: Antihypertensive therapy and the risk of coronary heart disease. J Cardiovasc Pharmacol 4:S206, 1982
24. Kaplan NM: Introduction to a symposium on initial therapy in hypertension. Am J Cardiol 51:619, 1983
25. Wright AD, Barber SG, Kendall MJ, Poole PH: Beta-adrenoceptor-blocking drugs and blood sugar control in diabetes mellitus. Br Med J 1:159, 1979
26. Garrett BN, Raskin P, Kaplan NM: Metoprolol in diabetes mellitus: effect on glucose homeostasis. Clin Sci 59:469S, 1980
27. Lauridsen UB, Christensen NJ, Lyngsoe J: Effects of nonselective and β_1-selective blockade on glucose metabolism and hormone responses during insulin-induced hypoglycemia in normal man. J Clin Endocrinol Metab 56:876, 1983
28. DeFeo P, Bolli G, Perriello G, et al: The adrenergic contribution to glucose counterregulation in type I diabetes mellitus: dependency on A-cell function and mediation through β_2-adrenergic receptors. Diabetes 32:887, 1983
29. Cutler R: Effects of antihypertensive agents on lipid metabolism. Am J Cardiol 51:628, 1983
30. Okun R: Effectiveness of prazosin as initial antihypertensive therapy. Am J Cardiol 51:644, 1983
31. Metz SA, Halter JB, Robertson RP: Induction of defective insulin secretion and impaired glucose tolerance by clonidine: selective stimulation of metabolic alpha-adrenergic pathways. Diabetes 27:554, 1978
32. Houston MC: Clonidine hydrochloride: review of pharmacologic and clinical aspects. Prog Cardiovas Dis 23:337, 1981

10 Management of the Pregnant Diabetic

Donald R. Coustan

Over the past 60 years a remarkable evolution has occurred in the approach to pregnancy management in the diabetic, with a concomitant progressive improvement in outcome for both the mother and her child. Prior to the availability of insulin in the early 1920s, reports of pregnancy among diabetics were rare; maternal mortality rates approached 50 percent, and perinatal mortality (stillbirths plus neonatal deaths) was similarly high. The first two decades after the isolation of insulin saw a rapid drop in maternal death rates, such that more than 99 percent of diabetic women survived their pregnancies by the early 1950s. Currently, with the exception of women with known coronary artery disease, pregnancy does not seem to increase the mortality risk for diabetic women more than for women in the general population. Perinatal mortality declined much more slowly. It is only during the past 20 years that rates below 10 percent have been attainable; during the past decade most reports from tertiary perinatal centers have described perinatal mortality among diabetic pregnancies below 5 percent (compared to 1–2 percent in the general population). As death rates have diminished, the increased incidence of congenital anomalies among infants of diabetic mothers has come to the forefront as the single most important remaining problem. Efforts are currently under way throughout the world to try to solve this problem, and some success has been achieved. This chapter outlines an approach to the management of pregnancy in the diabetic woman. The organization of the approach is chronological, starting with preconceptional counseling and ending in the postpartum period.

MANAGEMENT PRIOR TO CONCEPTION

Congenital anomalies occur in infants of diabetic mothers two to three times more frequently than in the general population. The cause of this increased incidence of birth defects remains to be established, but it is clear that whatever is causing them must be operating prior to 8 weeks after the last menstrual period (i.e., 6 weeks after conception), as fetal development has by then progressed beyond the point when commonly described anomalous structures have differentiated.[1] The likelihood of a genetic cause is considered to be low, as the offspring of diabetic fathers and non-diabetic mothers do not have more abnormalities than the general population. Thus some factor in the intrauterine environment, present during the first 8 weeks of gestation (or perhaps prior to conception), is probably responsible. Unfortunately, this critical time period in human gestation is difficult to study, as most pregnant women do not present for care until after the second missed menstrual period. The availability of tests measuring glycosylated hemoglobin (a reflection of glycemic control over the past few months) made it possible to assess glucose control prior to the time diabetic pregnant women consult their physicians. Researchers in England[2] and then at the Joslin Clinic[3] reported an increased incidence of congenital anomalies among offspring of diabetic mothers whose glycosylated hemoglobin levels were particularly high during the first trimester compared with those of offspring of diabetic mothers with more nearly normal glycosylated hemoglobin levels. These findings suggested, but did not prove, that poor diabetic control with hyperglycemia during early pregnancy (or prior to conception) may be related to the high incidence of birth defects described above. More recently (Table 10-1) a group of East German investigators[4] reported that among 128 overt diabetics registering for care and starting on a program of strict metabolic control (goals = plasma glucose of 60–130 mg/dl with a 24-hr mean of 80–90 mg/dl) prior to conception only one anomalous baby was born (0.8 percent). Among a group of 292 diabetics beginning intensive metabolic control after 8 weeks, 22 anomalous babies were born (7.5 percent). Although this was not a prospective randomized trial, it is a powerful demonstration of the importance of diabetic control prior to conception and/or during the first 8 weeks of gestation in preventing birth defects.

Recommendation: Diabetic women of childbearing age should be counseled about pregnancy prior to conception. They should be encouraged to consult a specialist in diabetes and/or high-risk pregnancies to discuss the implications of their diabetic con-

Table 10-1. Congenital Malformations Related to White's Classes and to the Onset of Strict Metabolic Control

White's Class	Registered Prepregnancy		Registered After 8 Weeks' Gestation		Total	
	Anomalies	No Anomalies	Anomalies	No Anomalies	Anomalies	No Anomalies
B	1	35	2 (2.3%)	85	3	120
C	0	35	9 (12.2%)	75	9	110
D	0	49	9 (9.1%)	90	9	139
R	0	8	2 (9.1%)	20	2	28
Total	1	127	22	270	23	397
	(0.8%)		(7.5%)		(5.5%)	

Source: Fuhrmann K, Reiher H, Semmler K, et al: Prevention of congenital malformations in infants of insulin dependent diabetic mothers. Diabetes Care 6:219, 1983.

$\chi^2 = 7.84 p < 0.01$, for anomalies in group (all classes) with onset of metablic control before conception compared with group (all classes) with onset of control after 8 weeks' gestation.

dition on pregnancy. Finally, they should be encouraged to begin a regimen of intensive metabolic control, including frequent home blood glucose monitoring, before becoming pregnant. It is reasonable to suggest that pregnancy be deferred until glysosylated hemoglobin levels are in or near the normal nondiabetic range.

METABOLIC MANAGEMENT DURING PREGNANCY

There is a strong correlation between the adequacy of maternal metabolic control during the third trimester and perinatal survival[5] (Fig. 10-1). During the mid-1960s and early 1970s, retrospective studies from Ireland[6] and Sweden[7] pointed out this relationship; since that time series from all over the world have reported perinatal mortality rates below 5 percent when intensive maternal metabolic control was attempted. The single series[8] in which no significant improvement in perinatal survival could be shown in tightly controlled pregnant diabetics reported perinatal mortality rates of 0 percent in the most euglycemic group, 3.5 percent in the intermediate group, and 12.5 percent in the group whose control was poorest. The series was too small for statistical significance.

Goals for Metabolic Control

The previously mentioned retrospective series, as well as metabolic studies of normal pregnant women, suggested that plasma glucose levels between 60 and 120 mg/dl are associated with the lowest perinatal mortality rates in diabetic pregnancies

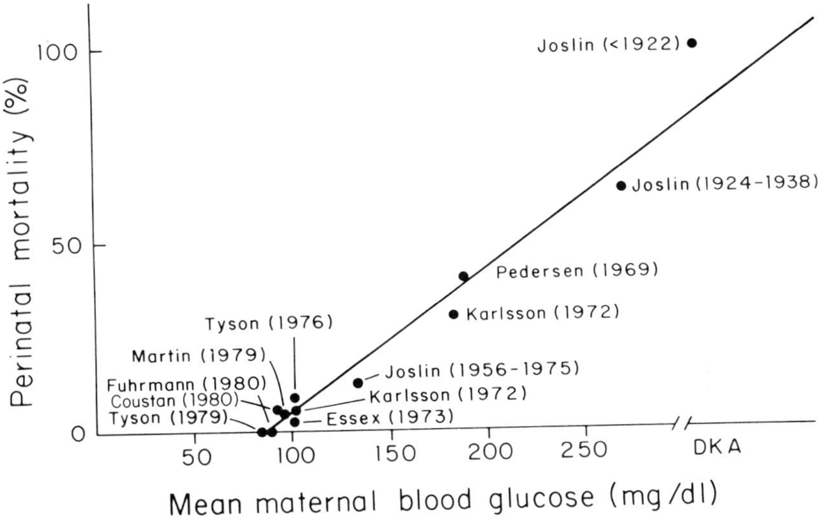

Fig. 10-1. Correlation of mean maternal blood glucose during the third trimester with perinatal mortality. (Adapted with permission from Jovanovic L, Peterson CM: Management of the pregnant, insulin-dependent diabetic woman. Diabetes Care 3:63, 1980.)

and represent the normal range for nondiabetic pregnancies. These, then, are the goals that are most appropriate for the plasma glucose levels of the pregnant diabetic. However, because goals tend to become "self-fulfilling prophecies" (i.e., plasma glucose values over the long run tend to cluster around whatever goals are set because the insulin dose is increased only if the goals are exceeded), we adjust our insulin regimen upward if plasma glucose levels exceed 100 mg/dl.

Recommendation: Aim for plasma glucose values of 60–120 mg/dl throughout the day.

Measurement of Glucose

Measurement of the urinary glucose concentration is of little value in managing the pregnant diabetic. In the first place, renal thresholds for glucose are constantly changing during pregnancy (indeed during the course of each day renal plasma flow increases and decreases with positional changes), rendering urine glucose results meaningless. Secondly, with plasma glucose between 60 and 120 mg/dl, urine glucose is negative most of the time. Thus it was clear as long as 10 years ago that blood glucose measurements, done frequently, were necessary to achieve the kind of excellent metabolic control associated with a favorable outcome. The need for frequent blood glucose determinations caused a multitude of logistic problems for pregnant diabetic women. Commercial laboratories were open only during business hours, so that early morning or evening glucose values were difficult to obtain. The patient's normal activities were interrupted by frequent trips to and from the laboratory. Thus the blood glucose levels obtained were not even representative of a normal day. Long-term hospitalization was often necessary. Over the past 5 years, home blood glucose monitoring, with or without a reflectance meter, has become widely available and less expensive. Currently, home monitoring is the standard for glucose measurement in the diabetic pregnancy. The advantages of such home monitoring include its greater accuracy and relevance (compared to urine testing), its convenience and portability, and its lower cost (as compared to laboratory blood glucose determination).

When home blood glucose monitoring first became available, we thought it would be difficult to convince our patients to test their blood three times in a day at least once or twice a week. In fact, they appreciated the newly found ability to gain some control over and understanding of their own glucose metabolism and tested much more often than we had requested. Many schemes for glucose testing are currently being used. We ask our patients to test a minimum of four times each day: (1) fasting; (2) 2 hr after breakfast; (3) late afternoon; and (4) 2 hr after dinner. Other published protocols call for testing at each premeal time, or six times daily. The important thing is that blood glucose be tested throughout the day to get a "profile" of metabolic control. All too often we encounter the pregnant diabetic woman who tells us that she has been in "very good control with all blood sugars under 120 mg/dl." On closer questioning we find that her blood glucose was being checked every week or two at her physician's office, at 3 P.M. We find out that this "excellent control" has been accomplished with one injection of intermediate-acting insulin each morning. What has been accomplished is that the patient is euglycemic once each day, at the peak of absorption of her intermediate-acting insulin. Throughout the rest of the day, her control is undocumented. Jovanovic and Peterson[9] aptly described three types of diabetic control: (1) good control; (2) poor control; and (3) undocumented control, which is the same as poor control.

As mentioned earlier in this chapter, glycosylated hemoglobin measurement is a useful way to assess control over the previous 1–2 months if blood glucose measurements are not available. It might be tempting to substitute glycosylated hemoglobin measurements for the frequent blood glucose determinations described above. Unfortunately, glycosylated hemoglobin determinations are not discriminative enough to differentiate between, for example, a patient with an average glucose level of 90 mg/dl and another averaging 135 mg/dl. This may be due to the fact that most laboratories use a relatively nonspecific method which measures hemoglobin A_1 rather than A_{1C}, or it may be inherent in the measurement itself. The fact is that in most of our pregnant diabetic patients *daily* adjustments of insulin dosage (based on blood glucose determinations) are necessary. No test done monthly, or even weekly, would allow that sort of "fine tuning." We obtain a glycosylated hemoglobin measurement at monthly intervals, but only as additional documentation of control, not as the primary variable to be followed.

Recommendation: Home blood glucose monitoring, performed at least four times daily, is the method of choice for assessing control in diabetic pregnancies.

Diet

Numerous dietary prescriptions have been proposed for the diabetic pregnancy. We use a scheme[10] (Table 10-2) in which total caloric intake is based on ideal body weight. Although the usual dietary protein intake recommended for pregnant women is 75–90 g/day, we suggest 125 g (500 claories) in an attempt to smooth out the peaks and valleys of glucose excursions throughout the day (protein being absorbed and transformed into glucose more slowly than carbohydrate). In order to ingest 125 g of protein in a palatable form, fat intake must also be increased (most high-protein foods also being high in fat). The caloric content of the meals is increased from breakfast to lunch to dinner, in keeping with typical American dietary habits. In addition to the bedtime snack, mid-morning or mid-afternoon snacks are added as necessary. During the second half of pregnancy, no patient is prescribed fewer than 1800 calories a day

Table 10-2. Composition of a Sample 2000-Calorie Diet[a]

					Total diet	
Constituent	Breakfast	Lunch	Dinner	Snack	g	%
Protein	22	40	45	16	123	25
Carbohydrate	57	57	57	19	190	37.5
Fat	18	24	28	12	82	37.5
Percent of total calories	24	30	33	13		100

Source: Lewis SB, Murray WK, Wallin JB, et al: Improved glucose control in non-hospitalized pregnant diabetic patients. Obstet Gynecol 48:260, 1976.

[a] All diet prescriptions were based on 125 g protein; fat and carbohydrate were equally divided for the remainder of calories. Calories were 30–35 kcal/kg/day.

and it is rare to suggest more than 2800 calories a day. During the first half of pregnancy, many women find it difficult to ingest 30–35kcal/kg ideal body weight, and lower intake is permissible so long as weight gain occurs at a normal rate. Similarly, later in pregnancy, if weight gain (not merely fluid retention) is excessive, the caloric intake can be adjusted downward.

Other equally appropriate dietary schemes exist. What is probably much more important than the particular prescription for diet is the acceptance of that diet by the patient and her constancy in following it. Roversi et al.[11] used a plan in which the pregnant diabetic woman tells the nutritionist what she would like to eat (without particular regard for dietary principles), and the nutritionist then helps the patient work out a plan for using that diet, the contract being that the patient will continue to eat the same diet (or its equivalent) at the same time of day each day throughout the pregnancy. If the patient decides to change the diet, she is brought back into the hospital and her insulin dosage is readjusted to the new diet. Using this plan, the outcomes in diabetic pregnancies reported by Roversi et al. are comparable to the best reported throughout the world. What is especially interesting is that their patients generally request a diet that turns out to be fairly close to what would be recommended using commonly employed nutritional principles. We have found Roversi's experience to be very helpful to us, especially when dealing with the various cultural differences in approach to diet we encounter. We encourage our nutritionists to be quite flexible in arriving at a dietary plan, with the knowledge that our patients are much more likely to follow the diet consistently if it is based on their nutritional habits and desires than if it is suited only to our perception of an ideal diet. It is clear that our efforts at meticulous metabolic control are doomed to failure if the patient varies the timing and content of her diet (and/or exercise periods) each day, and that, conversely, we can tailor our insulin dosage to fit just about any diet plan, so long as it is taken consistently with respect to timing and content each day.

Recommendation: Prescribe a diet that is acceptable to the patient, even if not 100 percent compatible with a predetermined scheme; emphasize to the patient that constancy is the cornerstone of her care.

Insulin

It is generally believed that most of the morbidity seen in the infant of a diabetic mother is related to fetal hyperinsulinemia. According to the widely accepted "Pedersen hypothesis,"[12] sustained or intermittent maternal hyperglycemia is associated with fetal hyperglycemia, as glucose crosses the placenta rapidly by a process of facilitated diffusion. Fetal hyperglycemia induces the fetal pancreas to produce insulin in greater than average quantities. Insulin crosses the placenta poorly or not at all, so that the increased fetal insulin cannot lower maternal blood glucose levels and thus cannot lower fetal blood glucose levels. Fetal insulin acts as a "growth hormone," and high levels are associated with macrosomia.[13] Some experimental evidence suggests that high fetal insulin levels can delay maturation of the fetal lungs. Neonatal hypoglycemia can occur if fetal insulin levels are high at the time of delivery, when clamping the umbilical cord suddenly shuts off the abundant supply of glucose coming from the mother. The possibility that fetal hyperinsulinemia and/or hyperglycemia can cause chronic asphyxia *in utero* is currently being investigated; if this turns out to be the case, it is likely that the asphyxia is responsible for the higher than normal levels of erythropoietin[14] seen in the umbilical cord blood of some infants of diabetic mothers. Those elevated levels of erythropoietin are likely responsible for the increased incidence of plethora and neonatal jaundice seen in such infants.

The above description of the deleterious effects of high fetal insulin levels is meant to explain why oral hypoglycemic agents are contraindicated in the pregnant diabetic. One of the mechanisms of action of such agents is to stimulate pancreatic insulin production. Because the available oral agents cross the placenta, their use might be associated with augmentation of fetal insulin production and/or release, an effect which would accentuate the presumed pathophysiology seen in such pregnancies. In fact, there have been case reports of prolonged neonatal hypoglycemia in some infants whose diabetic mothers were treated with oral hypoglycemic agents (although other series have described no such ill effects). For the time being, it seems most reasonable to avoid these agents in treating the pregnant diabetic woman.

Insulin is the treatment of choice for normalizing blood glucose levels in the pregnant diabetic woman. Because it does not cross the placenta, insulin administered to the mother does not raise fetal insulin levels. In fact, preventing maternal hyperglycemia results in lower fetal insulin levels. Numerous schemes for insulin administration have been suggested, and those in which multiple injections throughout the day are utilized seem to be successful. Although it may be theoretically ideal to use an injection of short-acting insulin before each meal and snack and with intermediate-acting insulin added at bedtime, we find that most (but not all) patients can be managed with two injections a day of mixed short-acting and intermediate-acting insulin.

We previously published[10] a formula for prescribing insulin based on studies of insulin release throughout the day in nondiabetic pregnant women[15] (Fig. 10-2). The proportions of NPH and regular insulin (2:1 before breafast; 1:1 before dinner; total morning dose is twice the total evening dose) should be considered a starting point and based on the assumption that the patient has no endogenous insulin release. Such is not always the case, and it is a rare patient who continues to take insulin in the same proportions throughout her pregnancy. Each component of the insulin formula is varied in proportion to the blood glucose level at the time of day closest to its peak of action. For example, the morning regular insulin dose is increased to cover high values during the mid-morning. The morning NPH dose covers the mid-afternoon glucose level. The evening regular insulin covers the evening value, and the evening NPH dose is responsible for the next morning's fasting blood sugar. In general, we respond to today's high glucose value by increasing the appropriate insulin dose *tomorrow,* rather than by adding an extra *ad hoc* insulin dose at the time of the high value. For example, if a patient reports a blood glucose level of 150 mg/dl at 10 AM, we do not have her take supplementary regular insulin at 10 AM. If we did, that insulin would be peaking in the afternoon, at the same time her morning NPH is most active. Instead, we suggest increasing tomorrow morning's regular insulin dosage on the assumption that the increased blood sugar was related to the normal increasing insulin requirements of pregnancy. (If, however, the patient knows why her glucose

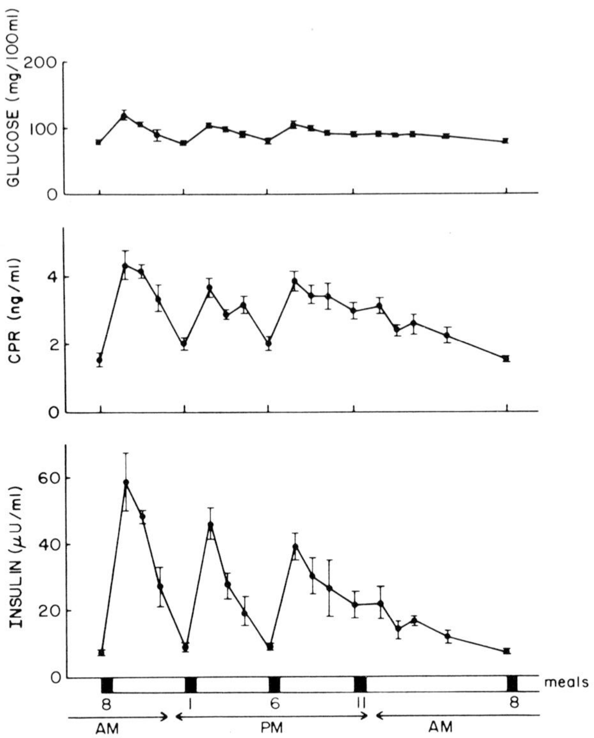

Serum glucose, insulin, and CPR levels in six normal women in the 3rd trimester of pregnancy (mean ± SEM)

Fig. 10-2. (Reprinted with permission from Lewis SB, Wallin JD, Kuzuya H, et al: Circadian variation of serum glucose, C-peptide immunoreactivity and free insulin in normal and insulin-treated diabetic pregnant subjects. Diabetologia 12:343, 1976.)

level was high—perhaps a dietary indiscretion—we do not change the insulin dose unless the same thing occurs on two consecutive days.) The exception would be if a blood glucose level is quite high, e.g., above 200 mg/dl, in which case we would add some supplemental insulin in order to avoid ketoacidosis, which may occur at lower blood sugar levels during pregnancy than in the nonpregnant state.

On the above two-injection mixed insulin schedule, some patients may require additional injections to attain euglycemia. For example, many patients experience the "dawn phenomenon": a relatively low or normal blood sugar in the very early morning but hyperglycemia upon awakening. Previously ascribed to the Somogyi effect, it is clear that most of these incidents are related to the predinner NPH insulin peaking in the early morning hours and then wearing off. When this situation is encountered, it is best to split the evening dose, giving the regular insulin at dinner time and the NPH at bedtime. The most important thing is to be flexible and arrange the insulin schedule to most easily maintain euglycemia and the patient's life style.

The portable subcutaneous insulin infusion pump has become increasingly popular as a method of administering insulin to diabetics. It has the advantage of closely mimicking normal pancreatic insulin release, with a continuous low basal infusion rate and mealtime boluses. Euglycemia has been achieved in many diabetics who were quite difficult to control without the pump. Its use in pregnancy has been associated with favorable results.[16] However, there is as yet no evidence that the insulin pump is necessary for every pregnant diabetic, or that its use gives uniformly superior results to intensive conventional insulin treatment with home glucose monitoring. The insulin pump is expensive and requires a high level of motivation on the part of both patient and physician. Because only short-acting insulin is used, accidental discontinuation of the infusion may be associated with the relatively rapid development of ketoacidosis. As should be clear from earlier sections of this chapter, pregnancy is a time when superb glucose control is worthwhile. If intensive conventional therapy is not adequate to achieve this goal in a particular patient, it is logical to turn to the insulin pump—but only if the patient is highly motivated, can do home glucose monitoring, and is in all other ways a candidate for this form of treatment. Further details of patient selection and use of insulin pumps are found elsewhere in this book.

Recommendation: In order to attain relatively normal glood glucose levels in the pregnant diabetic, prescribe at least two injections of mixed intermediate- and short-acting insulin each day; do not hesitate to use more frequent injections if necessary. Daily modifications of dosage are often necessary, so frequent communication with the patient is essential.

Hypoglycemia

When intensive metabolic control is attempted, maternal hypoglycemia is likely to occur with greater frequency than is seen in other circumstances. This side effect is clearly undesirable from the maternal point of view. Not only are there concerns about maternal neurological damage from chronic or recurrent hypoglycemia, but the more immediate welfare of the patient can be put in jeopardy from hypoglycemia. Activities such as driving a car, operating machinery, and even child care can have disastrous results if the patient's judgment is diminished or she suddenly loses consciousness. For this reason, we caution our patients, especially those who are prone to hypoglycemia, that they should not drive alone and that a support system of husband, parents, friends, and/or neighbors should be set up to check on their well-being throughout the day. These support personnel are to be well versed in the treatmeht of hypoglycemia, including the administration of glucagon if necessary. Our usual instructions are for the patient to take a mixed carbohydrate and protein snack (e.g., a glass of milk and a serving of cheese and crackers or peanut butter), wait 10–15 min, and then repeat the snack if not feeling better. We ask that she check the blood glucose at the time of the reaction and again after 15 min. If the patient is too hypoglycemic to take a snack of her own volition, the support person is to attempt to convince her to eat, and under these circumstances a snack higher in glucose is useful (i.e., orange juice or soda). Most of these patients have learned over the years to treat hypoglycemic symptons by ingesting carbohydrates continuously until they are feeling better. With this method, because of the lag time between ingestion of calories and their absorption into the bloodstream, the patient has a copious supply of yet-to-be-absorbed carbohydrates in her stomach by the time her hypoglycemic symptoms have abated, and the continued absorption of these calories often results in an overshoot of her blood sugar to hyperglycemic levels. We prefer that our pregnant diabetic women not become hyperglycemic, and that is the reason for the above recommendation. If the support person is unable to get the patient to ingest calories orally, we recommend that half of an ampule (0.5 U) of glucagon be given subcutaneously. Generally, the patient is alert enough to eat within 15 min of the glucagon injection. If not, the other half-ampule is given and the patient taken to an emergency facility, usually by ambulance. It must be emphasized that the effects of glucagon are evanescent, so the patient must eat and/or drink as soon as she is able, lest the glucagon wear off and she lose consciousness again.

When a hypoglycemic diabetic woman is brought to a hospital in an unconscious or semiconscious state, the usual treatment is to administer 25 g of glucose (50 cc of a 50 percent solution) rapidly intravenously. Because we like to avoid the "overshoot" of hyperglycemia in a pregnant diabetic woman, we prefer to infuse 10 g of glucose (200 cc of a 5 percent dextrose solution) rapidly. An alternative would be to give 12.5 g (half the 50-cc ampule of 50 percent glucose). Either of these two methods is usually successful; if not, more glucose can be given. The home glucose meter is quite useful in such situations, as it allows rapid bedside titration of blood glucose.

The focus of concern around hypoglycemia should be the diabetic woman herself, rather than her fetus. Although there is no evidence that maternal hypoglycemia is particularly good for the fetus, there is much anecdotal evidence to suggest that episodes of low blood glucose do not negatively affect fetal outcome. In addition, data from the Collaborative Perinatal Project[17] failed to demonstrate an effect of maternal hypoglycemic *coma* on mental and motor function during the first few years of life. In one study[18] of 2000 apparently normal pregnant women with *nondiabetic* glucose tolerance tests during the third trimester, those women with one or more of the four glucose tolerance test values below the fifth percentile (of the group as a whole) had an increased perinatal loss rate. However, those women with one or more values above the 95th percentile (even though not in the diabetic range) had an even higher perinatal mortality rate. This study suggests that, as far as the glucose tolerance test is concerned, to be in the "normal" range is best for the fetus, and low values are no worse than slightly high values. Although we do not believe that hypoglycemia is desirable from the standpoint of the fetus, neither do we believe that hyperglycemia is a safe alternative.

COMPLICATIONS OF DIABETES

Retinopathy

It has long been taught that proliferative retinopathy is likely to worsen during pregnancy, and many experts have suggested that severe proliferative retinopathy, especially if near the optic disc and/or macula, is a contraindication to pregnancy. However, adequate data comparing diabetic women who have similar degrees of proliferative retinopathy followed prospectively through a pregnancy and through a similar period of time in the nonpregnant state are not yet available. The deterioration of retinopathy reported in some pregnant diabetics may have been wrongly ascribed to the influence of pregnancy. With the advent of laser photocoagulation, treatment for proliferative retinopathy has become practical. Therefore every pregnant diabetic woman should be evaluated early in the course of her pregnancy by an ophthalmologist well versed in the diagnosis and management of diabetic eye disease. If laser therapy is deemed necessary, it can and should be carried out. The presence of proliferative retinopathy suggests that the patient is likely to have vascular disease in other parts of her body and thus puts the fetus at risk for intrauterine growth retardation and other complications. Therefore diabetic pregnant women with proliferative retinopathy need to be followed throughout pregnancy with the greatest of diligence; they are in the highest-risk category.

Nephropathy

Although the increased renal plasma flow in pregnancy tends to exaggerate the amount of proteinuria seen in women with nephropathy, there is no convincing evidence that pregnancy permanently accelerates the natural history of deteriorating renal function in such patients. Hypertension is quite common with nephropathy, and the prognosis for a favorable pregnancy outcome is diminished in those women who start out pregnancy with hypertension and a serum creatinine level above 1.5–2 mg/dl. The Joslin Clinic group[19] reported a perinatal survival rate of 89 percent for pregnancies complicated by diabetic nephropathy (defined as proteinuria of >400 mg/24 h).

COMPLICATIONS OF PREGNANCY

Hypertensive Disorders

Hypertensive disorders occur in diabetic pregnancies with a frequency two to four times greater than in other pregnancies. The development of hypertension or the worsening of preexisting chronic hypertension is associated with an increased risk of fetoplacental deterioration. An appropriate response (during the third trimester) is to hospitalize the patient for bed rest and careful observation, and to increase the frequency and intensity of efforts to assess fetal well-being (see below).

Maternal Edema

Generalized edema has been reported to occur in up to 22 percent of diabetic pregnancies and may be severe. It carries no particularly adverse prognosis. The best treatment is bed rest in a lateral position.

Hydramnios

Clinically apparent increased amniotic fluid has been reported in up to 30 percent of pregnant diabetic women. Although it is tempting to postulate that fetal hyperglycemia leads to fetal polyuria and thus hydramnios, this mechanism is as yet unproved. The presence of hydramnios is associated with an increased risk of preterm delivery.

MONITORING FETAL WELL-BEING

Because of the increased risk of sudden unexplained intrauterine fetal demise in diabetic pregnancies, numerous methods of assessing fetal well-being have been proposed. The more commonly employed methods are discussed below.

Estriol

Estriol is produced by enzymes located in the placenta, fetal adrenal glands, and fetal liver. Once synthesized, estriol appears in the maternal circulation, is conjugated in the maternal liver, and is then excreted in the urine. Estriol production can be measured in 24-hr urine specimens or as free estriol in plasma. Estriol levels normally show a gradual increase throughout the second half of pregnancy but may also stay relatively constant without fetal jeopardy. In diabetics estriol production has been demonstrated to fall abruptly prior to some cases of intrauterine fetal demise. For this reason, it has been standard in many centers to measure *daily* 24-hr urine estriol or *daily* serum-free estriol as a measure of fetal well-being; if the estriol falls 35–40 percent of the mean of the three previous days' values, fetal compromise is likely. Estriol measurement has the disadvantage of being expensive and cumbersome, with daily visits to the laboratory for blood tests or the delivery of 24-hr urine specimens. Many hospital laboratories find it difficult or impossible to provide the test on a daily basis (including weekends). Finally, because the likelihood of fetal demise is considerably lessened with tight metabolic control, we have found estriol measurement to be less useful in recent years than in the past. We still follow daily estriol levels during the last 6–8 weeks of pregnancy in diabetic women with less than optimal or undocumented metabolic control and in those with hypertensive complications.

Antepartum Fetal Heart Rate Monitoring

In recent years emphasis has shifted toward utilization of either the contraction stress test or the nonstress test as predictors of fetal well-being. In the former, a fetal heart rate and uterine activity monitor are applied to the maternal abdomen, and uterine contractions are induced by intravenous administration of a dilute solution of oxytocin or by stimulation of the mother's nipples (resulting in endogenous oxytocin release by the "milk let-down reflex"). If the fetal heart does not respond adversely to adequate contractions (at least three within a 10-min period) it is highly likely that the fetus is not asphyxiated. The nonstress test involves monitoring the fetal heart rate continuously, with the mother signifying the time that each fetal movement is felt. The presence of accelerations of the fetal heart rate in association with fetal movement is similarly a good indication of fetal well-being. Whichever test is chosen at a particular center (there are pros and cons for either type of test) is repeated at least weekly and in some situations more often. An abnormal test may require early delivery or may suggest closer observation, depending on the clinical situation. Because neonatal survival now occurs with some regularity as early as 26–28 weeks' gestation, diabetic pregnancies at particularly high risk (i.e., those complicated by hypertension, nephropathy, or ultrasonic evidence of intrauterine growth retardation) may be monitored beginning as early as 26 weeks. The majority of diabetic pregnancies are begun on antepartum monitoring at 30–34 weeks, depending on the severity of the diabetes.

Ultrasound

Diagnostic ultrasound is useful in assessing the well-being of the fetus of the diabetic mother in a number of ways. Early in pregnancy, accurate dating is best established ultrasonically. Some congenital anomalies can be diagnosed by ultrasound early enough to allow termination of an abnormal pregnancy. Fetal growth can be assessed by serial ultrasound examinations, making it possible to diagnose the extremes of intrauterine growth retardation or macrosomia early enough to allow timely intervention. Hydramnios (see above) can be detected, as can oligohydramnios, the state of diminished amniotic fluid volume often being seen with chronic asphyxia, growth retardation, or certain anomalies of the urinary tract. Some centers employ weekly real-time ultrasound evaluation along with fetal heart rate monitoring as a "fetal biophysical profile." Such parameters as fetal breathing, fetal muscle tone and reactivity, and placental texture give added information about fetal well-being.

TIMING OF DELIVERY

It is no longer necessary to deliver all infants of diabetic mothers at some arbitrary number of weeks before term. Although in the past this practice was responsible for dramatically lowering the incidence of stillbirths, the frequently observed delay in pulmonic maturation combined with early delivery was responsible for a good deal of neonatal morbidity and some neonatal mortality from respiratory distress syndrome (RDS). The utilization of previously described methods of antepartum surveillance of fetal well-being has allowed obstetricians to allow diabetic pregnancies to proceed closer to term with confidence that the fetus is unlikely to die *in utero,* provided the test results are consistently reassuring. Improvements in metabolic control of diabetes have lowered the frequency of fetal compromise. Finally, the advent of specific biochemical tests of amniotic fluid has made possible the accurate assessment of fetal pulmonic maturity. The two substances most commonly measured in this context are the lecithin/sphingomyelin (L/S) ratio and phosphatidylglycerol (PG). The L/S ratio is the more easily tested but suffers from a small but significant incidence of false-positive results (i.e., the test suggests maturity but the baby develops RDS), especially in diabetics delivered before 38 weeks' gestation. The presence of PG in amniotic fluid is an extremely reliable predictor of fetal pulmonic maturity, but this measurement is more complicated than the L/S ratio. Recently developed immunoassay techniques for PG may obviate this problem. Delivery may be necessary prior to documented fetal pulmonic maturity if maternal or fetal compromise are detected; it is here that the presence of a tertiary neonatal nursery is imperative so that the neonate has the optimal chance of survival and normalcy.

Recommendation: Amniocentesis for measurement of the L/S ration and/or PG should be performed prior to elective delivery (whether by induction of labor or cesarean section) in any diabetic pregnancy.

MODE OF DELIVERY

Maternal diabetes mellitus is not an indication for cesarean section. However, because maternal diabetes predisposes to a number of complications which may necessitate cesarean section, this mode of delivery is more common among diabetics than in the general population. Such complications include fetal macrosomia (causing failure to progress in labor), hypertensive disorders of pregnancy (which may necessitate early intervention at a time in gestation when the cervix is not yet "ripe" for labor), and fetal compromise (in which the stress of labor is not tolerated, giving "fetal distress" patterns on the fetal monitor). Moreover, because it has been traditional for many obstetricians to arbitrarily deliver all diabetics by cesarean, we encounter many such patients who desire a repeat cesarean section. Finally, many diabetics are referred for care relatively late in pregnancy and have been told repeatedly by their caregivers that they will be delivered by cesarean. It is not always possible to persuade these patients to attempt vaginal delivery. Our total (primary plus repeat) cesarean section rate is currently approximately 50 percent for diabetic pregnancies.

METABOLIC MANAGEMENT AT DELIVERY

It is clear that the infant of the diabetic mother has a pancreas that is more responsive to secretagogues (e.g., glucose) than the more-normal pancreas. Maternal hyperglycemia (and thus fetal hyperglycemia) at the time of delivery can evoke a fetal insulin surge. If fetal insulin levels are high at delivery, when the umbilical cord is clamped and the copious supply of glucose coming from the mother is suddenly interrupted neonatal hypoglycemia is likely to result. It is therefore important to maintain euglycemia meticulously during labor and delivery.

Planned Cesarean Section

A planned cesarean section is the most straightforward situation in which to ensure euglycemia at delivery. If the patient has been in excellent metabolic control and has been doing home glucose monitoring, her fasting blood glucose is between 50 and 100 mg/dl each morning. If her usual routine of diet and insulin is followed until the time she falls asleep on the night before delivery, she should have a normal blood glucose level upon arising. It is necessary to fast preoperative patients, generally after midnight, prior to surgery. Thus she cannot eat breakfast (and should not take any insulin) on the morning of surgery. If very much time elapses between her usual breakfast (and insulin) hour and her delivery, a whole new metabolic equilibrium will need to be reached. For this reason, it is essential to perform the cesarean section as early in the morning as possible; we generally schedule it for 7:30 AM. An intravenous line is established at about 6:30 AM, and normal saline is infused. Blood sugar is measured with a bedside reflectance meter. If it is in the normal range (as it should be), no glucose or insulin is added before delivery. Once the umbilical cord is clamped, we generally infuse 5 percent dextrose, about 100 ml/hr, to the mother in order to avoid the hypoglycemia which often occurs during the 24 hr after delivery (as fetal and placental factors causing insulin resistance are abruptly withdrawn). Once the postoperative cesarean section patient is able to eat, her nonpregnant insulin dose can be gradually titrated.

Induction of Labor

If labor is to be induced, the patient is instructed to take her usual evening insulin dose and eat a normal dinner and snack, but to fast from midnight on. No breakfast or morning insulin is taken on the day of induction. Early in the morning, an intravenous line is established and 5 percent dextrose in 0.5 N saline is infused by a pump at 125 ml/hr. Some investigators[20,21] have shown that many diabetics require no insulin at all during the induction of labor and so would not add insulin to the intraveous fluid unless hyperglycemia occurs. We prefer to begin by adding 10 U of regular insulin to a liter of the D5½NS, so that patients receive *approximately* 1.25 U of insulin per hour. If the blood glucose falls below 70 mg/dl, we mix a new solution containing 5 U of regular insulin per liter, and infuse at the same 125 ml/hr. Similarly, if the blood sugar exceeds 100 mg/dl we double the insulin concentration, always keeping the infusion *rate* constant. Thus we know that the patient will receive 6.25 g of dextrose per hour (and thus receive enough to avoid ketosis). The most important part of this protocol is the *hourly* measurement of blood glucose at the bedside. It generally takes about 6 hr to reach a steady state with the constant glucose–insulin infusion, but the trend of blood glucose levels during the first 2–3 hr is useful in predicting whether the insulin dose is too high or low. The use of intermittent injections of subcutaneous insulin for diabetics in labor has, in our experience, been totally unsatisfactory. The delay between injection and absorption forces one to guess what the blood glucose level will be a few hours later; the resultant wide fluctuation in blood glucose during labor may have adverse effects on the fetus and newborn.

Spontaneous Labor

Spontaneous labor is managed similarly to induction of labor, except that the patient may have already taken her usual dose of intermediate-acting insulin, so that a constant glucose infusion is used, with insulin added only if the blood glucose exceeds 100 mg/dl. Again hourly blood glucose determinations, done at the bedside, make metabolic management considerably easier than it used to be.

MANAGEMENT OF THE INFANT OF THE DIABETIC MOTHER

Ideally, every infant of a diabetic mother should be delivered in a center with neonatal intensive care facilities. Whatever the setting, those caring for diabetic pregnancy should be well prepared to deal with the following complications.

Hypoglycemia

Although neonatal hypoglycemia is particularly common among infants of diabetic mothers whose metabolic control has been less than optimal, it occurs in approximately 15 percent of infants whose mothers have been intensively managed with tight metabolic control. Neonatal hypoglycemia is generally defined as a blood glucose level of less than 30 mg/dl in the term infant or less than 20 mg/dl in the premature. We generally measure the capillary blood glucose (from a "heel stick"), using a Dextrostix test strip, at about 45 min of age and again at hourly intervals until it is clear that hypoglycemia is not present. In general, this problem becomes evident within the first 3 hr of life if it is going to happen at all. Many centers institute oral feeding early (at about 90 min of life) in infants of diabetic mothers in order to prevent hypoglycemia.

If the capillary blood glucose by Dextrostix is between 25 and 45 mg/dl, we confirm its accuracy with a laboratory blood glucose level, meanwhile instituting oral or gavage feeding of 10–15 ml of 10 percent glucose to be followed by normal formula. If the Dextrostix glucose is less than 25 mg/dl, we again confirm the result in the laboratory but may institute intravenous 10 percent dextrose (at 6 mg/kg/min) in the meantime. We do not advocate giving a large bolus of intravenous glucose, as it may stimulate the already "overactive" fetal pancreas to secrete more insulin and add to the problem.

We have found it useful to measure the glucose level in umbilical cord blood at the time of delivery. A comparison of this value with that obtained from the neonate at 45 min of age gives a general idea of the rapidity with which the glucose level is falling. A cord glucose level of 50 mg/dl falling to 35 mg/dl at 45 min of life is perfectly compatible with a normal neonate. On the other hand, a cord value of 180 mg/dl falling to 35 mg/dl suggests a high likelihood of hyperinsulinism and hypoglycemia.

Polycythemia

A central hematrocrit greater than 65 percent or a hemoglobin greater than 20 g/dl is considered diagnostic of neonatal polycythemia. This plethora may be associated with hyperviscosity of the blood, which may be seen with renal vein thrombosis and central nervous system and pulmonary complications. Partial exchange transfusion is often necessary for symptomatic polycythemia; some advocate this treatment for asymptomatic polycythemia as well.

Hyperbilirubinemia

Hyperbilirubinemia occurs with greater frequency among infants of diabetic mothers than in the general population, probably because of the greater bilirubin load presented to the liver in these relatively plethoric newborns. Treatment is the same as for other forms of neonatal jaundice.

Hypocalcemia

The mechanism of neonatal hypocalcemia in infants of diabetic mothers is unclear, but the phenomenon is real. It generally occurs on the second or third day of life and is treated with oral or intravenous calcium.

Respiratory Distress Syndrome

The respiratory distress syndrome (RDS) is clearly more common in infants of diabetics than in the normal population. As mentioned earlier in the chapter, fetal hyperinsulinism may delay pulmonic maturation. The striking thing about RDS in the infant of the diabetic mother is that the baby often seems too large to have such a problem; this is due to fetal macrosomia and should not delay the diagnosis. Treatment is the same as for other infants with RDS.

Congenital Malformations

As stated earlier in this chapter, congenital malformations occur with increased frequency among infants of diabetic mothers. Although many birth defects can be diagnosed before delivery, the majority are not evident until the affected child is born. For this reason, facilities should be available for diagnosis, management, and where feasible correction of congenital anomalies.

CLASSIFICATION OF DIABETES IN PREGNANCY

Most chapters on the subject of the pregnant diabetic begin with a table such as Table 10-3 outlining White's[22] classification. I have purposely deferred such a discussion to the end of this chapter in order to deemphasize the importance of assigning a class to pregnant diabetics. The White classes are useful when comparing various series reported in the literature, and there is a correlation between class of diabetes and the likelihood of vascular disease; but it would be a mistake to treat a class B diabetic any less meticulously than a class D patient. All overt diabetics should be considered at high risk and managed by a team with expertise and much experience with the problems of diabetic pregnancy.

Other classification schemes have been proposed and are in use. Pedersen's[12] "prognostically bad signs in pregnancy" (PBSP) (Table 10-4), attempt to predict poor

Table 10-3. White's Classification of Pregnant Diabetic Women

Class	Onset		Duration	Insulin or Oral Agent Needed	Vascular Disease
A (Abnormal GTT)	Any		Any	0	0
B	>20	*and*	<10	+	0
C	10–19	*or*	10–19	+	0
D	<10	*or*	>20	+	Background retinopathy
E	Any		Any	+	Calcified pelvic arteries
F	Any		Any	+	Nephropathy
R	Any		Any	+	Proliferative Retinopathy

Source: White P: Pregnancy and diabetes. In Marbel A, White P, Bradley RF, Krall LP (eds): Joslin's Diabetes Mellitus. 11th ed. Lea & Febiger, Philadelphia, 1971

outcome. It should be noted that the worse prognosis for outcome is a diabetic pregnancy associated with diabetic ketoacidosis; this complication is associated with a perinatal mortality rate as high as 85 percent.[22,23] Hollingsworth[24] suggested that the metabolic differences between type I (IDDM) and type II (NIDDM) diabetes may be significant in determining the type of morbidity likely to be encountered in the pregnancy.

SUMMARY

This chapter has dealt with the management of pregnancy in the *overt* diabetic. Space limitations preclude a complete discussion of the pregnant woman with an abnormal glucose tolerance test but normal fasting and postprandial blood glucose values, the class A diabetic in White's classification. However, critical to the care of the class A diabetic is the measurement of appropriate blood glucose values at appropriate intervals in order to make certain that the patient is not hyperglycemic. Once the diagnosis of abnormal carbohydrate tolerance is made, we obtain a "set" of blood glucose measurements (fasting, 2 hr after breakfast, late afternoon) weekly. If the fasting value exceeds 100 mg/dl or either of the other two exceed 120 mg/dl, we treat the patient as an overt diabetic.

A number of recent advances in diabetes, maternal-fetal medicine, and neona-

Table 10-4. Pedersen's Prognostically Bad Signs in Pregnancy

1. Clinical pyelonephritis (fever>39°C: urine culture)
2. Precoma (venous standard bicarbonate<10 mmol/L) or severe acidosis (venous standard bicarbonate 10–17 mmol/L)
3. Toxemia
4. "Neglectors" (failure to follow the recommended regimen, irrespective of the cause, including late registration for care)

Source: Pedersen J: The Pregnant Diabetic and Her Newborn. 2nd ed. Williams & Wilkins, Baltimore, 1977

tology have made it possible to reduce the perinatal mortality rate for diabetic pregnancy to levels approaching those seen in the general population. Population-based data from four states[25] have shown a declining perinatal mortality for diabetic pregnancies in recent years. However, these perinatal mortality rates are still 2.5–7 times higher than in the normal population. This suggests that the advances in understanding and management described herein have not yet been uniformly applied to clinical practice.

REFERENCES

1. Mills JL, Baker L, Goldman AS: Malformations in infants of diabetic mothers occur before the seventh gestational week: implications for treatment. Diabetes 28:292, 1979
2. Leslie RDG, Pike DA, John PN, White JM: Hemoglobin A_1 in diabetic pregnancy. Lancet 2:958, 1978
3. Miller E, Hare JW, Cloherty JP, et al: Elevated maternal hemoglobin A_{1C} in early pregnancy and major congenital anomalies in infants of diabetic mothers. N Engl J M 304:1331, 1981
4. Fuhrmann K, Reiher H, Semmler K, et al: Prevention of congenital malformationsi in infants of insulin dependent diabetic mothers. Diabetes Care 6:219, 1983
5. Jovanovic L, Peterson CM: Management of the pregnant, insulin-dependent diabetic woman. Diabetes Care 3:63, 1980
6. Harley JMG, Montgomery DAD: Management of pregnancy complicated by diabetes. Br Med J 1:14, 1965
7. Karlsson K, Kjellmer I: The outcome of diabetic pregnancies in relation to the mother's blood sugar level. Am J Obstet Gynecol, 112:213, 1972
8. Leveno KJ, Hauth JC, Gilstrap LZ, Whalley PJ: Appraisal of "rigid" blood glucose control during pregnancy in the overtly diabetic woman. Am J Obstet Gynecol 135:853, 1979
9. Jovanovic L, Peterson CM: Optimal insulin delivery for the pregnant diabetic patient. Diabetes Care, suppl. 1, 5:24, 1982
10. Lewis SB, Murray WK, Wallin JD, et al: Improved glucose control in non-hospitalized pregnant diabetic patients. Obstet Gynecol 48:260, 1976
11. Roversi GD, Gargiulo M, Nicolini U, et al: A new approach to the treatment of diabetic pregnant women. Am J Obstet Gynecol 135:567, 1979
12. Pedersen J: The Pregnant Diabetic and Her Newborn. 2nd ed. Williams & Wilkins, Baltimore, 1977
13. Susa JB, McCormick KL, Widness JA, et al: Chronic hyperinsulinemia in the fetal rhesus monkey: effects on fetal growth and composition. Diabetes 28:1058, 1979
14. Widness JA, Susa JB, Garcia JF, et al: Increased erythropoiesis and elevated erythropoietin in infants born to diabetic mothers and in hyperinsulinemic rhesus fetuses. J Clin Invest 67:637, 1981
15. Lewis SB, Wallin JD, Kuzuya H, et al: Circadian variation of serum glucose, C-peptide immunoreactivity and free insulin in normal and insulin-treated diabetic pregnant subjects. Diabetologia 12:343, 1976
16. Rudolf MCJ, Coustan DR, Sherwin RS, et al: Efficacy of the insulin pump in the home treatment of pregnant diabetics. Diabetes 30:891, 1981
17. Churchill JA, Berendes HW, Nemore J: Neuropsychological deficits in children of diabetic mothers. Am J Obstet Gynecol 105:257, 1969
18. Abell DA, Beischer NA, Pappas AJ, Willis MN: The association between abnormal glu-

cose tolerance (hyperglycemia and hypoglycemia) and estriol excretion in pregnancy. Am J Obstet Gynecol 124:388, 1976

19. Kitzmiller JL, Brown ER, Phillippe M, et al: Diabetic nephropathy and perinatal outcome. Am J Obstet Gynecol 141:741, 1981
20. Golde SH, Good-Anderson B, Montoro M, Artal R: Insulin requirements during labor: a reappraisal. Am J Obstet Gynecol 144:556, 1982
21. Jovanovic L, Peterson CM: Insulin and glucose requirements during the first stage of labor in insulin-dependent diabetic women. Am J Med 75:607, 1983
22. White P: Pregnancy and diabetes. In Marbel A, White P, Bradley RF, Krall LP (eds): Joslin's Diabetes Mellitus. 11th ed. Lea & Febiger, Philadelphia, 1971
23. Drury MI, Greene AT, Stronge JM: Pregnancy complicated by clinical diabetes mellitus—a study of 600 pregnancies. Obstet Gynecol 49:519, 1977
24. Hollingsworth DR: Alterations of maternal metabolism in normal and diabetic pregnancies: differences in insulin-dependent, non-insulin-dependent, and gestational diabetes. Am J Obstet Gynecol 146:417, 1983
25. Morbidity and Mortality Weekly Report, Center for Disease Control. Vol. 34. p. 49. CDC, Atlanta, 16 December 1983

SUGGESTED READINGS

Felig P, Coustan DR: Diabetes mellitus. In Burrow GN, Ferris TF (eds): Medical Complications During Pregnancy. Saunders, Philadelphia, 1982

Merkatz IR, Adam PAJ (eds): The Diabetic Pregnancy: A Perinatal Perspective. Grune & Stratton, New York, 1979

11 Acute Medical Illness and Surgery in the Diabetic Patient

David S. Schade

Acute medical illness induces a rapid change in homeostatic mechanisms in normal man. Such physiological changes as fever, tachycardia, and diaphoresis are outward manifestations of inward alterations in hormones and substrates. In nondiabetic man there may be significant increases in blood glucose as well as ketone body changes, but because of the multiple feedback factors that regulate insulin secretion severe hyperglycemia and/or ketoacidosis do not occur. In insulin-dependent diabetic patients, these homeostatic changes induced by illness can result in metabolic decompensation which, if not properly treated, can lead to diabetic ketoacidosis and death. Therefore it is not surprising that infection is the most common cause of diabetic ketoacidosis.[1] With proper medical management, diabetic ketoacidosis can be avoided, although in some cases prevention requires hospitalization. Proper therapy of acute medical illness requires both a knowledgeable patient and a readily available physician.

Surgery in the diabetic patient may be considered as a planned assault on body tissues, and substrate and hormonal physiological responses may be expected. Because the anesthetized patient is not able to directly assist the physician, careful management of blood glucose and insulin dosages are essential. Thus an understanding of normal homeostatic mechanisms by the physician is required if severe hypo- and hyperglycemia are to be avoided during or after surgery.

NORMAL HOMEOSTATIC MECHANISMS

To treat acute medical illness in the diabetic patient correctly, it is necessary to understand how nondiabetic man responds to illness and maintains homeostasis (normal glucose and ketone body concentrations). It should be emphasized that the major difference between diabetic and nondiabetic individuals undergoing illness is the ability to secrete insulin. The roles of other hormonal abnormalities in diabetic subjects, e.g., glucagon and epinephrine nonresponsiveness, are also of importance if hypoglycemia occurs.

Secretion of insulin in nondiabetic man involes two important variables: quantity and timing. As shown in Figure 11-1, the daily pattern of insulin secretion in normal man is complex, closely mimicking the changes in blood glucose concentration. The matching of insulin secretion to changes in blood glucose concentration is essential to maintain homeostasis.[2] In diabetic man, both of these variables must simulate, as closely as possible, that of the nondiabetic patient to maintain homeostasis. A third variable (which is not yet possible to correct in the diabetic patient) is the secretion of insulin preferentially into the portal venous system so that the liver is exposed to a higher concentration of insulin than the peripheral tissues. The importance of this factor is not yet resolved, although in dogs it has been shown that glucose recycling (the amount of lactate that is resynthesized into glucose) cannot be normalized without direct portal vein insulin infusion.[3] However, for the markedly ill diabetic patient, the consequences of hyperglycemia and hyperketonemia far exceed those of abnormal glucose recycling.

In nondiabetic man, both glucose and ketone bodies induce insulin secretion,

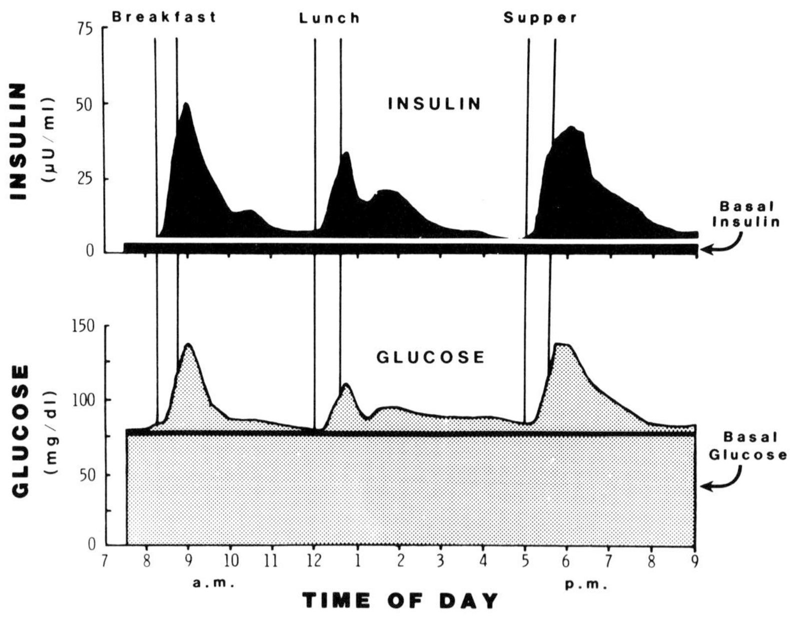

Fig. 11-1 Mean peripheral plasma insulin and glucose profiles in five nondiabetic subjects ingesting 630-kcal meals composed of 40 percent carbohydrate, 40 percent fat, and 20 percent protein. The meals took 15 min to ingest. The pattern of the rise in plasma insulin concentration closely matches that of the rise in plasma glucose concentration. (Reprinted with permission from Intensive Insulin Therapy. Excerpta Medica, New York, 1983, p. 24.)

thereby providing a self-regulating feedback mechanism.[4] Quantitatively, however, glucose is by far the most important, as exemplified by prolonged fasting in nondiabetic man, in which the glucose concentration is reduced but ketone body concentration greatly increased. In this state, insulin secretion is also suppressed; otherwise hypoglycemia would be severe. However, the goal of the physician in treating acute medical illness in the diabetic patient is to normalize, as much as possible, both glucose and ketone body concentrations, as abnormalities in either of these substrates can result in death of the patient.

GLUCOSE

Glucose is a six-carbon non-ionized molecule. Because it does not release hydrogen ions, it does not cause acidosis, even at very high blood concentrations. The tendency to develop hyperglycemia during acute illness is due to several mechanisms, including increased production, decreased tissue utilization, and decreased renal clearance (Fig. 11-2). Its acute detrimental effects are secondary to its activity as an

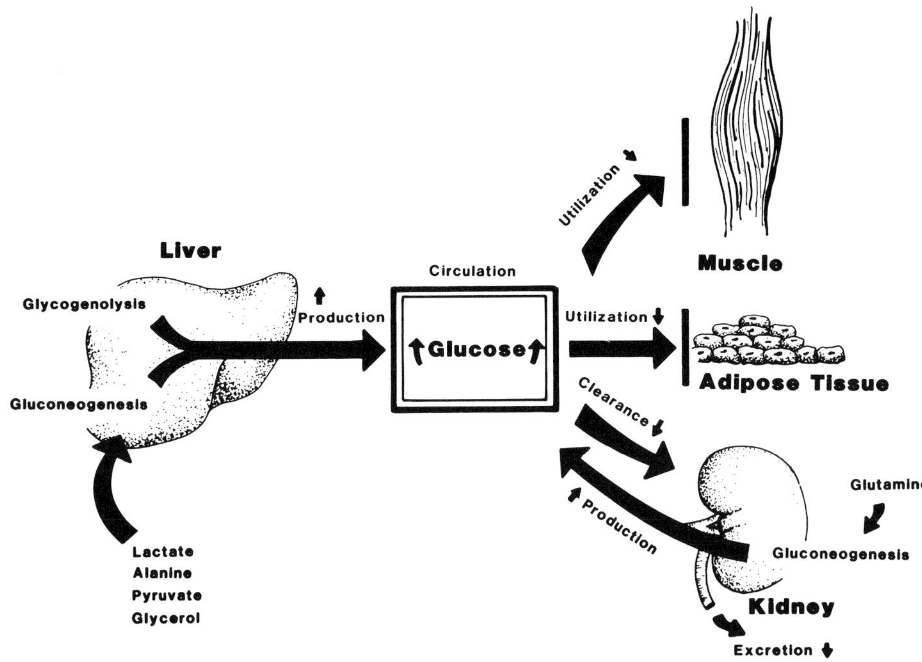

Fig. 11-2 Factors raising the blood glucose concentration during acute illness. Increased production is secondary to enhanced glycogenolysis and gluconeogenesis in the liver, and to gluconeogenesis in the kidney. Clearance of glucose from the circulation is decreased as the relative insulin deficiency inhibits entry of glucose into both muscle and fat tissue. If dehydration is severe, renal excretion of glucose also decreases. (Reprinted with permission from Schade DS, Eaton RP, Alberti KGMM, et al: Diabetic Coma, Ketoacidotic and Hyperosmolar. University of New Mexico Press, Albuquerque, 1981, p. 30.)

Table 11-1. General Principles in Treating the Diabetic Patient During Acute Illness or Surgery

Point 1:	Prolonged glucose concentrations above 250 mg/dl must be prevented by administration of rapid-acting (regular) insulin.
Point 2:	Urinary ketone bodies in the ill diabetic patient indicate that additional insulin is needed and carbohydrate may have to be ingested to permit insulin to be safely administered.
Point 3:	The most important role of the physician in treating the ill diabetic patient is his or her ready availability to the patient.
Point 4:	In the ill diabetic patient, the following parameters must be monitored: (1) weight; (2) mental function; (3) respiratory rate; (4) pulse; (5) temperature; (6) glucose; (7) urine ketone bodies; (8) insulin dose; and (9) oral intake.
Point 5:	All diabetic patients should be in good metabolic balance prior to surgery.
Point 6:	At least 12 hr should elapse between food intake and surgery in the diabetic patient.
Point 7:	The best index of fluid status in the surgical diabetic patient is the patient's stable preoperative weight.

osmotic particle, causing water shifts between body compartments. These shifts occur because water moves freely throughout the body tissues, whereas glucose transport across cellular membranes depends on multiple factors, not the least of which is insulin.

In addition to inducing acute fluid shifts, glucose may also cause one very important adverse effect: osmotic diuresis. Significant diuresis occurs in all individuals whenever the plasma glucose concentration exceeds the renal glucose threshold (approximately 200–250 mg/dl). Osmotic diuresis can be detrimental for two reasons: (1) it induces a loss of water (resulting in dehydration); and (2) multiple ions are excreted with the water (sodium, potassium, chloride, magnesium, phosphate, etc.) which may have detrimental effects on vascular volume and cellular membrane function. Thus the first general principle (Table 11-1) in treating the acutely ill diabetic patient is:

Point 1: Prolonged glucose concentrations above 250 mg/dl must be prevented by administration of rapid-acting (regular) insulin. In fact, the dose of insulin given to the medically ill diabetic patient is determined primarily by the plasma glucose concentration.

KETONE BODIES

All diabetic patients are familiar with ketone bodies, as various diabetic urine tests are available to monitor them (Acetest tablets or Ketostix). However, in our experience, few diabetic patients understand the meaning of the presence of ketone bodies in the urine or how to respond therapeutically to them.

The term "ketone bodies" commonly refers to three different but related molecules: acetone, acetoacetic acid, and beta-hydroxybutyric acid. These compounds are related in that acetoacetic acid and beta-hydroxybutyric acid are interconvertible, the reaction involving the enzyme beta-hydroxybutyrate dehydrogenase and the cofactors DPNH and hydrogen ions (H^+). Acetone is formed by the spontaneous decarboxy-

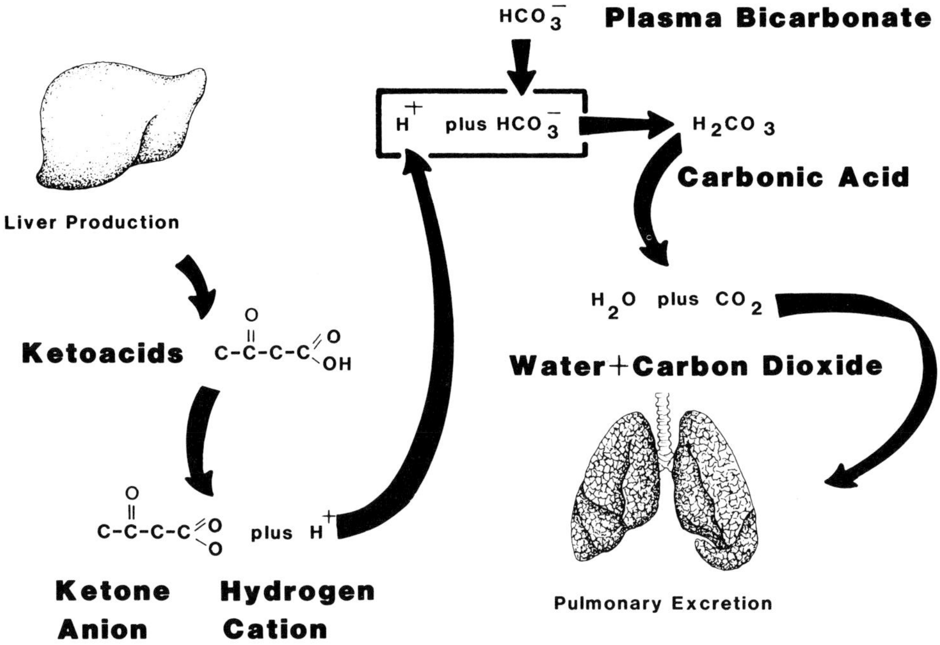

Fig. 11-3 The development of acidosis during acute medical illness. The ketoacids (aceto-acetate and 3-hydroxybutyrate) are released by the liver at an increased rate and dissociate into hydrogen ions (H^+) and ketone anions. The hydrogen ion combines with plasma bicarbonate to form carbonic acid, which is converted to water and carbon dioxide. Both of these molecules are then excreted by the lungs. As a result of this sequence of events, the plasma becomes more acidotic (increased hydrogen ions) and the plasma bicarbonate concentration decreases. Eventually, severe acidosis results in association with a markedly reduced bicarbonate concentration. (Reprinted with permission from Schade DS, Eaton RP, Alberti KGMM, et al: Diabetic Coma, Ketoacidotic and Hyperosmolar. University of New Mexico Press, Albuquerque, 1981, p. 172.)

lation of acetoacetic acid in an irreversible reaction with the liberation of carbon dioxide and water. Details of the pathophysiology of these compounds are described elsewhere.[5] Acetoacetic acid and beta-hydroxybutyric acid are not toxic per se but induce harmful effects by their dissociation (ionization) at body pH (i.e., 7.4) into hydrogen ions and the anions acetoacetate and betahydroxybutyrate (Fig. 11-3). If allowed to accumulate, the hydrogen ions lower the blood pH, resulting in systemic acidosis, which has multiple detrimental effects on cellular function, eventually inducing cardiovascular collapse.

Because insulin is the only circulating hormone which directly suppresses ketone body formation, its administration in the acutely ill diabetic patient is necessary for preventing ketoacidosis. However, in order to administer insulin without inducing hypoglycemia, it may be necessary to administer carbohydrate orally or parenterally. Thus the second general principle to be made in treating the acutely ill diabetic patient is:

Point 2: Urinary ketone bodies in the ill diabetic patient indicate that additional insulin is needed and carbohydrate may have to be ingested to permit insulin to be safely administered.

EFFECT OF ACUTE ILLNESS IN DIABETIC PATIENTS

Acute illness in the diabetic patient can lead to metabolic decompensation by several mechanisms: (1) fasting; (2) dehydration; (3) insulin deficiency; and (4) stress hormone excess. When these mechanisms are considered individually, therapy to correct these pathophysiological conditions is easily understood (Fig. 11-4).

Fasting

Acute medical illness is often accompanied by nausea and anorexia, resulting in a decrease in appetite. Because certain tissues cannot utilize fat for energy (e.g., central nervous system, red blood cells, and adrenal medulla), a sudden decrease in glucose ingestion results in stimulation of hormones to enhance endogenous production of glucose (by glycogenolysis and/or gluconeogenesis). Of importance is the fact that these catabolic hormones also result in mobilization of fatty acids from fat tissue and enhance hepatic ketone body production to provide noncarbohydrate-dependent tissues with an energy source. The relative deficiency of insulin decreases the peripheral utilization of ketone bodies, further increasing their plasma concentration. Thus the

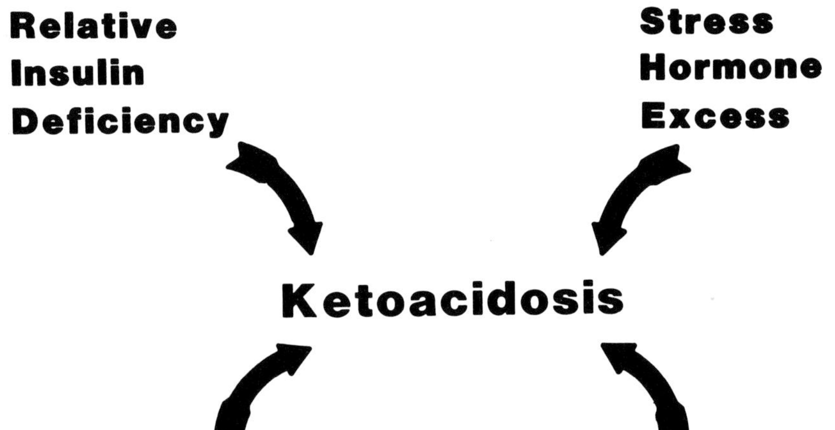

Fig. 11-4 Mechanisms resulting in metabolic decompensation in the sick diabetic patient. Two or more of the following factors are always present in diabetic ketoacidosis: (1) relative insulin deficiency; (2) stress hormone excess; (3) dehydration; and (4) fasting. (Reprinted with permission from Schade DS, Eaton RP, Alberti KGMM, et al: Diabetic Coma, Ketoacidotic and Hyperosmolar. University of New Mexico Press, Albuquerque, 1981, p. 107.)

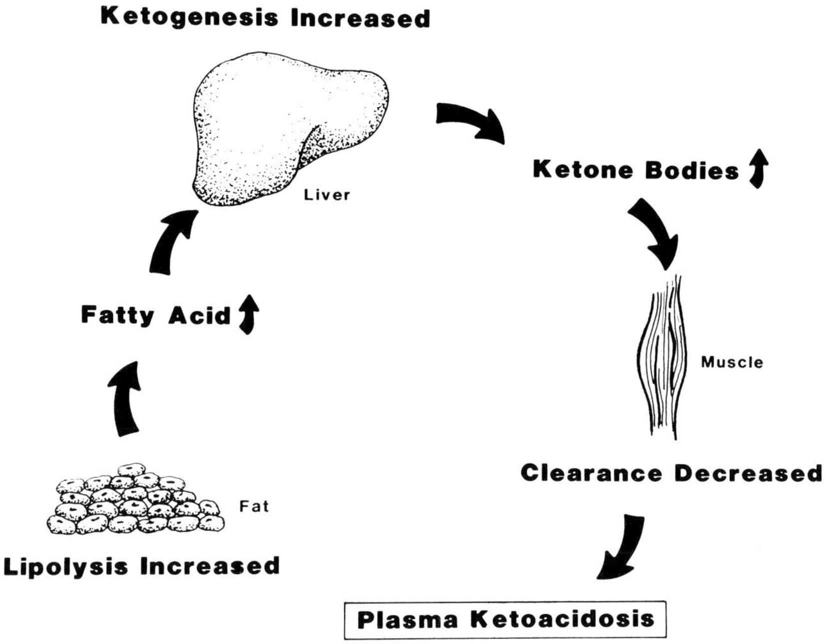

Fig. 11-5 Direct and indirect effects of fasting which may result in ketoacidosis. Increased fat cell lipolysis elevates the concentration of fatty acids in the plasma which are utilized by the liver for ketone body production. The liver, independent of the increase in fatty acid availability, also increases its rate of fatty acid oxidation to ketone bodies. These two metabolic alterations result in an increased release of ketoacids into the peripheral circulation, which are then cleared by tissue at a decreased rate, causing a profound decrease in the plasma pH. (Reprinted with permission from Schade DS, Eaton RP, Alberti KGMM, et al: Diabetic Coma, Ketoacidotic and Hyperosmolar. University of New Mexico Press, Albuquerque, 1981, p. 45.)

decrease in food intake sets the stage for the development of ketoacidosis (Fig. 11-5).

The correct approach to the acutely ill diabetic patient is to continue to ingest carbohydrate in preference to fat and protein. Fortunately, this is readily done if the patient consumes fruit juices or electrolyte-containing fluids, e.g., Gatorade. It should be emphasized that the diabetic patient is normally taught to avoid these foodstuffs and does not usually ingest them unless so instructed. The reason the diabetic patient usually does not require simple carbohydrate is that most foods contain sufficient complex carbohydrates to satisfy energy requirements of glucose-dependent tissues. However, when ill and nauseated, simple carbohydrates (mono- and disaccharides) are often better tolerated than complex carbohydrates and are therefore the energy source of choice. However, it must be emphasized that if the patient's blood glucose concentration is greater than his renal threshold (i.e., greater than 250 mg/dl) the ingestion of carbohydrates should be delayed until sufficient insulin is given to reduce blood glucose to below his renal threshold. Furthermore, ingestion of carbohydrate should be accompanied by small amounts of insulin to prevent hyperglycemia.

Dehydration

Dehydration occurs almost invariable during acute illness in normal man and is accentuated in diabetic man. The sites of fluid loss are multiple (Fig. 11-6), and attempts must be made to reduce the loss as much as possible. Fortunately, the site of greatest fluid loss is the kidney, and the deficit can be corrected if sufficient insulin is given to prevent hyperglycemia. The magnitude of fluid loss from the other sites depends on the etiology of the acute medical illness. If viral gastroenteritis is present, diarrhea may be severe, resulting in major loss of water and electrolytes. Fever and diaphoresis also increase fluid loss from the skin, encouraging the physician to prescribe antipyretics. Insensible water loss may also occur via the lungs, especially if hyperventilation is present. Because acidosis increases the respiratory rate, ketogenesis (i.e., ketoacid production) must be suppressed with insulin if fluid losses are to be controlled.

Fluid losses are detrimental for two reasons. First, loss of water itself results in cellular dehydration, which may alter cerebral function. Second, except for respiratory loss of water, all other sites of fluid loss are also accompanied by loss of electrolytes. Massive loss of sodium results in intravascular contraction, with consequent

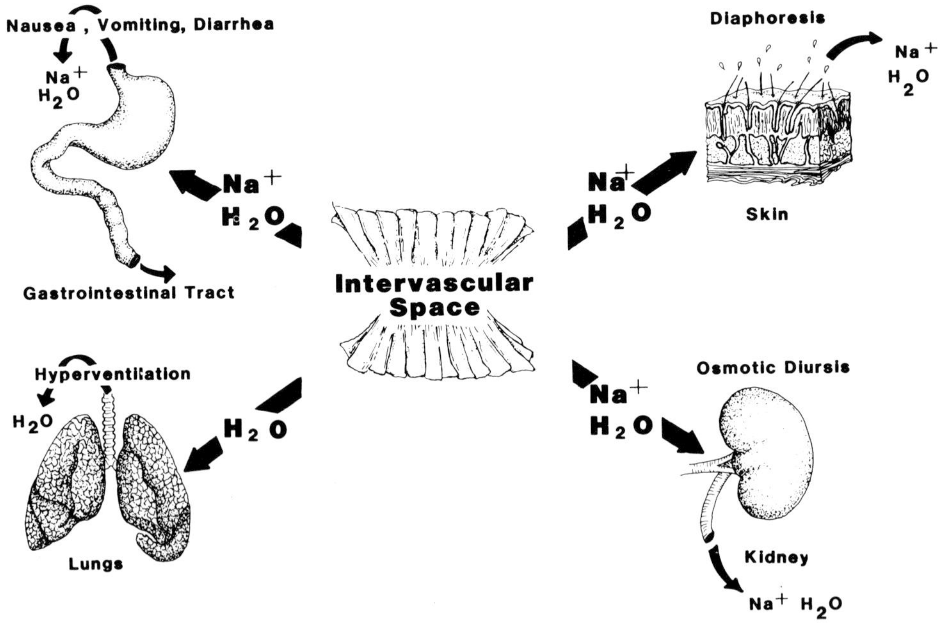

Fig. 11-6 Sources of fluid loss in the sick diabetic patient. Severe volume contraction occurs secondary to several mechanisms. Sodium (and other electrolytes) and water are lost via the gastrointestinal tract, skin, and kidneys. The acidosis-induced hyperventilation results in water loss. In spite of the hyperglycemia, the loss of sodium and water results in severe volume contraction, which may lead to shock and vascular collapse. (Reprinted with permission from Schade DS, Eaton RP, Alberti KGMM, et al: Diabetic Coma, Ketoacidotic and Hyperosmolar. University of New Mexico Press, Albuquerque, 1981, p. 162.)

decreased cardiac output. The most significant result of this effect is a decrease in glomerular filtration rate (prerenal azotemia). Although this kidney dysfunction eventually results in oliguria and thus restricts the loss of water, the real consequence is a further increase in glycemia, as large quantities of glucose can no longer be removed by the kidney. In fact, in the well-hydrated patient it is almost impossible to induce severe hyperglycemia (blood glucose greater than 350 mg/dl), even with severe insulin deficiency, as the kidney acts as a major site of glucose removal from the blood.[6] Dehydration also increases counterregulatory hormone secretion, which in turn potentiates the metabolic disturbance. In summary, because of the multiple mechanisms of fluid loss, patients admitted to the hospital in diabetic ketoacidosis are almost invariably dehydrated, with an average loss of 10 percent of body weight (7 L fluid in a 70-kg male).[7]

Insulin Deficiency

During periods of illness, nondiabetic man increases his basal insulin requirements to counteract the hyperglycemic effects of stress hormones. However, his total insulin requirements (basal plus meal-induced) may decrease, depending on his alterations in food intake. Thus if anorexia is present total insulin requirements may decrease, whereas if food ingestion continues total insulin secretion increases. In the diabetic patient changes in insulin requirements also occur, and the patient must make the correct decision as to whether to increase or decrease his insulin dose. Because

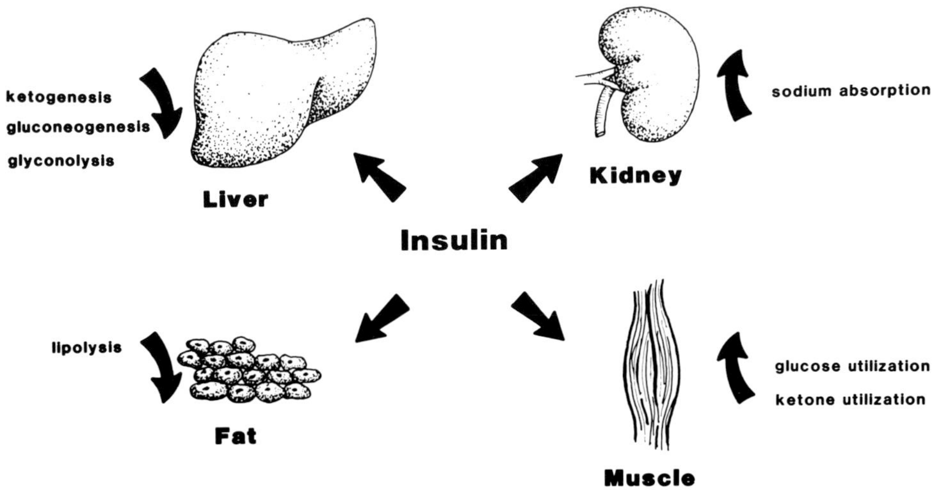

Fig. 11-7 Beneficial effects of insulin. Insulin exerts beneficial metabolic activity at several organs to inhibit the onset of diabetic ketoacidosis. At the adipocyte, hepatocyte, and myocyte, its activity prevents hyperglycemia and hyperketonemia, whereas at the kidney its activity prevents dehydration. (Reprinted with permission from Schade DS, Eaton RP, Alberti KGMM, et al: Diabetic Coma, Ketoacidotic and Hyperosmolar. University of New Mexico Press, Albuquerque, 1981, p. 61)

all individuals respond differently to insulin, it is not feasible to prescribe a set change in dosage. In this setting, the diabetic patient must monitor his blood glucose concentration, preferably directly by capillary blood glucose monitoring techniques, or indirectly by repeated urinalysis for glucose. Furthermore, because the presence of intermediate- or long-acting insulin (lente, NPH, ultralente, or PZI) prevents the diabetic patient from rapidly increasing or decreasing his circulating insulin concentration, the use of these insulins should be discontinued during an acute illness.

The beneficial effects of insulin are multiple, and during acute illness its regulatory effects on glucose and ketone body concentration are of prime importance (Fig. 11-7). Frequently overlooked, however, is insulin's role at the kidney to enhance conservation of sodium to counteract the natriuretic effect of glucagon.[8,9]

Stress Hormone Excess

Acute medical illness in normal man induces the secretion of stress hormones (glucagon, epinephrine, norepinephrine, cortisol, and growth hormone), which counteract the effects of circulating insulin.[10] The mechanism(s) whereby the secretion of these hormones increases is undoubtedly complex, involving not only changes in circulating substrates but also central nervous system mediation. Fever, which accompanies most types of acute illness, has been studied in detail, and secretion of the stress hormones precedes the rise in blood glucose and ketone body concentration.[11] Even in nondiabetic man, the synergistic effects of the stress hormones may induce hyperglycemia.[12] Because these hormones may rapidly change in concentration, frequent changes in insulin dosage are needed to maintain the diabetic patient in metabolic balance.

The relatively unopposed actions of the stress hormones in diabetic man result in enhanced glucose and ketone body concentrations by multiple mechanisms (Fig. 11-8). Lipolysis is stimulated in adipose tissue primarily by catecholamines. Glucagon enhances gluconeogenesis and ketogenesis in the liver from nonesterified fatty acids and other substrates. Utilization of glucose and ketone bodies (?) in peripheral tissues is decreased by cortisol and insulin deficiency. Glucagon excess and insulin deficiency enhance sodium loss and dehydration, further enchancing the hyperglycemia.

MANAGEMENT OF ACUTE MEDICAL ILLNESS

The goal of management of the acutely ill diabetic patient is twofold: (1) most important, to prevent metabolic decompensation; and (2) to prevent hospitalization. In some cases hospitalization may be required to attain the first goal, but appropriate timing of hospitalization results in a minimal hospital stay. (If in doubt, hospitalize the patient.) To achieve these two goals, a cooperative effort is needed between the physician and the patient. In our experience, patient cooperation is readily obtainable so long as he clearly understands the reason for the medical management and the benefits of correct therapy.

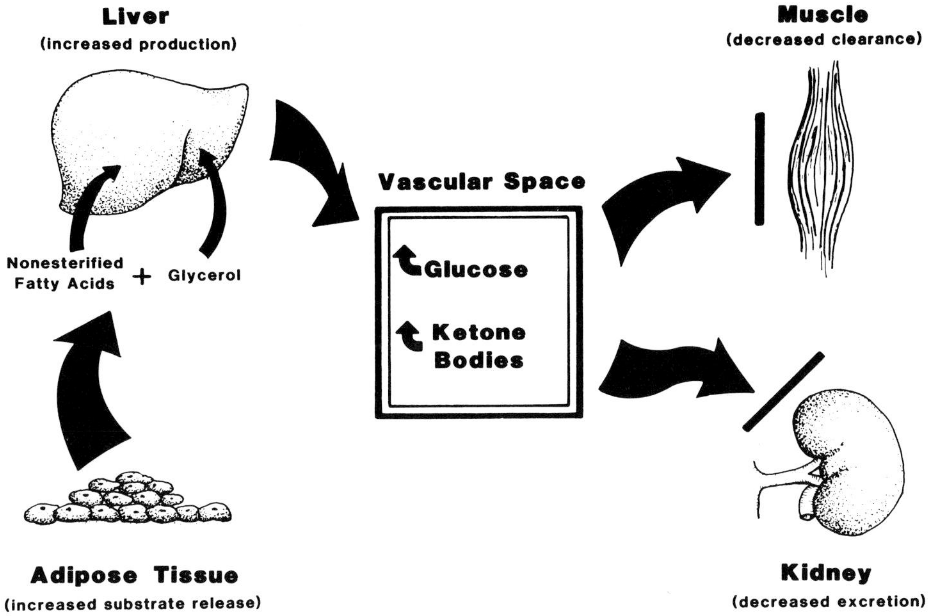

Fig. 11-8 Effects of stress hormone secretion in the acutely ill diabetic patient. Adipose tissue liberates increased quantities of glycerol and nonesterified fatty acids, which are converted in the liver to glucose and ketone bodies, respectively. Clearance of both glucose and ketone bodies by peripheral tissue and excretion by the kidney are decreased, augmenting the hyperglycemia and hyperketonemia. (Reprinted with permission from Schade DS, Eaton RP, Alberti KGMM, et al: Diabetic Coma, Ketoacidotic and Hyperosmolar. University of New Mexico Press, Albuquerque, 1981, p. 11.)

Role of the Physician

The importance of the physician in the management of acute medical illness cannot be overemphasized. Alberti and co-workers have shown that when diabetic patients are taught only to perform capillary blood glucose monitoring without additional physician input and encouragement no improvement in blood glucose concentration occurs.[13] Thus the third general principle to be emphasized in treating the ill diabetic patient is the essential role of the physician.

Point 3: The most important role of the physician in treating the ill diabetic patient is his or her ready availability to the patient. If the patient cannot easily reach the physician for advice and decision-making, the ill diabetic patient should be hospitalized immediately.

Once the physician has identified an ill diabetic patient, sequential monitoring of specific parameters must be performed, as the appropriate time for hospitalization is determined by these parameters (Table 11-2).

Point 4: In the ill diabetic patient, the following parameters must be monitored: (1) weight; (2) mental function; (3) respiratory rate; (4) pulse; (5) temperature; (6) glucose; (7) urine ketone bodies; (8) insulin dose; and (9) oral intake. Of these nine

Table 11-2. Patients Flow Sheet for Prevention of Ketoacidosis

Parameter	Hours after Patient Contact With the Physician						
	0	+4	+8	+12	+16	+20	+24
Body weight							
Mental function							
Respirations/min							
Pulse/min							
Temperature							
Blood glucose							
Urine glucose							
Urine ketones							
Insulin dose (rapid acting) (units)							
Oral Intake (volume)							
Physician instructions							
Comments							

parameters, the most important are the first three (weight, mental function, and respiratory rate) as they are used to determine the necessity of hospitalization.

Even if the patient is already hospitalized, these parameters need to be monitored, although nursing care can substitute for patient participation. Until the hospitalized patient is able to ingest fluids without nausea and vomiting, insulin should be administered intravenously according to the sliding scale given in Table 11-3. If the patient's blood glucose level is less than 100–150 mg/dl, the insulin infusion should be accompanied by an infusion of glucose aimed at delivering about 7.5 g/hr (150 ml of D5W/hr). Although it is certainly possible to treat patients with subcutaneous insulin injections in the hospital, the ease of an intravenous insulin infusion, with frequent blood glucose monitoring, makes this approach the treatment of choice, as episodes of hyper- and hypoglycemia are rare, and development of ketoacidosis should never occur. Obviously the sliding scale presented here is intended as a guideline. Insulin dosages must be adjusted on the basis of the response of each patient.

Because many physicians have not utilized a continuous insulin infusion except to treat diabetic ketoacidosis, initial reluctance is to be expected. The reason this approach is safe (probably safer than subcutaneous insulin injections) is that extremely reliable peristaltic fluid pumps are now universally available in hospitals in the United States to carefully monitor fluid administration (e.g., IVAC, IMED). If the insulin is made up in a dilute solution (Table 11-3), large amounts of insulin are never unexpectedly delivered to the patient. We do not recommend the use of concentrated insulin in small, syringe-driven infusion pumps,[14] as pump malfunction can result in overinsulinization and severe hypoglycemia.

Role of the Patient

The parameters which need to be monitored by the ill diabetic patient are listed in Table 11-2. These parameters must be measured at least every 4 hr and an accurate record kept of each reading. First, the weight of the patient is critical for determining

Table 11-3. Intravenous Insulin Infusion Rate To Maintain Metabolic Homeostasis

PATIENT	
"A"	"B"
Thin Minimum illness Usually insulin requirement <50 U/day Infusion fluid: 1 liter sodium chloride (0.45 mol/L) plus potassium chloride 20 mEq/L plus 500 U heparin[a] plus 50 U rapid-acting insulin.	Obese Severe illness Usually insulin requirement >50 U/day Infusion fluid: 1 liter sodium chloride (0.45 mol/L) plus potassium chloride plus 500 U heparin[a] plus 100 U rapid-acting insulin.

Blood Glucose Conc. (mg/dl)	Infusion Rate (ml/hr)	"A" Insulin (U/hr)	"B" Insulin (U/hr)
0–50	5	0.25	0.50
5–100	10	0.50	1.00
100–150	15	0.75	1.50
150–200	20	1.00	2.00
200–250	25	1.25	2.50
250–300	30	1.50	3.00
300–350	35	1.75	3.50
350–400	40	2.00	4.00
>400	50	3.00	6.00

Insulin should always be delivered by a reliable self-regulating fluid pump, e.g., an IVAC or IMED.

Blood glucose should be measured (by fingerprick and BG Chemstrips or Visidex) every 4 hr to readjust the insulin infusion rate.

[a]Does not anticoagulate patient but does maintain the intravenous line patent.

hydration status. Although records of oral input and urinary output of fluid are possible, this approach to monitoring hydration is fraught with error. Furthermore, input and output fluid monitoring ignores losses secondary to diarrhea, vomiting, diaphoresis, and respiration. To monitor weight, the patient must have a bathroom scale available, even if he must purchae it at the time of illness. Weight loss in excess of 5 percent of body weight is indicative of severe dehydration (i.e., loss of 3 kg in a 60-kg individual) and is reason to immediately hospitalize the patient. Furthermore, if the patient cannot ingest fluids to maintain his weight, rehydration is indicated, either in the physician's office, the hospital emergency room, in in the hospital itself. Thus the ninth parameter measured (Table 11-2) is oral intake, which indicates whether it is possible for the patient to remain hydrated. Unless this is possible, management at home is fruitless and immediate hospitalization is mandatory.

The second parameter to be monitored is the patient's mental status. Because the ability to keep accurate records is essential, inability to do this is indication of confusion and reason for hospitalization. Furthermore, telephone contact with the physician every 4 hr is required and permits the physician to assess the mental acuity of the patient. Excessive drowsiness or fatigue also indicates that mental status has deteriorated, and immediate hospitalization is indicated.

The third parameter for the patient to monitor is respiratory rate. Because the respiratory rate is in part voluntary, it is most helpful if another member of the patient's family monitors this for him without his knowledge. Acidosis stimulates respiration, and so an increase above 24 breaths/min is reason to hospitalize the patient. Hypernea also suggests the presence of pneumonia, for which hospitalization is mandatory.

Thus the three most important parameters on which the decision to hospitalize the patient are based are weight, mental status, and respiratory rate. Conversely, the last two parameters to monitor (blood glucose and ketone bodies) are not used to decide on hospitalization but are needed to determine the insulin dosage and the need for additional carbohydrate intake.

The fourth parameter, pulse, is easy for the patient to monitor and a good assessment of the degree of stress he is undergoing. Although an increase in pulse rate may be observed secondary to fever, dehydration, and infection, if it is within the normal range it is extremely reassuring to the physician that the patient is tolerating his acute illness well. Obviously, the pulse must be monitored after the patient has been recumbent for several minutes. Standing and lying pulses are not reliable as a sign of dehydration in the diabetic patient, as autonomic neuropathy may be present.

The fifth parameter, body temperature, is important in assessing the need for antipyretics. If fever accompanies the illness, antipyretic medication should be taken every 4 hr for at least 24 hr to prevent hyperthermia. Acetaminophen and aspirin are useful antipyretics, the former not causing stomach upset. Fever should be avoided because not only does it induce dehydration but it also augments the secretion of stress hormones.[11] The presence of fever should raise concerns about its nature and should signal the need for physician attention if no obvious cause is apparent.

Blood glucose concentration is utilized to determine the quantity of regular insulin needed. There is no role for intermediate- and long-acting insulin preparations in the treatment of acute medical illness in the diabetic patient. Subcutaneous injection of regular insulin should be administered every 4 hr as dictated by the physician, not the patient. More frequent administration of insulin (i.e., every 2 hr) is not necessary unless severe hyperlgycemia is present (i.e., blood glucose greater than 500 mg/dl), as the kinetics of subcutaneous insulin are such that maximum effects occur at 2 hr and are still present at 4 hr. However, insulin injection should not be delayed longer than 4 hr, as the danger of insulin deficiency becomes imminent with the consequence of severe metabolic decompensation. Even if the blood glucose concentration is low (<100 mg/dl), a small dose of regular insulin (3–5 U) is indicated in conjunction with the ingestion of liquids containing carbohydrate.

Although the insulin dose will need to be adjusted according to the degree of stress of the patient, his body weight, and his inherent sensitivity to insulin, we begin with the following sliding scale with insulin injection every 4 hr: For the usual patient who requires approximately 40 U of insulin per day, we recommend that 20 U be given for blood glucose concentration greater than 300 mg/dl (repeat every 2 hr until the blood glucose concentration is less than 300 mg/dl), 15 U for blood glucose concentration between 300 and 200 mg/dl, and 10 U for blood glucose concentration between 200 and 150 mg/dl. For blood glucose concentration below 150 mg/dl, 5 U of insulin should be given, otherwise relative insulin deficiency may occur and ketogenesis augmented. Obviously, this regimen has to be adjusted for both the degree of stress that the patient is experiencing and his degree of obesity or inherent insulin resistance.

The seventh parameter to monitor is urinary ketone bodies. The presence of ketone bodies in the urine (Ketostix, Acetest tablets) must be interpreted in light of the clinical condition of the patient. Thus the physician must remember that as the patient is improving the quantitative estimate of ketone bodies in the urine may actually increase because of the conversion of beta-hydroxybutyrate to acetoacetate and the fact that tests for ketone bodies measure only acetoacetate[5] (Fig. 11-9). However, if ketone bodies are present in the urine prior to initiation of therapy, two conclusions can be made: (1) The patient is mobilizing fat secondary to a rise in stress hormones and a relative deficiency of insulin; and (2) the possibility of ketoacidosis developing is significant. Because the only circulating hormone known to suppress ketogenesis is insulin, regular insulin injections must be continued even if the blood glucose concentration is not elevated. In this case, ingestion of carbohydrate is required to pre-

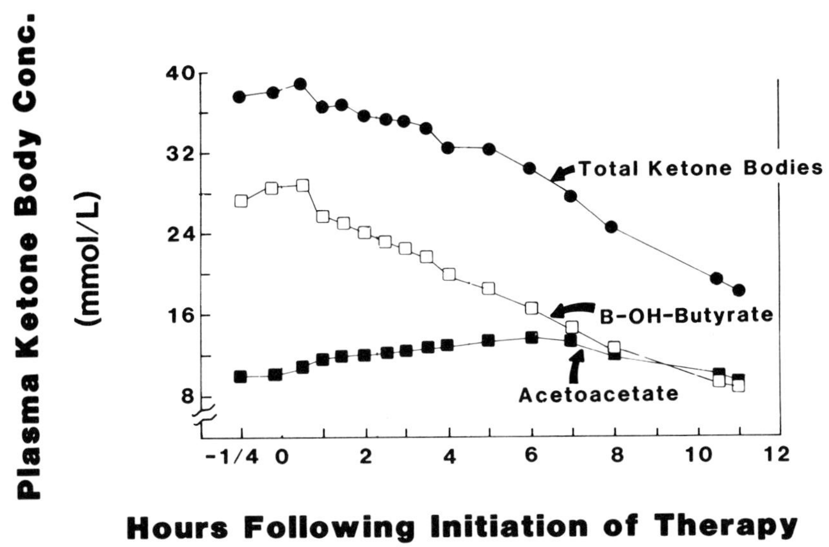

Fig. 11-9 Sequential changes in plasma ketone bodies during therapy of diabetic ketoacidosis. During the administration of insulin and rehydration in diabetic ketoacidosis, the total plasma ketone body concentration progressively falls. However, the individual ketones (acetoacetate and beta-hydroxybutyrate) demonstrate a differential response as metabolic improvement continues. Acetoacetate shows an initial rise as total ketone bodies decline, whereas beta-hydroxybutyrate progressively declines throughout the hospital course. The rise in acetoacetate is due to interconversion of beta-hydroxybutyrate to acetoacetate as the acidosis is corrected. Because the semiquantitative tests (Acetest tablets) measure only acetoacetate (and to a small extent acetone), it seems that the acidosis is becoming worse during therapy when in fact the patient is improving. (Reprinted with permission from Schade DS, Eaton RP, Alberti KGMM, et al: Diabetic Coma, Ketoacidotic and Hyperosmolar. University of New Mexico Press, Albuquerque, 1981, p. 244.)

vent hypoglycemia. Of importance is the fact that hyperglycemia and hyperketonemia do not have to coexist as evidenced by the syndromes of alcoholic ketoacidosis,[15] euglycemic ketoacidosis,[16] and hyperosmotic, nonketotic coma.[17]

Full cooperation of the patient is essential to prevent hospitalization during acute medical illness. If the patient has nausea and vomiting, two alternatives are available, assuming the patient is not in metabolic decompensation. First, the patient can be hospitalized for a short period of time until the vomiting terminates, or rehydration can be accomplished in the physician's office or the emergency room, at least once per day. Obviously, the choice of these two alternatives depends on the patient. Hospitalization is recommended if he (1) lives far from the hospital and physician, (2) has no transportation or telephone available, (3) is unreliable or noncompliant, or (4) has extremely brittle diabetes. However, if the patient is able to ingest fluid, rehydration in his home is feasible by ingestion of fluids and electrolytes such as juices, beef bouillon, or electrolyte-containing fluids, e.g., Gatorade.

Monitoring by the patient of the parameters in Table 11-2 is mandatory, and frequent physician contact is necessary. For monitoring, all diabetic patients should have the following items available: (1) an oral thermometer; (2) a bathroom scale; (3) acetaminophen tablets (antipyretics); (4) regular insulin; (5) beef bouillon cubes; (6) glucagon (1-mg vial); and (7) fruit juice. These items not only permit the diabetic patient to monitor his clinical condition but also allow him to respond to dehydration and hypoglycemia. All diabetic patients should be encouraged to obtain these items before becoming ill.

PHYSICIAN MANAGEMENT OF SURGERY

When the diabetic patient undergoes surgery, the physician has one major advantage over treating acute illness in the diabetic patient at home—the patient is always hospitalized. Therefore frequent monitoring is possible, and the physician only has to know what parameters to monitor and what fluids and insulin to administer. The goals of the physician are the same as in treating acute medical illness, i.e., to prevent diabetic ketoacidosis, hyperglycemic coma, and hypoglycemia.

There are numerous published regimens on treating the diabetic patient undergoing surgery.[14,18–22] Few of these are comparative studies of different regimens but, rather, descriptive approaches utilized in a particular hospital. Thus there is no one "best" regimen, and practically any rational approach works so long as the patient is monitored frequently enough to make changes in insulin and fluids. However, there are general principles which make the care of the patient undergoing surgery much easier.

Point 5: All diabetic patients should be in good metabolic balance prior to surgery. Good metabolic balance means normal vital signs and electrolytes (sodium, potassium, chloride, and carbon dioxide) and a blood glucose concentration of 100–200 mg/dl. The reason for stabilizing the patient preoperatively seems self-evident, as metabolic deterioration takes longer to occur when starting at eumetabolism. Although this approach has been emphasized by Alberti and Thomas,[21] examination of published series of patients undergoing surgery indicates that a large fraction of them are significantly hyperglycemic immediately before surgery.[18,20] The easiest approach to achieving eumetabolism is to admit the patient to the hospital the day before surgery and to discontinue all intermediate- and long-acting insulins and oral antidiabetic agents (chlorpropamide should be discontinued at least 36 hr before surgery because of its long half-life). After admission, the patient is placed on a sliding scale using intravenous insulin as outlined in Table 11-3 with appropriate adjustments individualized to the patient. The disadvantage of this approach—that the patient is admitted 1 day before surgery—is offset by the improved safety and ease of diabetic control which results.

Another general principle relative to surgery in the diabetic patient is the timing of food ingestion. Standard procedure for most patients undergoing surgery is usually no food or drink after midnight; however, this is not appropriate for the diabetic patient.

Point 6: At least 12 hr should elapse between food intake and surgery in the diabetic patient. The reason for this approach is that the diabetic patient may have gastroparesis which is not known at the time of surgery, and thus prolonged retention of food in the stomach may occur with the danger of aspiration pneumonia during anesthesia induction. Furthermore, the meal should be light and easily digestible, liquids being passed more easily than solids through the stomach.[23] Obviously, if the diabetic patient is continued on long-acting insulin or oral hypoglycemic agents prior to surgery, a 12-hr fast may induce hypoglycemia. Thus discontinuation of these agents and initiation of intravenous insulin utilizing a sliding scale with intravenous glucose as needed is the approach of choice. Another advantage of using intravenous insulin is to permit continued metabolic control of the diabetic patient, even if the surgery is delayed. This is not an infrequent event, as the time of surgery can be altered by several unanticipated factors, e.g., the duration of the operation immediately before the diabetic patient's surgery or the sudden occurrence of emergency surgery necessitating the use of the operating room facilities. When an intravenous insulin infusion is used to maintain homeostasis, no major changes in diabetic management are needed during an unanticipated delay. It should be emphasized that the use of the approach outlined necessitates frequent blood glucose monitoring (every 2–3 hr) to adjust the insulin infusion rate. Furthermore, in those patients with relatively low blood glucose levels ($<$100 mg/dl) it is advisable to add glucose to the intravenous fluid regimen ($\sim$5g/hr).

Management During Routine Surgery

As referenced above, there are many "successful" regimens which can be used to treat the diabetic patient undergoing surgery. These range from giving one-half the dose of subcutaneous insulin on the day of surgery[18] to the continuous intravenous infusion of insulin, glucose, and potassium. The latter regimen makes physiological sense and has been successfully used by Alberti and colleagues.[21] The theory is that by supplying glucose the need for protein catabolism to meet gluconeogenic needs in the diabetic patient is reduced, and a less negative nitrogen balance results. In our experience, infusion of this solution is more complex than necessary, and we prefer to continue the same preoperative treatment of the diabetic patient through surgery

(Table 11-3) and then to meet his caloric needs postoperatively. Furthermore, for practical purposes, blood sampling for glucose determinations can be done via a three-way stopcock from the same intravenous access site through which the insulin is being infused if glucose is not in the infusion fluid. Because we recommend that blood glucose concentration be monitored every hour during surgery (by use of glucose reagent strips such as Chemstrip BG or Visidex), the use of a three-way stopcock attached to an intravenous access site precludes the necessity of capillary blood glucose monitoring in the operating room (although this is not difficult if the anethesiologist has a fingerprick device). Thus no changes need to be made in the preoperative regimen until the patient returns from the recovery room, when his caloric needs must be considered. Depending on the nature of the surgery, this may range from a clear liquid diet to total parenteral nutrition. We do not recommend that a fixed intravenous dose of insulin be used during surgery as the development of hypo- or hyperglycemia is possible.

The most difficult aspect of diabetic care before, during, and after surgery is undoubtedly correct fluid management. The reason for this difficulty is not only that many diabetic patients have compromised renal function preoperatively but that cardiovascular insufficiency (manifested by angina or congestive heart failure) is common. In this age of expensive laboratory tests and equipment, the best assessment of fluid status is frequently forgotten.

Point 7: The best index of fluid status in the surgical diabetic patient is the patient's stable, preoperative weight. Thus daily weights are a necessity in all diabetic patients undergoing surgery, even if a bed scale must be used. Other indices of hydration, e.g., dry skin, dry mucous membranes, and records of fluid intake and output are not nearly as reliable as the patient's weight.

The fluid regimen must be individualized to the patient. For minor surgery in which the patient is ingesting fluid orally within hours after surgery, 5 percent glucose in 0.45 M sodium chloride (D5½NS) is acceptable at 100 ml/hr postoperatively. In contrast, for the diabetic patient who undergoes abdominal surgery and will not be ingesting fluid for several days, a more variable regimen is needed. In this patient, serum electrolytes must be measured at least daily and more often if potassium abnormalities are present. In general, 2–3 L of fluid (i.e., approximately 100 ml/hr) should be infused to replace insensible losses and to provide a urine output of at least 40 ml/hr. Obviously, additional fluid may also be needed if nasogastric suction or wound drainage is significant. Furthermore, sufficient glucose must be given to prevent ketosis (approximately 150–200 g/day). This amount of carbohydrate can be given by having all fluids infused contain 5 percent glucose. Thus if the patient receives 3 L of fluid per day, he will also receive 150 g of glucose. It should be remembered that more "free" water is lost than isotonic saline, and so hypotonic fluids (i.e., relative to sodium, as 5 percent glucose in water is isotonic) are indicated. An acceptable (and easy) fluid regimen in the diabetic patient is to alternate 1 L of 5 percent dextrose in water (D5W) with 1 L of D5 0.5N saline, remembering to add 20 meq of potassium chloride to each liter of fluid infused. This regimen will maintain a diabetic patient in balance for several days if intravenous insulin is also infused according to Table 11-3. For more prolonged therapy, total parenteral nutrition will be required which is described elsewhere.[24]

Management During Emergency Surgery

Infrequently, the diabetic patient may require emergency surgery. If he is in metabolic balance upon admission (e.g., after an automobile accident), the same rules apply as if the patient were admitted for surgery electively; that is, all subcutaneous insulin is discontinued, and intravenous insulin infusion is begun. It must be remembered, however, that the patient has probably already injected his insulin for that day, and hypoglycemia may occur. Thus not only should an insulin infusion be begun, but intravenous glucose may need to be administered if the blood glucose concentration is less than 100 mg/dl. The easiest method to administer glucose to the hypoglycemic patient is to rapidly give 10 ml of 50 percent glucose intravenously and to repeat as necessary. This solution is available commercially and is utilized routinely in all emergency rooms. Blood glucose concentration will transiently increase approximately 50 mg/dl after this dosage.

In contrast, emergency surgery may need to be performed in the unstable diabetic patient admitted in diabetic ketoacidosis with an abdominal catastrophe, e.g., a ruptured appendix. In this condition, aggressive fluid and insulin must be immediately begun utilizing standardized therapy for diabetic ketoacidosis. Although an in-depth description of the treatment of this condition is beyond the scope of this chapter, Table 11-4 summarizes an acceptable approach. The reader is referred to several recent monographs on this subject.[25–27] In this situation, we strongly urge that the patient's physician accompany the patient to the operating room and make the therapeutic decisions during surgery relative to the patient's metabolic state. Because of the complexity of the patient's condition, a team approach is required, and the patient's physician must assume responsibility for the patient's metabolic condition. Consultation with an endocrinologist or diabetologist should be obtained if possible.

Postoperative Therapy

The treatment of the patient in the postoperative period is dependent on the surgery involved. In the majority of patients, a progressive diet from liquids to solids if feasible within 48 hr. Until the patient is taking solid foods, the insulin infusion should be continued utilizing a sliding scale (Table 11-3). Once the patient can ingest solid foods, he is begun on his usual dose of subcutaneous insulin, and the intravenous insulin infusion is terminated 30 min after the insulin injection is given. This delay in termination prevents a period of acute insulin deficiency, as 30 min may be required before subcutaneous insulin is absorbed and exerts significant hypoglycemic activity.[28] It must also be remembered that during the postoperative period insulin resistance due to surgical stress is still present, and adjustments in the subcutaneous dose will be needed as determined by the patient's blood glucose concentration, food intake, and presence of surgical complications, e.g., fever and infection. If infection is present, maintenance of the insulin infusion is the easiest method to ensure the eumetabolic state. If major abdominal surgery is performed and weeks of no oral ingestion of food are anticipated, total parenteral nutrition must be begun according to standard guidelines.[24] Again, an infusion of intravenous insulin is the best approach to ensure reasonable metabolic control.

Table 11-4. Diabetic Ketoacidosis: Initial Therapy

1. Isotonic saline (NaCl 0.9%; 150 mmol/L): 1.5 L for 1st hour of therapy, 1 L for 2nd–4th hours. Thereafter 0.5 L/hr in 8 hr. If the patient is elderly or has cardiovascular disease, titrate fluid according to central venous or pulmonary wedge pressure. For severe hypotension infuse plasma expanders.
2. Short-acting insulin (regular): Intravenous 5–10 U/hr stat. then adjust dosage as necessary. See Table 11-3.
3. Potassium (K^+): 20 mmol/hr intravenously (20 meq/hr).
   a. Use ECG to monitor throughout as a guide to potassium theory.
   b. Start 20 mmol/hr from time of first fluid and insulin therapy. Keep plasma potassium between 4 and 5 mmol/L.
   c. If at any stage plasma potassium is:
      3 mmol/L—increase infusion to 40–60 mmol/hr
      3–4 mmol/L—increase infusion to 30 mmol/hr
      5–6 mmol/L—slow infusion to 10 mmol/hr
      6 mmol/L—stop potassium infusion
   d. First plasma potassium result must be available within 1 hr.
4. Diagnostic procedures.
   a. Rapid clinical examination; confirm diagnosis and establish cause. Weigh patient.
   b. Reagent strip blood glucose and serum acetoacetate level (Acetest).
   c. Send blood to laboratory for glucose, electrolytes, calcium, phosphate, magnesium, urea, arterial pH, pO_2, pCO_2, Hgb, Hct, and WBC. Culture blood and urine; chest x-ray.
5. Repeat plasma glucose, pH, and potassium measurements at 2 and 4 hr and as required thereafter.
6. Use syringe pump or pediatric infusion set to deliver intravenous insulin. Run at least 10 ml insulin-saline through the infusion set before connecting to the patient. If no response in plasma glucose and pH after 2 hr, double dose every 2 hr until a satisfactory response is achieved.
7. If pH <7.0 and clinical condition is unstable, give 500 ml of 2.6% sodium bicarbonate ($NaHCO_3$) (125 mmol; 3 ampules) + an additional 20 mmol potassium over 60 min. Check arterial pH 30 min after bicarbonate administration finishes and give further 50 mmol bicarbonate infusions until pH above 7.0.
8. Other considerations.
   a. Continuous stomach aspiration if patient unconscious or semiconscious.
   b. If no urine passed by 4 hr, catheterize.
   c. Give antibiotics early if any evidence of infection or if invasive procedures used.
   d. Give oxygen if pO_2 below 80 mm Hg.
   e. Consider low-dose heparinization in the elderly, the totally unconscious, or the severely hyperosmolar (>380 mOsm/L).
   f. Consider phosphate replacement—2.5 mmol/hr.

Adapted from Schade DS, Eaton RP: Diabetic ketoacidosis—pathogenesis, prevention and therapy. Clin Endocrinol Metab 12;321, 1983.

SUMMARY

This chapter has attempted to demonstrate that the management of acute medical illness and surgery in the diabetic patient is based not only on an understanding of glucose and ketone body metabolism but also on appropriate cooperation between the patient and physician. During acute medical illness, metabolic decompensation is preventable if the factors which regulate blood glucose and ketone body concentration are controlled by appropriate therapy. In most cases hospitalization can also be avoided, but not at the expense of patient welfare. Management of the diabetic patient undergoing surgery is also not difficult so long as insulin is appropriately administered. Because rapid changes in insulin dosage can best be made with the infusion of intravenous insulin, this is the method of choice for the patient undergoing surgery. With the present availability of glucose reagent strips to rapidly monitor blood glucose concentration, treatment of the diabetic patient with acute medical illness or who is undergoing surgery has been greatly simplified.

ACKNOWLEDGMENTS

The writing of this chapter was made possible by grants from the NIH (1 RO1 AM31973, 1 RO1 AM26129, 1 P50 HD11327), the General Clinical Research Center (grant RR-997), and the KROC Foundation.

REFERENCES

1. Hockaday TD, Alberti KGMM: Diabetic coma. Br J Hosp Med 7:183, 1972
2. Eaton R, Spencer W, Schade DS, et al: Diabetic glucose control: matching plasma concentration to dietary and stress hyperglycemia. Diabetes Care 1:40, 1978
3. Stevenson RW, Parsons JA, Alberti KGMM: Effect of intraportal and peripheral insulin on glucose turnover and recycling in diabetic dogs. Am J Physiol 244:E190, 1983
4. Miles J, Haymond M, Gerich J: Suppression of glucose production and stimulation of insulin secretion by physiological concentrations of ketone bodies in man. J Clin Endocrinol Metab 52:34, 1981
5. Schade DS, Eaton RP: Differential diagnosis and therapy of hyperketonemic state. JAMA 241:2064, 1979
6. Clements RS Jr, Vourganti B: Fatal diabetic ketoacidosis: major causes and approaches to their prevention. Diabetes Care 1:314, 1978
7. Martin HE, Smith K, Wilson ML: The fluid and electrolyte therapy of severe diabetic acidosis and ketosis: study of 29 episodes (26 patients). Am J Med 24:376, 1958
8. DeFronzo RA: The effect of insulin on renal sodium metabolism: a review with clinical implications. Diabetologia 21:165, 1981
9. Spark RF, Arky RA, Boulter PR, et al: Renin, aldosterone, and glucagon in the natriuresis of fasting. N Engl J Med 292:1135, 1975
10. Schade DS, Eaton RP: The controversy concerning counterregulatory hormone secretion: an hypothesis for the prevention of diabetic ketoacidosis? Diabetes 26:596, 1977
11. Schade DS, Eaton RP: The temporal relationship between endogenously secreted stress hormones and metabolic decompensation in diabetic man. J Clin Endocrinol Metab 50:131, 1980
12. Shamoon H, Hendler R, Sherwin RS: Synergistic interactions among antiinsulin hormones in the pathogenesis of stress hyperglycemia in humans. J Clin Endocrinol Metab 52:1235, 1981
13. Alberti KGMM, Worth R, Home PD, et al: Home blood glucose monitoring: does it improve diabetic control per se? In Petersmn CM (ed): Diabetes Management in the '80's: The Role of Home Blood Glucose Monitoring and New Insulin Delivery Systems. Praeger, New York, 1982
14. Barnett AH, Robinson MH, Harrison JH, Watkins PJ: Mini-pump: method of diabetic control during minor surgery under general anaesthesia. Br Med J 280:78, 1980

15. Levy LJ, Duga J, Girgis M, Gordon EE: Ketoacidosis associated with alcoholism in non-diabetic subject. Ann Intern Med 78:213, 1973
16. Munro JR, Campbell IW, McCuish AC, Duncan LJP: Euglycaemic diabetic ketoacidosis. Br Med J 2:578, 1973
17. Rosenberg SA, Brief DK, Kinney JM, et al: The syndrome of dehydration, coma and severe hyperglycemia without ketosis in patients convalescing from burns. N Engl J Med 272:931, 1965
18. Galloway JA, Shuman CR: Diabetes and surgery: a study of 667 cases. Am J Med 34:177, 1963
19. Fletcher J, Langman MJS, Kellock TD: Effect of surgery on blood sugar levels in diabetes mellitus. Lancet 2:52, 1965
20. Taitelman U, Reece EA, Bessman AN: Insulin in the management of the diabetic surgical patient: continuous intravenous infusion vs. subcutaneous administration. JAMA 237:658, 1977
21. Alberti KGMM, Thomas DJ: The management of diabetes during surgery. Br J Anaesth 51:693, 1979
22. Johnston DG, Alberti KGMM: Diabetic emergencies: practical aspects of the management of diabetic ketoacidosis and diabetes during surgery. Clin Endocrinol Metab 9:437, 1980
23. Rock E, Malmud L, Fisher RS: Motor disorders of the stomach. Med Clin North Am 65:1269, 1981
24. Grant JP: Handbook of Total Parenteral Nutrition. Saunders, Philadelphia, 1980
25. Schade DS, Eaton RP: Diabetic ketoacidosis—pathogenesis, prevention and therapy. Clin Endocrinol Metab 12:321, 1983
26. Foster DW, McGarry JD: The metabolic derangements and treatment of diabetic ketoacidosis. Semin Med Beth Israel Hosp Boston 309:159, 1983
27. Schade DS, Eaton RP, Alberti KGMM, Johnston DG: Diabetic Coma, Ketoacidotic and Hyperosmolar. University of New Mexico Press, Albuquerque, 1981
28. Dimitriadis GD, Gerich JE: Importance of timing of preprandial subcutaneous insulin administration in the management of diabetes mellitus. Diabetes Care 6:374, 1983

12 Diabetes Mellitus: Psychological Issues in Patient Management

Alan M. Jacobson
Joan Leibovich

Clinicians and investigators have had a longstanding interest in the psychosocial aspects of diabetes mellitus. This has stemmed from clinical experiences of trying to foster patient cooperation in following prescribed regimens, the obvious role of overeating and obesity in the etiology of adult-onset diabetes, concerns about the influence of treatment programs on the psychological development of children, and recognition that many patients experience difficulties in learning and using diabetes-related information. Awareness of psychosocial issues has increased recently and has stimulated several reviews and numerous research reports of relevance to the clinician.[1–7] In this chapter the authors review some features of the clinical and research literature and explore some approaches to patient problems useful for the physician caring for the patient with diabetes. Because diabetes is an illness affecting all age groups with varying intensity, we focus the discussion on young patients with insulin-dependent diabetes and, where meaningful, discuss parallels with the older noninsulin-dependent patient.

A MODEL FOR UNDERSTANDING PSYCHOSOCIAL FACTORS IN DIABETES

Figure 12-1 depicts a model for thinking about the interactions of diabetes and psychosocial influences based on a similar schema presented by Mattson[8] previously. As suggested by the model, we can consider several forces impinging on the vulnerable individual. The movement from being at risk or vulnerable to becoming symptomatic is equally relevant whether we consider the individual before diabetes has been diagnosed or the patient with longstanding illness. Among individuals without diabetes, this model provides a way of conceptualizing psychosocial influences on the onset of diabetes: a psychosomatic model of etiology which we discuss in more detail later. Among patients with diabetes this diagram provides a model for understanding how psychosocial factors might influence the course of diabetes. At this time we pursue the elements in this model as a general way to delineate potentially significant psychosocial factors for consideration in evaluating and following diabetic patients. In later sections particular elements of the model are discussed as they relate to developmental phases of the patient and diabetes. The model identifies three major influences on diabetic status: (1) environmental stresses; (2) environmental supports; and (3) the patient's coping ability.

Environmental stressors include problematic life events, e.g., job loss, and biological phenomena, e.g., infections or surgery. Supports can be thought of as cultural institutions in the environment which impact on the individual. These include family, church, friends, and the health care provider. Although theoretically positive in their influence, these supports can have negative effects as well; for example, the family in stress may undermine individual adaptation of a diabetic family member. Supports and stressors can modify the influence of one another on the patient "at risk" for becoming symptomatic.

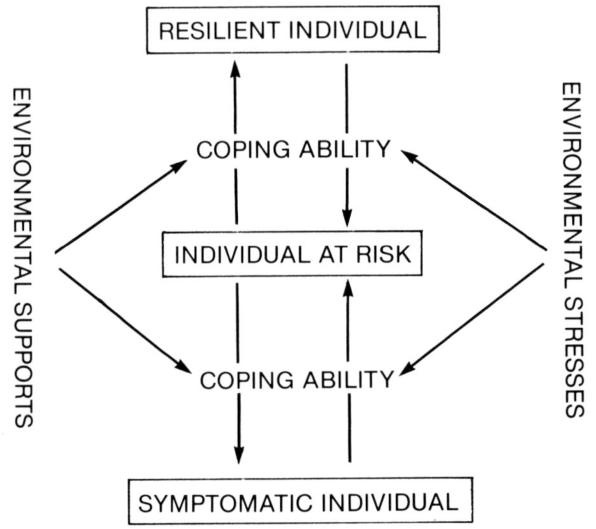

Fig. 12-1 A model for thinking about the interactions of diabetes and psychosocial influences.

Symptomatic refers to the development of personal, psychiatric, or medical problems, e.g., recurrent insulin reactions, ketoacidosis, or decreased success in caring for one's diabetes. The individual's own coping skills directly impact on this process. To the extent that the individual remains symptom-free and is able to function well, in the face of stressors, we can think of the individual "at risk" as being resilient to their influence. Studies of children of psychiatric parents demonstrate that some remarkably competent individuals are resilient in these high-stress low-support environments.[9] A clinical example may serve to highlight some of these interactions and influences.

> Jeanne is a 15-year-old living at home with her parents and a younger brother. She presents to her physician with increased problems controlling her blood glucose levels. He also notes that she seems upset but refuses to discuss anything about this apparent change in mood or her diabetes. Further history gathered from the parents reveals that her father has been experiencing increased problems at work and is threatened with a layoff because of recent business failures. This pressure has led to an increase in arguing between parents, because (as becomes apparent later) the father had always been insecure about his capacities and feared that eventually he would be shown to be a failure. The mother has little tolerance for the father's insecurities, which accentuates the arguments. Both children become upset by the change in their parents, which affects them in several ways. For Jeanne this manifests as a depressed mood and lack of interest in handling her life that includes her diabetic regimen. Excessive eating was one way in which she soothed her depression, leading to increasingly problematic glycemic control.

In this instance the added distress caused by work failure turned a reasonably supportive family environment into one of hostility and distance. Jeanne's capacity to cope decreased, and she became symptomatic. Intervention on the part of the medical and psychiatric staff focused on strengthening the family's cohesion, which indirectly helped Jeanne's depression and her coping ability, so she could again control her eating and other diabetes-relevant behaviors. This vignette depicts how an environmental stressor disturbs available supports and individual coping and how the medical team serves as an additional support.

Psychosocial Stress and Diabetic Control

Schade and Eaton,[10] among others, emphasized the importance of stress, especially physiological stress, e.g., infections, in triggering ketoacidosis. As Mason[11] suggested, psychosocial stress can be just as powerful an influence on hormonal shifts. Several studies document the possible effects of psychosocial stressors on the course of diabetes. For example, Jacobson et al.,[12] Grant et al.,[13] and Barglow et al.[5] found that life changes tend to coincide with periods of diabetic metabolic instability in at least some patients. Stress can influence diabetic control by several mechanisms: (1) As in the above example, commonly stressful experiences may lead to changed behaviors including those of diet management, exercise, and insulin monitoring. (2) During stressful periods, metabolically influential agents, e.g., alcohol, may be used to quell upsets. (3) Psychiatric illness may be accompanied by different hormone secretion patterns, thus influencing diabetic brittleness. For example, severe depressions are often accompanied by shifts in the diurnal variation in cortisol production. (4) Emotional arousal in response to stress may lead to changed production of hormone groups which can influence glucose and fat metabolism. This stress effect has been examined by several researchers. They have demonstrated that several hormone groups have counterregulatory effects on glucose and fat metabolism.[10,14,15] Intravenous infusion of these hormones in physiological ranges can elevate plasma ketone body and glucose levels among insulin-deficient individuals.[14] Such counterregulatory hormones include catecholamines, cortisol, glucagon, and growth hormone. These hormones are secreted in response to environmental stress. For example, Schade and Eaton demonstrated that fever produced by infusion of pyrogen stimulates the production of counterregulatory hormones in levels sufficient to elevate plasma levels of glucose, ketone bodies, and free fatty acids among diabetic patients.[15]

Other work has suggested that diabetic individuals differ from those without diabetes in that they are particularly sensitive to the counterregulation of these hormones. Even patients whose blood glucose has been normalized for up to 26 weeks using an open-loop delivery system seem to demonstrate this increased sensitivity to counterregulatory hormones.[16]

This work therefore establishes a theoretical physiological bridge linking stressful life events, emotional arousal, and management difficulties among insulin-dependent diabetics. However, although stress stimulation studies utilizing hormone infusions and physical stressors demonstrate the potential importance of counterregulatory hormone influence on diabetic metabolic control, few studies have examined the specific effects of psychosocial stress on diabetic metabolic activity.

The few studies that have specifically examined psychosocial stress among diabetics suggest some interesting relationships between emotionally stressful experience and the diabetic metabolic state. The earliest work of this kind was performed by Hinkle and Wolf.[17] They demonstrated that interviews which focused on personal problems and conflicts identified during prior psychotherapy sessions usually provoked decreases in blood glucose. However, blood glucose changes seemed to vary with the type of emotions that were elicited during these sessions. Experiences of anxiety and tension during the interviews were associated with decreases in blood glucose, while anger was associated with increased blood glucose. Vandenbergh et al.,[18] using hypnotic suggestion to induce a stressful experience, found that blood glucose levels usually dropped in response to stress. Strikingly, the usual effect of stress interviews, i.e., a decrease in blood glucose, contradicts the experimentally known effect of stress hormones on blood glucose.

In sum, this research suggests a complex interaction between psychosocial stress and blood glucose levels. In implies that patients may experience wide fluctuations in blood glucose up or down under emotionally upsetting conditions. Indeed, Hinkle and Wolf's findings of a correlation between specific emotional states and the direction of a glucose fluctuation suggest an interesting hypothesis: that different emotional states stimulate release of different combinations of stress-related hormones, thus leading to variability in levels.

Research on the effect of psychosocial stress on free fatty acid and ketone body levels have more consistently matched the hypothesized expectations. For example, Vandenbergh,[18] using hypnosis, and Baker et al.,[19] using stress-eliciting family interviews, demonstrated regular increases in free fatty acids. Baker et al. also reported that extremely brittle diabetic children with major family problems could be differentiated from children with easily managed diabetes as well as from children whose difficulties controlling their diabetes were caused by problems with regimen adherence. Plasma free fatty acids levels in these extremely brittle children were more elevated and returned more slowly to a baseline than in children from either control group. They concluded that for these psychosomatic children there was a direct effect of emotional state on free fatty acid release that was not found in the other two groups, and that family conflicts could induce emotional responses which led directly to recurrent ketoacidosis regardless of regimen adherence.

Overall, then, there is some systematic evidence of the presence of a linkage between emotional arousal and diabetic metabolic instability among some insulin-dependent diabetics. It suggests that in some patients "brittleness" may in part reflect psychosomatic processes outside the control of patient's behaviors—something important to recall in an illness where so much emphasis is placed on patient self-regulation.

Environmental Supports

Among the potentially important environmental supports, two of the most important were introduced by our previous patient vignette: the family and the health care professional.

Family. Increasing research has focused on the role of the family in diabetes management. Several studies highlight this issue.[20–23] For example, Koski et al., in their follow-up of a group of diabetic children and their families, suggested that the emotional tone in the family was associated with the level of diabetes control. Changes in some families—either to improved cohesion and stability or to a worsened state—were associated with shifts in the control of the child's diabetes.[20] Anderson and Auslander also found a modest association of family environment with diabetes control.[21] Simmonds found that children whose diabetes was in good to excellent control had stronger family units in comparison to the families of children in poor control.[22,23] Two issues limit the value of these observations: (1) The investigations were largely cross-sectional and, with the exception of the study by Koski et al., did not include any follow-up. Thus directionality of the relationship between family functioning and diabetic control of the child is unclear. (2) The studies utilized subject reports for their information about family functioning rather than direct observation of the family unit.

Health Care Provider. The physician and nurse are in a unique position to influence the family as a group and the individual patient. By listening to patient concerns they can provide a sense of caring that at the very least gives support at times of distress. At the next level the health care provider is often the first person outside the family to learn of problems. Consequently, he or she can serve as an important source of referrals to mental health providers and outside social agencies. This means that the interval history takes on a broader scope than the gathering of medical information. A short amount of time during each session for more open-ended questions may identify problems impinging on the patient's capacity to handle his or her diabetes. Lazare's approach emphasizes the value of viewing the patient as a customer who may have hidden requests. If successfully elicited, Lazare et al. suggested that the health care provider will be in a better position to treat the patient's medical problems.[24] They assume that the nature of the doctor–patient relationship is such that patients often hide certain concerns, but that careful listening and questions designed to show that the health care provider wants to know about all concerns which the patient brings to the appointment, will lead to revelation of covert requests. In many instances these requests and concerns have direct relevance to the medical illness.[24]

Coping Ability

Differences in coping ability and in the appraisal of what is stressful may be important in determining when an individual "at risk" becomes symptomatic. As described by Jacobson and Hauser[1] and Hamburg and Inoff,[6] diabetes presents the patient with a series of predictable phases or life crises. Each individual appraises these differently and, depending on his or her coping ability, deals with them more or less successfully. Lazarus and others have described a useful way of describing the coping process and understanding individual differences in coping.[25–28] From this perspective, stress occurs when there is no automatic way of responding to a given situation. The individual begins by appraising the situation to identify that a response to the stimulus is required and that no simple automatic response will entirely resolve the situation. The coping response affects the situation, which in turn is reevaluated for further response. Lazarus et al. also described a taxonomy for categorizing the various coping responses or strategies taken. Coping responses can be assessed according to their mode. These modes include direct action, search for further information, action inhibition, and intrapsychic activity. Coping strategies can also be categorized according to their function, i.e., whether they instrumentally alter the situation or palliatively regulate the emotional response.

From the perspective of this approach the clinician can understand how certain individuals might function well in situations which respond well to specific external direct actions but have distinct difficulty when direct action does not resolve the situation very successfully and instead the individual must cope with a situation in which his coping strategies must include palliation of difficult feelings. Alternatively, Lazarus[27] and others described research which shows that certain strategies work in one situation but not in others. For example, extensive use of denial (even to the extent of denying the reason for admission to a coronary care unit) is associated with better outcomes in response to myocardial infarction[29] but could be distinctly problematic in long-term management of diabetes. A milder level of denial which allows a patient to be optimistic about appraising the future may help an adolescent care for his diabetes, though it is not clear how this would affect the patient who later develops complications. Further research is needed to extend these types of observations by evaluating patients with diabetes at different points in their lives as patients.

PHASES OF DIABETES

The course of diabetes can be thought of as evolving through three distinct periods: onset, complication-free management, and complications. Each presents somewhat different stresses for the patient and family.

Onset

Although some early case reports[30] suggested that diabetes may be a psychosomatic illness in that psychosocial stressors may be influential in its etiology, little empirical research has examined this question. In one study, Stein and Charles[31] compared diabetic subjects with controls not having diabetes and found a higher than expected history of loss in the diabetes group. No other projects have explored this issue in a systematic fashion.

Recent evidence that insulin-dependent diabetes is an autoimmune process in which islet cell antibodies can be detected long before clinical manifestations of the disease process suggests that psychosocial influences could be important in two distinct ways. (1) Psychosocial environmental influences could affect the immune process, as has been suggested by research in other areas.[32] (2) Psychosocial stresses could serve as the proximate trigger for the development of clinically observable diabetes among individuals who already have islet cell destruction. In the second instance, psychosocial stress, like biological stress, increases insulin requirements, which cannot be met by a depleted group of beta cells. These two questions require different research strategies for their assessment.

At onset, the patient and family are faced with new and often totally unexpected problems. For a few families with a strong family history of diabetes, the onset may have been anticipated. For example, in one family the parents had been having their children's urine tested annually. When one of the children developed a flu syndrome in which he began urinating frequently, they went to the pediatrician with the diagnosis all but made. More typically, however, the change is more sudden and jarring. The event may be so tumultuous and the family so overwhelmed that initial information about diabetes management must be titrated to the individual capacities to learn. Remarkably, many families and patients seem relatively unflustered by the diagnosis of diabetes. They may even feel relieved because they had thought the symptoms were due to a more feared illness, e.g., cancer. Such individuals may express optimism about the future, feel that by having diabetes they will now have to live a more healthful life and launch into the new diet and recommended exercise regimens with a sense that this is a fortuitous event. Others may see themselves as essentially healthy and resent the fact that others may think of them as having an illness. Little research has been done to assess the prognostic implications of these differing responses to the onset of diabetes.

Management Years

Once a diagnosis has been made, patients and their families enter the world of diabetes: food exchanges, shots, urine tests, blood tests, and sick days. Later in the chapter we describe some of the basic themes in the lives of patients with diabetes, but during the years after diagnosis one issue underlies all others: the necessity for extensive education. Patients and families learn, forget, and learn again many of the basics of diabetes. Numerous studies in education and diabetes education emphasize the necessity for repetition and the likelihood that information will be forgotten quickly.[33,34] Consequently, diabetes education should be conceived of and explained to the patient and family as a cycle of continually refining their understanding of diabetes-related issues. Early, the information is simple and focused on the necessities, as family members are likely to be overwhelmed by the affective and procedural features of living with a chronic illness. Educational programs which are predominantly didactic are less likely to be effective.[7] Individualized programs which take into account developmental issues, provide the family with a sense of emotional support, and utilize behavioral approaches to maximize mastery are most likely to succeed. The development of entertaining and instructive video programs linked to computers provide one approach to disseminating knowledge which will require extensive work to develop. These approaches may be especially useful in rural areas or where centers of diabetes treatment are distant.

It is important for the health care provider to remember that patients forget or simply do not learn more frequently than might be anticipated. In some instances these failures to learn reflect underlying psychological problems or, in children, learning problems which may also be manifest in school performance. For example, Hauser and Jacobson found that adolescents with diabetes show arrests in ego development, which may mean that their capacity to learn and utilize many of the tasks of diabetes are more difficult.[4]

Studies of the impact of diabetes on children and adults during the management years have not found consistent evidence for distinct personality or psychiatric effects. Although some research suggests that diabetic children may be overly dependent,[35] other studies fail to show any such patterns.[36,37] Previous reviews have emphasized several methodological limitations to these studies, including sample bias and the use of idiosyncratic measures.[38] Although these studies do not show consistent evidence for such effects, they do strongly show a consistent relationship between the mental health of the patient and emotional tone in the family and the successful care of blood glucose levels.[20,22,23]

Complications

One of the common themes and concerns of the patient with diabetes has to do with anticipation of the development of complications. Both clinical reports and systematic research emphasize that worry about the future is a major concern for both parents and children with diabetes.[4,39] When complications arise, they may be met with intense and unexpected responses which are seemingly out of proportion to the complication that has been diagnosed. For example, one 26-year-old man became intensely anxious when the ophthalmologist informed him that he noted "a touch of retinopathy" which did not necessitate treatment. The patient was taken by surprise, having anticipated a normal examination. His worst fears—those of going blind—were activated by the information. Other patients feel betrayed by the development of complications. They may be angry because they believed that their good self-care would be rewarded and now every high blood glucose represented a demonstration of their failure. As noted earlier, these individual variations may also reflect differences in coping strategies that patients typically utilize.[25–28]

As the following case suggests, specific life circumstances determine the particular meaning of new complications for the patient.

> Mrs. R., 27 years old and married, has had diabetes for 15 years. During the prior year she had been under increasing stress from work and financial pressures. She wanted to change jobs but had to be very careful about this because she was currently supporting herself and her husband, who could get only occasional employment. At a time when she finally believed she could leave her current employment, her ophthalmologist recommended laser treatments for newly identified retinopathic changes. This was the first complication of diabetes she had experienced. Because of the cost of laser treatments she felt it necessary to remain at her present job. Her decreased vision made it difficult to perform the tasks with the required precision, leading to increased work conflicts and an added sense of pressure. For Mrs. R. it was this aspect of the complications that was most upsetting.

For some families the development of complications tips a former delicate balance in the direction of family dysfunction or disorganization. A fragile intrafamilial balance may not be able to withstand the assault of one more major stress.

One middle-aged woman attributed her husband's extramarital affair to the onset of her mild neuropathy. Further investigation revealed that the couple throughout their 25 years of marriage had tacitly agreed to ''ignore'' her diabetes. She feared that if she burdened her spouse with complaints, he might leave her. On his part, her husband had feared that the neuropathy signaled the ''beginning of the end'' and that he would soon be left a widower. Marital therapy resulted in more open and clear communication and in a greater sense of partnership.

The evolution of complications to levels of severity which interfere with personal functioning are likely accompanied by an increased perception of stress, more actual negative life events, and more psychological symptoms.[40] Thus the onset of proliferative retinopathy and impaired vision may lead to loss of work, added financial problems, and perceived stress, which adds to the burden of coping with the illness process. This can lead to decreased success in caring for one's health. For example, when her husband began on dialysis, Mrs. B. became overprotective and never left his side because she felt that she had to take care of him or he would die suddenly. They had no children and few friends, so her life revolved around him. He regressed and demanded all her attention, and to his detriment he decreased his activity level to the point where he came bedridden unnecessarily.

DEVELOPMENTAL ISSUES IN RESPONSES AND ADAPTATION TO DIABETES

Diabetes can emerge at any time during the life cycle. The impact of the condition on an individual's perception of himself, his understanding of its short- and long-range implications, and the manner in which these factors are integrated into his life are greatly influenced by his specific stage of psychosocial development. Because little empirical research has examined family experiences with an eye to these developmental differences, most of this discussion necessarily derives from clinical experiences and research from other areas.

Infants

When diabetes occurs in infants, it is the parents who necessarily shoulder the responsibility for care. They often feel initially concerned about the infant's survival and overwhelmed to monitor the condition when the baby cannot communicate his needs with words.

The primary developmental task for the infant lies in establishing a trusting relationship with his environment, mediated through his interaction with his parents and their responses to his needs. The infant may sense the added tensions in his parents in the ways they cuddle, nurse, and respond to crying and upset. Not being able to label or identify anything more than this change in their parents, this tension may lead to more upset on the part of the infant with diabetes. Parental anxieties are often focused on differentiating hypoglycemic reactions or high glucose levels from the usual distresses of infancy.

Another common source of discomfort for parents lies in the necessity to give insulin injections to and perform blood tests on a small baby who cannot understand their lifesaving functions. The arena of food, around which so much early parent–child interaction occurs, can also become tense as parents feel pressure to have their babies eat specific amounts at predictable times to prevent hypoglycemic episodes.

Toddlers (1.5–3 Years)

When the infant becomes a toddler he begins to take the first steps in asserting his ''separateness'' and individuality. This requires of parents some degree of ''letting go'' in acknowledgment of the child's need to explore his environment. Parental fear and tension about the well-being of their toddler with diabetes may result in an excessive focus on the youngster's helplessness and dependence, thereby inhibiting his beginning attempts at autonomy. The balkiness and temper tantrums characteristic of this age often makes it difficult to distinguish between behavior related to hypoglycemia and other causes.

Preschool (3–5 Years)

The preschool youngster is typically intensely concerned about his body's strength and intactness and is vulnerable to fearing its being damaged. He lacks the capacity to understand the cause and nature of his illness and tends to interpret the pain and discomforts of diabetes and its management procedures as punishment or retribution for real or imagined misbehavior. He may view diabetes as temporary. Parents and physicians can offer support and reassurance, and avoid blaming the child or punishing him for diabetes-relevant behaviors; this then counteracts his fears, especially around painful procedures.

School Age (6–11 Years)

During the primary grade school years, the child increasingly forms important attachments outside the immediate family. In his newly meaningful relationships with contemporaries, the youngster with diabetes may view himself as "different" or less "adequate" and may be prone to keep his illness a secret. Encouraging the child's participation in the typical activities of his age group and being sensitive to his having a choice about informing others about his condition (and telling other responsible adults privately) help to moderate his feelings of "differentness." Some children of this age wish to attend summer camp. Although special camps for diabetic youngsters can be an important resource, some children may balk at going because they feel confronted and forced to acknowledge the fact that they have diabetes.

The school-age child's growth is marked by increasing curiosity and learning about his inner and outer worlds. His energies are channeled into the mastery of intellectual, social, and physical skills. In seeking the cause of his illness, especially mysterious because it involves internal physical functions, he may blame himself (e.g., for eating excessive amounts of candy) or his parents (for somehow not protecting him). These distorted cause-and-effect interpretations flourish if they are not encouraged to surface and if the parents themselves have misconceptions about causality which have not come into the open.

The older grade school child is more able to comprehend the relation of the etiology, course, and treatment of diabetes as removed from the realm of personal punishment. He can also grasp the meaning of the genetic component which may have been identified. This understanding may generate spoken or unspoken accusations and resentments toward the parent(s) linked to the diabetic condition. If it occurs, it is helpful for parents to allow the expression of anger activated by this awareness of hereditary factors.

With the increasing motor skills and curiosity about management procedures, children of this age often demonstrate interest in participating in the regimen. Age-appropriate involvement, e.g., assisting with blood and urine testing, meal planning, drawing up and occasionally injecting insulin, can enhance the youngster's sense of mastery. Premature relinquishment of care may be a temptation for parents wishing to escape the burdens of the illness. This "underprotectiveness" or premature transfer of these responsibilities may lead to difficulties later in adolescence when the teenager, by mismanaging his self-care, may signal his inability to carry the emotionally laden burdens independently.

Adolescence (12–17 Years)

The development of increasing autonomy and independence is the major psychosocial task of adolescence. Typical strivings for less reliance on family may clash with the diabetic teenager's need for parental guidance in managing his illness, which may have a less stable course during this period of rapid physical growth.

In the service of evolving a sense of self-identity, many teenagers temporarily reject or question the values and standards of parents and other authorities. Diabetes care can become one ground for this struggle. Teenagers with diabetes may personally test the hypothesis that they actually have diabetes by not following medical instructions (e.g., overeating, omitting insulin, refusing to do blood and urine tests). In attempting to discover for themselves the very existence of diabetes and the limits of its dangers, teenagers may be expressing a preparation for impending separation from parents. Such "testing out" behavior can also create medical difficulties if carried to an extreme (e.g., frequent episodes of ketoacidosis or hypoglycemia, abuse of insulin). Optimally, teenagers can manage many aspects of their self-care but require overall parental supervision, just as they would for other activities.

A paramount feature of adolescence is the importance of peer attachments. Contemporaries can offer support, a sense of strength, and a feeling of "belonging." Diabetic teens may have problems with feeling "different" and unacceptable, with resulting depression, anxiety, and confusion. Attempts to gain social acceptance and demonstrate likeness to peers may translate into digressions from the prescribed regimen.

Adolescents are typically focused on and insecure about the dramatic physical changes of puberty. The diabetic teenager may experience his condition as a blow to his developing body image and sexual identity. The normal concerns about bodily functions can be intensified as he must concentrate constant vigilance and anxious attention on somatic events.

By adolescence, the youngster has gained the capacity to conceptualize the permanence of his chronic condition, the uncertainty about his future health status, and the threat of future complications and a possibly shortened life span. That recognition can make the teenager more prone to develop depressive symptoms as well as an overt major depression. In order to cope with these concerns some teenagers make secret "deals" with their illness. One girl decided that she would accept any and all complications, but she believed that this acceptance could be paired with a deal with her illness that it would not occur until she was 65.

By virtue of being outside the intense parent–adolescent dyad, professionals overseeing the health care of the adolescent with diabetes can provide an important positive influence. The promise of confidentiality between teenager and physician helps to foster a trusting relationship whereby the teenager feels safe in airing his worries. The adolescent may view guidelines drawn by professionals as less threatening to his growing self-sufficiency than those coming directly from parents. A noncritical, accessible, and flexible stance on the part of the physician increases the likelihood of having medical advice followed. It is important to recognize that many of the problems with diabetes experienced by teens and their families are temporary and parallel the other typical problems of adolescence.

Young Adults

More at ease with his own individuality as separate from his parents, the young adult may be more accepting of the realities of his chronic illness and have integrated its care more comfortably into his daily life. Planning and implementing educational and career goals and making meaningful interpersonal commitments are prime issues of this period. The threat of future or emerging diabetic complications may create reluctance on the one hand or urgency on the other to make long-range commitments to careers or marriage. Young women contemplating pregnancy must include the complex issues diabetes places on this planning. Anxious concerns may arise for young men as they can anticipate the possibility of future sexual dysfunction. Young men and women with diabetes wonder about placing additional economic and emotional burdens on their partners, especially if complications develop which impair their ability to work or fulfill family obligations.

Many patients as young adults recognize that they have previously been caring poorly for their diabetes and return to their physicians with renewed interest in managing the illness. This renewal may accompany the development of the first signs of long-term complications. Separation from parents may also mark the time that adolescent struggles around independence have begun to be resolved, thus allowing their taking a more positive attitude toward self-care and greater overall responsibility.

Parenting a Child with Diabetes

The child's adaptation to diabetes is closely tied to his parents' overall response to his disability. Several factors in parental response are particularly critical in determining the diabetic child's overall positive adaptation. In order to accept the realities of their child's chronic illness, parents must mourn the "loss" of their desired normal child and master their resentful and self-accusatory feelings about the condition. Parents who do not come to terms with these painful feelings tend to remain excessively anxious, fearful, and guilty and in some form transmit these emotions to their youngsters.

Parents who have successfully mastered the conflicting emotions aroused by the implications of diabetes are more able to encourage gradual self-care while promoting realistic age-appropriate activities and enforcing only the necessary restrictions. However, the complex daily tasks of diabetes can create stresses in balancing the encouragement of the child's independence and protecting him from dire health consequences. The following statements illustrate this.

1. "I can't let my 10-year-old go to a slumber party when no one will be there to monitor her insulin dose."
2. "How can my son play soccer when I cannot be there to watch for insulin reactions."
3. "Our daughter once had a severe reaction insulin in the middle of the night. My husband and I now take turns checking on her through the night."

Parenting a child with diabetes imposes worries and demands which may place extreme strain on all family members. If one parent (usually the mother) carries an inordinate share of the burdens of care, she may feel resentment toward her husband and isolated from him. On their part, husbands may feel jealousy and anger at their wives for channeling an excessive amount of energy into caring for their offspring with diabetes. One father remarked. "Even when we do go out alone for an occasional dinner, my wife talks only about diabetes."

Parents can benefit from an opportunity to communicate their dilemmas about sharing the care of their youngster. When both parents are involved in the responsibilities of care, they may feel closer to each other and the child reassured. When one parent avoids the responsibilities of care, the child senses this distance and wonders about the reasons behind this removal from such an important aspect of his life. One 9-year-old expressed, "My father is scared to death of my diabetes. He shakes when I get my injection." Indeed this father harbored great dread about diabetes and had not dealt with his personal fears about his son.

Siblings of children with diabetes are also greatly affected by the daily care and the family's emotional involvement. Jealousy and resentment may be felt by the healthy sibling as he experiences the "special" attention, time, and energy spent on his brother or sister. He may feel penalized by having his parents less available to him. Siblings may flaunt their good health (often with food not permitted to the child with diabetes). He may also harbor concerns about his brother's or sister's illness, guilt about having been spared the condition, or worry about developing it himself. As with other relatives, siblings need to be a part of the family's education about diabetes and benefit from expressing their anxious, resentful, and guilty, albeit expected emotions.

THERAPEUTIC CONSIDERATIONS FOR THE HEALTH CARE PROVIDER

The current state of technology in treating diabetes does not allow the complete normalization of glucose levels in individuals with insulin-dependent diabetes. Therefore both patient and physician must operate within the confines of this imperfect reality.

The patient with diabetes must make a multitude of independent decisions daily around the complex adjustments in balancing diet, insulin, and exercise. Therefore he must also be actively involved in the process of designing his individual realistic treatment goals and program. These aims vary widely among patients and even over time for an individual, and they may be influenced by many factors. When the patient does not participate in this goal-setting process he is less likely to follow through. The patient–physician model derived from the rather unique demands which diabetes imposes contrasts with the more traditional relationship wherein the physician determines the prescription and then expects the patient to follow through. For the individual with diabetes, the physician functions better as an expert consultant than an authoritarian figure. Working within the collaborative model, the physician and patient are less likely to become locked in a "compliance" bind. This type of bind can result in the physician's "blaming" the patient for not adhering to a plan which may, for multiple reasons, prove impossible for him to carry out. Patients sometimes complain that physicians convey accusations through such statements as "You must have done something wrong," when results are unacceptable. Indeed the terminology commonly used in diabetes care can communicate moral overtones: "good" and "bad" control, "cheating," and "poor compliance."

Holding the patient responsible, directly or through implication, for his "misdeeds" in achieving unacceptable treatment results may have negative psychological reverberations at such a time when diabetic complications may emerge. Many patients experience guilt and depression at having "transgressed" and "caused" the negative consequences of their illness when, rather, a complex interplay of variables is more likely involved.

Patients may feel judged as "good" or "bad" people depending on their achieving "good" or "bad" metabolic balance. When the physician's orientation is focused on the course of diabetes rather than including the total and complex individual, patients may feel slighted or unappreciated. Reinforcing patients' feelings that they are dealt with as an illness, rather than a person, is the rather common expression "He is a diabetic." Although some patients themselves use these terms, many object to the notion that they *are* their illness, rather than that diabetes is only one aspect of their total identity. One middle-aged woman with 30 years of diabetes said that when she had visited a new physician his gaze remained on the log of her blood glucose levels which she had brought, and that he did not make direct eye contact with her during the entire office visit. By not noticing her demeanor or inquiring about her life outside of diabetes, he could not have known that her less than successful glucose levels were reflective of her depression resulting from the recent loss of a close friend.

Treatment goals, mutually agreed on, must take into account both medical and psychosocial aspects. Approaches comprised solely of information transfer and medical care may be less effective than those where psychosocial orientations are incorporated.[41]

Including mental health professionals as a routine part of medical care can serve a preventive as well as a therapeutic function. Easy access to such professionals can permit early identification of personal problems which often surface around a patient's inability to accomplish inadequate self-care. Impaired capacity to learn basic skills at the onset may represent difficulties in the grief process. Problems in carrying out the medical regimen may relate to a wide variety of personal and interpersonal conflicts. Sensitive and nonjudgmental listening on the part of the physician may help identify the psychological road blocks to adequate self-care and allow for referral to specialized psychiatric assistance when more extensive exploration is indicated.

Several themes recur with some regularity in the lives of people with diabetes. These may present behaviorally in poor adherence to diabetic care or even by a rigid attachment to self-care, and so it is useful for the health care provider to listen for them during patient visits.

Not uncommon is the underlying fear of insulin reactions. The possibility of sudden drops in blood sugar may represent dreaded public exposure, especially when diabetes has been kept a secret.

> A 25-year-old successful, hard-working professional woman was able to achieve only a consistently rather high glucose level. Both she and her physician were puzzled by these results which resisted all management maneuvers. When her anxiety and frustration escalated and began to interfere with her work, she was referred for psychiatric evaluation. She herself had been unaware of the existence or power of her avoidance of hypoglycemia. Only after several months of psychotherapy did the personal meaning of hypoglycemic episodes emerge from her personal history. Behind the facade of a happy family life, her childhood was marked by abuse by her alcoholic father in unpredictable outbursts. Hypoglycemia represented to her a "loss of control" linked to her parent's hurtful rages.

After uncovering this hidden connection she was able to deal more realistically with the possibilities of insulin reactions and attain more satisfactory glucose levels. She actually came to feel more "in control" as a consequence of shedding her driving, albeit unrecognized fear.

Another commonly motivating issue in poor adherence to diabetic management is the psychological denial of the existence of diabetes. The recognition of the implications of having this illness are warded off by means of behavior which seems to translate as: "If I behave as if I do not have diabetes, I will not have it." The variations on this theme are numerous, but the persistent inattention to the demands and signs of diabetes can reflect this type of denial.

A 20-year-old man developed frequent infections because of high glucose levels. Only when blurry vision occurred, creating panic, could he inform his physician of his fear of blindness, which was a complication in his older, deceased brother's diabetic course. Except for the obligatory daily insulin, this young man had not modified his previous life style with the onset of diabetes 2 years before. If anything, he had increased his alcohol and drug intake and drove his car more recklessly. His attempts to keep his anxieties about diabetes at bay resulted in his defiant and dangerous activities. Only over time with the gentle uncovering of his fears was he able to recognize and tolerate his anxiety and sadness, confront his maladaptive behavior, and begin to move toward gradual change.

The preceding vignette reflects an extreme use of the mechanism of denial which may exist in many patients to a lesser degree. The case also demonstrates how fear of the future can constitute an underlying force in behavior, even when it is unacknowledged by the individual or his family.

In addition to individual, couple, and family therapy, another modality, the discussion or therapy group, may prove especially helpful to some patients and their families. This type of resource can uniquely offer the support of other people in shared circumstances and is best organized around common attributes (e.g., young adults with diabetes, diabetic teenagers, parents of diabetic youngsters, newly diagnosed adults). This type of group setting can provide a "safe," supportive, and accepting forum for the airing of mutual concerns and dilemmas. When led by a trained professional who guides the discussion, participants can gain important validation for the universality of many of their worries as well as a fresh perspective on those concerns which may be distorted by their own personal histories or styles of coping. Identification of their own excessive responses may lead some group members to request referral for individual or family counseling. Successful group endeavors tend to decrease the sense of isolation and aloneness experienced by many patients and their families in handling the enormous burdens of diabetes.

SPECIFIC MANAGEMENT ISSUES

Pumps and Home Glucose Monitoring

The advent of newer, rapidly developing treatment tools, e.g., the open-loop insulin pump and home glucose monitoring, offers the hope of improved glucose balance and the possible lessening or delay of diabetic complications. Without the benefit of long-term study, questions continue to arise regarding the importance of specific psychosocial factors which may contribute to outcomes of these treatment approaches. Two studies of small numbers of selected adolescents and adults evaluated over short periods (less than 1 year) do not demonstrate any negative effects of intensive treatment regimens.[42,43] Unfortunately, neither study evaluated these patients over a longer time frame, and neither assessed a wide range of representative patients. As volunteers who were carefully selected for insulin pump therapy, they do not reflect the wide range of patients whose experience might be considerably different. For example, one adolescent who had been experiencing mixed feelings about caring for his diabetes found that pump treatment forced him to think of himself as a diabetic, something he secretly tried to forget. Consequently, he undermined the intensive treatment, forcing an abrupt termination while still an inpatient.

In contemplating pump therapy, the health care team must carefully assess a particular patient's prior adjustment to diabetes and its management as well as his expectations for the results of pump therapy. Underlying psychological issues in the failure of more traditional management techniques may likewise come into play with the pump. Some patients initially request the pump technique as a "substitute pancreas" which will do the work for them or even "cure" their diabetes. They will of course be disappointed, as operating a pump requires extensive education and demands more careful monitoring of blood glucose and the timing of exercise and meals. Patients remain the activators of the device and make frequent decisions about its actions. Patients who have success with pump therapy seem to view it as an extension of the tools which *they* can utilize in mastering the fluctuations of the course of diabetes. They continue to be "in charge."

Public acknowledgment of diabetes, derived from the wearing of an insulin pump, necessitates that the patient have come to terms with accepting himself as a person with diabetes. One adolescent felt it was too humiliating to have to explain repeatedly to her classmates the reasons for the pump and believed that in the eyes of her friends her attractiveness was diminished. One middle-aged lawyer stopped pump use when he felt it put him at a disadvantage with his clients. Another professional man, more at peace with his diabetes, felt he was making a strong positive statement about caring for and about himself and saw this as bolstering his own confidence in himself as well as in the eyes of others.

Careful advance preparation for the predictable mechanical hitches or ultimate results is beneficial in avoiding frustrations, and disappointments arising from the expectation of unrealistic goals. A young woman felt she had exhausted all hope and "gave up" on self-care when the pump failed to help her attain near-normal glucose levels. Underneath this stated goal was her wish to become pregnant, which did not occur and was in fact more the source of her hopelessness.

As with the initiation of pump therapy, home glucose monitoring (HGM) must be evaluated with an eye toward the added demands but potentially more satisfactory treatment outcomes. The patient must be an active participant in choosing the technique and in understanding it use and potential benefit. Because HGM can improve the accuracy of measuring transient glucose levels, many patients experience a decrease in previous feelings of helplessness, vulnerability, and frustration when they were making decisions without this more precise measure. Those individuals who successfully execute HGM feel an added sense of mastery and self-confidence.

For some patients HGM can result in an even more anxious and rigid focus on their condition to the exclusion of other aspects of their lives. For example, an 18-year-old boy used HGM to test seven times per day and incorporated this technique into his ritualized attempts to over-control his illness. These rituals included running 10 miles per day and filling every moment with activities to keep from binge eating. The HGM was one added technique in this style of fearful adaptation. Such individuals sometimes have to be advised to let up on their exhaustive efforts, which can themselves come to be anxiety-producing. Others initially feel resentment about incorporating additional time- and attention-consuming diabetes-related activities into their lives.

Obesity

Among the most challenging and problematic clinical dilemmas is treatment of the chronically overweight patient.[44] Diabetes, when coupled with obesity, may provide greater incentive for weight reduction, but it also complicates metabolic balance and dietary choices.

Successful initial weight loss has been reported in programs emphasizing behavioral and cognitive strategies socially reinforced by group participation. These treatment approaches include self-monitoring of food intake, learning techniques for stimulus control, family involvement, and the patient's active participation in building realistic, attainable goals with the expectation that there will be inevitable lapses.

Maintenance of desired weight often proves more difficult to attain than initial weight reduction. Those approaches which include follow-up sessions, are flexible and responsive to individual needs, and encourage the involvement of relatives effect the most lasting results.

The psychological portrait of the obese individual varies along a spectrum from the overweight, normal person to the severely emotionally disturbed patient. Consequently, no one treatment package can be effective for all, and each must be tailored according to individualized needs. Treatment of these patients must be tempered in that many patients do not lose weight but still need their physician's interest and involvement. The particular meaning of eating or the conflicts contributing to compulsive overeating are highly variable. These personal issues may need to be identified and addressed, sometimes through psychotherapy or counseling, before lasting changes in eating patterns can be sustained. For some people, psychotherapy focused around issues of self-esteem has produced sustained weight loss as one offshoot of increased personal self-confidence.

Insulin Misuse

Individuals with diabetes have at their disposal a lifesaving substance in insulin. For some, insulin can also become a tool utilized to attain disturbed psychological aims that can constitute threats to health. Such distortions of the use of insulin run the gamut from: (1) overeating without sufficient insulin coverage in order to lose weight; to (2) omission of insulin altogether or sporadically; to (3) taking excessive insulin to cover binge eating with resultant weight gain; to (4) using insulin amounts beyond physical need to produce severe hypoglycemia, unconsciousness, or even death, reflecting a self-destructive intention. Although the general prevalence of extreme maneuvers may be low, these do occur and involve the most complex medical and psychological challenges. Among the most difficult of these patients are those who surreptitiously and repeatedly over- and under-use insulin, leading to repeated diabetic ketoacidosis or frequent, severe insulin reactions. An approach to the medical assessment of these patients has been described previously,[45] so we focus on some psychosocial issues in their diagnosis and initial management.

Those people who resort to omitting insulin altogether or to deliberate overinsulinization comprise a group of greatest medical and psychological risk. Various personality factors may produce such distortions.

> Mary, a 16-year-old and the youngest of six children, was closely tied to her father as his ''little girl.'' When she developed diabetes he resisted accepting the need for insulin treatment as his own elderly mother was able to treat her diabetes without it. He himself had hypertension and refused the physician's recommendation of medication. He also devalued the physician's efforts with Mary, as they threatened his control over his daughter. Mary did begin insulin therapy with her mother's support, but this created stress for her in defying her father. Over a 1-year period she had a series of severe, unconscious reactions but denied the deliberate overuse of insulin. Only after several near-fatal episodes and the establishment of a trusting relationship with a therapist was Mary able to ''admit'' to her manipulation and to her confusions about the need for insulin. Her hospitalizations served to place her in a dependent, child-like position where she could again be her father's special little girl. Over time, elucidation of the meaning for her of low blood glucose evolved: ''If my blood sugar is low enough. I can't/don't have diabetes.''

Review of our recent case records revealed 9 patients who persistently and secretly misused insulin. Unlike many patients who may miss doses occasionally, misreport urine and blood glucose results, and ''cheat'' with their diets, these patients secretly manipulated insulin and, like Mary, only under great duress would they acknowledge the acts.

Table 12-1 shows the characteristics of these patients. All but one were women,

Table 12-1. Characteristics of Nine Patients Who Misused Insulin

Patient	Sex	Age (years)	Marital Status	Occupation	Living Arrangement	Psychiatric Diagnosis	Comments
B.L.	M	11	S	Student, grade school	With parents	Adjustment reaction	Parents are Christian Scientists
D.R.	F	34	M	Secretary	With husband and children		Began after onset of severe gastroparesis—also induced subcutaneous abscesses
C.D.	F	17	S	Student high school	With parents	Depression	Began after a move to a new community
R.A.	F	21	S	Security guard	With parents	Borderline character disorder	No clear precipitant—severe family problems
D.J.	F	22	S	Health aide	With mother	Borderline character disorder	No clear precipitant—severe family problems
L.S.	F	20	S	Student college	With father	Depression	Major family problems
M.D.	F	16	S	Student high school	With parents	Hysterical character	Began after illness in father
H.P.	F	16	S	Student high school	With parents	Hysterical character	Major family problems—to outsiders looked like "perfect diabetic"
H.C.	F	23	S	Registered nurse	With roommate	Borderline character disorder—depression	Began after onset of complications—past history of suicide attempt—major family problems

and most were in their second or third decade. They usually exhibited notable psychiatric problems, most typically of a characterological nature. All had repeated insulin reactions and ketoacidosis requiring hospitalization. Unlike Mary, most did not accept psychiatric follow-up and demonstrated problems over many years. By history, many came from families in which there had been longstanding serious emotional problems in their parents. Unlike reports of patients with Munchausen's syndrome, these patients often had reasonably stable current living arrangements, held jobs, or went to school. In two instances (D.R., H.C.) the episodes came on after the development of diabetic complications. Only one patient had other problems of a factitial nature (D.R., who induced repeated subcutaneous absesses). The one male in our series was prepubertal and seemed to want to deny his illness for religious reasons.

The physician who has spent time attempting to track down the medical reasons for such episodes may understandably feel frustrated, angry, or embarrassed to discover the patient's deliberate actions. It is, however, best to present this suspicion in a neutral and direct fashion, as free as possible from accusation. Many patients still deny the problem, and it may be only after repeated episodes that an acknowledgment is made. If follow-up with the medical/psychiatric team can be maintained over a long time frame, the patient may eventually be able to confront and contain the need to misuse insulin.

Bulimia

One specific problem in which insulin can be misused is that of the eating disorder termed bulimia. The coexistence of bulimia and diabetes increases the difficulties of the clinician and the patient. Bulimia, described as recurrent episodes of binge eating followed by self-induced vomiting or purging by laxatives or diuretics, may be difficult to identify, as the behavior is often hidden and the patient may not be noticeably over- or underweight. While bulimia may occur in patients with clear cases of anorexia nervosa, many patients do not demonstrate symptoms of the condition. Although only a few epidemiological studies have been performed, they suggest that bulimia is far more common in women than men and most are 15–30 years of age. The prevalence in women is probably 1:20.[46] No studies have examined the prevalence of bulimia in patients with diabetes. The nature of the bulimic syndrome may vary in diabetics, as they may use underinsulinization instead of vomiting or laxatives. Menstrual irregularities and significant fluctuations in weight may be primarily related to bulimic behaviors and secondarily affect diabetes balance. The potential for dangerous electrolyte imbalances creates a medical risk, increased for individuals with diabetes. Characteristic of these patients is their abnormal beliefs about their shape and weight. Purgatives and decreased insulin dose are the methods used to affect their weight and counteract their uncontrolled food intake. Diabetes is not necessarily a prime determinant of bulimia, but the consequences of the binge/purge cycles bring these patients to the attention of their physicians more frequently. Some research suggests that many bulimics have a primary affective disorder, and as a consequence antidepressants may be helpful in combination with psychotherapeutic intervention.[47]

Bulimia in diabetics may be especially difficult to treat because conflicts over the diabetes may enhance misuse of insulin. In addition, diabetic patients may find that weight gain, due to water retention from reinstituting insulin after a purgative phase, so upsetting that the patient reenters a purgative phase without even becoming bulimic. For example, one patient reported being less depressed and felt less of an urge to eat, but when she restarted regular twice-daily insulin injections she retained fluids and gained weight. She became frightened and felt out of control so cut back on insulin again without even binging.

SUMMARY

The patient, the family, and the health care providers jointly face a series of predictable crises with which they must cope in treating diabetes. To the extent that each person recognizes the nature of these situations, the dilemmas they pose, and the difficulty that any individual would have with them, the more likely is the treatment to be successful in both biomedical terms and in a personal sense of well-being.

The health care provider is in a unique position for treating a chronic condition like diabetes. By understanding important issues, e.g., individual coping strategies and personal development, he or she can influence positively the patient and family, and facilitate their adaptation to diabetes.

ACKNOWLEDGMENT

This was supported in part by Department of Health and Human Services grant AM 27845.

REFERENCES

1. Jacobson AM, Hauser ST: Behavioral and psychological aspects of diabetes. In Ellenberg M, Rifkin H (eds): Medical Examination Publishers, New York, 1982
2. Johnson SB: Psychosocial factors in juvenile diabetes: a review. J Behav Med 3:96, 1980
3. Surwit RS, Scovern AW, Feinglos MN: The role of behavior in diabetes care. Diabetes Care 5:337, 1982
4. Hauser ST, Jacobson AM, Powers S, Noam G: Ego development and self-image complexity in early adolscence: longitudinal studies of psychiatric and diabetic patients. Arch Gen Psychiatry 40:325, 1983
5. Barglow P, Edidin D, Budlong-Springer A, et al: Diabetic control in children and adolescents: psychosocial factors and therapeutic efficacy. J Youth Adol 12:77, 1983
6. Hamburg BA, Inoff GE: Coping with predictable crises of diabetes. Diabetes Care 6:409, 1983
7. Anderson RM: Defining and evaluating diabetes patient education. Diabetes Care 6:619, 1983 (letter to the editor)
8. Mattson A: In Hamburg BA, Lipsett LF, Inoff GE, Drash AL (eds): Behavioral and Psychosocial Issues in Diabetes: Proceedings of the National Conference. DHHS Publ. No. 80-993. Government Printing Office, Washington, DC, 1980

9. Garmezy N: Children under stress: perspectives on antecedents and correlates of vulnerability and resistance to psychopathology. In Rabin A (ed): Further Explorations in Personality. Wiley, New York, 1981
10. Schade DS, Eaton RP: Diabetic ketoacidosis—pathogenesis, prevention and therapy. Clin Endocrinol Metab 12:321, 1983
11. Mason J: A review of psychoendocrine research on the sympathetic-adrenal medullary system. Psychosom Med 30:631, 1968
12. Jacobson AM, Rand L, Hauser ST: Psychosocial stress and metabolic control in diabetics. Diabetes, suppl. 2, 40:5a, 1983
13. Grant I, Kyle GC, Teichman A, Mendels J: Recent life events and diabetes in adults. Psychosom Med 36:121, 1974
14. Eigler N, Sacca L, Sherwin RJ: Synergistic interactions of physiologic increments of glucagon, epinephrine and cortisol in the dog. Clin Invest 63:114, 1979
15. Schade D, Eaton R: The temporal relationship between endogenously secreted stress hormones and metabolic decompensation in diabetic man. J Clin Endocrinol Metab 50:131, 1980
16. Shamoon H, Hendler R, Sherwin RS: Altered responsiveness to cortisol, epinephrine, and glucagon in insulin-infused juvenile-onset diabetes. Diabetes 29:284, 1980
17. Hinkle LE, Wolf S: Experimental study of life situations, emotions and the occurrence of acidosis in a juvenile diabetic. Am J Med Sci 217:130, 1949
18. Vandenbergh R, Sussman K, Titus C: Effects of hypnotically induced acute emotional stress on carbohydrate and lipid metabolism in patients with diabetes mellitus. Psychosom Med 28:382, 1966
19. Baker C, Barcai A, Kay R, Hague N: Beta adrenergic blockage and juvenile diabetes: acute studies and long-term therapeutic trial. J Pediatr 75:19–29, 1969
20. Koski M-L, Atlas A, Kumento A: A psychosomatic follow-up study of childhood diabetics. Acta Paedopsychiatr (Basel) 42:12, 1976
21. Anderson B, Auslander W: Research on Diabetes Management and the Family. Diabetes Care 3:696, 1980
22. Simmonds JF: Psychiatric status of diabetic youth matched with a control group. Diabetes 26:921, 1977
23. Simmonds JF: Psychiatric status of diabetic youth in good and poor control. Int J Psychiatry Med 7:133, 1976
24. Lazare A, Cohen F, Jacobson AM, et al: The walk-in patient as a customer: a key dimension in evaluation and treatment. Am J Orthopsychiatry 42:872, 1972
25. Lazarus RS, Launier R: Stress-related transactions between person and environment. In Peruin LA (ed): Perspectives in Interactional Psychology. Plenum, New York, 1978
26. Cohen F, Lazarus RS: Active coping processes, coping dispositions, and recovery from surgery. Psychsom Med 35:375, 1973
27. Lazarus R: The costs and benefits of denial. In Breznitz S (ed): Denial and Stress. International Universities Press, New York, 1980
28. Moos RH, Tsu VD: The crisis of physical illness. In Moos, RH (ed): Coping with Physical Illness, Plenum, New York, 1977
29. Hackett TP, Cassem N: Development of a quantitative rating scale to assess denial. J Psychosom Res 18:93, 1974
30. Menninger WC: Psychological factors in the etiology of diabetes. J Nerv Ment Dis 81:1, 1935
31. Stein S, Charles E: Emotional factors in juvenile diabetes mellitus: a study of the early life experiences of eight diabetic children. Psychosom Med 37:237, 1975
32. Srikarta S, Ganda O, Eisenbarth G, Soeldner JS: Islet-cell antibodies and beta cell func-

tion in monozygotic triplets and twins initially discordant for type I diabetes mellitus. N Engl J Med 308:322, 1983
33. Johnson S, Pollak T, Silverstein J, et al: Cognitive and behavioral knowledge about insulin-dependent diabetes among children and parents. Pediatrics, 69:708–713, 1982
34. Collier G, Etzwiler D: Comparative study of diabetes knowledge among juvenile diabetics and their parents. Diabetes. 21:51, 1971
35. Swift C, Seidman F, Stein H: Adjustment problems in juvenile diabetes. Psychosom Med 29:555, 1967
36. Olatawera M: The psychiatric complications of diabetes mellitus in children. Afr J Med Sci 2:231, 1972
37. Dunn S, Tuttle J: The myth of the diabetic personality. Diabetes Care 4:640, 1981
38. Hauser ST, Pollets D: Psychological aspects of diabetes mellitus: a critical review. 2:227, 1979
39. Barrion C, Miles M, Carter M: Problems of mothers in management of children with diabetes. Diabetes Care 6:548, 1983
40. Jacobson AM, Rand L, Hauser ST: Psychological stress and glycemic control in patients with and without proliferative diabetic retinopathy. Psychosom Med (in press)
41. Laron Z, Galatzer A, et al: A Multidisciplinary comprehensive ambulatory treatment scheme for diabetes mellitus in children. Diabetes Care 2:342, 1979
42. Siegler D, LaGreca A, Citrin W, et al: Psychological effects of intensification of diabetic control. Diabetes Care 5:19, 1982
43. Rudolf M, Ahern J, Genel M, et al: Optimal insulin delivery in adolescents with diabetes, impact of intensive treatment on psychosocial adjustment. Diabetes Care 5:53, 1982
44. Abrams DB: Clinical developments in the behavioral treatment of obesity. Clin Behav Ther Rev 1:1, 1979
45. Service RJ (ed): Hypoglycemic Disorders: Pathogenesis, Diagnosis and Treatment. G.K. Hall, Boston, 1983
46. Fairburn C: Bulimia: its epidemiology and management. Psychiatr Ann 13:953, 1983
47. Hudson J, Pope H, Jonas J: Treatment of bulimia with antidepressants: theoretical considerations and clinical findings. Psychiatr Ann 13:965, 1983

13 Economic Impact of Diabetes Mellitus

John A. Galloway
Pomeroy Sinnock
Jaime A. Davidson

Until quite recently a symposium on diabetes mellitus covering the diagnosis, pathophysiology, and treatment of the disease would have been considered complete. Today, however, when the cost of treating diabetes can have an enormous impact on therapeutic outcomes, such a symposium would have to deal with the economic implications of the disease as well. Rising health care costs and the federal government's recent attempts to contain health care expenditures[1,2] make understanding the economics of diabetes a *sine qua non* for proper patient management. Just as an appreciation of factors affecting metabolism is required for designing prescription diets and insulin regimens, knowledge of the economic forces which may affect diabetic patients in their long-term life planning is essential for providing counsel on where to obtain medical care, drugs, and expendables and how to choose the right type of insurance. To enable health care professionals to gain understanding of the economic implications of diabetes mellitus, this chapter: (1) presents an overview of the total cost of diabetes mellitus to the United States as a society; (2) describes how having diabetes mellitus affects an individual's eligibility for and coverage by health insurance; (3) reviews the various effects having diabetes mellitus may have on an individual's employability, work performance, and longevity; (4) delineates current day-to-day costs to selected types of patients with diabetes; and (5) suggests prospective strategies which can reduce the economic impact of diabetes mellitus.

The use of trademarks is for identification purposes only and does not constitute endorsement by the Public Health Service or the US Department of Health and Human Services.

PREVALENCE OF DIABETES MELLITUS AND COST TO SOCIETY

To appreciate the total cost of diabetes to American society, one must be aware of statistics on the prevalence of the disease, recent trends in health care expenditures in the United States, and the fraction of the total attributable to diabetes mellitus.

Data from the federal government[3,4] indicate that in 1979 there were 5.5 million persons with diagnosed diabetes mellitus in the United States. Of this number, 300,000–500,000 were classified as having type I diabetes mellitus [insulin-dependent diabetes mellitus (IDDM)]. About 50 percent of this group were under age 19. Another 5.0–5.2 million persons were estimated to have type II diabetes mellitus [noninsulin-dependent diabetes mellitus (NIDDM)]. Of this group, 45 percent were estimated to be on oral agents, 15–25 percent on insulin, and the remainder on diet alone. In 1978, 34,000 persons died of diabetes mellitus, a finding which placed diabetes mellitus as the sixth leading cause of death in the United States. In 1979 an estimated 2.4 percent of persons living outside institutions were estimated to have diabetes mellitus. The frequency of diabetes is significantly higher among the elderly; it is prevalent in one out of six persons over age 65. Diabetes mellitus is more frequent among certain ethnic and gender groups. Thus middle-aged black women have a higher frequency than whites of both sexes of comparable age. The incidence of diabetes mellitus has increased significantly during the past 45 years, with data from national household interview surveys showing a rise from 0.4 percent in 1936 to 2.4 percent in 1979. The frequency of diabetes mellitus in younger patients has also increased, having tripled between 1958–1960 and 1978 for persons age 44 and under.

TRENDS IN OVERALL U.S. HEALTH COSTS

In 1980 the total bill for all goods and services related to health care was $247.2 billion.[5,6] Health care expenditures rose at an annual rate of 13.2 percent over the 1975–1980 period. In 1982 the United States spent $322.4 billion (or 10.5 percent) or its gross national product for health care.[7] Of the $247.2 billion spent in 1980, 40 percent went to hospitals and 19 percent to physicians.[8] It is estimated that of the $247.2 billion consumers paid approximately $80 billion and the remaining $167.2 billion came from third-party payers.[9]

Entmacher[10] estimated that of the $247.2 billion approximately 2 percent (slightly less than $5 billion) went to the direct care of patients with diabetes mellitus. Although current data are not available on the total cost of diabetes mellitus, which includes direct costs (expenditures for medical and related expenses) and indirect costs (loss of productivity due to morbidity and mortality), the National Diabetes Commission in their 1975 report estimated the cost to be over $5 billion.[11] In a 1979 report, Platt and Sudovar[12] estimated the overall costs of diabetes mellitus to be almost $16 billion. Another survey (Table 13-1) indicated that the total cost rose from $2.6 billion in 1969 to $9.7 billion in 1980[9,13] (P. Entmacher, personal communication).

Because of a lack of current data, estimates of the economic impact of the complications of diabetes are not readily available. However, trends on the use of Medicare-

Table 13-1. National Diabetes Data Group: Trends in the Cost of Diabetes, 1969–1980

	Millions of Dollars				
Parameter	1969	1973	1975	1977	1980
Total	$2,589	$4,015	$5,270	$6,780	$9,700
Mobidity	1,460	2,630	4,200	5,740	8,240
Direct[a]	996	1,650	2,520	3,400	4,800
Indirect[b]	464	980	1,680	2,340	3,440
Mortality[c]	1,129	1,385	1,070	1,040	1,460
No. of deaths	38,530	38,208	37,000	33,570	33,000 (est.)
Prevalence (millions)	3.2	4.2	4.8	5.0	5.3 (est.)

Sources: Paul Entmacher (Metropolitan Life Insurance Co. and NDDG member); Sinnock P, Bauer DW: Reimbursement issues in diabetes: a review. Diabetes Care, 7:291–96, 1984.

[a] Includes costs of care in short-stay hospitals, physician's services, drugs, nursing home care, and other medical professional services. Does not include medical costs incurred by diabetics for conditions other than diabetes.

[b] Includes the dollar equivalent of man-years lost from work and keeping house due to disability caused by diabetes. Does not include losses due to other diseases in diabetics.

[c] Includes the dollar equivalent of man-years lost due to death from diabetes as the underlying cause of death. Does not include such losses due to diabetes as a contributing cause of death or deaths of diabetics in which diabetes was not listed on the death certificate.

supported programs[14] for the treatment of diabetic patients with end-stage renal disease provide a clear indicator for just one complication of diabetes. For instance, in 1980 diabetic patients accounted for over 20 percent of the persons entering the Medicare end-stage renal disease (ESRD) program.[15] The total cost of the ESRD program in 1982 was $2 billion.[16] Given the facts that the prevalence of diabetes mellitus is increasing and health care is becoming more expensive, an extrapolation of the above trends would easily support the conclusion that the total cost of diabetes mellitus to U.S. society in 1984 will reach $20 billion and possibly $25 billion.

INSURANCE FOR THE DIABETIC PATIENT

The patient's ability to obtain and keep health care insurance, maintain a good work record, and obtain life insurance at reasonable rates is crucial to reducing the lifetime economic impact of diabetes mellitus.[17]

In their review, Sinnock and Bauer[9] found that 92 percent of persons with diabetes were covered to some extent by health insurance. As indicated in Table 13-2 (based on their report), 70.8 percent have private insurance (there are over 700 private insurance carriers, including over 100 Blue Cross/Blue Shield plans); 41.3 percent Medicare; and 11 percent Medicaid. Overall, 80 percent of all health insurance is covered under group policies.[9] According to Entmacher[18] 8 percent of the known diabetics in the United States (about 440,000) do not have health care insurance and are not eligible for group plans. This proportion corresponds to that of the U.S. population in general. The only option for these persons is to seek a plan under which they can be covered on an individual basis. Seven states (Florida, Connecticut, Indiana, Minnesota, North Dakota, Rhode Island, and Wisconsin) have pooled-risk insurance plans to assist their residents who cannot obtain satisfactory coverage from

Table 13-2. Diabetic Population with Health Insurance by Selected Demographic Characteristics

Demographic Characteristic	Percent with Insurance			
	Private	Medicare	Medicaid	Total
Age				
<65	71.6	3.7	10.6	87.1
>65	69.4	95.9	11.6	99.4
Sex				
Male	75.4	37.8	6.9	93.2
Female	67.7	43.8	13.8	90.7
Race				
White	74.7	40.8	8.2	92.8
Nonwhite	48.9	44.4	27.4	86.0
All diabetics	70.8	41.3	11.0	91.7

Source: National Center for Health Statistics, 1978. National Health Interview Survey.

Note: Because of overlapping coverage, the sum of each row does not add to the total coverage.

private insurers. The Indiana pooled-insurance plan, which went into effect 1 July 1982, is administered by Mutual of Omaha and funded by contributions from the public health insurers in the state. The maximum premium cannot exceed 150 percent of the state's standard premium rate.

Substantial variations exist in private health care plans made available to employees. These have been reviewed by Taylor,[19] who found that approximately 88 percent of U.S. workers were employed by companies that offered health insurance. However, the workers' likelihood of having health care insurance depended on several factors. For instance, firms having less than 26 employees were least likely to offer health insurance programs. (In this subgroup 45 percent of employees, accounting for 9 million persons, worked for firms that failed to offer health insurance.) In addition, unionized workplaces were more likely to have health insurance benefits than nonunion shops. Employer–employee contributions to the health insurance plans also varied. Data from 1977 disclosed that the overall health insurance premium was about $590 annually per insured employee, with employers paying 80 percent. However, the amount varied by about 10 percent depending on company size, region (southern employers paid the least—59 percent of the premium), and whether the company was unionized. About one-third of the companies with health insurance paid all of the premium. A recent survey indicates that the total health insurance premium was about $959 annually of which employers pay about 71%.[20]

EMPLOYABILITY OF DIABETIC PATIENTS

Entmacher has reviewed many issues related to employability and insurability of persons with diabetes mellitus.[17] Two factors which adversely affect the employability of diabetics compared to nondiabetic individuals are inherent risks to themselves and others resulting from diminished consciousness as a consequence of hypoglycemia, and the reluctance of employers to assume the potential increase in liability for diabetes-related absenteeism. Obvious jobs from which diabetics on insulin or oral agents are excluded are: (1) construction where the worker is near moving equipment or working on a scaffold; (2) commercial flying; and (3) operating commercial vehicles in interstate or foreign commerce.

Concerning the performance of diabetic patients at several large companies, Entmacher[17] found attendance records of the majority of diabetic workers to be as good as and frequently better than those of nondiabetics. However, because of the adverse effect of a small percentage of diabetic employees, the mean attendance rate for the group was reduced. Based on his review, Entmacher recommended screening diabetics prior to employment in order to enhance the likelihood of hiring those whose disease would not detract significantly from their work performance.[17]

To reduce discrimination against the diabetic as well as other handicapped persons, Congress passed the Rehabilitation Act of 1973.[21] The Act applies to the federal government, employers having federal contracts for $2500 or more, and recipients of federal grants. In addition, to offset employers' reluctance to hire diabetic patients because of possible injury proneness on the job which could increase unemployment compensation insurance rates, most states have "second injury" laws which make available funds to reduce the burden on employers of extended disability of a handicapped employee, the handicap having been recorded at the time of employment.[17]

LIFE INSURANCE FOR THE DIABETIC PATIENT

A review of mortality data from large corporations who employ significant numbers of diabetic patients disclosed the mortality rate to be 2.6 times greater among diabetics than among nondiabetics. Also, when compared with nondiabetic controls, more diabetics were drawing pensions.[22] This being the case, insurance company medical directors carefully review applications received from diabetic patients.

The actuarial basis on which rates are established for diabetics and the specific factors affecting those rates are exemplified by studies such as that by Goodkin.[22] This observer reported a prospective study of 10,538 diabetics who applied for life insurance with the Equitable Life Assurance Society of the United States. Eighty-nine percent of the applicants were male. The mortality ratio for declined applicants was four times the norm, and for those who were issued insurance it was 1.67 times the norm. Applicants who became diabetic at age 15 could be expected to live to age 47, compared to age 74 for nondiabetic applicants. If diabetes is discovered at age 25, the diabetic applicant would be expected to live another 33 years, where as the nondiabetic would be expected to live another 49 years. The mortality ratio for poorly controlled patients (2-hr postprandial blood glucose over 250 mg/dl, a history of a recent bout of hyperglycemia, or an insulin reaction) was four times the norm, compared with 1.67 times the norm for the "fairly well controlled" group.

Hypertension associated with diabetes mellitus has a substantial adverse effect on mortality.[22] For instance, diabetic applicants with a diastolic blood pressure <90 mm and a systolic pressure <140 mm Hg had a mortality rate 2.67 times that of the nondiabetic. Those with a systolic pressure of 140–159 mm Hg had a mortality rate 3.34 times that of the nondiabetic, and those with a systolic blood pressure of ≥ 160

mm Hg five times that of the nondiabetic. Finally, albuminuria (≥20 mg in a random urine sample) in early-onset diabetic applicants resulted in a 10-fold increase in mortality over nondiabetic subjects.[22] These findings illustrate why life insurance companies examine carefully the data received on applicants with diabetes mellitus and indicate the importance of control of hyperglycemia and hypertension for all persons with diabetes mellitus.

In most if not all cases in which a diabetic patient applies for life insurance, a statement by the attending physician is requested. The quality and detail of this statement can be of great assistance to the diabetic patient who controls his/her diabetes and follows medical advice in obtaining the lowest possible premium.

DAY-TO-DAY COSTS OF DIABETES MELLITUS

The direct costs for health care and treatment for diabetes mellitus depend on several factors: the type and severity of the disease, how it is treated, the frequency of professional visits, the costs of drugs and expendables, and the extent to which various costs are covered by health care insurance. Estimates of the annual cost of outpatient care and expendables for three typical patients are shown in Table 13-3. These projections assume usual rates for professional charges (determined by a telephone survey of 11 diabetologists), frequency of professional visits, costs of drugs and expendables, and other charges. Based on these data, the usual annual cost of diabetes to the patient may range from about $900 for an uncomplicated type II patient to $2800 for a type I patient on continuous subcutaneous insulin infusion (CSII) treatment.

Not included in these estimates are the initial costs of an intensive educational experience, which may cost $350 to $1200 depending on the scope, duration, and intensity of the course, and extras which may be offered, e.g., psychological testing and counseling and exercise training (considering the potential long-term benefits of such programs we regard these educational programs to be significant bargains in the health care field). In addition, the table does not include the cost of glucose-monitoring devices (which now cost about $150 each) or insulin infusion pumps (which cost $900–$3600 each, with the most popular units costing about $2500).[23]

We have not listed diabetic diet as a special expense because the foods required by most diabetic diets are the same as those ingested by nondiabetics with the exception that concentrated carbohydrates are to be avoided. This is not to say that certain "dietetic" foods are not preferred by some patients. However, the nutritional benefit of using such foods has not been clearly established.[24]

Since pharmacy purchases have been estimated to account for about 9 percent[25] to 13 percent[9] of the average total economic impact (direct and indirect costs) of diabetes mellitus, consumers are interested in comparative costs of various drugs and expendables and in knowing where the best prices can be obtained. Table 13-4 presents the results of a limited survey we conducted in seven large metropolitan cities and four smaller cities (population under 50,000). This survey demonstrates that prices vary to some extent in both small cities and in large metropolitan areas.

Finally, the Connecticut Affiliate of the American Diabetes Association[26] has formed a buying group to purchase for its members certain expendable items in bulk

Table 13-3. Annual Direct Costs of Care

A. Type I patient taking two doses daily of human or purified pork insulin (total dose 50 U). Patient uses disposable insulin syringes (one time only) and performs self glucose monitoring twice daily.		
Professional visits		
Initial $150; follow-up every 3 months at $40 each	$ 270	
Outpatient laboratory tests	$ 180	$450
Insulin $12.95/vial	$ 240	
Disposable syringes 19 cents each	$ 139	
Alcohol swabs (6/day)	$ 45	
Blood glucose test strips 50 cents each	$ 365	
Lancets 5 cents each	$ 40	
Ketone body test (2/week)	$ 9	
Miscellaneous	$ 162	$1000
Grand Total		$1450
B. Type II diabetic patient on oral agent (1 tablet per day). Performs self glucose monitoring four times per week. Patient is taking a diuretic and an antihypertensive medication.		
Professional visits		
Initial $150; follow-up every 3 months at $40 each	$270	
Outpatient laboratory tests	$180	$450
Oral agent		
Chlorpropamide 250 mg $30/100	$100	
Dyazide 1 daily $15.45/100	$ 56	
Aldomet (250 mg b.i.d.) $15.85/100	$113	
Self glucose monitoring (test strips $104; lancets $11)	$115	
Miscellaneous	$ 56	$440
Grand Total		$890
C. Type I diabetic patient on continuous subcutaneous insulin infusion. Changes catheter and syringes every day. Performs self glucose monitoring four times daily. Uses purified pork or human insulin, 50 U/day.		
Professional visits		
Initial $150; follow-up every 2 months (× 5) at $40 each ($200)		$350
Insulin ($12.95/vial)	$ 360[a]	
Catheters (box of 150 costs $275 or $1.83 each)	$ 670	
Syringes (box of 30 costs $20 or 66 cents each)	$ 241	
Blood glucose test strips 50 cents each	$ 730	
Lancets 5 cents each	$ 73	
Alcohol swabs 6/day	$ 45	
Miscellaneous	$ 151	
Outpatient laboratory work	$ 180	$2450
Grand Total		$2800

Note: These estimates do not include fees for consultants (e.g., podiatrists, otorhinolaryngologists, gynecologists, urologists, or surgeons).

[a] Estimates for total cost of insulin for patients on pumps are about 50 percent greater than those on the same total daily dose of insulin administered by conventional syringe (see "A" above). The reason for this is that substantial quantities of insulin are lost in the catheters and syringes of pump systems.

Table 13-4. Patient Cost for Diabetes-Related Pharmaceuticals and Accessories

Drugs/Equipment	Large City (n=7)			Small City (n=4)		
	Low	High	Mean	Low	High	Mean
Lente Iletin II (purified pork insulin zink suspension—Lilly)	$12.18	$14.90	$13.52	$12.43	$16.75	$14.75
NPH Iletin I (isophane insulin suspension—Lilly)	6.69	9.13	7.93	6.85	10.30	8.11
Humulin N (NPH human insulin of recombinant DNA origin—Lilly)	12.18	14.90	13.38	12.42	15.80	14.51
Dyazide (50 mg triamterene + 25 mg hydrochlorthiazide—SK&F), n = 100	14.39	23.80	18.46	16.30	23.75	19.33
Aldomet (methyldopa—MSD), 250 mg, n = 100	14.89	25.54	19.20	15.90	24.95	19.51
Inderal (propranolol hydrochloride—Ayerst), 40 mg, n = 100	15.69	22.26	17.92	15.90	20.95	18.01
B-D Lo-Dose Disposable Syringes, N = 100	16.68	27.35	21.83	16.50	23.00	19.61
Monoject U = 100 Syringes, n = 100	17.98	24.62	21.70	16.68	20.16	18.11
Autolet Lancets, n = 100	10.89	12.50	11.75	6.88	11.95	10.03
Dymelor (Acetohexamide—Lilly), 500 mg n = 100	24.49	30.05	26.56	22.50	27.50	25.12
Orinase (tolbutamide tablets, USP—Upjohn), 0.5 g, n = 100	6.25	14.89	10.26	9.85	20.95	14.89
Diabinese (chlorpropamide—Pfizer), 250 mg, n = 100	27.39	41.74	33.37	26.30	34.21	29.85
Tolinase (tolazamide tablets, USP—Upjohn), 250 mg, n = 100	26.82	40.31	32.99	27.80	38.95	32.82
Ames Ketostix, one bottle or package = 50	3.55	5.30	4.35	3.55	4.69	4.18
Bio-Dynamics Chemstrip, package = 25	13.30	17.71	15.00	11.82	15.98	13.77
Tes-Tape (glucose enzymatic test strip—Lilly), single roll	4.54	6.30	5.06	4.38	5.59	5.12

quantities and therefore at reduced prices. The Affiliate provides, for a nominal charge, instructional services for patients for whom self glucose monitoring has been prescribed. The Board of Directors of the American Diabetes Association has gone on record as opposing this activity by affiliates of the organization.

DIAGNOSIS-RELATED GROUPS

A discussion of the economic impact of diabetes mellitus, or any other common and potentially serious disease, would be incomplete without mention of the recently promulgated plan of the Health Care Finance Administration to control hospital costs by prospectively establishing a rate schedule for reimbursement for hospital care by Medicare.[1,2] Alarmed by spiraling hospital costs, which for instance in 1982 were three times the inflation rate,[27] and determined to reduce health care costs, the Reagan administration and Congress enacted P.L. 98-21. This legislation includes a detailed plan, called the Medicare Prospective Payment System, by which hospitals are reimbursed using a predetermined rate based on the patient's admitting diagnosis.

Four hundred sixty-seven disease categories are listed, and a formula based on the number of hospital days and resources needed to treat these disease categories is used to determine the Medicare reimbursement. Bransome[28] summarized the application of this reimbursement method to the hospital care of patients with diabetes mellitus, but it is beyond the scope of this chapter to detail the application of the DRG system. However, it is appropriate to include certain general statements concerning the impact of these rules on diabetic patients.

First, generally speaking, if a patient enters the hospital with a urinary tract infection and is placed in DRG 321 (kidney and urinary tract infection in a patient age 18 to 69 without a co-morbid complication) which allows for an average hospital stay of 5.6 days, and the patient is discharged sooner than the 5.6 days called for by the DRG reimbursement formula, the hospital profits. On the other hand, if the patient stays longer, the hospital loses money. (Provisions are made for "outliers," hospital stays that are longer than the DRG allows; however, only a small percentage of a hospital's admissions can be submitted for review under these rules.) Second, good medical practice dictates that some conditions require longer hospitalization than is permitted by the DRGs. For instance, Bransome points out that pregnancy in diabetes, which may require prolonged hospitalization for adequate control, will not be adequately served by the Prospective Payment System. A corollary disadvantage of the DRGs is the possibility of underservice to the patient to cut hospital costs. Third, since at this time the rules apply only to Medicare, as hospitals attempt to reduce their Medicare billings there is the distinct likelihood that a portion of the costs will be shifted to patients who are covered by private plans,[29] a process which in the short run could increase the cost of private health insurance. Finally, DRGs specifically exclude health education, which in the case of diabetes has been shown to be effective in reducing hospital utilization.[9,30] Thus while the Prospective Payment System will reduce hospital costs by compelling health care providers (hospitals and physicians) to combine their efforts to reduce utilization of hospital resources, the implementation of DRGs will inevitably result in modifications of health care delivery as a consequence of changes in modes of practice (the chief one being a greater amount of service delivered in the outpatient setting) and deletion of optional services. The extent and impact of the Medicare Prospective Payment System probably will not be appreciated for another 3–4 years when the plan is fully implemented.

STRATEGIES TO REDUCE THE ECONOMIC IMPACT OF DIABETES MELLITUS

A number of strategies can be invoked to reduce the economic impact of diabetes mellitus (Table 13-5). Some are obvious, but others are not and therefore deserve elucidation. First, because emotional stress is a common cause not only of episodic but sustained hyperglycemia, psychological counseling for the patient and/or family can be of immense value in improving diabetic control. Over the past 20 years federal legislation[31–33] has made counseling and other psychiatric services available at affordable prices for virtually all patients. The recognition by physicians of the deleterious effects of psychic stress on metabolic control and the referral of patients

Table 13-5. How Patients and Families of Patients May Reduce the Economic Impact of Diabetes Mellitus

Preventive or anticipatory strategies
1. Adopt life styles which can promote good health. Maintain normal body weight; avoid smoking, drugs, excessive alcoholic intake, and life stress; utilize techniques to reduce stress, e.g., psychological intervention.
2. In families with strong family histories, consider HLA type to identify high-risk family members and purchase life insurance with an additional purchase benefit (rider with guaranteed issue).
3. Obtain career counseling.
4. Maintain group health insurance.
After diabetes has been discovered
1. Obtain medical care from a physician or association of physicians or clinic with interest and expertise in the field of diabetes. These clinics should include or have ready access to patients education services (dietitian, nurse educators).
2. Become well educated in the management of the disease. As soon as possible after developing diabetes, become adept at performing self glucose monitoring.
3. Invoke strategies for personal life style that reduce the stress of living, maintain job performance, and overall offset the liabilities of diabetes mellitus.
4. Seek medical attention promptly for all health problems, including those related, as well as those unrelated, to diabetes mellitus.
5. If a change in employment is considered, anticipate the effect of diabetes on obtaining health insurance.

for psychological evaluation when other causes of poor control have been ruled out can often be a highly cost-effective procedure.

Second, life insurance for persons at risk for diabetes mellitus should be purchased before hyperglycemia occurs. It is human nature to deny the presence of diabetes when the condition has been diagnosed, but it is even more difficult to face the prospect of an apparently healthy family member developing the disorder. HLA haplotyping in families at risk for diabetes may identify relatives of diabetic probands who are likely to become affected. For instance, Gorsuch et al.[34] have found that the risk of developing Type I diabetes may be 100 times greater in a nondiabetic HLA haplotype identical sibling than in nondiabetic families, with 30 percent of HLA identical siblings developing diabetes by the age of 30. Life insurance can be purchased for such individuals at about 10 percent above the standard rates with the guarantee that additional insurance can be purchased at standard rates at established intervals in the future.

PATIENT EDUCATION AND DIABETES

In our view, education for the diabetic patient and his or her family is perhaps one of the most cost-effective procedures to reduce the economic impact of the disease. The available data clearly indicate that education reduces utilization of expensive inpatient and outpatient services.[30]

MAINTENANCE OF HEALTH CARE INSURANCE

Whereas the nondiabetic patient may consider changing jobs with impunity, the diabetic patient or the breadwinner with a diabetic family member should exercise caution when considering a new position. The insurance benefits of the current and the prospective employer should be carefully compared, and the individual should be absolutely certain that no hiatus in insurance coverage occurs during the transition.

Finally, diabetic patients and their families should be advised on their rights as patients[35] so they can deal effectively if their insurance carriers deny claims.[36] Excellent sources of information on life management, e.g., publications by the American Diabetes Association, the federal government, and other agencies, provide a unique offering of options for the patient to utilize in altering his/her economic destiny.

In summary, the economic impact of diabetes mellitus is a significant factor not only for the affected patient and the patient's family but for society in general. Careful consideration of the possibilities for reducing the fiscal effects of the disease can result in significant reductions in not only the financial but the psychic and physical trauma of the disorder.

ACKNOWLEDGMENTS

We wish to express appreciation to Irene M. Brandt, Government Relations Division, Eli Lilly and Company, Washington, DC, and to Caroline I. Hart for her assistance in preparing the manuscript.

REFERENCES

1. Department of Health and Human Services, Health Care Financing Administration, Medicare Program: Federal Register, 1 September 1983, Part IV. Prospective Payments for Medicare Inpatient Hospital Services; Interim Final Rule with Comment Period, pp. 39752–39890
2. Department of Health and Human Services, Health Care Financing Administration, Medicare Program: Federal Register, 3 January 1984, Part IV. Prospective Payment for Medicare Inpatient Hospital Services; Final Rule, pp. 234–340
3. Drury TF, Harris M, Lipsett LF: Prevalence and Management of diabetes mellitus. In: Health: United States. pp. 25–31. DHSS Publication No. PHS 82-1232. U.S. Department of Health and Human Services, Public Health Service, Office of Health Research, Statistics and Technology, Hyattsville, MD, December 1981
4. National Diabetes Data Group: Data Sheet on the Prevalence and Incidence of Diabetes Mellitus in the U.S. NIADDK, NIH, Bethesda, MD, 18 November 1982
5. U.S. Department of Health and Human Services, Public Health Service: Health: United States, 1981. DHSS Publication No. PHS 82-1232. Hyattsville, MD, December 1981
6. Health United States and Prevention Profile. p. 9. Government Printing Office, Washington, DC, 1983
7. Heckler MM: H.H.S. News, U.S. Department of Health and Human Services. Government Printing Office, Washington, DC, 17 January 1984
8. Health Insurance Association of America: Source Book of Health Insurance Data; 1981–82. HIAA, Washington, DC, 1982

9. Sinnock P, Bauer DW: Reimbursement issues in diabetes: a review. Diabetes Care Volume 7, Number 3, pp. 291–296, May/June 1984
10. Entmacher P: Personal communication
11. Report of the National Diabetes Commission to the Congress of the U.S. Vol. III: Reports of Committees, Subcommittees and Workgroups. Part 2. p. 307
12. Platt WG, Sudovar SG: The social and economic costs of diabetes mellitus: an estimate for 1979. Home Healthcare Group, Ames Division, Miles Laboratories, Elkhart, IN
13. Entmacher P: Metropolitan Life Insurance Company and NDDG member
14. P.L. 92-603
15. The Medicare Experience with End-Stage Renal Disease; Trends in Incidence, Prevalence, and Survival. Department of Health and Human Services, Health Care Financing Administration, Office of Research and Demonstrations, Washington, DC, 1980
16. Davis CK: Statement before Subcommittee on Health, Committee on Ways and Means, United States House of Representatives, 9 February 1984
17. Entmacher PS: Economic aspects (of diabetes mellitus); employability and insurability. In Ellenberg M, Rifkin (eds): Diabetes Mellitus. p. 1053. Medical Examination Publishers, New York, 1983
18. Entmacher PS: Perosnal communication
19. Taylor AK: Employment-related health insurance. In: Health: United States. p. 87. U.S. Department of Health and Human Services, Public Health Service, Office of Health, Research, Statistics and Technology, Hyattsville, MD, 1981
20. Private Insurance: Premium Expenditures and Sources of Payment, Data Preview 17, National Center for Health Services Research, DHHS Publication No. (DHS) 84-3364, November, 1983
21. P.L. 93-112
22. Goodkin G: Mortality factors in diabetes: a 20 year mortality study. J Occup Med 17:716, 1975
23. White N, Santiago J: What can be achieved with insulin pumps and what are the complications of such therapy? (in press)
24. Wunschel IM, Sheikholislam BM: Is there a role for dietetic foods in the management of diabetes and/or obesity? Diabetes Care 1:247, 1978
25. Marks RG: Diabetes: the expensive disease. In: Drug Topics. p. 55. 2 September 1980
26. Stewart WA: Personal communication
27. Health: United States, 1982. Public Health Service Publication No. 82-1232. Government Printing Office, Washington, DC, December 1982
28. Bransome ED: Diabaetes, doctors and DRG's. In: What's New, Clinical Diabetes. pp. 11–16. 1984
29. Iglehart JK: Medicare begins prospective payment of hospitals. N Engl J Med 308:1428, 1983
30. Davidson JK, Delcher HK, Englund A: Spin-off cost benefits of expanded nutritional care. J Am Diet Assoc 75:250, 1979
31. Community Mental Health Centers Act (P.L. 88-164), 1964
32. Community Mental Health Centers Act (P.L. 91-211), 1970
33. Omnibus Budget Reconciliation Act of 1981 (P.L. 97-35)
34. Gorsuch AN, Spencer KM, Lister J, et al: Can future type I diabetes be predicted? A study of families of affected children. Diabetes 31:862, 1982
35. Bill of Rights for People with Diabetes Mellitus. Approved by the American Diabetes Association Board of Directors, June 1983. In: Diabetes Forecast. pp. 34–35. November–December 1983
36. Weinrauch S: Claim denied. In: Diabetes Forecast. pp. 34–35. September–October 1983

Index

Page numbers followed by (t) represent tables.